Thomson's Concise
Medical Dictionary

Thomson's Concise Medical Dictionary

WILLIAM A. R. THOMSON, M.D.

CHURCHILL LIVINGSTONE 1973
Edinburgh and London

ISBN 0 443 00940 6

Printed in Great Britain
by Cox & Wyman Ltd,
London, Reading and Fakenham

Preface

WHEN I was working on this labour of love—for such it has been—I was telephoned one day by a colleague. He had heard that I was working on a dictionary, and he wanted to know what my 'philosophy' was. For a moment I was mystified. To my old-fashioned mind 'philosophy' automatically suggested what the *Shorter Oxford English Dictionary* so nicely describes as 'the system which a person forms for the conduct of life'. Then it quickly dawned on me what my well-meaning colleague—an expert on dictionaries I learned subsequently—meant was the theoretical basis on which I was planning my dictionary.

When I confessed that, in my ignorance, it had never occurred to me that I ought to have a 'philosophy' if I was going to prepare a dictionary, he was obviously rather upset. He would have been more upset if I had dared to tell him that my approach was almost entirely empirical. In others words, that I was working on that system of hunches that, combined with a smattering of science, has for so long formed the sound basis of the successful practice of medicine. If he had wished me to develop my theme I should have told him that it was the same principle that I had followed in editing *The Practitioner*—to the satisfaction, apparently, of a not inconsiderable number of readers scattered throughout all five continents.

In short, the aim of this dictionary is to provide the doctor, and all those who work with him—whether secretary, nurse, or technician, as well as medical students, pharmacists and scientists in the medical field—with a short concise dictionary containing definitions of the vast majority of words with which they will come in contact during the course of their daily duties. There are several first-class large medical dictionaries in the English language (even though all but one come from the United States of America), but there is no concise dictionary written and produced in Britain suitable for the day-to-day quick reference which the busy clinician so often needs.

The choice of words has been purely empirical, and based upon my own predilection as a result of my personal experience, whether as the reader, or the editor, of medical journals. I am bound to have omitted words that some readers would like to see included, just as I am bound to have included some that may be considered supernumerary.

This latter criticism may appear to be particularly applicable to what some may consider the excessive space allotted to anatomical terms. The reason for this is the current tendency to reduce the amount of anatomical detail which students are expected to memorize. I have every sympathy with this move, it makes it all the more important that the doctor should have a quick method of discovering what is meant by some anatomical phrase he may happen to encounter. Equally is this true of the nurse and any other member of the medical team. Hence the apparent superfluity of anatomical terms.

To the etymologist the book will appear characterless and forlorn. The explanation, however, is quite simple. I have gone on the principle that, like myself, the vast majority of doctors today have, as Ben Jonson said of Shakespeare, 'small Latin, and less Greek'. What I have therefore done is to include merely the derivation of some of the more important of the prefixes and suffixes used in medical terms. These have served me well, and, based largely upon my editorial experience, I have assumed that they will be sufficient for the vast majority of clinicians. I have also given the plural form of most of the commonly used terms that do not merely take an 's' to signify the plural form.

Abbreviations I have reduced to a minimum—and for two reasons. They can be so misleading as to be dangerous, and the memorizing of them puts an unnecessary strain on the doctor's memory. Honesty also compels me to add that they are the ruination of style. Where they are useful, and where they have been shown in the dictionary, is when they represent measurements and certain well-recognized entities with cumbersome names such as some of the hormones. The only other abbreviations used are in the derivations of prefixes and suffixes: Gk, Greek; L, Latin; Ger, German; Fr, French; Ital, Italian; OE, Old English.

Eponyms have been eschewed for the same reasons as abbreviations, although I am afraid the occasional one may have slipped in. Proprietary names of drugs have not been included in order to save space, and for the same reason pronunciations have not been indicated. Apart from anything else, I often wonder how many doctors understand phonetic symbols.

'To make dictionaries is dull work', according to the great lexicographer himself. I have certainly not found this to be the case. It has been a fascinating task, and it was with mixed feelings that I found that the assignment was completed. It now goes forth in the hope that it will do something to lighten the task of the practitioner and allow him to get even more interest out of his daily work.

While immersed in preparing this dictionary I have learned much of the 'mystery of words'. It is a mystery that has oft held me entranced. I only trust that, in the words of St Paul, I have deceived no man with vain words. Mistakes I must have made. For these I pray forgiveness— and ask for correction. The beauty of the English language is its flexibility. I only trust that I have not been too flexible in interpreting it to my many friends at home and overseas.

William A. R. Thomson

Contents

A

A-, An- (Gk *an:* without). Prefixes indicating lack of, without.

Ab- (L *ab:* off, from). Prefix signifying off, away from.

Abacterial. Free from bacteria.

Abarognosis. Inability to recognize the quality of weight.

Abasia. Inability to walk as a result of motor incoordination.

Abdomen. The region of the trunk that lies below the diaphragm.

Abducent nerve. The 6th cranial nerve, which innervates the lateral rectus muscle of the eye.

Abduct. To draw away from the median line or from a neighbouring part.

Aberrant. Deviating from the normal course, structure or appearance.

Abiatrophy. Premature loss of vitality.

Abiogenesis. Spontaneous generation.

Abiosis. The state of being lifeless.

Abiotrophy. Loss of vitality or degeneration of certain tissues, usually genetic in origin. Sometimes used as a generic term for hereditary degenerative diseases.

Ablatio. Removal, detachment. **Ablatio placentae,** premature detachment of a normal placenta.

Ablation. Removal of a part, such as a tumour, by a surgical operation.

Ablepharia. Congenital absence, partial or complete, of the eyelids.

Ablepsia. Blindness.

Abortifacient. A drug or agent that induces abortion.

Abortion. Expulsion of the foetus before the 28th week of pregnancy. **Complete abortion,** one in which all the products of conception have been expelled. **Habitual abortion,** any case in which three or more consecutive spontaneous abortions have occurred. **Incomplete abortion,** an abortion in which only parts of the products of conception have been expelled. **Inevitable abortion,** an abortion in progress which cannot be arrested. **Missed abortion,** retention of the dead ovum or foetus for more than two weeks (carneous mole). **Septic abortion,** abortion from an infected uterus.

Threatened abortion, arrest of the process before abortion becomes inevitable.

Abrachiocephalus. A headless and armless monster.

Abrasion. An area of skin, mucous membrane (or tooth) worn away by friction or some other abnormal mechanical process.

Abrasor. An instrument used for abrasion; a rasp.

Abreaction. The release of pent-up, repressed emotions, as evoked in the process of psychoanalysis.

Abrosia. Fasting, or the state induced thereby.

Abruptio. A tearing away. **Abruptio placentae,** premature separation of the placenta.

Abscess. A localized collection of pus.

Abscissa. The horizontal coordinate in a graph illustrating the interrelationship of two sets of data. (*Plural*: abscissae.)

Abscission. Cutting away.

Absinth. A liqueur, consisting of an alcoholic solution of wormwood, anise, marjoram oils and oil of thuja. This last is a cerebral convulsant.

Absorption. The taking up of fluids, gases or other substances by the skin, mucous membranes, blood vessels, lymphatics and other tissues of the body.

Abstract. A powder produced by extracting the active principles of a crude drug with alcohol. A summary of an article or book.

Abulia. Impairment or loss of will power.

Acacia. B.P. 1968. The dried gummy exudation from the stem and branches of *Acacia senegal* (L.) and of some other species of Acacia. It is used as a suspending agent, usually with tragacanth, in mixtures containing resinous tinctures or powders which do not readily disperse.

Acantha. The spine. The spinous process of a vertebra.

Acanthaesthesia. A perverted sensation, as of being pricked with needles.

Acanthion. The tip of the anterior nasal spine.

Acanthosis. An increase in thickness of the prickle-cell layer of the epidermis. *Acanthosis nigricans*, a form of acanthosis characterized by pigmented warty growths. In adults associated often with carcinoma of the internal organs.

Acapnia. The condition of diminished carbon dioxide in the blood.

Acardiacus. A foetal monster without a heart; usually a parasitic twin.

Acarophobia. A morbid fear of becoming infested with mites or other insects.

Accessory nerve. The 11th cranial nerve, which innervates the sternocleidomastoid and trapezius muscles and most of the muscles of the soft palate.

Acclimatization. The process of becoming adjusted to a new climate or natural conditions, whether it be height, heat or cold.

Accommodation. Adaptation or adjustment, especially of the eye. The faculty of the eye of altering its refractive power so that rays of light are brought accurately to a focus on the retina.

Accoucheur. Obstetrician.

Accretio cordis. Adhesive pericarditis.

Acephalus. A foetal monster without a head.

Acepifylline. The B.P. Commission approved name for piperazine theophyllin-7-ylacetate. A spasmolytic drug.

Acepromazine maleate. B.P.C. 1968. $C_{23}H_{26}N_2O_5S$. A tranquillizing drug.

Acetabulum. The cup-shaped socket on the outer aspect of the innominate bone in which the head of the femur articulates.

Acetanilide. An acetyl derivative of aniline, once widely prescribed as an analgesic and antirheumatic. Now largely discarded because of its toxicity, particularly its tendency to produce methaemoglobinaemia.

Acetarsol. B.P. 1968. $C_2H_{10}AsNO_5$. A drug used in the treatment of amoebiasis and *Trichomonas vaginalis* vaginitis.

Acetazolamide. B.P. 1968. $C_4H_6N_4O_3S_2$. A specific inhibitor of carbonic anhydrase which is used as a diuretic and in the treatment of glaucoma.

Acetic acid. $C_2H_4O_2$. The *British Pharmacopoeia* 1968 preparation contains 32·5 to 33·5 per cent $C_2H_4O_2$. It has a mild expectorant action taken internally. Externally it has an irritant action and is used in liniments.

Acetoacetic acid. $CH_3COCH_2.COOH$. One of the ketone bodies which are formed in excess in starvation and uncontrolled diabetes mellitus.

Acetohexamide. The B.P. Commission approved name for *N*-4-acetylbenzenesulphonyl-N'-cyclohexylurea. An oral hypoglycaemic agent.

Acetomenaphthone. B.P. 1968. $C_{15}H_{14}O_4$. A drug with the same action as phytomenadione (vitamin K_1), but acts more slowly.

Acetone. Dimethyl ketone. A highly inflammable fluid that is used as a solvent for organic substances. Minute amounts are present in normal blood and urine. Increased amounts appear in the urine of uncontrolled diabetic patients.

Acetonuria. An excess of acetone bodies in the urine.

Acetorphine. The B.P. Commission approved name for a narcotic analgesic.

Acetrizoic acid. B.P. 1968. $C_9H_6I_3NO_3$. A radiographic contrast medium.

Acetum. Vinegar.

Acetylcholine. The mediator of impulses at all autonomic ganglia, parasympathetic postganglionic endings, sympathetic postganglionic endings in sweat glands and motor nerve endings in skeletal muscles.

Acetylcysteine. The B.P. Commission approved name for N-acetyl-L-cysteine. A drug used for the liquefaction of bronchial secretion.

Acetylsalicylic acid. Aspirin.

Achalasia. Failure or inability to relax.

Acheilia. Congenital absence of one or both lips.

Acheiria. Congenital absence of one or both hands.

Achlorhydria. Absence of hydrochloric acid from the gastric juice.

Achloropsia. Inability to recognize or distinguish green tints.

Acholia. Lack or absence of secretion of bile.

Acholuria. Absence of bile pigments from the urine.

Achondroplasia. The form of dwarfism resulting from a hereditary abnormality characterized by faulty endochondral ossification.

Achor. A papular eruption on the hairy parts of the skin. Popularly known as milk crust when it occurs in infants.

Achrestic. Indicating lack of utilization.

Achromatic. Colourless. Staining with difficulty.

Achromatopsia. Colour blindness.

Achromobacteraceae. A family of bacteria of the order Eubacteriales found chiefly in soil and water.

Achylia. Absence of chyle. **Achylia gastrica,** complete absence of hydrochloric acid and ferments from the gastric juice.

Acid. A compound of electronegative elements or groups plus ionizable hydrogen (H^+). For individual acids see specific names.

Acidaemia. A lowered pH of the blood.

Acid-fast. A term used to describe bacteria which are not decolorized by acid after staining with aniline dyes: e.g. *Mycobacterium tuberculosis.*

Acidophil. Having an affinity for acid stains.

Acidosis. The state characterized by increase in hydrogen ion concentration, resulting from accumulation of acid or loss of base from the body.

Acinitrazole. The B.P. Commission approved name for 2-acetamido-5-nitrothiazole. A drug used in the treatment of trichomoniasis.

Acinus. A sac-like dilatation which tends to occur in grape-like clusters in certain compound glands. (*Plural:* acini.)

Acladiosis. A chronic ulcerative skin condition caused by *Acladium castellani,* which occurs in South-east Asia and Macedonia.

Aclasis. Pathological continuity of growth. **Diaphysial aclasis,** failure of normal growth in the metaphysial region of bone, in which the extremities of the shaft become irregularly thickened.

Acne. A chronic inflammatory disease of the sebaceous glands. **Acne vulgaris,** the commonest form of acne. It is a chronic inflammatory condition, in which retention of excessive sebum secreted by overactive sebaceous glands leads to a characteristic eruption.

Aconite. B.P.C. 1968. The dried root of *Aconitum napellus* (L.). Used as a liniment for the relief of rheumatic pains, it produces tingling followed by numbness.

Aconitine. The active constituent of aconite.

Acoustic. Pertaining to the organs or sense of hearing.

Acoustics. The science of sound.

Acrania. The developmental abnormality characterized by partial or complete absence of the skull (or cranium).

Acridine. A hydrocarbon ($C_{13}H_9N$) derived from coal tar, from which came the acridine dyes once used widely as antiseptics.

Acriflavine. An acridine dye used as a non-irritant antiseptic.

Acrocyanosis. Persistent blueness of the extremities.

Acrodermatitis. Inflammation of the skin of the extremities.

Acrodynia. A toxic affection of the autonomic nervous system characterized by redness or cyanosis of the extremities, anorexia, sweating, photophobia and mental changes. Also known as pink disease and erythroedema.

Acrogeria. Premature ageing of the skin.

Acromegaly. A chronic disease characterized by hypertrophy of the bones of the head, chest, hands and feet, as well as of the soft tissues. It is due to hyperplasia of the eosinophilic cells of the adenohypophysis with consequent over-production of growth hormone.

Acromion. The outer end of the spine of the scapula.

Acromphalus. Undue prominence of the umbilicus. Also the centre point of the umbilicus.

Acroparaesthesia. Numbness, tingling and stiffness in the extremities.

Acrophobia. Morbid fear of heights.

Acrosclerosis. Sclerotic changes in the hands and feet. Characteristically found in Raynaud's phenomenon.

Acrosome. The head cap of a spermatozoon.

Acrotic. When referring to the pulse indicates weakness or absence of the pulse.

Acrylic. Relating to synthetic plastic resins derived from acrylic acid.

Actin. One of the protein constituents of the muscle fibre.

Actinic. Pertaining to the ultraviolet rays of the spectrum.

Actinium. A chemical element with radioactive properties. Symbol Ac. Atomic weight 227. Atomic number 89.

Actinobacillus. A genus of small, gram-negative, non-motile organisms, one of which, *A. actinomycetemcomitans,* is found in human cases of actinomycosis.

Actinomyces. A genus of anaerobic or micro-aerophilic non-acid-fast organisms within the family Actinomycetaceae.

Actinomycetaceae. One of the three families constituting the order Actinomycetales.

Actinomycetales. An order of the class Schizomycetes, which consists of three families: Mycobacteriaceae, Actinomycetaceae, and Streptomycetaceae.

Actinomycin. The B.P. Commission approved name for a group of anti-microbial substances with anti-tumour activity, produced by *Streptomyces antibioticus* and *S. chrysomallus*. They are differentiated by a terminal letter. Actinomycin C and actinomycin D are proving of value in the treatment of new growths.

Actinomycosis. A chronic infectious disease of cattle, caused by *Actinomyces bovis*, and sometimes transmitted to man, causing granulomatous growths in the mouth and elsewhere in the body, which break down and discharge yellow granules.

Actinotherapy. The therapeutic use of light rays, especially violet and ultra-violet rays.

Actomyosin. A complex formed by actin and myosin which plays an important part in the physiology of muscular contraction.

Acuminate. Pointed, tapering.

Acupuncture. The insertion of needles as a form of counter-irritation.

Acyanotic. Characterized by lack of cyanosis.

Adactylia. Congenital absence of fingers and toes.

Adamantine. Pertaining to dental enamel.

Adamantinoma. A slowly growing, locally malignant tumour of the jaw, derived from the epithelial residues of the enamel organ; it does not form enamel.

Adam's apple. A widely used popular term for the laryngeal prominence.

Addiction. The state of being surrendered to a habit. **Drug addiction,** the state of being so addicted to a drug that it is impossible to give up the habit voluntarily.

Addison's disease. A disease characterized by extreme weakness, pigmentation of the skin, wasting and low blood pressure, due to destruction of the cortex of the suprarenal glands. Named after Thomas Addison (1793–1860), the physician at Guy's Hospital, London, who first described it.

Additive. A substance deliberately added to fulfil some specific purpose: e.g. *food additive*.

Adduct. To draw towards the median line.

Adductor. A muscle which draws a part towards the midline of the body.

Adenine. An amino purine base produced by the decomposition of nucleic acid.

Adenitis. Inflammation of a gland.

Adeno- (Gk *adēn:* gland). Prefix denoting relation to a gland or glands.

Adenocarcinoma. A columnar-cell carcinoma with formation of glandular spaces.

Adenohypophysis. The anterior part of the hypophysis cerebri (or pituitary gland).

Adenoids. Hypertrophy of the lymphoid (or adenoid) tissue on the posterior wall of the nasopharynx.

Adenoma. A benign tumour of glandular tissue.

Adenosarcoma. A tumour with the combined characteristics of an adenoma and a sarcoma.

Adenosine. A mononucleoside produced by the hydrolysis of nucleic acid and adenine nucleotides.

Adenosine phosphate. The B.P. Commission approved name for adenosine monophosphate, which is found in muscle and yeast, and which is an intermediate product in the release of energy for muscular work.

Adenosine triphosphate (ATP). A compound that plays an important part in the contraction of voluntary muscle and also in sugar metabolism.

Adenosis. Any chronic disorder or disease of the glands, particularly the lymphatic glands.

Adenotome. An instrument for excising glands, particularly adenoids.

Adenovirus. One of a group of viruses which derive their name from the fact that they were first isolated from fragments of adenoid tissue. They cause a wide variety of upper respiratory tract infections.

Adeps. The purified omental fat of pigs used in the making of ointments.

Adhesion. The uniting together of structures which should normally be separate and freely movable, usually the result of inflammation. **Interthalamic adhesion,** the flattened grey band that connects the medial walls of the third ventricle.

Adiadochokinesia. The inability to perform rapid, alternating movements.

Adicillin. The B.P. Commission approved name for 6-[D(+)-5-amino-5-carboxyvaleramido] penicillanic acid.

Adipectomy. Excision of adipose tissue.

Adipocere. The wax-like substance

which develops in corpses in the presence of moisture and at favourable temperatures in the absence of air, as under earth or water.

Adipose. Fatty. Fatty to an excessive degree.

Adiposis. An excessive accumulation of fat in the body. **Adiposis dolorosa,** a disease, usually in women, characterized by painful, localized, fatty swellings and nerve lesions.

Aditus. An opening or passage.

Adjuvant. A substance administered to assist or modify the action of some other substance: e.g. a drug or an antigenic agent.

Adnexa. Appendages or accessory parts.

Adolescence. The period of life between childhood and adulthood.

Adrenalectomy. Removal of a suprarenal gland.

Adrenal glands. The suprarenal glands.

Adrenaline. B.P. 1968. $C_9H_{13}NO_3$. The active principle of the medulla of the suprarenal gland, which may be obtained from the glands of certain animals or prepared synthetically. It acts on the effector cells of the sympathetic system. Its main therapeutic use is in the treatment of allergic conditions, particularly bronchial asthma and anaphylactic shock. Because of its vasoconstrictor action it is used to diminish the absorption of local anaesthetics and to reduce local haemorrhage.

Adrenaline acid tartrate. B.P. 1968. The hydrogen tartrate of adrenaline. It has the same action and therapeutic use as adrenaline, 1·8 mg. being equivalent to 1 mg. of adrenaline. It is the constituent of **Adrenaline injection,** B.P. 1968, and **Adrenaline solution,** B.P. 1968.

Adrenergic. Having an adrenaline-like action.

Adrenochrome. The red oxidation product of adrenaline.

Adrenocorticotrophic. Having a hormonal influence on the cortex of the suprarenal glands.

Adrenocorticotrophin. Adrenocorticotrophic hormone. Corticotrophin. (*Abbreviation:* ACTH.)

Adrenogenital. Referring to the adrenal glands and the gonads. **Adrenogenital syndrome,** a condition characterized by virilization in the female and precocious puberty in the male, due to excessive production of androgens.

Adrenolytic. Inhibiting the action of adrenergic nerves; inhibiting the response to adrenaline.

Advancement. The operation of moving forward the insertion of a muscle or tendon; most commonly performed in eye surgery.

Adventitia. The outer covering of an organ, more particularly an artery.

Adventitious. Accidental or acquired, as opposed to natural or hereditary; out of the normal situation; referring to the adventitia.

Aedes. A genus of culicine mosquito, the most important of which, medically, is *A. aegypti,* which is the carrier of yellow fever and dengue.

Aegophony. The bleating quality of the voice as heard on auscultation over a thin layer of pleural fluid.

Aer-, Aero- (Gk *aēr:* air). Prefixes indicating a relationship to air or gas.

Aerobe. A micro-organism that requires oxygen or air in order to live and grow. **Facultative aerobe,** a micro-organism which can grow in the absence or presence of oxygen.

Aerodontalgia. Dental pain induced by air locked in the pulp canal at high altitude as when flying.

Aerogen. A gas-producing micro-organism.

Aerophagy. Swallowing of air.

Aerophobia. Morbid fear of fresh air and/or draughts.

Aerosol. A suspension of very fine liquid (or, rarely, solid) particles in a gas, used mainly for sterilizing or therapeutic purposes.

Aesthesiometer. An instrument for measuring the sensation of touch.

Afebrile. Without fever.

Affect. Feeling, emotion, especially as it influences a mental state.

Afferent. Conducting towards the centre.

Affusion. A method of treatment by pouring water on the body.

Afibrinogenaemia. Absence or deficiency of fibrinogen in the blood. Fibrinogenopenia.

Aflatoxin. A toxic constituent of the fungus, *Aspergillus flavus,* which is a common contaminant of ground nuts. Aflatoxin is a potent liver toxin and produces hepatomas in ducklings. It may well have a carcinogenic action in man.

Afterbirth. The placenta and associated membranes expelled from the uterus after the birth of the child.

Afterdamp. The irrespirable gases, carbon dioxide, nitrogen and carbon monoxide, left in a coalmine after an explosion of firedamp.

After-image. The visual impression remaining after stimulation of the retina has ceased.

After-pains. The cramplike painful contractions of the uterus following childbirth.

Agammaglobulinaemia. The condition characterized by absence or gross deficiency of gamma-globulin in human serum.

Aganglionosis. Congenital absence of ganglion cells. **Intestinal aganglionosis,** megacolon.

Agar. The solid residue obtained by concentrating a concoction prepared from various species of seaweed of the genus Gelidium. Its main use is as the basis of bacteriological culture media and as a thickening agent in the food industry. Medicinally it is used in the treatment of constipation.

Agene. Nitrogen trichloride, once used widely as a flour improver, but now banned for this purpose on account of the toxic effects it produces in dogs.

Agenesis. Absence or imperfect development of an organ of the body; sterility.

Agglutination. The clumping together of cells in a fluid, applied particularly to red blood cells and bacteria.

Agglutinin. An antibody that causes the clumping together, or agglutination, of bacteria or other cells. **Cold agglutinins,** agglutinins that will only react at low temperatures.

Agglutinogen. A substance which, when injected into the blood stream, evokes the product of a specific agglutinin.

Agitographia. Excessive speed of writing, with omission of words or parts of words.

Agitophasia. Excessive speed of speech, with slurring or omission of syllables or words.

Aglossia. Congenital absence of the tongue.

Agnathia. Total or virtual absence of the lower jaw.

Agnosia. Inability to recognize objects through the senses.

Agonal. Pertaining to death. Terminal.

Agonist. A contracting muscle, as opposed to an antagonist muscle.

Agoraphobia. Morbid fear of open spaces.

Agranulocyte. A non-granular leucocyte.

Agranulocytopenia. Agranulocytosis.

Agranulocytosis. The condition charac-

terized by marked diminution in the number of polymorphonuclear leucocytes.

Agraphia. Loss of the ability to write.

Agromania. Morbid desire for the country or to be alone.

Ague. Old term for malaria, a chill, or certain forms of neuralgia.

Agyria. Congenital absence of the cerebral convolutions or gyri.

Aichmophobia. Obsessional fear of sharp-pointed objects.

Ainhum. A disease in male Negroes, of unknown etiology, characterized by the slow, painless, spontaneous amputation of a toe (usually the fifth) by a constricting fibrous ring.

Air. The mixture of gases constituting the earth's atmosphere. At sea level the average constitution by volume is 78·08 per cent nitrogen, 20·95 per cent oxygen, 0·93 per cent argon, 0·03 per cent carbon dioxide, 0·0018 per cent neon, 0·0005 per cent helium, 0·00001 per cent xenon.

Air-bed. A rubber bed inflated with air.

Air-sickness. The form of motion sickness induced by flying.

Akinaesthesia. Lack of muscle sense or sense of movement.

Akinesia. Loss of, or impaired, motor function.

Ala. A winglike process. (*Plural:* alae.)

Alalia. Impairment of speech or lack of ability to talk.

Alanine. $C_3H_7NO_2$. One of the non-essential amino-acids.

Alastrim. A mild form of smallpox. Also known as variola minor.

Albinism. Congenital absence of pigment from the skin, hair and eyes.

Albino. A person afflicted with albinism.

Albumin. One of a group of simple proteins, which is present in both animal and plant tissues, and is soluble in water and coagulable by heat.

Albuminuria. The presence of serum albumin (and globulin) in the urine. In fact, a misnomer for proteinuria.

Albumose. One of the products of digestion of protein. It is not coagulable by heat.

Alcohol. A derivative of a hydrocarbon, in which one or more of the hydrogen ions is replaced by a hydroxyl group. **Absolute alcohol,** dehydrated alcohol, B.P. **Alcohol (95 per cent),** B.P. 1968, a mixture of ethyl alcohol and water, which contains not less than 94·7 per cent v/v or 92 per cent w/w, and not more than 95·2 per cent v/v or

92·7 per cent w/w of ethyl alcohol. **Dehydrated alcohol, B.P.** 1968, or absolute alcohol, contains not less than 99·4 per cent v/v or 99 per cent w/w, and not more than 100 per cent v/v or 100 per cent w/w of ethyl alcohol. **Denatured alcohol,** ethyl alcohol used for industrial purposes, to which contaminants have been added to render it unfit for human consumption. **Dilute alcohols, B.P.** 1968, prepared by diluting alcohol (95 per cent) with purified water, B.P. 1968, to dilutions ranging from 90 per cent v/v (rectified spirit) to 20 per cent v/v. **Ethyl alcohol,** C_2H_6O, ethanol, obtained by the fermentation of starches. The constituent of alcoholic liquors. **Methyl alcohol,** CH_4O, methanol, wood alcohol, used as a fuel and to denature ethyl alcohol, highly toxic to man. **Industrial methylated spirit, B.P.** 1968, a mixture of 19 volumes of alcohol (95 per cent) with 1 volume of approved wood naphtha. **Rectified spirit,** a synonym for the B.P. dilute alcohol containing 90 per cent alcohol. **Surgical spirit, B.P.C.** 1968, 25ml. of castor oil, 20ml. of diethyl phthalate, and 5ml. of methyl salicylate in 1000ml. of industrial methylated spirit.

Alcoholism. Acute alcoholism, the state induced by excessive ingestion of alcoholic liquors. **Chronic alcoholism,** drinking of alcoholic liquors which is out of the drinker's control, usually unrecognized by the victim until external events finally compel him to admit it to himself (or herself).

Alcuronium chloride. The B.P. Commission approved name for diallyl-dinortoxiferin dichloride, a muscle relaxant used by anaesthetists in relatively short operations of around twenty minutes' duration.

Aldosterone. The B.P. Commission approved name for 11β,21-dihydroxy-3,20-dioxopregn-4-en-18-al. The major electrolyte-controlling steroid secreted by the adrenal cortex.

Aldosteronism. The syndrome produced by excessive production of aldosterone, and characterized by hypokalaemia, alkalosis, hypertension and muscular weakness.

Aldrin. A chlorinated hydrocarbon insecticide.

Aleukaemia. Absence of leucocytes in the blood.

Alexia. Word blindness.

Alexin. Complement.

Algesimeter. An instrument for measuring the degree of sensitivity to pain.

Algid. Chilly, cold.

Alginic acid. B.P.C. 1968. A polyuronic acid obtained from seaweed, and used in pharmacy as a tablet disintegrant and binder.

Alienation. Insanity.

Alienist. A psychiatrist.

Aliment. Food, or nutritive substance.

Alimentary. Pertaining to food or nutrition.

Alimentation. The process of giving or taking nutriment.

Aliphatic. Fatty. Pertaining to the open-chain series of hydrocarbons.

Aliquot. A part; any portion that bears a known quantitative relationship to a whole.

Alizarin. A red dye obtained from the root of madder, and used as a pH indicator.

Alkalaemia. A state characterized by decrease in the hydrogen ion concentration of the blood.

Alkali. A substance that neutralizes an acid to form a salt, and turns red litmus blue.

Alkaloid. One of a large group of basic nitrogenous substances found widely distributed in plants. They include such well-known drugs as atropine, morphine and strychnine.

Alkalosis. The condition characterized by alkalaemia.

Alkaptonuria. An inborn error of metabolism characterized by the excretion of homogentisic acid in the urine as a result of the incomplete oxidation of phenylalanine and tyrosine.

Allachaesthesia. Touch sensation experienced at a point other than that touched.

Allantiasis. Sausage poisoning.

Allantoin. The diureide of glyoxylic acid, present in allantoic fluid and foetal fluid. It is used to stimulate epithelial growth in wounds and ulcers.

Allantois. The foetal membrane which in mammals contributes to the formation of the umbilical cord and placenta.

Allele. One of two or more forms of a gene that occur at a given locus on a chromosome.

Allelomorph. Allele.

Allergen. Any substance capable of producing a state of allergy.

Allergy. The hypersensitive state resulting in an abnormal reaction to a given allergen.

Allocheiria. The condition in which sensation is experienced on the opposite side of the body to that in which it was induced.

Allomorphism. Change of shape of cells due to pressure or metaplasia.

Allopurinol. B.P. Addendum 1969. $C_5H_4N_4O$. A drug used in the treatment of gout. It acts by suppressing the formation of uric acid.

Alloxan. A substance used widely for the production of diabetes mellitus in experimental animals. This it does by destroying the islets of Langerhans in the pancreas.

Allyloestrenol. The B.P. Commission approved name for 17α-allyloestr-4-en-17β-ol. A progestational steroid.

Allylprodine. The B.P. Commission approved name for 3-allyl-1-methyl-4-phenyl-4-propionyloxypiperidine. An analgesic.

Almond oil. B.P. 1968. The fixed oil obtained by cold expression from the seeds of bitter almond (or sweet almond). It is used in emollient preparations for the skin and as a vehicle for oily injections.

Aloes. B.P. 1968. The solid residue obtained by evaporating the liquid which drains from the cut leaves from various species of *Aloë*. It is a purgative, and is contraindicated in pregnant women and nursing mothers.

Aloin. B.P.C. 1968. A crystalline substance obtained chiefly from Curaçao aloes. It has the same action as aloes.

Alopecia. Baldness. **Alopecia areata,** patchy, usually reversible, baldness.

Aloxiprin. The B.P. Commission approved name for a polymeric condensation product of aluminium oxide and O-acetylsalicylic acid. An antirheumatic preparation.

Alphacetylmethadol. The B.P. Commission approved name for 4-dimethylamino-1-ethyl-2,2-diphenylpentyl acetate. An analgesic.

Alphameprodine. The B.P. Commission approved name for 3-ethyl-1-methyl-4-phenyl-4-propionyloxypiperidine. An analgesic.

Alphamethadol. The B.P. Commission approved name for 6-dimethylamino-4,4-diphenylheptan-3-ol. An analgesic.

Alphaprodine. The B.P. Commission approved name for 1,3-dimethyl-4-phenyl-4-propionyloxypiperidine. An analgesic.

Alprenolol hydrochloride. B.P. Addendum 1971. $C_{15}H_{23}NO_2$,HCl. An adrenergicbeta-receptor blocking agent.

Alum. B.P. 1968. The double sulphate of potassium and aluminium, or ammonium and aluminium. It is a powerful astringent, used as a mouthwash, to reduce excessive perspiration, and to harden the skin.

Aluminium. A light, whitish, malleable and ductile metal. Symbol Al. Atomic weight 26·98. Atomic number 13.

Aluminium hydroxide gel. B.P. 1968. An aqueous suspension of hydrated aluminium oxide together with varying quantities of basic aluminium carbonate, used as a slow-acting antacid. **Dried aluminium hydroxide gel,** B.P. 1968, the dried product of the interaction in aqueous solution of an aluminium salt with ammonium carbonate or sodium carbonate. It has the same action as aluminium hydroxide gel B.P. **Aluminium hydroxide tablets,** B.P. 1968, 500 mg of dried aluminium hydroxide gel with peppermint oil.

Aluminium powder. B.P.C. 1968. A protective dusting powder, used, for instance, around a colostomy.

Aluminium sulphate. B.P.C. 1968. A hydrated mixture of the normal salt, $Al_2(SO_4)_3$, with a small proportion of basic aluminium sulphate. It is a more potent astringent than alum.

Alveolus. A small sac-like dilatation, such as the air cells of the lungs, the depressions in the mucous lining of the stomach, and the sockets of the jaws into which the teeth fit. (*Plural:* alveoli.)

Alveus. A channel or trough. **Alveus hippocampi,** a bundle of nerve fibres investing the convexity of the hippocampus.

Alvine. Pertaining to the abdomen or intestines.

Amanita. A genus of mushroom, which contains several of the most toxic mushrooms, such as *Amanita muscaria* (the fly agaric), *Amanita phalloides* (the death-head), and *Amanita virosa* (the destroying angel).

Amaurosis. Complete blindness in one eye or both eyes in the absence of ophthalmoscopic or other marked objective signs.

Ambazone. The B.P. Commission approved name for 1,4-benzoquinone amidinohydrazone thiosemicarbazone hydrate. An antiseptic active against haemolytic streptococci, *Streptococcus viridans* and pneumococci. Used mainly in oral and tonsillar infections.

Ambenonium chloride. The B.P. Commission approved name for *NN'*-di-(2-diethylaminoethyl) oxamide bis-2-chlorobenzylochloride. A cholinesterase inhibitor.

Ambenoxan. The B.P. Commission approved name for 2-(2-methoxy-ethoxyethylaminomethyl)-1,4-benzodioxan. A muscle relaxant.

Ambidextrous. Able to use both hands equally well.

Ambivalence. In psychiatry, the state in which an individual concurrently hates and loves the same person or object.

Amblyopia. Partial loss of sight in one or both eyes in the absence of ophthalmoscopic or other marked objective signs.

Amblyoscope. An instrument to train an amblyopic eye to participate in binocular vision.

Ambucetamide. The B.P. Commission approved name for α-dibutylamino-4-methoxyphenylacetamide. A uterine antispasmodic.

Ambutonium bromide. The B.P. Commission approved name for (3-carbamoyl-3,3-diphenylpropyl) ethyldimethylammonium bromide. An antispasmodic.

Amelia. Congenital absence of the limbs.

Ameloblast. An enamel-forming cell.

Ameloblastoma. A tumour occurring in the lower molar region and derived from the tooth-forming epithelial cells.

Amenorrhoea. Absence of menstruation.

Amentia. An obsolete term, still used to denote mental deficiency.

Ametazole. The B.P. Commission approved name for 3-(2-aminoethyl) pyrazole. A stimulant of gastric secretion used in fractional gastric analysis.

Amethocaine hydrochloride. B.P. 1968. $C_{15}H_{25}ClN_2O_2$. A local anaesthetic suitable for infiltration, surface, or spinal anaesthesia.

Ametropia. The condition in which incident parallel rays of light do not come to a focus on the light-sensitive layer of the retina, due to abnormal length of the globe, abnormal curvature of the refracting surfaces of the cornea or lens, or abnormal refractive indices of the media.

Amfonelic acid. The B.P. Commission approved name for 7-benzyl-1-ethyl-4-oxo-1, 8-naphthyridine-3-carboxylic acid. A central nervous system stimulant.

Amiculum. A capsule of myelinated fibres surrounding the olivary nucleus.

Amide. An organic compound containing the univalent radical $CONH_2$.

Amiloride. The B.P. Commission approved name for *N*-amidino-3,5-diamino-6-chloropyrazinamide. A diuretic.

Aminacrine hydrochloride. B.P. 1968. $C_{13}H_{11}ClN_2,H_2O$. A non-staining acridine derivative which is used as an antiseptic, being active against many gram-positive and gram-negative bacteria.

Amino-acid. A derivative of the saturated fatty acid series, in which the alpha hydrogen atom has been replaced by an amino (NH_2) group. From amino-acids the body synthesizes proteins. Ten of them are essential to life.

Aminocaproic acid. B.P. Addendum 1971. $C_6H_{13}NO_2$. An antifibrinolytic agent which acts by inhibiting plasmin and plasminogen inhibitors which have fibrinolytic properties. It is used in the treatment of severe haemorrhage associated with excessive fibrinolysis.

Aminometradine. The B.P. Commission approved name for 1-allyl-6-amino-3-ethylpyrimidine-2,4-dione. A relatively weak diuretic used to control oedema in patients with mild congestive heart failure.

Aminophylline. B.P. 1968. Theophylline with ethylenediamine. A smooth muscle relaxant used for the relief of bronchospasm in asthma, for the relief of Cheyne-Stokes respiration and as a diuretic. Preferably given by intravenous or intramuscular injection, or as a suppository.

Aminopterin sodium. The B.P. Commission approved name for sodium *N*-[4-(2, 4-diaminopteridin-6-yl methyl) amino-benzoyl]-L-glutamate. A folic acid antagonist which is proving of value in the treatment of acute leukaemia.

Aminorex. The B.P. Commission approved name for 2-amino-5-phenyl-2-oxazoline. An appetite suppressant.

Amiphenazole. The B.P. Commission approved name for 2,4-diamino-5-phenylthiazole. A respiratory stimulant.

Amisometradine. The B.P. Commission approved name for 6-amino-1-methallyl-3-methylpyrimidine-2,4-dione. A diuretic.

Amitosis. The process of direct division of a cell, in which the nucleus divides in two, followed by division of the rest of the cell, thus producing two daughter cells, each with a nucleus.

Amitriptyline embonate. B.P.C. Supplement 1971. $C_{63}H_{62}N_2O_6$. An antidepressant with the same action as amitriptyline hydrochloride but, being tasteless, is preferred for liquid preparations for oral administration.

Amitriptyline hydrochloride. B.P. 1968. $C_{20}H_{24}ClN$. An antidepressant drug with anticholinergic activity, which does not inhibit monoamine oxidase.

Ammonia. NH_3. A colourless, pungent, alkaline gas. **Strong ammonia solution,** B.P.C. 1968, an aqueous solution of ammonia. This is the basis of several B.P.C. 1968 preparations, including **Aromatic ammonia solution** (sal volatile solution), and **Aromatic ammonia spirit** (spirit of sal volatile).

Ammoniated mercury. B.P. 1968. White precipitate. In the form of **Ammoniated mercury ointment,** B.P. 1968, 2·5 per cent of ammoniated mercury in simple ointment B.P., this preparation is used to a diminishing extent in the treatment of certain skin diseases such as impetigo.

Ammonium. The monovalent radical NH_4.

Ammonium bicarbonate. B.P.C. 1968. NH_4HCO_3. An irritant to mucous membranes, still used in small doses as a reflex expectorant.

Ammonium chloride. B.P. 1968. NH_4Cl. On account of the mild acidosis it produces, used to enhance the diuretic action of mercurial diuretics. It has also still a clinical reputation as an expectorant.

Amnesia. Loss or lack of memory.

Amniocentesis. Aspiration of amniotic fluid.

Amniography. Radiological visualization of the amniotic sac.

Amnion. The innermost of the membranes enwrapping the foetus.

Amnioscopy. The method whereby the volume and the colour of the amniotic fluid can be assessed without interfering with the pregnancy.

Amodiaquine hydrochloride. B.P. 1968. $C_{20}H_{24}Cl_3N_3O,2H_2O$. A quinoline derivative used as an antimalarial drug.

Amoeba. A member of the family Amoebidae, which in turn is a member of the class Rhizopoda. It is a unicellular organism, the main characteristic of which is that it puts out pseudopodia. (*Plural:* amoebae.)

Amoebiasis. The state of being infected with amoeba, especially *Entamoeba histolytica*.

Amoeboma. A granulomatous mass, or amoebic granuloma, that may develop anywhere in the large intestine during the course of intestinal amoebiasis.

Ampere. The electric current produced by one volt passing through a resistance of one ohm. (*Abbreviation:* A.)

Amphetamine sulphate. B.P. 1968. $C_{18}H_{28}N_2O_4S$. A sympathomimetic drug with marked stimulant effects. In view of the dangers of its abuse, it should only be prescribed when definitely indicated and under careful supervision.

Amphomycin. The B.P. Commission approved name for an antibiotic produced by *Streptomyces canus*.

Amphoric. The term used to describe the quality of the resonance or respiration when it resembles the sound produced by blowing over the mouth of an empty bottle. A cavity in the lung is the classical cause.

Amphoteric. Capable of acting as either an acid or a base.

Amphotericin. B.P. Addendum 1969. An antibiotic derived from *Streptomyces nodosus*, which is of value in the treatment of deep-seated mycotic infections, but must be used with extreme care because of its toxicity.

Ampicillin. B.P. 1968. A semi-synthetic penicillin salt which is acid resistant and is effective when given by mouth. It is destroyed by penicillinase. It has a wider spectrum than benzylpenicillin, being active against many gram-negative bacteria. **Ampicillin sodium** can be given intramuscularly or by slow intravenous injection.

Ampoule. A glass container, with one end drawn out to a point so as to be capable of easy, efficient sealing. It is used to contain sterile drugs for injection.

Ampulla. A flask-like dilatation of a canal or tubular structure. (*Plural:* ampullae.) **Ampulla of ductus deferens,** the dilated, tortuous section of the ductus deferens at the base of the bladder. **Hepatopancreatic ampulla,** the dilated duct formed by the junction of the bile duct and the pancreatic duct in the wall of the descending part of the duodenum. **Rectal ampulla,** the dilated lower part of the rectum. **Ampulla of the semicircular canal,** the dilatation at one end of each semicircular canal.

Ampulla of the semicircular duct, an ampulla corresponding to the one in the semicircular canal. **Ampulla of the uterine tube,** the tortuous lateral half of the uterine tube lying between the infundibulum and the isthmus.

Amputation. The removal of a limb or any other appendage of the body, whether complete or partial.

Amygdaloid body (nucleus). A nuclear mass, above and in front of the inferior horn of the lateral ventricle, which receives afferent fibres from the olfactory tract.

Amylase. An enzyme found in saliva and pancreatic juice, which hydrolyses starch to maltose.

Amyl nitrite. B.P.C. 1968. $C_5H_{11}NO_2$. A volatile oily liquid, used by inhalation for relief of the pain of angina pectoris.

Amylobarbitone. B.P. 1968. $C_{11}H_{18}N_2O_3$. An intermediate acting barbiturate, which is given by mouth. **Amylobarbitone sodium,** B.P. 1968, $C_{11}H_{17}N_2NaO_3$, can be given intravenously or orally.

Amyloid. A complex protein deposited in the tissues as a result of degenerative changes.

Amyloidosis. The condition characterized by the deposit of amyloid in the tissues.

Amylose. The soluble constituent of starch.

Amyotonia. Atony of the muscles. **Amytonia congenita,** a rare disease of infancy characterized by progressive muscular weakness and atrophy.

Amyotrophy. Muscular atrophy. **Amyotrophic lateral sclerosis,** a disease of the motor neurones, characterized by wasting of the muscles of the arm and spasticity of the legs.

Anabolism. Constructive metabolism. The assimilation of nutritive matter and its conversion into protoplasm.

Anacidity. Lack of acidity.

Anacrotism. An abnormality of the pulse, characterized by one or more notches on the ascending limb of the pulse tracing. Seen in some cases of aortic stenosis.

Anaemia. The condition characterized by diminution in the number of circulating red cells and/or their content of haemoglobin. **Achrestic anaemia,** a rare form of megaloblastic anaemia, due to failure to utilize the anti-anaemic factor. **Addisonian anaemia,** pernicious anaemia. **Aplastic anaemia,** anaemia due to complete failure of blood regeneration due to

aplasia of the bone marrow. It may be idiopathic or due to toxic agents such as drugs. **Auto-immune haemolytic anaemia,** an acquired haemolytic anaemia associated with the formation of auto-antibodies against the patient's own erythrocytes. **Cooley's anaemia,** thalassaemia. **Dyshaemopoietic anaemia,** a generic term used to describe those forms of anaemia resulting from a disturbance in growth of the erythrocyte due to defective supply of raw materials, whether iron, folic acid or vitamin B_{12}. **Haemolytic anaemia,** anaemia due to excessive destruction, or haemolysis, of erythrocytes. It may be hereditary or acquired. Important forms of haemolytic anaemia are *congenital* (or *hereditary*) *spherocytosis* (*acholuric family jaundice*), *haemolytic disease of the newborn,* and *paroxysmal haemoglobinuria.* **Hypochromic anaemia,** an anaemia characterized by a microcytic, hypochromic blood picture due to an absolute or relative lack of iron, or an inability to utilize it. **Hypoplastic anaemia,** anaemia due to hypoplasia of the bone marrow. **Iron-deficiency anaemia,** hypochromic, microcytic anaemia due to absolute or relative lack of iron, most commonly due to lack of iron in the diet or to haemorrhage. **Mediterranean anaemia,** thalassaemia. **Megaloblastic anaemia,** an anaemia characterized by hyperchromic macrocytes in the blood, due to arrest of formation of erythrocytes in the bone marrow at the stage of megaloblasts, as a result of a lack of vitamin B_{12} and/or folic acid. **Megaloblastic anaemia of infancy,** an anaemia in infants fed on dried milk, due to lack of folic acid and ascorbic acid. **Megaloblastic anaemia of pregnancy,** an anaemia which may occur in the last trimester of pregnancy or the puerpenum, due to lack of folic acid. **Nutritional anaemia,** the anaemia which occurs in premature infants, and sometimes in twins, due to lack of iron. **Nutritional hypochromic anaemia,** a form of iron-deficiency anaemia, due to lack of iron in the diet, most common in women, particularly in pregnancy, and in infants who are premature or twins. **Nutritional megaloblastic anaemia,** an anaemia due to prolonged ingestion of a diet poor in vitamin B_{12} and folic acid, and possibly other unknown factors, and widespread in tropical countries. **Pernicious anaemia,** a megaloblastic anaemia due to idiopathic failure of the stomach to secrete the intrinsic factor necessary for the absorption of vitamin B_{12} from the alimentary tract. **Post-haemorrhagic anaemia,** the microcytic, hypochromic anaemia resulting from haemorrhage. **Refractory anaemia,** an anaemia which fails to respond to any of the known haematinic agents. **Secondary anaemia,** an anaemia which arises in the course of some other disease, such as uraemia or rheumatoid arthritis. **Sickle-cell anaemia,** a severe anaemia due to inheritance of an abnormal haemoglobin, and characterized by the presence of sickle-shaped erythrocytes in the blood.

Anaerobe. A micro-organism capable of growing in the absence of oxygen.

Anaesthesia. Loss of feeling or sensation. **Basal anaesthesia,** the partial anaesthesia often induced, as by the injection of barbiturates, as a preliminary to general anaesthesia. **Block anaesthesia,** anaesthesia induced by injecting the anaesthetic solution into or around the nerve trunks supplying the area of operation. **Caudal anaesthesia,** a method used in obstetrics, by injecting the anaesthetic solution into the caudal canal. **Endotracheal anaesthesia,** anaesthesia induced by passing the anaesthetic direct into the lungs by an endotracheal tube. **Epidural anaesthesia,** anaesthesia induced by injecting the anaesthetic solution through a catheter in the epidural space, and used in obstetrics. **General anaesthesia,** anaesthesia of all parts of the body. **Glove and stocking anaesthesia,** anaesthesia of the parts of the body covered by gloves and stockings; a manifestation of hysteria. **Inhalation anaesthesia,** anaesthesia induced by the inhalation of anaesthetic gases such as ether and chloroform. **Intravenous anaesthesia,** anaesthesia induced by the intravenous injection of drugs such as thiopentone, of short duration and usually a preliminary to general anaesthesia. **Local anaesthesia,** anaesthesia of the part to be operated on, induced by local injection of the anaesthetic solution. **Refrigeration anaesthesia,** anaesthesia induced by intense cold, using either a volatile spray such as ethyl chloride, or ice packs. **Regional anaesthesia,** anaesthesia of part only of the body. **Spinal anaesthesia,** anaesthesia induced by injection of the anaesthetic solution into the subarachnoid space.

Anaesthetic. Without feeling. A drug used to induce anaesthesia.

Anaesthetist. An expert, or specialist, in administering anaesthetics.

Anagen. Growth phase of hair cycle.

Anal. Pertaining to the anus.

Analeptic. A restorative medicine. A drug that stimulates the central nervous system.

Analgesia. Loss of the power to feel pain without the loss of consciousness.

Analgesic. A drug that causes loss of pain without loss of consciousness. Insensitive to pain. Causing analgesia.

Analogue. An organ, or part of an organism, similar in function but different in structure and origin. In chemistry, a compound of similar structure to another but different in respect of a certain atomic component.

Analysand. The subject being psychoanalysed.

Analysis. Separation into component parts by determination of the chemical constitution of a substance. An abbreviation for psychoanalysis.

Anamnesis. The medical history of a patient.

Ananabasia. Inability to ascend heights.

Anaphase. The phase of mitosis between metaphase and telophase in which the centromeres split into two halves and the two constituent chromatids of each chromosome separate to group around the centrosomes.

Anaphylaxis. A condition of exaggerated reaction, or hypersensitiveness, to the injection of foreign protein.

Anaplasia. Reversion in a cell to more primitive, or embryonic, form such as may occur in malignant disease. Loss of structural differentiation.

Anasarca. Generalized oedema.

Anastomosis. An intercommunication between two blood vessels or other tubular structures. (*Plural:* anastomoses.) **Arteriovenous anastomosis,** an intercommunication between an artery and a vein.

Anatomy. The science of the structure or morphology of the body.

Anatoxin. A toxin which has been rendered non-toxic, but is still capable of inducing the production of antitoxin.

Ancylostoma. A genus of nematodes or roundworms, responsible for hookworm. *Ancylostoma braziliense,* the species responsible for larva migrans. *Ancylostoma duodenale,* the major species responsible for hookworm.

Ancylostomiasis. Hookworm disease,

caused by *Ancylostoma duodenale* or *Necator americanus*, which is rampant throughout the tropics and subtropics. It is responsible for a high incidence of morbidity and tends to run a long chronic course.

Androgen. A substance that governs the development of the secondary sexual characteristics of the male.

Androgynoid. A pseudo-hermaphrodite. Possession of masculine characteristics by a genetically pure female.

Androsterone. An androgenic steroid found in the urine of men and women. It is not as potent as testosterone.

Anencephaly. Absence of the brain.

Aneurine. Thiamine. Vitamin B_1.

Aneurysm. A circumscribed dilatation of an artery. **Arteriovenous aneurysm,** an abnormal communication between an artery and a vein. **Berry aneurysm,** a small aneurysm of one of the branches of the internal carotid artery, rupture of which is often the cause of a subarachnoid haemorrhage. **Cirsoid aneurysm,** the condition produced by lengthening, dilatation and tortuosity of a length of artery, and sometimes the accompanying veins and capillaries. **Dissecting aneurysm,** an aneurysm in which the blood splits the coats of the arterial wall. **False aneurysm,** an aneurysm in which all the coats of the arterial wall are ruptured and the blood is contained by the peri-arterial tissues. **Mycotic aneurysm,** an aneurysm caused by an infected embolus, as in subacute bacterial endocarditis. **Traumatic aneurysm,** an aneurysm caused by a wound or trauma.

Angiitis. Inflammation of a blood vessel or lymphatic vessel.

Angina. A choking sensation in the throat, or the condition responsible for such a sensation. A strangling oppressive pain **Agranulocytic angina,** progressive ulceration of the pharynx and soft palate with severe diminution in the number of granular white cells in the blood. **Angina pectoris,** severe substernal pain occurring on exercise and due to coronary artery disease. **Vincent's angina,** ulcerative stomatitis, due to infection with the fusiform bacillus and *Borrelia vincenti.*

Angiocardiography. X-ray of the heart after the injection of a radio-opaque substance.

Angiography. X-ray of the blood vessels and lymphatic vessels after the injection of a radio-opaque substance.

Angioid. Pertaining to a blood vessel.

Angiokeratoma. A warty angioma that occurs in the extremities in young people.

Angiology. The study of the blood vessels and the lymphatics.

Angioma. A tumour composed of blood vessels or lymphatic vessels.

Angioneurotic oedema. A condition of unknown etiology, characterized by paroxysmal attacks of oedematous swelling of the skin, subcutaneous tissue and mucous membranes. It responds to adrenaline and/or antihistamines.

Angiospasm. Spasmodic contractions of the blood vessels.

Angiotensin. The polypeptide, produced by the proteolytic action of renin, which has a controlling influence on the blood pressure, probably by controlling the output of aldosterone from the adrenal cortex.

Angiotensin amide. The B.P. Commission approved name for Val$_5$-hypertensin II-asp-β-amide. A pressor agent about 10 times more potent than noradrenaline.

Angle. The meeting point of two lines of plane. The degree of inclination of two intersecting planes. **Acromial angle,** the subcutaneous landmark where the lower border of the crest of the spine of the acromion becomes continuous with the lateral border of the acromion. **Angle of the anterior chamber,** the peripheral recess of the anterior chamber of the eye, bordered posteriorly by the root of the iris and the ciliary body and anteriorly by the corneo-sclera. **Carrying angle,** the angle of around 163° formed by the forearm and the upper arm when the forearm is fully extended and the hand supinated. **Angle of deviation,** the angle made by the line joining the object of fixation and the nodal point and the visual line. **Angle of eye,** the outer and inner corner, or canthus, of the eye. **Gamma angle,** the angle formed where the visual axis, which passes through the nodal point and the fovea centralis, crosses the optic axis. **Infrasternal angle,** the angle at the thoracic outlet formed by the cartilages of the 10th to 7th costal cartilages and the lower end of the sternum. **Iridocorneal angle,** the part of the anterior chamber of the eye that lies between the trabecular tissue and scleral spur anteriorly and outwards and the periphery of the iris posteriorly and inwards. **Angle of mandible,** the angle formed by the inferior and posterior borders of the mandible. **Metre angle,** unit used in measuring convergence. **Angle of mouth,** the junction of the upper and lower lips. **Angle of rib,** situated on the shaft of the rib, 5 to 6cm. from the tubercle. **Sacrovertebral angle,** where the sacrum articulates with the 5th lumbar vertebra. **Angle of squint,** the angle between the axes of the squinting and the normal eye. **Sternal angle,** where the upper end of the sternum articulates with the manubrium. **Angle of torsion of femur,** the angle formed by the transverse axis of the head of the femur and the transverse axis of the lower end of the bone. **Angle of torsion of the humerus,** the angle made by the longest axes of the upper and lower articular surfaces of the humerus. **Visual angle,** the angle subtended at the nodal point of the eye by the extremities of the object looked at.

Angor. Extreme distress. **Angor animi,** fear of impending dissolution.

Angostura. The bark of *Galipea cusparia,* from which a bitter substance, angosturin, at one time widely used medicinally as a bitter tonic, is obtained.

Angstrom. The unit of measurement of wave-length; one ten-thousand millionth of a metre. (*Abbreviation:* Å.)

Anhydraemia. A deficiency of the water content of the blood.

Anhydrase. An enzyme that catalyses the removal of water from a compound.

Anicteric. No trace of jaundice.

Anidrosis. Deficiency in the secretion of sweat.

Anileridine. The B.P. Commission approved name for ethyl 1-(4-aminophenethyl)-4-phenylpiperidine-4-carboxylate. An analgesic.

Anion. An ion carrying a negative charge.

Aniridia. Absence of the iris.

Aniseikonia. The condition in which the size and shape of the images in the two eyes are unequal.

Anise oil. B.P. 1968. The oil obtained by distillation from the dried fruits of star anise, *Illicium verum,* or from the dried ripe fruits of *Pimpinella anisum* (L.), and used as a mild carminative and mild expectorant.

Anisindione. The B.P. Commission approved name for an anticoagulant which is active when taken by mouth.

Anisocytosis. Abnormal variation in the size of circulating erythrocytes.

Anisomelia. Inequality between two paired limbs.

Anisometropia. The condition in which the refractions of the two eyes show a considerable difference.

Ankle. The talocrural joint.

Ankylosis. Fixation or immobility of a joint.

Anlage. The area in the embryo from which the adult structure is developed.

Annulus. A ring or ring-like structure. (*Plural:* annuli.) **Annulus (Anulus) fibrosus,** the outer laminated portion of an intervertebral disc.

Anoci-association. A method of anaesthesia aimed at reducing surgical shock to a minimum by heavy premedication, light general anaesthesia and local anaesthesia.

Anode. The positive pole of a source of electricity.

Anodontia. Congenital absence of teeth.

Anodyne. A drug that relieves pain. Relieving or easing pain.

Anomalopia. Partial colour blindness.

Anomaloscope. An instrument for the detection of colour blindness.

Anomia. Inability to name objects or to recognize names.

Anonychia. Congenital absence of nails.

Anopheles. A genus of the tribe Anophelini, which is one of the three tribes in the subfamily Culicinae (comprising all the true mosquitoes.) More than 200 species and varieties of the genus Anopheles have been described. Their medical importance is as transmitters of malaria and, to a lesser extent, of filariasis.

Anophthalmos. Congenital absence of one or both eyeballs.

Anorchism. Absence of the testes. Anorchia.

Anorexia. Loss or absence of appetite. **Anorexia nervosa,** the condition characterized by severe and persisting anorexia, with accompanying gross loss of weight, usually in young women, and of psychiatric origin.

Anosmia. Loss of the sense of smell.

Anovulation. Cessation or suspension of ovulation.

Anoxaemia. Insufficient oxygenation of the blood.

Anoxia. Deficiency of oxygen in the tissues.

Ansa. A loop or arc. (*Plural:* ansae.) **Ansa cervicalis,** the loop formed by the descending branch of the hypoglossal nerve and branches from the 2nd and 3rd cervical nerves. **Ansa lenticularis**

the bundle of efferent fibres from the globus pallidus to the subthalamic region. **Ansa subclavia,** a loop of fibres which links the middle with the inferior cervical sympathetic ganglia.

Antacid. A substance that neutralizes acidity. Usually applied to medicaments used to neutralize gastric hyperacidity.

Antagonist. An agent that exerts an action opposite to another. Usually applied to a muscle or a drug.

Antazoline hydrochloride. B.P. 1968. $C_{17}H_{20}ClN_3$. A relatively weak antihistamine, given by mouth. **Antazoline mesylate,** the B.P.C. preparation for intramuscular or slow intravenous use.

Ante- (L *ante:* before). Prefix indicating before, in front of.

Antecubital. In front of the elbow.

Anteflexion. A bending forward, usually applied to the normal forward curvature of the uterus.

Ante-mortem. Before death.

Antenatal. Between conception and birth.

Antenna. The feeler of an arthropod. (*Plural:* antennae.)

Antepartum. Before birth.

Anterior. In front. Anatomically, used to describe the front of the body and limbs.

Anteversion. Inclined or displaced forward, usually applied to the uterus.

Anthelmintic. A preparation that destroys or eliminates worms.

Anthracosis. Blackening of the lungs due to the inhalation of coal dust.

Anthrax. An infectious disease of herbivora caused by *Bacillus anthracis,* and transmissible to man by infected carcasses, hides, skin, hair and wool. **Pulmonary anthrax** (*wool-sorters' disease*), the form of disease caused by inhalation of the bacillus and largely restricted to the lungs. **Intestinal anthrax,** a rare form due to eating contaminated meat.

Anthropo-, Anthrop- (Gk *anthrōpos:* man). Prefixes indicating a relation to man.

Anthropometry. The comparative measurement of the human body and its parts.

Anthroponomy. The study of the development of the human body with regard to its environment and its relations to other organisms.

Anti- (Gk *anti:* against). Prefix, indicating against, instead.

Antibacterial. Destroying bacteria.

Antibiotic. Inimical to life. A substance produced by micro-organisms which is inimical to other micro-organisms. Penicillin is the classical example.

Antibody. A specific immunoglobulin substance produced in the blood and tissues by contact with an antigen, which has the property of destroying the antigen, or the micro-organism producing the antigen. **Antibody, homocytotropic,** an antibody which sensitizes homologous skin for immediate hypersensitivity reactions.

Anticoagulant. A substance, or drug, that prevents coagulation of the blood.

Anticonvulsant. A substance that prevents or relieves convulsions, as in the treatment of epilepsy.

Antidepressant. Preventing depression. A drug that relieves depression.

Antidote. A substance that antagonizes or neutralizes the action of a poison.

Antidromic. Relating to impulses passing along a nerve in the direction opposite to normal.

Antigen. A substance that provokes the formation of antibodies.

Antihelix. The curved prominence between the outer rim, or helix, of the ear and the entrance to the ear.

Antihistamine. A substance that counteracts the effects of histamine.

Antiketogenic. Reducing, or preventing, the formation of ketones. The foods or drugs used for this purpose.

Antimetabolite. A substance with a comparable molecular structure, but an antagonistic pharmacological action, to an essential metabolite.

Antimitotic. Arresting mitosis. A substance which has such an action.

Antimony. A metallic element. Symbol Sb. Atomic weight 121·75. Atomic number 51.

Antimony potassium tartrate. B.P.C. 1968. $C_4H_4KO_7Sb$. Tartar emetic. Has the same action as the sodium salt, but is less soluble and more irritant.

Antimony sodium tartrate. B.P. 1968. $C_4H_4NaO_7Sb$. A drug used in the treatment of schistosomiasis.

Antimycotic. Inimical to the growth of fungi.

Antioxidant. A substance that prevents or delays oxidation, and thus, for example, prevents rancidity in fat.

Antiperistalsis. Reversed peristalsis.

Antiphlogistic. A substance which prevents or controls inflammation.

Antipruritic. A drug that prevents or controls pruritus, or itching.

Antiputrescent. Having an antiputrefactive action.

Antipyretic. A drug that allays fever.

Antisepsis. The prevention of sepsis by destruction of the causative microorganisms.

Antiseptic. A substance that inhibits the growth of bacteria.

Antiserum. A native (unconcentrated) serum, or a preparation from a native serum, containing substances that have a specific prophylactic or therapeutic action when injected into individuals exposed to, or suffering from, a disease due to a specific microorganism.

Antispasmodic. An agent or drug that relieves or diminishes spasm.

Antitoxin. A preparation from native serum containing the antitoxic globulin or its derivative that has the specific power of neutralizing the toxin formed by a specific microorganism.

Antitragus. The small tubercle on the lower rim of the outer ear.

Antitussive. A remedy that relieves or eases cough.

Antivenene. The active principle in snake venom antiserum.

Antivenom. An antitoxin against snake venom. **Snake venom antiserum,** B.P.C. 1968, native serum, or a preparation from native serum, containing the antitoxic globulins, or their derivatives, that have the power of neutralizing the venom of one or more kinds of snakes. The antigens and methods used vary from country to country.

Antoxidant. Antioxidant.

Antroscope. An instrument for examining the maxillary sinus (or antrum).

Antrostomy. The opening of an antrum for purposes of drainage.

Antrum. A cavity, usually within a bone. (*Plural:* antra.) **Mastoid antrum,** an air sinus in the petrous part of the temporal bone. **Pyloric antrum,** the part of the stomach immediately preceding the pylorus.

Anuria. Complete suppression of urine.

Anus. The lower terminal opening of the alimentary canal. **Imperforate anus,** absence, or closure, of the anus.

Anxiety. The state of being anxious: that is, depressed, worried and apprehensive. **Anxiety state,** the emotional syndrome, characterized by undue depression, worry and apprehension.

Aorta. The major artery of the body, which stretches from the left ventricle to the level of the lower border of the fourth lumbar vertebra, where it divides into the right and left common iliac arteries. **Abdominal aorta,** the lower stretch of the aorta, from the diaphragm to its termination at the level of the fourth lumbar vertebra. **Arch of the aorta,** the curved section of the aorta that connects the ascending and the descending aorta. **Ascending aorta,** the first part of the aorta, from the left ventricle to the arch of the aorta. **Descending aorta,** the thoracic and abdominal aorta. **Thoracic aorta,** the stretch of the aorta from the aortic arch to the diaphragm.

Aortitis. Inflammation of the aorta.

Aortography. Radiological visualization of the aorta by means of injection of a radio-opaque substance. **Arch aortography,** visualization of the thoracic aorta by transfemoral catheterization and passage of a catheter into the aortic arch. **Lumbar aortography,** visualization of the abdominal aorta by needle puncture of the aorta through the back.

Aperient. A laxative drug.

Aperitive. An appetizer, or stimulant of the appetite.

Apex. The pointed portion of a conical-shaped organ, such as the heart or lungs. (*Plural:* apexes.)

Aphakia. Absence of the lens of the eye.

Aphasia. Impairment or loss of the ability to understand or produce the symbols used in communicating with others—whether speech, reading or writing. Absence of speech. **Amnestic aphasia,** difficulty in finding, or inability to find, names. **Central amnesia,** difficulty in understanding speech, associated with gross disorder of thought and expression. **Cortical motor aphasia,** the form of aphasia in which the expressive aspect of speech suffers severely. **Developmental aphasia,** congenital word-deafness and developmental alexia. **Expressive aphasia,** cortical motor aphasia. **Motor aphasia,** inability to make speech movements. **Nominal aphasia,** amnestic aphasia. **Receptive aphasia,** inability to comprehend written or spoken words. **Sensory aphasia,** receptive amnesia. **Subcortical motor aphasia,** pure word-dumbness. **Syntactical aphasia,** central aphasia. **Total aphasia,** complete motor and sensory aphasia. **Transcortical aphasia,** preservation of the power of repetition, but with either spontaneous speech or comprehension severely affected. **Verbal aphasia,** expressive aphasia. **Visual aphasia,** word-blindness.

Aphemia. Motor aphasia.

Aphonia. Loss of voice.

Aphrenia. Dementia.

Aphrodisiac. Stimulating sexual desire. A drug that stimulates sexual desire.

Aphtha. A small white spot, usually in the mouth, caused by a fungal infection.

Apicolysis. Artificial collapse of the apex of the lung.

Aplasia. Lack of development, or congenital absence, of an organ.

Apnoea. Stoppage of respiration.

Apocrine. Pertaining to those cells that incorporate part of their protoplasm in their secretion.

Apodia. Congenital absence of the feet.

Apomorphine` hydrochloride. B.P. 1968. $C_{17}H_{18}ClNO_2,\frac{1}{2}H_2O$. A powerful emetic.

Aponeurosis. The white, fibrous, collagenous membrane which ensheathes muscle and acts as a means of attachment of the muscle to the parts which it moves. (*Plural*: aponeuroses.)

Apophysis. An outgrowth, or projection, especially of bone.

Apophysitis. Inflammation of an apophysis. **Calcanean apophysitis,** a form of osteochondritis affecting the posterior epiphysis of the calcaneus.

Apoplexy. The sudden loss of consciousness, followed by paralysis, resulting from a cerebral haemorrhage, or occlusion of the middle cerebral artery by thrombosis or embolism.

Appendicectomy. Surgical removal of the vermiform appendix.

Appendicitis. Inflammation of the vermiform appendix.

Appendicostomy. The operation of making an opening in the vermiform appendix for the purpose of draining or irrigating the caecum and ascending colon.

Appendix. An appendage, or small accessory part attached to the main part of an organ. **Vermiform appendix,** the worm-like tube which springs from the postero-medial wall of the caecum, 2cm. or so below the end of the ileum. The average length is 9cm. (range, 2 to 20cm.)

Apperception. Conscious perception.

Appetite. Desire or craving, usually for food.

Applicator. An instrument for making local applications.

Apposition. The state of being in contact.

Apraxia. The inability to perform a purposive movement, the nature of which is understood, in the absence of severe motor paralysis, sensory loss, and ataxia.

Aproctia. Imperforate, or absent, anus.

Aprosexia. Inability to fix attention, due to mental weakness, or defective hearing or vision.

Aprosody. Absence of the normal pitch and rhythm of the voice.

Aprosopia. Congenital absence of part or all of the face.

Aprotinin. The B.P. Commission approved name for a polypeptide proteinase inhibitor which inhibits the formation of trypsin and other proteolytic enzymes and is used in the treatment of acute pancreatitis.

Aptocaine. The B.P. Commission approved name for *N*-[2- (pyrrolidin-1-yl)propionyl]-*o*-toluidine. A local anaesthetic.

Apus. An individual lacking feet or the lower extremities.

Apyrexia. Absence of fever.

Aqua. The latin for water. In pharmacy used to describe solutions of volatile oils or other aromatic substances in water. Now replaced by the term water.

Aqueduct. A canal or channel. **Aqueduct of the cochlea,** a canal in the bony labyrinth of the internal ear, containing perilymph, which communicates, directly or indirectly, with the subarachnoid space. **Aqueduct of the mid-brain,** the narrow canal, about 15mm. long, connecting the third with the fourth ventricle. **Aqueduct of the vestibule,** a canal in the bony labyrinth of the internal ear, which carries the endolymphatic duct.

Aqueous. The aqueous humour of the eye.

Arachis. A genus of leguminous plants. **Arachis oil,** B.P. 1968, the refined fixed oil obtained from the seeds of *Arachis hypogaea* (L.). Used as a substitute for olive oil.

Arachnida. A class of the Arthropoda, which includes mites, scorpions, spiders and ticks.

Arachnidism. The condition induced by the bite of poisonous spiders.

Arachnodactyly. Abnormally long slender fingers and toes.

Arachnoid. The delicate membrane enveloping the brain and spinal cord, and lying between the dura mater externally and the pia mater internally. Also known as the arachnoid mater.

Arachnoiditis. Inflammation of the arachnoid.

Arbor. A tree-like structure. **Arbor vitae,** the term applied to the tree-like, branching appearance of the cut surface of the cerebellum, and of the canal of the cervix uteri.

Arboviruses. The group of viruses transmitted by arthropods. There are around 200 of them, and they include the viruses of dengue and of yellow fever.

Arc. Part of the circumference of a circle. **Carbon arc,** a maintained electric arc between two carbon electrodes. **Mercury arc,** an electric discharge through a vacuum tube with mercury electrodes. Both these are rich in ultra-violet radiation. **Reflex arc,** the nervous pathway for reflex action, consisting of at least a receptor or sensory neurone and an effector or motor neurone.

Arch. A structure with a curved, arch-like outline. **Alveolar (dental) arch,** the arch formed by the alveolar margins of the jaws. **Aortic arch,** the curved part of the aorta connecting the ascending with the descending aorta. **Arches of the foot,** the arched outline of the tarsal and metatarsal bones. These arches are longitudinal (medial and lateral) and transverse. **Hyoid arch,** the second visceral arch, in man only found in the embryo. **Lumbocostal arches,** the lateral is a tendinous arch over the quadratus lumborum; the medial is a tendinous arch over the psoas major. **Mandibular arch,** the first visceral arch, from which the lower jaw and much of the face are developed. **Palmar arches,** the deep is formed by the anastomosis of the terminal part of the radial artery with the deep palmar branch of the ulnar artery; the superficial is formed mainly by the ulnar artery, being completed usually by a branch of the radial index artery. **Plantar arch,** the arterial arch in the foot formed by the anastomosis of the lateral plantar artery and the dorsalis pedis artery. **Pubic arch,** the arch formed by the conjoined rami of the ischium and pubis on each side. **Superciliary arch,** the bony prominence above each orbit. **Vertebral arch,** the posterior or dorsal part of a vertebra, consisting of a pair of pedicles and a pair of laminae. **Visceral arches,** the embryonic structures from which the lower part of the face and the whole of the neck develop. There are six of them.

Arch-, Archi- (Gk *arcē:* origin). Prefixes signifying first or original.

Archenteron. The primitive gut cavity of the embryo.

Archicerebellum. The phylogenetically oldest part of the cerebellum, consisting of the flocculonodular lobe and the lingula.

Archipallium. The cortex of the dentate gyrus and hippocampus.

Arcuate. Arched, bow-shaped.

Arcus. An arch. (*Plural:* arcus.) **Arcus juvenilis,** a lipoid infiltration of the cornea met with in children. **Arcus parieto-occipitalis,** the arched gyrus that surrounds the end of the parieto-occipital sulcus. **Arcus senilis,** a lipoid infiltration of the cornea in old people.

Area. A circumscribed region. **Association area,** an area of the cerebral cortex concerned with the integration of afferent and efferent connexions. **Auditopsychic area,** that part of the cortex of the superior temporal gyrus, in which auditory impressions receive their interpretation. **Auditory area,** the cortex of the superior temporal gyrus and the transverse temporal gyri; it is divided into a sensory and a psychic part. **Auditosensory area,** that part of the cortex of the anterior transverse temporal gyrus and the superior temporal gyrus, in which auditory impressions reach consciousness. **Bare area of the liver,** the area on the posterior surface of the liver devoid of peritoneal covering and attached to the diaphragm by areolar tissue. **Area of superficial cardiac dullness,** the roughly triangular area, which can be mapped out by light percussion and corresponding to the portion of the heart not covered by the lungs. **Cingulate area,** the cingulate gyrus. **Embryonic area,** that part of the developing ovum from which the embryo is formed. **Extrapyramidal areas,** those areas of the cerebral cortex from which generalized movements may be evoked by stimulation, even after ablation of the motor area. **Intercondylar area,** the roughened strip on the superior surface of the tibia, between the articular surfaces of the two condyles. **Macular area,** the posterior portion of the visuosensory area, which is the cortical receiving centre for visual impressions from the macula. **Motor**

area, the cerebral cortex of the precentral gyrus and the adjoining part of the paracentral lobule, which initiates and organizes purposive movements. **Parastriate area,** part of the visuopsychic area. **Parietal area,** the cerebral cortex between the visual area behind and the postcentral area in front which constitutes one of the large association areas. **Parolfactory (subcallosal) area,** the cortex on the medial surface of the cerebral hemisphere, lying between the posterior parolfactory sulcus and the anterior parolfactory sulcus. **Peristriate area,** part of the visuopsychic area. **Piriform area,** the cortex of the uncus and the anterior part of the parahippocampal gyrus, in which olfactory impressions reach consciousness. **Postcentral area,** the cortex of all but the lowest part of the postcentral gyrus and continued into the adjoining part of the paracentral lobule, which receives afferent fibres from the thalamus, representing relays conveying exteroceptive and proprioceptive sensibilities. **Precentral area,** the precentral gyrus and the posterior portions of the superior, middle and inferior frontal gyri. **Premotor area,** the anterior part of the precentral area. **Temporal area,** the cortex of the middle and inferior temporal gyri, lesions of which are accompanied by disturbance of auditopsychic functions. **Visuopsychic area,** the area surrounding the visuosensory area, which is responsible for the correlation of visual impressions and their association with past experience. **Visuosensory area,** the cortical receiving centre for visual impressions, occupying the walls of the posterior part of the calcarine sulcus and extending on to the surface of the cuneus and the lingual gyrus.

Areflexia. Absence of reflexes.

Areola. A small space. (*Plural:* areolae.) The coloured area of skin encircling the nipple of the breast.

Argentaffinoma. A tumour, most often found in the appendix, terminal ileum and colon, and derived from the argentaffin cells of Kultschitzky; also known as argentaffin carcinoma.

Arginine. $C_6H_{14}N_4O_2$. One of the essential amino-acids.

Arginine glutamate. The B.P. Commission approved name for the L-arginine salt of L-glutamic acid. A nutrient sometimes of value in the management of hepatic coma.

Argipressin. The B.P. Commission approved name for 8-argininevasopressin. An antidiuretic hormone.

Argyll Robertson pupil, the pupil that responds to accommodation but not to light. Almost pathognomonic of syphilis. Named after the Edinburgh physician, D. M. C. L. Argyll Robertson (1837–1909).

Argyria. The condition induced by prolonged ingestion of silver salts, characterized predominantly by ashen-grey discoloration of the skin.

Ariboflavinosis. The condition resulting from lack of riboflavine in the diet, and characterized by cheilosis, stomatitis, eye changes, and seborrhoeic dermatitis.

Arm. The upper limb.

Armpit. The axilla.

Arrhenoblastoma. A masculinizing tumour of the ovary which arises from the primitive ovarian mesenchyme.

Arrhythmia. Any variation from the normal rhythm of the heart. **Sinus arrhythmia,** irregularity of the heart rate in accordance with the respiratory cycle, speeding up on inspiration and slowing on expiration.

Arrowroot. B.P.C. 1968. The starch granules of the rhizome of *Maranta arundinacea.* (L.) It has the general properties of starch, and is used as a gruel in the treatment of diarrhoea.

Arsenic. An element, symbol As, atomic weight 74·92, atomic number 33, certain salts of which have been widely used in medicine—and also in crime. Apart from certain organic preparations, there is none left in the 1968 *British Pharmacopoeia* or *British Pharmaceutical Codex.*

Arteri-, Arterio- (Gk *arteria:* artery). Prefixes indicating association with an artery.

Arteriectomy. Excision of a portion of an artery.

Arteriogram. An X-ray of an artery outlined by a radio-opaque substance.

Arteriography. The visualization by means of X-rays of an artery after injection of a radio-opaque substance.

Arteriole. A small artery.

Arteriolitis. An inflammatory or degenerative condition of the arterioles. **Necrotizing arteriolitis,** the degenerative condition of the arterioles characteristic of malignant hypertension.

Arteriopuncture. The obtaining of blood from an artery.

Arteriosclerosis. A condition characterized by thickening and hardening of the arterial wall, accompanied by loss of elasticity.

Arteriospasm. Spasm of an artery.

Arteriotomy. The cutting of an artery, usually for the purpose of blood-letting.

Arteriovenous. Involving both an artery and a vein. **Arteriovenous aneurysm,** an abnormal communication between an artery and a vein.

Arteritis. Inflammation of an artery. **Temporal arteritis,** an inflammatory disorder of unknown cause affecting particularly the temporal arteries. Also known as **cranial arteritis** and **giant-cell arteritis.**

Artery. A vessel that conveys blood away from the heart. (*Plural:* arteries.)

Arthr-, Arthro- (Gk *arthron:* joint). Prefixes indicating association with a joint or articulation.

Arthralgia. Pain in a joint.

Arthrectomy. Excision of a joint.

Arthritis. Inflammation of a joint. **Rheumatoid arthritis,** polyarthritis of unknown etiology, accompanied by constitutional disturbances.

Arthrodesis. Surgical fixation of a joint.

Arthrogram. X-ray of a joint.

Arthrolith. A calculus in a joint.

Arthropathy. Any disease affecting a joint.

Arthroplasty. The making of a new, artificial joint, or the loosening of a fixed or ankylosed joint.

Arthropoda. The phylum, the members of which are characterized externally by a segmented, hard exoskeleton, a proportion of the segments bearing paired appendages. Among the classes into which it is subdivided are the Insecta, Arachnida, Crustacea, Chilopoda, Diplopoda, and Pentastomida.

Arthroscope. An instrument for the visualization of the interior of a joint.

Arthrosis. Degenerative disease of a joint. A joint.

Arthrotomy. Incision into a joint.

Articular. Pertaining to a joint.

Articulation. A joint. The enunciation of words.

Arytenoid. Shaped like a ladle. Applied to two cartilages, and associated muscles, in the larynx.

Asaphia. Indistinct enunciation.

Asbestosis. A form of lung disease (pneumoconiosis) caused by the inhalation of asbestos particles.

Ascariasis. The disease caused by infestation with *Ascaris lumbricoides.*

Ascaricide. A drug which destroys roundworms (or ascarides).

Ascaris. A genus of intestinal Nematodes, also known as roundworms.

Ascites. A collection of serous fluid in the peritoneal cavity.

Ascorbic acid. B.P. 1968. $C_6H_8O_6$. The antiscorbutic vitamin which is either prepared synthetically or extracted from various fruits, including rose hips, blackcurrants, and citrus fruits, and is also known as vitamin C.

Asemia. Inability to understand or use writing, speech or signs.

Asepsis. Absence of infection.

Aspartic acid. $C_4H_7NO_4$. An aminoacid.

Aspergillosis. A fungus infection, usually involving the lungs in man, in whom it is usually due to *Aspergillus fumigatus.* It is a common disease in birds.

Aspergillus. A genus of fungi belonging to the family Ascomycetes. *Aspergillus fumigatus* is the common infecting member in aspergillosis in man and birds.

Aspermatogenesis. Failure of development of spermatozoa.

Aspermia. Absence of spermatozoa in seminal fluid.

Asphyxia. The condition characterized by lack of oxygen, and excess of carbon dioxide, in the tissues, and usually due to interference with respiration. **Asphyxia neonatorum,** asphyxia in the new-born infant, usually due to the infant never having breathed. **Asphyxia pallida,** the state of shock in the new-born infant characterized by asphyxia, pallid cold clammy skin and faint pulse.

Aspiration. The removal of fluids or gases from a cavity by means of suction. Inspiration.

Aspirator. An apparatus for removing fluid from a cavity by suction.

Aspirin. B.P. 1968. Acetylsalicylic acid. A potent analgesic and antipyretic.

Assay. Analysis or test of purity. **Biological assay,** estimation of the amount of a material in a given preparation by observation of its activity on a living population, usually animals, but occasionally micro-organisms, plants, men or tissue cells. **Microbiological assay,** assaying nutritional factors, such as vitamins, and antibiotics by studying their effect on the growth of micro-organisms.

Assimilation. The incorporation of nutritive material into the substance of the body.

Association. The coordination, linking, or union of the functions of similar parts, whether physical or psychological.

Assonance. A morbid use of alliteration.

Assuetude. Habituation.

Astasia. Inability to stand because of motor incoordination. **Astasia-abasia,** inability to walk or stand because of defective will-power.

Astereognosis. Inability to recognize objects by feeling or touching them.

Asthenia. Debility. Weakness.

Asthenopia. Sense of weakness in the eyes.

Asthma. Paroxysmal dyspnoea of expiratory type. **Bronchial asthma,** a paroxysmal condition characterized by attacks of expiratory dyspnoea due to bronchospasm evoked by allergic and other factors. **Cardiac asthma,** the paroxysmal dyspnoea that occurs in severe cases of left-sided heart failure.

Astigmatism. The error of refraction in which a point of light cannot be made to produce a punctate image on the retina by any spherical correcting lens.

Astringent. Causing contraction or drying up. A drug that produces these effects.

Astrocyte. One of the three main types of cells constituting neuroglia, the connective tissue of the central nervous system. Astrocytes are believed to be primarily concerned with the nutrition of nervous tissue.

Astrocytoma. A tumour composed of astrocytes.

Astrophobia. Fear of outer space and the stars.

Asyllabia. The form of aphasia in which letters are recognized but cannot be made into syllables or words.

Asymbolia. Loss of the ability to appreciate signs or gestures.

Asymptomatic. Without symptoms.

Asynchronism. Lack of coordination.

Asynclitism. Oblique presentation of the foetal head.

Asyndesis. A form of mental defect characterized by inability to relate or connect thoughts and ideas.

Asynechia. Absence of continuity of structure.

Asynergia. Absence of coordinated movements between muscles having opposite actions: e.g. the flexors and extensors of a joint.

Asystole. Arrest of contraction of the heart.

Ataractic. A drug that produces peace of mind. A tranquillizer.

Ataraxia. Peace of mind.

Atavism. The inheritance of some characteristic, trait, or disease from a grandparent or more remote ancestor, which is not present in the parents.

Ataxia. Loss of control over voluntary movements, or incoordination of muscular action. **Cerebellar ataxia,** the ataxia that follows loss of cerebellar function. **Hereditary ataxia,** a group of closely related hereditary or familial disorders characterized by degenerative changes in one or more of the optic nerves, the cerebellum, the olives and the long descending and ascending tracts of the spinal cord. None is common, but the most common is known as **Friedrich's ataxia.** **Locomotor ataxia,** tabes dorsalis. **Sensory ataxia,** ataxia induced by defective sensory information. **Spinal ataxia,** ataxia induced by disease of the spinal cord. **Vestibular ataxia,** ataxia induced by vestibular disease.

Ataxiadynamia. Incoordination combined with muscular weakness.

Ataxiophemia. Incoordination of the muscles of speech.

Ataxiophobia. A morbid fear of disorder.

Atel-, Atelo- (Gk *atelēs:* incomplete). Prefixes signifying incomplete or imperfect.

Atelectasis. Partial collapse of the lungs. Incomplete expansion of the lungs in the newborn.

Ateleiosis. Infantilism or dwarfism.

Atelocardia. Incomplete development of the heart.

Atelocheilia. Incomplete development of the lips.

Atelocheiria. Incomplete development of the hand.

Ateloglossia. Incomplete development of the tongue.

Atelognathia. Incomplete development of the mandible.

Atelopodia. Incomplete development of the foot.

Athelia. Absence of the nipples.

Atheroma. The condition characterized by fatty degeneration of the arterial intima.

Atherosclerosis. The condition characterized by a combination of atheroma and arteriosclerosis.

Athetoid. Pertaining to athetosis.

Athetosis. The slow, writhing, continuous, involuntary movements, usually of the hands, resulting from damage of the basal ganglia of the brain.

Athyreosis. The condition produced by lack, or absence, of the secretion of the thyroid gland.

Atlas. The first cervical vertebra.

Atom. The ultimate part of a molecule capable of separate existence and still retaining the properties of the element of which it is a part.

Atomic number. The number of protons in the nucleus of a given atom.

Atomizer. An instrument for producing a jet or spray.

Atony. Loss, or lack, of tone.

Atopen. An allergen or antigen.

Atopy. A form of hypersensitivity encountered in man, but not in animals, and characterized, amongst other features, by a familial tendency.

Atraumatic. Not causing any wound or harm.

Atremia. Absence of tremor.

Atresia. The absence, or closure by a membrane, of a natural orifice.

Atrioventricular. Pertaining to the atria and ventricles of the heart. **Atrioventricular bundle,** the muscular band which conducts the heart impulse from the atrioventricular node to the ventricles. **Atrioventricular node,** the node situated in the atrial septum above the orifice of the coronary sinus, continuous on the one hand with the atrial septal musculature and on the other with the fibres of the atrioventricular bundle.

Atrium. A vestibule. (*Plural:* atria.) **Atrium of the heart,** the chamber that receives the blood from the veins. **Atrium of the lungs,** the entrance to the terminal air saccule. **Atrium of the middle meatus of the nose,** a shallow depression in the vestibule of the nose.

Atropine. B.P. 1968. $C_{17}H_{23}NO_3$. An alkaloid, ($\pm$)-hyosycamine, obtained from Duboisia species, and other plants of the family Solanaceae or prepared synthetically. It has a parasympatholytic action, and antagonizes the muscarine-like actions of acetylcholine and similar drugs. It diminishes the rigidity and salivation of parkinsonism, diminishes the secretions of the salivary and sweat glands and of the bronchial and gastro-intestinal tracts, relaxes spasm of involuntary muscle, increases the heart rate, produces vasodilatation, dilates the pupil and paralyses accommodation. **Atropine methonitrate,** B.P. 1968, a drug mainly used in the treatment of congenital pyloric stenosis. **Atropine sulphate,** B.P. 1968, the generally used salt of atropine.

Atrophy. The state of wasting characterized by reduction in the size of an organ or tissue resulting from a reduction in the number and size of its individual cells. **Acute yellow atrophy of the liver,** the term at one time applied to a fulminating form of hepatitis. **Brown atrophy,** atrophy of the myocardium, so called because of the brown colour given to the myocardium by granules of a variety of lipofuscin. **Denervation atrophy,** the atrophy that follows denervation of muscle, as in poliomyelitis. **Disuse atrophy,** the atrophy that follows prolonged immobilization of muscle. **Ischaemic atrophy,** the atrophy that develops when a muscle is deprived of its blood supply. **Muscular atrophy,** the name applied to a group of diseases characterized by muscular wasting resulting from primary muscular disease. **Optic atrophy,** the condition of the optic disc resulting from degeneration of the optic nerve. **Peroneal muscular atrophy,** the form of muscular atrophy characterized by wasting of the muscles of the leg. **Progressive muscular atrophy,** the form of motor neurone disease in which the muscular wasting tends to remain localized for a long time to the muscles of the hand and forearm.

Attar. An essential volatile oil distilled from a plant.

Attenuation. Weakening or thinning.

Attrition. Wearing away by abrasion or rubbing.

Audioanalgesia. Analgesia induced by sound.

Audiogram. The graphic record of hearing acuity produced by an audiometer.

Audiometer. An instrument for recording the range and acuity of hearing.

Auditory. Pertaining to the sense of hearing.

Augnathus. A monster with a double lower jaw.

Aura. The premonitory sensation experienced before a convulsion—usually an epileptic convulsion.

Aural. Pertaining to the ear or sense of hearing, or an aura.

Aurantium. Orange.

Auricle. The pinna or flap of the ear. The small muscular pouch projecting from the upper part of each atrium of the heart.

Auride. A dermatitis due to gold therapy.

Auriscope. An instrument for examining the ear.

Auristillae. Ear-drops.

Aurum. Gold.

Auscultation. The method of diagnosis characterized by listening to the sounds produced in the organ of the body being examined, usually the heart or lungs.

Autism. The condition characterized by morbid self-absorption.

Auto- [(Gk *autos:* self). Prefix meaning self or same.

Auto-agglutination. Agglutination of an individual's red blood cells by his own serum.

Autochthonous. Indigenous. Found in the same place as originated.

Autoclave. An automatically controlled apparatus for sterilization by means of steam.

Autodigestion. Autolysis.

Autogamy. Self-fertilization.

Autogenesis. Self-generation.

Autogenous. Endogenous. Self generated.

Autograft. A graft taken from the same body as that in which it is to be grafted.

Autohypnosis. Self-induced hypnosis.

Auto-immunity. The process whereby an individual develops or acquires antibodies to his own tissues.

Auto-intoxication. Poisoning resulting from absorption of waste products produced in the body during the course of metabolism.

Autolysis. Self-digestion of tissues in the body by enzymes produced by the cells of the tissue concerned.

Automatism. The performance of acts without conscious will as in sleepwalking or after an epileptic fit.

Autonomic. Self-controlling. Independent. **Autonomic nervous system,** that part of the nervous system, made up of the sympathetic and the parasympathetic system, which functions independently of the will.

Autoploidy. The state of having two or more sets of chromosomes as a result of redoubling of a single haploid set.

Autopsy. Necropsy. Post-mortem examination.

Autoradiography. The method of producing a radiograph by means of radiations from within the object itself.

Autosome. A paired chromosome—as opposed to a sex chromosome.

Autosuggestion. The mental state, often encountered after accidents, in which the individual magnifies the import of minor injuries to such an extent that he believes he is affected by some major disability, such as paralysis of a limb.

Autotroph. A non-parasitic bacterium which, like plants, is able to utilize carbon dioxide as the main source of carbon, energy being obtained by the oxidation of inorganic compounds or from sunlight.

Autovaccine. Autogenous vaccine. A vaccine made from culture of microorganisms from the individual's own tissues or secretions.

Aux-, Auxo- (Gk *auxein:* to increase). Prefixes signifying relation to increase or growth.

Auxanology. The science of growth.

Auxin. A plant hormone that promotes growth.

Auxotroph. A micro-organism that can only grow on a simple medium if this is supplemented by a particular nutrient: e.g. a particular amino-acid or vitamin.

Avascular. Bloodless. Without blood vessels.

Avian. Pertaining to birds.

Avirulent. Not virulent.

Avitaminosis. The condition produced by lack of one or more vitamins.

Avulsion. The forceful tearing away or [wrenching of a part of the body.

Axilla. The armpit. (*Plural*: axillae.)

Axis. A line about which a body rotates, or the line drawn through the centre of a body. The 2nd cervical vertebra. (*Plural:* axes.) **Axis cylinder process,** axon. **Axis of lens,** the line connecting the anterior and posterior poles of the optic lens. **Optic axis,** the line joining the anterior and posterior poles of the eyeball. **Axis of the pelvis,** an imaginary line showing the position of the centre of the foetal head in its passage through the pelvis.

Axolemma. The membrane surrounding the axon, or axis cylinder.

Axon. The efferent process of a nerve cell.

Axoplasm. The semifluid substance within the axolemma of an axon.

Azacyclonol. The B.P. Commission approved name for 1α-4-piperidylbenzhydrol. A tranquillizer.

Azamethonium bromide. The B.P. Commission approved name for 3-methyl-3-azapentamethylenedi (ethyldimethylammonium bromide). A ganglionic blocking agent.

Azapetine. The B.P. Commission approved name for 1-allyl-2,7-dihydro-3, 4 : 5, 6-dibenzazepine. A vasodilator.

Azaserine. An anti-tumour antibiotic, produced by a strain of streptomyces and also by chemical synthesis. It is used in the treatment of chronic lymphatic leukaemia.

Azathioprine. B.P. Addendum 1969. $C_9H_7N_7O_2S$. An immunosuppressive agent widely used in organ transplantation.

Azetepa. The B.P. Commission approved name for *PP*-diaziridin-1-yl-*N*-ethyl-1,3,4-thiadiazol-2-yl-phosphinamide. An antimetabolite.

Azidocillin. The B.P. Commission approved name for 6-[D(—)-α-azidophenylacetamido] penicillanic acid. An antibiotic.

Azoospermia. Absence of spermatozoa in the semen.

Azotaemia. The accumulation of nitrogenous substances, especially urea, in the blood.

Azovan blue. The B.P. Commission approved name for the tetrasodium salt of 4,4'-di-(8-amino-1-hydroxy-5,7-disulpho-2-naphthylazo)-3,3'-bitolyl. Also known as Evans Blue. A diagnostic agent.

Azote. Nitrogen.

Azygos. Unpaired.

Azuresin. A cation-exchange compound used for the detection of free hydrochloric acid in the gastric juice.

B

Bacillaemia. The presence of bacilli in the bloodstream.

Bacilluria. The presence of bacilli in the urine.

Bacillus. A member of the Bacillaceae genus of the Bacteroidacae family of the order of Eubacteriales. (*Plural:* bacilli.)

Bacitracin. B.P. 1968. An antibiotic produced by certain strains of *Bacillus licheniformis* and by *B. subtilis* var. *Tracy*, which is active against a wide range of gram-positive organisms, spirochaetes and some gram-negative cocci. **Bacitracin zinc,** B.P.C. 1968, a zinc salt of bacitracin, with the same action, uses and side-effects, and used in lozenges, ointments and dusting-powders.

Back. A term loosely applied to the dorsum of the trunk.

Bacteraemia. The presence of bacteria in the bloodstream.

Bacteria. Small micro-organisms, usually unicellular, with a simple and primitive form of cellular organization. (*Singular:* bacterium.)

Bactericidal. Causing the death of bacteria.

Bactericide. An agent that kills bacteria.

Bacteriology. The study of bacteria.

Bacteriophage. A virus that infects and parasitizes bacteria.

Bacteriostatic. An agent that inhibits the growth of bacteria.

Bacterium. The singular of bacteria.

Bacteroidaceae. A family of the order of Eubacteriales. Most are strict anaerobes and parasites of the alimentary tract.

Bacteroides. A genus of the family of Bacteroidaceae. It contains 30 species, all of which are gram negative.

Bagassosis. The industrial lung disease liable to develop in those who work with bagasse, the broken sugar cane after the sugar has been extracted from it.

B.A.L. Dimercaprol.

Balance. An instrument for weighing. A state of equilibrium. **Acid-base balance,** the normal ratio of acid and base in the body. **Fluid balance,** the ratio between fluid intake and fluid output. **Nitrogen balance,** the balance between the intake and output of nitrogen.

Balanitis. Inflammation of the glans penis.

Balanoposthitis. Inflammation of the glans penis and the prepuce.

Balantidiasis. A form of dysentery due to infection with *Balantidium coli.*

Balantidium. A genus of ciliated protozoa.

Balbuties. Stammering.

Baldness. Lack, or absence, of hair.

Ballismus. The violent, flinging, involuntary movements that may accompany damage to the basal ganglia.

Ballistocardiogram. The record produced by a ballistocardiograph.

Ballistocardiograph. An instrument for measuring cardiac output by recording the movements of the body caused by the impact and recoil of the blood after ejection from the ventricles.

Ballottement. The diagnostic procedure based on the movement of a solid organ in fluid by flicking it. Most commonly applied to the method of diagnosing the presence of the foetus in the uterus.

Balneology. The science of the therapeutic uses of baths.

Balneotherapy. The treatment of disease by baths.

Balsam. A mixture of oleo-resins with benzoic acid, cinnemic acid, or both. **Analgesic balsam,** a synonym for compound methyl salicylate ointment, B.P.C. 1968. **Friar's balsam,** a synonym for compound benzoin tincture, B.P.C. 1968. **Peru balsam,** B.P.C. 1968, a viscous balsam exuded from the scorched and wounded trunk of *Myroxylon pereirae.* **Tolu balsam,** B.P. 1968, a balsam obtained from the trunk of *Myroxylon balsamum.*

Bamethan. The B.P. Commission approved name for 2-butylamino-1-(4-hydroxyphenyl) ethanol. A vasodilator.

Bamifylline. The B.P. Commission approved name for 8-benzyl-7-[2-(*N*-ethyl-2-hydroxyethylamino)ethyl]-theophylline. A bronchodilator.

Bamipine. The B.P. Commission approved name for 4-(*N*-benzylanilino)-1-methylpiperidine. An antihistamine

Band. A structure or appliance that binds. **Moderator band,** a muscular band that extends from the ventricular septum to the base of the anterior papillary muscle of the heart, and may help to prevent over-distension of the ventricle.

Bandage. A strip of material used to apply pressure, prevent movement, or retain dressings in position. **Adhesive bandage,** one of two types: a self-adhesive bandage which is normally sticky, and diachylon adhesive bandage which needs to be warmed before application. **Barrel bandage,** a bandage for the support of the injured jaw. **Capeline bandage,** a bandage to cover the head. **Cotton and rubber elastic bandage,** B.P.C. 1968, a bandage in which the warp threads are of cotton and combined cotton and rubber yarn and the weft threads are of cotton. **Cotton and rubber elastic net bandage,** B.P.C. 1968, a bandage of characteristic net fabric of lace construction, in which the warp threads are of combined cotton and rubber yarn and the bobbin threads are of cotton. **Cotton stretch bandage,** B.P.C. 1968, a bandage of plain weave, in which both the warp and weft threads are of cotton. **Crêpe bandage,** B.P.C. 1968, a bandage of plain weave, in which the warp threads are of cotton and wool and the weft threads are of cotton. **Diachylon elastic adhesive bandage,** B.P.C. 1968, a bandage of elastic cloth spread evenly with a diachylon mass. **Domette bandage,** B.P.C. 1968, a bandage of union fabric of plain weave, in which the warp threads are of cotton and the weft threads are of wool. **Figure-of-eight bandage,** a roller bandage applied in such a way that it resembles the figure 8. **Four-tailed bandage,** a bandage split at both ends. **Half-spread zinc oxide elastic self-adhesive bandage,** B.P.C. 1968, an elastic adhesive bandage with half the width of fabric unspread. **Many-tailed bandage,** a bandage composed of several strips of material sewn together lengthwise and over-lapping. **Open-wove bandage,** B.P.C.

1968, a bandage of cotton cloth of plain weave. **Plaster of Paris bandage,** B.P.C. 1968, a bandage of cotton cloth impregnated with dried calcium sulphate and suitable adhesives so that the dried calcium sulphate is adherent to the fabric. **Pressure bandage,** a bandage that exerts continuous pressure. **Rayon and rubber elastic bandage,** B.P.C. 1968, a bandage of plain weave, in which the warp threads are of rayon and combined cotton and rubber yarn and the weft threads are of rayon. **Roller bandage,** strips of bandage material 3 to 4 metres long rolled from one end. **Spica bandage,** a figure-of-eight bandage in which the successive strips overlap, giving a fancied appearance of an ear of wheat. **Spiral bandage,** a roller bandage applied to a limb, with successive strips overlapping. **T-bandage,** a bandage composed of two strips of material sewn together in a T-shape. **Triangular calico bandage,** B.P.C. 1968, a triangular-shaped piece of unbleached calico. **Zinc oxide elastic self-adhesive bandage,** B.P.C. 1968, a bandage of elastic cloth spread evenly with a self-adhesive plaster mass containing zinc oxide. **Zinc paste bandage,** B.P.C. 1968, a bandage of open-wove cloth impregnated with a paste containing zinc oxide. **Zinc paste and coal tar bandage,** B.P.C. 1968, a bandage of open-wove cotton cloth impregnated with a paste containing zinc oxide and prepared coal tar. **Zinc paste and ichthammol bandage,** B.P.C. 1968, a bandage of open-wove cotton cloth impregnated with a paste containing zinc oxide and ichthammol. **Ventilated diachylon elastic adhesive bandage,** B.P.C. 1968, a bandage of elastic cloth spread evenly with a diachylon mass so as to leave strips of unspread fabric along its length. **Ventilated zinc oxide elastic self-adhesive bandage,** B.P.C. 1968, an elastic adhesive bandage spread so as to leave strips of unspread fabric along its length.

Baragnosis. Inability to recognize, or appreciate, weight.

Barbitone sodium. B.P. 1968. $C_8H_{11}N_2NaO_3$. A long-acting barbiturate.

Barbiturate. A derivative of barbituric acid. The barbiturates are hypnotics that in therapeutic doses have little or no effect on the medullary centres and therefore do not affect respiration or blood pressure. They have no analgesic action.

Barbiturism. The condition induced by barbiturate intoxication and characterized by pyrexia, headache and skin eruptions.

Baritosis. A type of benign pneumoconiosis resulting from the inhalation of finely ground particles of barium sulphate.

Barium. A metallic element. Symbol Ba. Atomic weight 137·34. Atomic number 56.

Barium sulphate. B.P. 1968. $BaSO_4$. Used as a contrast medium in radiological examination of the gastro-intestinal tract.

Barley. A cereal grain obtained from *Hordeum vulgare* and *Hordeum distichon*, and used as a food and for malting. **Barley water**, a beverage made by allowing 57 grammes of pearl barley to simmer for two hours in 1 litre of water, straining and adding sugar and lemon to flavour. **Pearl barley**, the polished whole grain of barley after removal of the husk. It contains 0·12mg. of thiamine per 100 grammes.

Baroceptor. The name of the receptors in the walls of the aorta and the carotid arteries which respond to stretching and are stimulated by changes in blood pressure.

Barograph. A self-registering barometer.

Barometer. An instrument for recording changes in atmospheric pressure.

Barotrauma. Injury to the middle ear or paranasal sinuses caused by changes in atmospheric (or water) pressure. **Otitic barotrauma**, injury to the ear by gross inequality of pressure within and without the middle ear. **Sinus barotrauma**, injury to the paranasal sinuses resulting from gross inequality between the pressure inside and outside the affected sinus.

Bartholinitis. Inflammation of the greater vestibular (Bartholin's) glands.

Bartonella. A genus of the family Bartonellaceae, now included in the order Rickettsiales. *Bartonella bacilliformis*, the causative organism of Oroya fever and verruga peruana.

Bartonellosis. A disease caused by *Bartonella bacilliformis*, transmitted by the bite of female sandflies (Phlebotomus), which occurs in the mountainous districts of South America.

Barylalia. Indistinct speech due to imperfect articulation.

Base. The bottom or foundation of a structure. The chief ingredient of a mixture or compound. A compound that yields hydroxyl ions in aqueous solution, and unites with an acid to form a salt.

Basilar. Relating to a base, or basal point. **Basilar artery**, the artery formed by the junction of the two vertebral arteries, which supplies the pons, the temporal and occipital lobes of the cerebrum and the cerebellum. **Basilar membrane**, the membrane in the cochlea that stretches from the tympanic tip of the osseous spiral lamina to the crista basilaris.

Basilemma. Basement membrane.

Basilic. Prominent, or important. **Basilic vein**, the vein which begins in the ulnar part of the dorsal venous network of the hand, and runs up the arm to be continued as the axillary vein.

Basion. The midpoint of the anterior margin of the foramen magnum.

Basophil. A granulocyte with large, coarse granules that stain deeply with methylene blue. Basophils normally constitute 1·5 to 2 per cent or less of the circulating polymorph leucocytes in the blood. The cell of the anterior lobe of the pituitary that has an affinity for basic stains.

Basophilia. An excess of basophil leucocytes in the blood. The bluish appearance of immature red blood cells when stained with certain dyes. **Punctate basophilia**, the stippled appearance of stained red blood cells in certain degenerating or toxic conditions such as lead poisoning.

Bat ears. Prominent ears.

Bath. The immersion of the body or part of it in water or some other medium for cleaning or therapeutic purposes. The receptacle or room containing such a medium. **Alkaline bath**, a bath containing sodium carbonate, used in the treatment of certain skin conditions. **Aromatic bath**, a medicated bath scented with volatile oils. **Bran bath**, a bath containing bran, used to soothe general irritation of the skin. **Carbonic acid bath**, a bath containing naturally effervescent spa water or water with carbonic acid bubbling through it, used to stimulate the skin. **Cold water bath**, a bath in which the water is at a temperature of around 16°C. **Electric bath**, a bath of tepid water with an electrode hanging in the water at either end, not touching the patient. **Foam bath**, a bath rendered foamy by aeration and the addition of a surface tension-reducing agent. **Hot-air bath,** a bath in hot air: e.g. a Turkish bath. **Light bath,** exposure of the body to the sun or to artificially produced ultra-violet rays. **Medicinal bath,** a bath containing some medicinal substance: e.g mustard. **Mud bath,** immersion of the patient in warmed mud for the alleviation of rheumatism. **Mustard bath,** a bath containing mustard, usually used as a foot-bath. **Peat bath,** immersion of the patient in water containing peat. **Pine-needle bath,** a bath containing water in which fresh pine needles have been boiled. **Russian bath,** a hot vapour bath. **Sand bath,** immersion of the body, or part of it, in hot dry sand for the alleviation of rheumatism. **Sauna bath,** a sweat bath followed by beating with twigs and a cold plunge. **Sea-water bath,** a bath in sea-water or artificial brine, for the alleviation of rheumatism. **Sitz bath,** a hip bath. **Sulphur bath,** a bath in spa water containing sulphuretted hydrogen or in water containing sulphur. Used in the treatment of certain skin conditions and rheumatism. **Tepid bath,** a bath in which the water is slightly below body temperature. **Turkish bath,** a process in which the individual passes from room to room of increasing temperature, ending up with a form of massage and then a cold dip. **Vapour bath,** the exposure of the body to some form of vapour, medicated or otherwise. **Warm bath,** a bath in which the temperature of the water ranges from 37° to 43°C. **Wax bath,** the immersion of part of the body in molten wax for the relief of rheumatism.

Bathophobia. Morbid fear of depth and deep places.

Bathyaesthesia. Deep sensation.

Beat. A pulsation or stroke. **Apex beat,** the visible and/or palpable impulse of the apex of the heart on the chest wall. **Dropped beat,** a heart beat that fails to appear, as in partial heart block. **Ectopic beat,** a contraction of the heart that has its origin elsewhere than in the sinu-atrial node.

Beclamide. The B.P. Commission approved name for *N*-benzyl-3-chloropropionamide. An anticonvulsant.

Beclomethasone. B.P. Addendum 1969. $C_{28}H_{37}ClO_7$. A corticosteroid for topical application.

Bed. A structure in which to rest or sleep. A supporting structure. **Air bed,** a mattress inflated with air.

Capillary bed, the network of capillaries. **Fracture bed,** a non-sagging bed for a patient with a fractured limb or spine. **Nail bed,** the germinative zone and corium underlying the nail. **Water bed,** a mattress filled with water.

Bed bug. *Cimex lectularius,* which inhabits insanitary houses and comes out of its hiding place at night to feed on man. It is not a disease vector. *Cimex hemipterus* is its tropical opposite number.

Bed pan. A shallow receptacle for the reception of the urine and/or faeces of a patient confined to bed.

Bedsore. An area of inflamed skin, which tends to ulcerate, and occurs on the skin overlying bony prominences, such as the heels, buttocks and elbows, in patients confined to bed for long periods.

Beef. The flesh of the ox or cow. **Beef extract,** a non-protein extract of beef which has no food value but aids digestion by stimulating gastric secretion. **Beef tea,** a form of beef extract popular as a gastric stimulant in convalescence.

Beer. The product of the fermentation of malt and hops. The content of ethyl alcohol ranges from around 3 to 8 per cent. The caloric value is 30 to 60kcal./100ml. and it contains significant amounts of nicotinic acid and riboflavine.

Beeswax. A secretion of the honey bee. **White beeswax,** B.P. 1968, prepared by bleaching the wax obtained from the honeycomb of the bee *Apis mellifera.* **Yellow beeswax,** B.P.C. 1968, the secretion of *Apis mellifera.* Both are used in the preparation of ointments.

Behaviourism. The psychological doctrine that all man's activities, mental as well as physical, are trained reflex actions, with mind and consciousness of secondary importance.

Bejel. A form of non-venereal syphilis usually acquired in young childhood, and endemic among Bedouin Arabs in the Middle East.

Bel. The unit of intensity of sound.

Belch. Eructation of gas from the stomach.

Belladonna. *Atropa belladonna.* Deadly nightshade. Of pharmacological interest because it is the source of atropine. **Belladonna herb,** B.P.1968, the dried leaves, or leaves and other aerial parts, of *Atropa belladonna,* collected when the plants are in flower. **Belladonna dry extract,** B.P. 1968, a preparation containing 1 per cent of the alkaloids of belladonna herb. **Belladonna root**, B.P.C. 1968, the dried root of *Atropa belladonna*, used chiefly in preparations for external application. **Belladonna tincture**, B.P. 1968, a preparation containing 0·03 per cent w/v of the alkaloids of belladonna herb. **Prepared belladonna herb**, B.P. 1968, belladonna herb reduced to a fine powder and adjusted to contain 0·3 per cent of alkaloids.

Belly, The abdomen.

Belt. A supporting girdle.

Bemegride. B.P. 1968. $C_8H_{13}NO_2$. A general analeptic used as a stimulant in respiratory failure. It is given intravenously.

Benactyzine. The B.P. Commission approved name for 2-diethylaminoethyl benzilate. A tranquillizer.

Bendrofluazide. B.P. 1968. $C_{15}H_{14}F_3N_3O_4S_2$. A non-mercurial diuretic.

Bends. The pains characteristic of caisson disease, and induced by the release of nitrogen bubbles in different parts of the body as a result of too rapid decompression of divers or caisson workers.

Benethamine penicillin. B.P.C. 1968. The *N*-benzylphenethylamine salt of benzylpenicillin. As it is only slightly soluble in water, it releases penicillin slowly into the circulation after intramuscular injection.

Benign. A medical synonym for non-malignant.

Benorylate. The B.P. Commission approved name for 4-acetamidophenyl *O*-acetylsalicylate. An analgesic.

Bentonite. B.P. 1968. A native colloidal hydrated aluminium silicate, used for suspending powders in aqueous preparations, and as gels for ointment and cream bases.

Benzaldehyde. B.P.C. 1968. C_7H_6O. A flavouring agent.

Benzalkonium bromide solution. B.P.C. 1968. An aqueous solution containing a mixture of alkylbenzyldimethylammonium bromides, which has the actions and uses of benzalkonium chloride solution.

Benzalkonium chloride solution. B.P. 1968. An aqueous solution of a mixture of alkylbenzyldimethylammonium chlorides, which is a relatively non-toxic antiseptic with detergent properties, active against gram-positive organisms, less so against gram-negative organisms.

Benzathine penicillin. B.P. 1968. The *NN'*-dibenzylethylenediamine salt of benzylpenicillin, which is relatively stable in the presence of gastric juice or serum, and from which penicillin is slowly released when it is given by mouth or intramuscularly.

Benzethidine. The B.P. approved name for ethyl 1-(2-benzyloxyethyl)-4-phenylpiperidine-4-carboxylate. A narcotic analgesic.

Benzethonium chloride. The B.P. Commission approved name for benzyldimethyl-2-{ 2-[4-(1,1,3,3-tetramethylbutyl)-phenoxy]ethoxy }ethylammonium chloride. A disinfectant.

Benzhexol hydrochloride. B.P. 1968. $C_{20}H_{32}ClNO$. An antagonist of some of the actions of acetylcholine. Used in the treatment of parkinsonism.

Benzilonium bromide. The B.P. Commission approved name for 3-benziloyloxy-1,1-diethylpyrrolidinium bromide. An inhibitor of gastric secretion.

Benziodarone. The B.P. Commission approved name for 2-ethyl-3-(4-hydroxy-3,5-di-iodobenzoyl)coumarone. A coronary vasodilator.

Benzocaine. B.P. 1968. $C_9H_{11}NO_2$. A local anaesthetic.

Benzoic acid. B.P. 1968. $C_7H_6O_2$. A preservative for acid preparations in virtue of its antibacterial and antifungal properties. **Compound benzoic acid ointment**, B.P.C. 1968, an ointment used in the treatment of fungous infections of the skin.

Benzoin B.P.C. 1968. A balsamic resin obtained from *Styrax benzoin* and *Styrax paralleloneurus*, and used as an ingredient of inhalants for catarrh of the upper respiratory tract.

Benzonatate. The B.P. Commission approved name for 2-(ω-methoxypolyethyleneoxy) ethyl 4-butylaminobenzoate. A cough suppressant.

Benzphetamine. The B.P. Commission approved name for (+)-*N*-benzyl-*N*α-dimethylphenethylamine. An appetite suppressant.

Benzpyrene. A strongly carcinogenic hydrocarbon present in coal-tar pitch.

Benzquinamide. The B.P. Commission approved name for 2-acetoxy-3-diethylcarbamoyl-1,3,4,6,7,11b-hexahydro-9,10-dimethoxy-2*H*-benzo[*a*]quinolizine. A tranquillizer.

Benzthiazide. The B.P. Commission approved name for 3-benzylthiomethyl-6-chloro-1, 2,4-benzothiadiazine-7-sulphonamide 1,1-dioxide. A diuretic.

Benztropine mesylate. B.P. 1968. $C_{22}H_{29}NO_4S$. A depressant of the motor cortex, with antihistamine and atropine-like actions, used in the treatment of parkinsonism.

Benzydamine. The B.P. Commission approved name for 1-benzyl-3-(3-dimethylaminopropoxy)indazole. An anti-inflammatory agent and analgesic.

Benzyl alcohol. B.P. 1968. C_7H_8O. A weak local anaesthetic with strong antiseptic properties.

Benzyl benzoate. B.P. 1968. $C_{14}H_{12}O_2$. An acaricide used in the treatment of scabies.

Benzylpenicillin. B.P. 1968. The sodium or potassium salt of 6-phenylacet-amidopenicillanic acid, usually administered by intramuscular injection of an aqueous solution.

Bephenium hydroxynaphthoate. B.P.C. 1968. $C_{28}H_{29}NO_4$. An anthelmintic which is proving effective in the treatment of hookworm infestations.

Berberi. A deficiency disease caused by lack of thiamine, and characterized by peripheral neuritis and/or oedema with heart failure.

Bergamot oil. The oil obtained from the rind of *Citrus bergamia*, a widely used perfume which may be responsible for photosensitization reactions in the skin.

Beryllium. A metallic element. Symbol Be. Atomic weight 9. Atomic number 4.

Beryllosis. A disease of the lungs caused by inhalation of particles of beryllium oxide.

Betacetylmethadol. The B.P. Commission approved name for 4-dimethylamino-1-ethyl-2,2-phenylpentyl acetate. A narcotic analgesic.

Betahistine. The B.P. Commission approved name for 2-(2-methylaminoethyl)pyridine. A diamine oxidase inhibitor used in the treatment of Menière's syndrome.

Betamethadol. The B.P. Commission approved name for 6-dimethylamino-4,4-diphenylheptan-3-ol. A narcotic analgesic.

Betamethasone. B.P. 1968. $C_{22}H_{29}FO_5$. A corticosteroid with a similar action to that of cortisone acetate but in much lower dosage. **Betamethasone sodium phosphate,** B.P. 1968, $C_2H_{28}FNa_2O_8P$, a preparation used as a local application and for intra-articular and intra-muscular injection, having an action comparable with betamethasone. **Betamethasone valerate,** B.P. 1968, used for topical application.

Betaprodine. The B.P. Commission approved name for 1,3-dimethyl-4-phenyl-4-propionyloxypiperidine. A narcotic analgesic.

Betatron. A circular electron accelerator, the electron beam of which can be used either directly or indirectly in the treatment of cancer.

Betel. The dried leaves of *Piper betle,* which, wrapped round the betel nut (the nut of *Areca catechu*) and lime, is a popular masticatory in India, and responsible for a certain number of cases of cancer of the mouth.

Bethanidine sulphate. B.P. Addendum 1969. $(C_{10}H_{15}N_3)_2,H_2SO_4$. A hypotensive agent.

Bevonium methylsulphate. The B.P. Commission approved name for 2-benziloyloxymethyl-1,1-dimethylpiperidinium methylsulphate. An antispasmodic.

Bezitramide. The B.P. Commission approved name for 1-(3-cyano-3, 3-diphenylpropyl)-4-(2-oxo-3-propionyl-1-benzimidazolinyl) piperidine. A narcotic analgesic.

Bezoar. A concretion found in the stomach or intestines.

Bi- (L *bi:* twice). Prefix indicating twice or double.

Bialamicol. The B.P. Commission approved name for 3,3'-diallyl-5, 5'-bisdiethylaminomethyl-4,4'-dihydroxybiphenyl. An amoebicide.

Bibenzonium bromide. The B.P. Commission approved name for 2-(1,2-diphenylethoxy)ethyltrimethylammonium bromide. A cough suppressant.

Bicameral. Having two cavities or divisions.

Bicaudal. Having two tails.

Biceps. A muscle having two heads: e.g. biceps brachii and biceps femoris.

Biconcave. Concave on two surfaces, usually applied to a lens.

Biconvex. Convex on two surfaces, usually applied to a lens.

Bicornuate. Having two horns.

Bicuspid. Having two cusps or prongs. A premolar tooth.

Bidet. A sitz (hip) bath with an attachment for giving vaginal douches or rectal enemas.

Bifid. Split in two parts.

Bifocal. Having two foci. Applied to spectacles in which there are lenses adjusted for both near and distance reading.

Bifurcation. Division into two branches.

Bigeminal. Occurring in pairs.

Bigeminy. The condition of occurring in pairs, applied particularly to the occurrence of two pulse beats in quick succession.

Bilateral. Relating to, or having, two sides.

Bile. The fluid secreted by the liver and stored in the gall-bladder.

Bilharzia. The old term for Schistosoma.

Biliary. Pertaining to bile.

Bilious. Pertaining to bile. Popular term for dyspeptic.

Biliousness. A meaningless popular term for a state of ill health characterized by headache, nausea, loss of appetite and abdominal discomfort.

Bilirubin. $C_{33}H_{36}O_6N_4$. The principal, red pigment in bile derived from the breakdown of haemoglobin.

Bilirubinaemia. Excess of bilirubin in the blood.

Biliuria. The presence of bile in the urine.

Biliverdin. The green bile pigment produced by the oxidation of bilirubin.

Bilobular. Having two lobules.

Bilocular. Divided into two compartments.

Bimanual. Pertaining to, or done by, two hands.

Bimodal. A frequency curve characterized by two peaks.

Binary. Consisting of two parts or elements.

Binaural. Relating to two ears.

Binder. A wide bandage or girdle.

Binocular. Having two eyes. Adapted to the use of two eyes: e.g. a binocular microscope.

Binovular. Derived from two ova.

Bio- (Gk *bios:* life). Prefix denoting life.

Bioassay. The determination of the activity or amount of a substance by its effect on living tissue and comparing this with an internationally accepted standard.

Biochemistry. The chemistry of living organisms and of vital processes.

Biology. The science of life.

Biometrics. Biometry.

Biometry. The science of the application of statistics to biological science.

Bionomics. The study of the relation of organisms to their environment.

Biophysics. The physics of life processes.

Biopsy. The examination of living tissue removed from the body for diagnostic purposes.

Biotin. A constituent of the vitamin B complex which is essential for the growth of yeasts and micro-organisms, and probably essential for normal growth in man.

Biparietal. Relating to both parietal bones of the skull.

Biparous. Producing two at one birth.

Biped. Having two feet. An animal with two feet.

Biperiden. The B.P. Commission approved name for 1-(bicyclo[2,2,1] hept-5-en-2-yl)-1-phenyl-3-piperidino-propan-1-ol. A drug for the treatment of parkinsonism.

Bipolar. Having two poles.

Bipp. A widely used abbreviation for an antiseptic paste, containing bismuth subnitrate, iodoform and paraffin.

Bird fancier's lung. A form of pneumonia due to sensitization to pigeons.

Birefringence. The property possessed by certain biological materials of doubly refracting a beam of plane polarized light.

Birth. The process of being born.

Birthmark. A circumscribed discoloration of the skin present at birth, usually a naevus.

Bisacodyl. B.P. 1968. $C_{22}H_{19}NO_4$. A laxative with little or no action on the small intestine.

Bisacromial. Relating to both acromions.

Biseptate. Divided into two by a septum.

Bisexual. Hermaphrodite. Equally attracted to the two sexes.

Bismuth. A chemical element. Symbol Bi. Atomic weight 208·98. Atomic number 83.

Bismuth carbonate. B.P.C. 1968. A weak antacid.

Bismuth glycollylarsanilate. The B.P. Commission approved name for bismuthyl *N*-glycollylarsanilate. An amoebicide.

Bismuth subgallate. B.P.C. 1968. An ingredient of dusting-powders, and used in the form of suppositories for the treatment of haemorrhoids.

Bismuth subnitrate. B.P.C. 1968. A weak antacid.

Bisoxatin. The B.P. Commission approved name for 2,3-dihydro-2,2-di-(4-hydroxyphenyl) - 1,4-benzoxazin-3-one. A laxative.

Bistoury. A long, narrow, straight or curved, knife, with pointed or blunted end, used in opening abscesses, sinuses or fistulae.

Bite. A skin puncture produced by the teeth of a mammal or by an insect or snake. To bring the teeth together. In dental prosthetics a plastic impression of the closure of the upper and lower teeth.

Bitemporal. Pertaining to both temporal bones.

Bithionol. The B.P. Commission approved name for 2,2'-thiobis-(4,6-dichlorophenol). An antiseptic.

Bitrochanteric. Pertaining to both greater trochanters.

Bitropic. Having affinity for two tissues or organisms.

Bitters. Substances, quite unrelated chemically, which have the common property of an intensely bitter taste and are used to stimulate appetite.

Bivalent. Having a combining power equal to two atoms of hydrogen.

Black currant. B.P.C. 1968. The fresh ripe fruits of *Ribes nigrum*, together with their pedicels and rachides. A rich source of ascorbic acid: 100 to 300mg. per 100G.

Blackdamp. The mixture of predominantly nitrogen, with some carbon dioxide, that tends to collect in mines, deep wells and the like.

Blackhead. A comedo.

Blackout. Temporary loss of consciousness.

Blackwater fever. A particularly virulent form of malaria, characterized by the presence of gross haematuria. Hence the name.

Bladder. A membranous or musculo-membranous, distensible sac for the collecting or storage of fluids or gases. **Gall-bladder,** a pear-shaped sac, with a capacity of 30 to 50ml., situated on the under-surface of the right lobe of the liver, which acts as a reservoir for bile. **Urinary bladder,** the reservoir for urine, with a mean capacity of around 220ml., situated in the pelvis anterior to the bowel.

Blastema. The primitive, or primordial, substance from which cells are formed.

Blasto- (Gk *blastos:* germ). Prefix indicating relationship to budding

Blastocoele. The fluid-filled cavity, bounded by trophoblast cells, which occupies the whole of the interior of the blastocyst.

Blastocyst. The second stage in the development of the fertilized ovum, formed by the end of the fourth, or the beginning of the fifth, day after ovulation. It lies free in the uterine cavity.

Blastomere. One of the cells into which the fertilized ovum divides.

Blastomyces. A genus of budding yeastlike fungi.

Blastomycosis. A chronic, suppurative, granulomatuos infection of man caused by Blastomyces.

Blastopore. The opening in the embryo through which the archenteron of the gastrula communicates with the exterior.

Bleeder. A lay term for a haemophiliac.

Blenn-, Blenno- (Gk *blenna:* mucus). Prefixes indicating association with mucus.

Blennorrhagia. A discharge of mucus.

Blennorrhoea. An excessive discharge of mucus.

Blephar-, Blepharo- (Gk *blepharon:* eyelid). Prefixes indicating a relationship with an eyelid.

Blepharitis. Inflammation of the eyelids.

Blepharophimosis. Narrowing of the palpebral fissure.

Blepharoplasty. An operation for plastic repair of an eyelid.

Blepharospasm. Spasm of the eyelids.

Blindness. Loss of the power of vision. **Blue blindness,** inability to distinguish the colour blue. **Colour blindness,** inability to recognize one or more of the seven fundamental colours of the spectrum. **Eclipse blindness,** blindness induced by looking at the eclipsed sun with unprotected eyes. **Green blindness,** the inability to recognize the colour green. **Night blindness,** the inability to see at night or in the darkness. **Red blindness,** the inability to recognize the colour red. **Snow blindness,** blindness induced by exposing the unprotected eyes to the glare of snow and ice. **Word blindness,** inability to recognize written words.

Blister. A collection of fluid beneath the epidermis. An agent that induces the formation of such a collection of fluid.

Block. A stoppage or obstruction **Arborization block,** the form of heart block induced by interference with conduction in the finer ramifications of the atrioventriculear bundle. **Atrioventricular block,** the form of heart block induced by interference with conduction in the atrioventricular bundle. **Bundle-branch block,** the form of heart block induced by interference with conduction in one of the two bundles into which the atrioventricular bundle divides. **Epidural block,** anaesthesia induced by injection of the anaesthetic solution into the vertebral canal underneath the dura mater. **Field block,** anaesthesia of an area by infiltration of the surrounding tissues with the anaesthetic solution. **Heart block,** interference with the conducting tissues of the heart. **Nerve block,** blocking of sensory impulses by local anaesthesia of nerve endings, plexuses or roots. **Pudendal block,** a form of local anaesthesia used in obstetrics. **Stellate block,** inactivation of the stellate ganglion by local anaesthesia.

Blood. The red, opaque fluid that circulates within the cardiovascular system and which carries nutriments and oxygen to all parts of the body and removes waste products including carbon dioxide. In health there is around 85ml. of blood per kg. body weight: i.e. around 5 litres in the adult male and 3·5 litres in the adult female. The *British Pharmacopoeia* 1968 and *Addendum* 1969 contain the following preparations of human blood. **Human albumin,** a solution in water of human albumin obtained from pooled liquid human plasma. **Dried human albumin,** prepared by freeze-drying human albumin of protein concentration not exceeding 10 per cent w/v. **Whole human blood,** blood withdrawn from adult human beings and mixed with an anticoagulant solution, usually water for injections B.P. 1968, containing 1·7 to 2·1 per cent of sodium acid citrate and 2·5 per cent of dextrose. **Concentrated human red blood corpuscles,** whole human blood from which part of the plasma and anticoagulant solution have been removed. **Human fibrin foam,** a dry artificial sponge of human fibrin, prepared by clotting with human fibrin a foam of a solution of human fibrinogen. It is used, in conjunction with human fibrin, as a haemostatic agent in surgery in sites in which bleeding cannot easily be controlled by the commoner methods of haemostasis. **Human fibrinogen,** a sterile dried preparation of the soluble component of liquid human plasma which, on addition of human thrombin, is transformed into fibrin. It is used in conjunction with human thrombin to fix nerve sutures and to assist the adhesion of skin and mucous membrane grafts, and given intravenously for the treatment of fibrinogen deficiency, particularly that associated with pregnancy. **Human normal immunoglobulin injection,** a sterile preparation containing almost all the gamma-G globulins of human plasma together with smaller amounts of other plasma proteins. It is used for the protection of susceptible contacts of rubella, measles, poliomyelitis and infectious hepatitis. **Dried human plasma,** prepared by drying a pool of the supernatant fluids which are separated, by centrifuging or by standing, from quantities of whole human blood. Reconstituted it is used for the restoration of plasma volume. **Human plasma protein fraction,** a solution of the protein of liquid human plasma containing certain globulins that retain their solubility on heating. Used in the same way as dried human plasma. **Dried human plasma protein fraction,** a sterile freeze-dried preparation of human plasma dried fraction, used in the same way as dried human plasma. **Dried human serum,** prepared by drying a pool of the fluid which separates from human blood which has clotted in the absence of any anticoagulant. It is used as is dried human plasma. **Human thrombin,** the enzyme which transforms human fibrinogen into fibrin, and prepared from human plasma.

Blood bank. A store of blood for therapeutic use.

Blood cell. One of the cellular components of blood, subdivided into three main groups: red blood cells, or erythrocytes; white blood cells, or leucocytes; platelets.

Blood corpuscle. A blood cell.

Blood count. The number of red or white blood cells in a cubic millimetre of blood. The normal adult red cell count varies from 4,200,000 to 6,400,000 per c.mm., with an average of 5,500,000 for men and 4,800,000 for women. The normal white cell count ranges from 4,000 to 11,000 per c.mm.

Blood donor. One who gives blood for therapeutic purposes.

Blood group. One of the genetically determined, immunologically distinct series into which the blood is divided, and which is of outstanding importance in blood transfusion. It is also of medico-legal significance.

Blood pressure. The pressure of the circulating blood, usually restricted to the arterial blood pressure. **Diastolic blood pressure,** the minimal arterial pressure. **Pulse pressure,** the difference between the systolic and diastolic pressures. **Systolic blood pressure,** the maximal arterial pressure. The upper normal limit of blood pressure in the adult is usually taken to be 140 millimetres of mercury systolic, and 90 diastolic.

Blood vessel. One of the peripheral

system of tubes through which the blood circulates, consisting of arteries, arterioles, capillaries, venules and veins.

Body. The trunk. The major part of an organ. Any discrete mass. **Amygdaloid body,** a nuclear mass lying above and in front of the inferior horn of the lateral ventricle. **Amyloid bodies,** small colloid masses in the prostate. **Aschoff body,** the characteristic pathological lesion of acute rheumatism. **Carotid body,** an ellipsoidal structure, lying deep to the bifurcation of the common carotid artery, and concerned with the control of the circulation. **Chromaffin body,** paraganglion. **Ciliary body,** the ciliary ring, the ciliary processes and the ciliaris. **Coccygeal body,** a mass of epithelioid cells, immediately below the tip of the coccyx, of unknown function. **Cortical bodies,** small masses, identical with the suprarenal cortex, found in the neighbourhood of the suprarenal glands or elsewhere. **Geniculate body, lateral,** an oval elevation on the surface of the brain inferior to the posterior end of the thalamus. **Geniculate body, medial,** an oval structure underlying the thalamus. **Howell-Jolly bodies,** nuclear fragments formed by karyorrhexis of the nucleus of the normoblast, and evidence of immaturity of the erythrocytes. **Inclusion bodies.** distinctive structures found in body cells in association with viruses. **Mamillary bodies,** two round masses situated below the floor of the third ventricle. **Negri body** the acidophilic inclusion body, the presence of which in the hippocampus is presumptive diagnosis of rabies. **Nissl bodies,** large, basic-staining granules in the cytoplasm of nerve cells. **Para-aortic bodies,** two masses of chromaffin cells, situated on either side of the abdominal aorta, which undergo progressive atrophy during childhood and are completely disintegrated by the age of 14 years. **Pararenal (paranephric) body,** a collection of fat behind the renal fascia. **Perineal body,** a fibromuscular node just anterior to the anus to which most of the muscles in this area are attached. **Pineal body,** a conical body, 8mm. long, lying between the superior colliculi. **Pituitary body,** hypophysis cerebri. **Polar bodies,** the two small bodies extruded by the oocyte in the early process of maturation. **Trapezoid**

body, formed by fibres derived from the cochlear nuclei and the nuclei of the corpus trapezoideum. **Tympanic body,** jugular glomus. **Vertebral body,** the part of a vertebra lying anterior to the vertebral foramen. **Vitreous body,** a colourless, transparent gel that occupies about four-fifths of the eyeball, and the meshes of which are filled with the vitreous humour. **Wolffian body,** mesonephros.

Boil. Furuncle. An abscess in the skin, usually caused by *Staphylococcus aureus*, and sited around a hair root.

Boldenone. The B.P. Commission approved name for 17β-hydroxyandrosta-1,4-dien-3-one. An anabolic steroid.

Bolmantalate. The B.P. Commission approved name for 17β-hydroxyoestr-4-en-3-one adamantane-1-carboxylate. An anabolic steroid.

Bolus. A mass of masticated food. A mass of food passing through the intestine. A large pill.

Bone. The supporting form of connective tissue in which the intercellular system of collagen fibres and matrix has become ossified by the deposition of mineral salts. **Flat bone,** a bone, as in the skull and shoulder blades, composed of two thin layers of compact bone separated by spongy bone. **Irregular bone,** bone of irregular form that cannot be fitted into any of the other categories of bone. **Long bone,** a bone consisting of a shaft and two ends, as in the bones of the limbs. **Pneumatic bone,** a bone containing air cells, such as the ethmoid. **Sesamoid bone,** a rounded nodule of bone embedded in certain tendons, such as the patella. **Short bone,** a term used to describe the bones of the carpus and tarsus. **Sutural bone,** a supernumerary bone occurring in a suture of the skull.

Borax. B.P. 1968. Sodium borate. A weak antibacterial agent used in gargles and eye-washes.

Borborygmus. Rumbling intestinal flatulence.

Bordetella. A genus of gram-negative coccobacilli. (*Abbreviation: Bord.*) *Bordetella pertussis,* the causative organism of whooping-cough.

Boric acid. B.P. 1968. H_3BO_3. A feeble antibacterial and antifungal preparation, used in irrigating lotions and as a dusting powder.

Bornholm disease. Epidemic myalgia. An acute infective disease of viral origin (usually a Coxsackie virus), characterized by pain around the lower margin of the ribs, headache and fever.

Boron. A non-metallic element. Symbol B. Atomic weight 10·81. Atomic number 5.

Borrelia. A genus of spirochaetes, with relatively few, irregular, wide and open coils. (*Abbreviation: Borr.*) *Borrelia duttoni*, the causative organism of West Africa relapsing fever. *Borrelia recurrentis*, the causative organism of European relapsing fever. *Borrelia vincenti*, in association with *Fusobacterium fusiforme*, commonly found in ulcerative and necrotic lesions in the mouth and elsewhere in the body.

Boss. A rounded protuberance.

Botryoid. Resembling a bunch of grapes.

Botulism. A rare but fatal form of food poisoning induced by contamination of food with *Clostridium botulinum*.

Bougie. A cylindrical instrument for introduction into natural passages of the body in order to dilate a stricture or to apply some medication which it contains.

Bouillon. Broth. A nutriment medium for the growth of micro-organisms.

Bowel. The intestine.

Brachial. Pertaining to the arm.

Brachialgia. Pain in the arm.

Brachium. An arm-like structure. **Brachium of the inferior colliculus,** fibres from the lateral lemniscus and the inferior colliculus to the medial geniculate body. **Brachium of the superior colliculus,** visual fibres from the retina and the optic radiation to the superior colliculus.

Brachy- (Gk *brachys:* short). Prefix indicating short.

Brachycephaly. The state of having a disproportionately short head.

Brachydactyly. The state of having disproportionately short fingers or toes.

Brady- (Gk *bradys:* slow). Prefix indicating slow.

Bradycardia. A slow heart rate (usually taken to be under 60 per minute).

Bradykinesia. Extreme slowness in movement.

Bradykinin. A polypeptide which is a powerful vasodilator.

Braidism. Hypnotism.

Braille. The system of printing by means of raised points introduced by Louis Braille to enable the blind to read by touch.

Brain. That part of the central nervous system lying within the cranial cavity and consisting of the cerebrum, the midbrain, pons, cerebellum and medulla oblongata.

Bran. The meal derived from the outer covering of a cereal grain.

Branchial. Relating to the branchia, or arches and clefts of the foetus.

Brandy. The product of the distillation of fermented grape juice, containing between 48 and 54 per cent of ethyl alcohol.

Bread. A staple article of diet made from flour mixed with water, kneaded with or without yeast, and then baked.

Breakbone fever. Dengue.

Breast. The front of the chest One of the mammary glands.

Breath. The respired air.

Breathing. The inspiration and exhalation of air. **Amphoric breathing,** the sound, like that heard on blowing over a carafe, heard in auscultation over a cavity in the lungs and at times over a pneumothorax. **Bronchial breathing,** the sound normally heard on auscultation over the larynx and trachea and in disease over consolidated lung. **Bronchovesicular breathing,** the mixture of bronchial and vesicular breathing heard normally over the primary bronchi and at the apex of the right lung, and over early and incomplete consolidation of the lung. **Vesicular breathing,** the type of breath sounds produced over normal lung tissue.

Breech. The buttocks.

Bregma. The meeting place of the coronal and sagittal sutures in the skull.

Bretylium tosylate. The B.P. Commission approved name for 2-bromo-benzylethyldimethylammonium tolu-ene-*p*-sulphonate. A hypotensive agent.

Brilliant green. B.P. 1968. $C_{27}H_{34}N_2O_4S$. An antiseptic used in the treatment of infected wounds and burns.

Broca's area. The motor speech centre.

Brocresine. The B.P. Commission approved name for *O*-(4-bromo-3-hydroxybenzyl)hydroxylamine. A histidine decarboxylase inhibitor.

Bromelains. The B.P. Commission approved name for a concentrate of proteolytic enzymes derived from *Ananas comosus* Merr. Used in the treatment of soft tissue injuries and traumatic oedema.

Bromhexine. The B.P. Commission approved name for *N*-(2-amino-3,5-dibromobenzyl)-*N*-cyclohexylmethylamine. A bronchial mucolytic.

Bromide. A salt of hydrobromic acid. Bromides were at one time widely used in the treatment of epilepsy and as sedatives.

Bromidrosis. Evil-smelling perspiration.

Bromindione. The B.P. Commission approved name for 2-(4-bromophenyl) indane-1,3-dione. An anticoagulant.

Bromine. A volatile liquid element. Symbol Br. Atomic weight 79·9. Atomic number 35.

Bromism. Chronic bromide intoxication, characterized by acne, mental dullness, unsteady gait and halitosis.

Bromodiphenhydramine. The B.P. Commission approved name for N-2-(4-bromobenzhydryloxy) ethyldimethylamine. An antihistamine.

Brompheniramine. The B.P. Commission approved name for 1-(4-bromophenyl)-3-dimethylamino-1-(2-pyridyl)-propane. An antihistamine.

Brompton mixture. A mixture, containing morphine, cocaine and whisky (or rum), which enjoys a high reputation as a pain-reliever—particularly in the terminal stages of malignant disease.

Bromsulphthalein. A dye used as the basis of a test of liver function. Injected intravenously, it is excreted in the bile. Retention therefore indicates failure of biliary excretion.

Bronchial. Pertaining to the bronchi.

Bronchiectasis. A disease characterized by dilatation of the bronchi and bronchioles.

Bronchiole. A smaller branch of a bronchus.

Bronchiolitis. Inflammation of the bronchioles.

Bronchitis. Inflammation of the bronchi.

Bronchoconstrictor. An agent that constricts the bronchi.

Bronchodilator. An agent that dilates the bronchi.

Bronchogenic. Pertaining to the bronchi.

Bronchogram. The X-ray picture of the lung after the injection of a radio-opaque dye.

Bronchography. The method of examining the lungs by the intra-bronchial injection of a radio-opaque dye.

Bronchophony. The exaggerated vocal resonance heard over consolidated lung.

Bronchopneumonia. Infection of the terminal bronchioles, which spreads to the surrounding alveoli, producing a patchy consolidation of the lungs.

Bronchoscope. An instrument for the examination of the interior of the tracheobronchial tree.

Bronchospasm. Spasm of the bronchial tree, such as occurs in asthma.

Bronchospirometry. Estimation of ventilatory function by means of a bronchospirometer, which is essentially a double bronchoscope, and allows of samples of air being obtained from each lung.

Bronchus. Any part of the air passages of the lungs between the trachea and the bronchioles. (*Plural:* bronchi.)

Bronopol. The B.P. Commission approved name for 2-bromo-2-nitropropane-1,3-diol. An antiseptic and preservative.

Broth. A thin soup. A culture medium for the growth of micro-organisms.

Brow. The forehead. The superciliary arch.

Brucella. A genus of the family Brucellaceae, consisting of gram-negative coccobacilli. (*Abbreviation: Br.*) Three species are recognized: *Brucella abortus*, which occurs mainly in cattle; *Brucella mellitensis*, which occurs in goats and sheep; *Brucella suris*, which occurs in pigs.

Brucellin. A purified extract of Brucella administered intradermally in the diagnosis of brucellosis.

Brucellosis. A disease caused by infection with species of Brucella. In man it is also known as undulant fever, Malta fever, Mediterranean fever.

Bruise. Contusion.

Bruit. A murmur, or abnormal sound, heard on auscultation.

Bruxism. Grinding of the teeth, especially during sleep.

Bubo. An inflammatory swelling of a lymphatic gland.

Bubonic. Pertaining to a bubo.

Bubonocele. Swelling in the groin due to an incomplete inguinal hernia.

Buccal. Relating to the mouth.

Bucetin. The B.P. Commission approved name for N-3-hydroxybutyryl-p-phenetidine. An analgesic.

Buclizine. The B.P. Commission approved name for 1-(4-t-butylbenzyl)-4-(4-chlorobenzhydryl)piperazine. An anti-emetic.

Buclosamide. The B.P. Commission approved name for N-butyl-4-chloro-salicylamide. An antimycotic.

Bud. A small outgrowth resembling the bud of a plant. **Taste buds,** the peripheral organs of Taste.

Buffer. A substance which reduces the

extent or speed of a reaction, as, for instance, between acid and alkali.

Bufylline. The B.P. Commission approved name for theophylline-2-amino-2-methylpropan-1-ol. A bronchodilator.

Buggery. Sodomy.

Bulb. Any rounded organ or mass. **Aortic bulb,** the dilatation at the union of the ascending aorta with the arch of the aorta. **Hair bulb,** the enlargement at the root of a hair. **Jugular bulbs,** dilatations at the origin (*superior bulb*) and at the termination (*inferior bulb*) of the internal jugular vein. **Olfactory bulb,** the enlarged distal end of the olfactory tract, in which the primary olfactory neurones end and the secondary neurones begin. **Bulb of the penis,** the enlarged proximal part of the corpus spongiosum.

Bulimia. Insatiable appetite.

Bulla. A large bleb or blister.

Bundle. A collection of fibres or strands. **Atrioventricular bundle,** the part of the conducting path in the heart that carries the impulse from the atrioventricular node to the ventricles. **Ciliary bundle,** a small bundle of very fine fibres, lying close to the edge of the eyelid behind the eyelash.

Buniodyl. The B.P. Commission approved name for 3-(3-butyramido-2,4,6-tri-iodophenyl)-2-ethylacrylic acid. A radio-opaque substance.

Bunion. A swelling, usually inflammatory, of a bursa (usually that of the metatarsophalangeal joint of the big toe).

Buphenine. The B.P. Commission approved name for 1-(4-hydroxyphenyl)-2-(1-methyl-3-phenylpropylamino)propan-1-ol. A peripheral vasodilator.

Buphthalmos. Infantile glaucoma.

Bupivacaine hydrochloride. B.P. Addendum 1969. $C_{18}H_{28}N_2O,HCl,H_2O$. A local anaesthetic.

Burn. An injury caused by heat or any cauterizing agent, whether physical or chemical.

Burning feet. A syndrome characterized by a burning sensation of the feet, probably due to some vitamin deficiency which is widespread in India and the Far East.

Bursa. A closed sac, lined with synovial membrane and containing a viscid fluid, found in areas of the body exposed to friction, as between two structures that move relative to each other. (*Plural:* bursae.) **Adventitious bursa,** a bursa that develops after

birth as a result of unusual pressure or muscular activity. **Interligamentous bursa,** a bursa between two ligaments. **Subcutaneous synovial bursa,** a bursa lying between the skin and a bony prominence. **Subfascial synovial bursa,** a bursa beneath a fascial or aponeurotic sheet. **Submuscular synovial bursa,** a bursa lying between a muscle and bone, tendon or ligament. **Subtendinous synovial bursa,** a bursa lying between a tendon and bone, tendon and ligaments, or two tendons. **Omental bursa,** the portion of the peritoneal cavity lying behind the stomach.

Burr. A rotatory instrument for the cutting of bone or teeth.

Bursitis. Inflammation of a bursa.

Bursolith. A concretion or calculus in a bursa.

Busulphan. B.P. 1968. $C_6H_{14}O_6S_2$. A cytotoxic agent, used principally in the treatment of chronic myelogenous leukaemia.

Butacaine sulphate. B.P.C. 1968. $C_{36}H_{62}N_4O_8S$. A local anaesthetic.

Butalamine. The B.P. Commission approved name for 3-phenyl-5-(2-dibutylaminoethyl)amino-1,2,4-oxadiazole. A vasodilator.

Butamyrate. The B.P. Commission approved name for 2-(2-diethylaminoethoxy)ethyl 2-phenylbutyrate. A cough suppressant.

Butanilicaine. The B.P. Commission approved name for *N*-butylaminoacetyl-6-chloro-*o*-toluidine. A local anaesthetic.

Butethamate. The B.P. Commission approved name for 2-diethylaminoethyl 2-phenylbutyrate. An antispasmodic.

Buthalitone sodium. The B.P. Commission approved name for a mixture of 100 parts by weight of the monosodium derivative of 5-allyl-5-isobutyl-2-thiobarbituric acid and 6 parts by weight of dried sodium carbonate. A hypnotic.

Butobarbitone. B.P. 1968. $C_{10}H_{16}N_2O_3$. An intermediate-acting barbiturate.

Butoxamine. The B.P. Commission approved name for ($\pm$)-*erythro*-1-(2,5-dimethoxyphenyl)-2-t-butylaminopropan-1-ol. An inhibitor of fatty acid mobilization.

Butylated hydroxyanisole. B.P. 1968. $C_{11}H_{16}O_2$. An antioxidant for preserving fats and oils.

Butylated hydroxytoluene. B.P. 1968. $C_{15}H_{24}O$. An antioxidant for preserving fats and oils.

Butter. The fatty part of milk obtained by churning cream.

Buttermilk. The fluid containing casein and lactic acid, left after the churning of milk.

Buttock. The gluteal prominence.

Byssinosis. The form of pneumoconiosis due to the inhalation of cotton dust.

C

Cabbage. *Brassica oleracea.* A widely used vegetable which contains about 5 per cent of carbohydrate and, when properly cooked, is a reasonably rich source of vitamin C.

Cacao. The seeds of *Theobroma cacao* (L.), from which chocolate and cocoa are made.

Cacation. Defaecation.

Cachectic. Wasted.

Cachet. An oral capsule, generally made of rice paper, for enclosing a dose of unpleasant tasting medicine.

Cachexia. An extreme state of malnutrition and wasting.

Cachou. An aromatic pill for sweetening of the breath.

Caco- [(Gk *kakos:* bad). Prefix indicating bad or unpleasant.

Cacogeusia. Bad taste.

Cacomelia. Congenital deformity of a limb.

Cacophony. Discordant sound.

Cacosmia. A stench.

Cadaver. A corpse.

Cade oil. B.P.C. 1968. The oil obtained from *Juniperus oxycedrus* (L.), and used in dermatological preparations.

Cadmium. A metallic element widely used in the making of alloys. Symbol Cd. Atomic weight 112·40. Atomic number 48. Prolonged inhalation of its salts can produce an extreme form of emphysema.

Caecectomy. Surgical excision of the caecum.

Caecum. The first part of the large intestine, situated in the right iliac fossa. Its average length is 6cm., and its average breadth 7·5cm.

Caeruloplasmin. The copper-containing α_2-globulin of the blood.

Caesarean section. Delivery of a child by surgical opening of the uterus.

Caesium. A rare metallic element. Symbol Cs. Atomic weight 132·91. Atomic number 55.

Cafedrine. The B.P. Commission approved name for L-7-[2-(β-hydroxy-α-methylphenylamino)ethyl]theophylline. An analeptic.

Caffeine. B.P. 1968. $C_8H_{10}N_4O_2$. A cerebral stimulant and a diuretic derived from tea waste, or coffee, or the dried leaves of *Camellia sinensis* (L.), or by synthesis. **Caffeine hydrate,** B.P. 1968, the monohydrate of caffeine, with the same action and uses. **Caffeine and sodium iodide,** B.P.C. 1968, a diuretic.

Caisson disease. The name commonly given to compressed air illness when it occurs in caisson workers.

Cajuput oil. B.P.C. 1968. The oil obtained by distillation from the fresh leaves and twigs of certain species of Melaleuca. It is a mild counter-irritant.

Calamine. B.P. 1968. A basic zinc carbonate suitably coloured with ferric oxide. It has a mild astringent action on the skin and is widely used in topical applications to relieve the discomfort of irritable skin conditions. **Calamine lotion,** B.P. 1968, a lotion containing 150 grammes of calamine and 50 grammes of zinc oxide per 1000 ml., which cools the skin by evaporation. **Oily calamine lotion,** B.P.C. 1968, a soothing application for the skin.

Calc-, Calci-, Calco- (L *calx, calcis:* lime). Prefixes indicating association with lime or calcium.

Calcaneus. The heel-bone, which articulates with the talus above and the cuboid anteriorly.

Calcar. A spur or spur-like process. **Calcar avis,** a projection in the medial wall of the lateral ventricle. **Calcar femorale,** a bony spur on the shaft of the femur anterior to the lesser trochanter.

Calcicosis. The form of pneumonoconiosis induced by the inhalation of marble dust.

Calciferol. B.P. 1968. Vitamin D_2, which may be prepared by the ultraviolet irradiation of ergosterol. It has all the actions and uses of naturally occurring vitamin D, which is necessary for the absorption of calcium and phosphorus. Deficiency causes rickets in children and osteomalacia in adults. **Calciferol**

solution, B.P. 1968, a solution of calciferol in a suitable vegetable oil, containing 0·075mg. in 1ml. **Strong calciferol tablets,** B.P. 1968, each tablet contains 1·25mg. of calciferol.

Calcification. The process of depositing of lime salts in the tissues.

Calcinosis. The condition characterized by the deposition of calcium salts in the tissues. **Calcinosis cutis,** widespread deposition of calcium salts in the skin.

Calcitonin. The B.P. Commission approved name for a hormone extractable from the mammalian thyroid gland which lowers the calcium concentration in the circulating plasma.

Calcium. The element which is a major constituent of bone. Symbol Ca. Atomic weight 40·08. Atomic number 20.

Calcium alginate. B.P.C. 1968. An absorbable haemostatic.

Calcium aminosalicylate. B.P. 1968. $C_{14}H_{12}CaN_2O_6$,3 H_2O. A drug used in the treatment of tuberculosis, in conjunction with streptomycin nd/or isoniazid.

Calcium benzamidosalicylate. The B.P. Commission approved name for calcium 4-benzamido-2-hydroxybenzoate, an anti-tuberculosis drug.

Calcium carbonate. B.P. 1968. $CaCO_3$. An antacid.

Calcium chloride. B.P. 1968. $CaCl_2$, $6H_2O$. A soluble calcium salt used in the preparation of solutions for injection.

Calcium cyclamate. B.P. 1968. $C_{12}H_{24}CaN_2O_6S_2$,2H_2O. A sweetening agent.

Calcium gluconate. B.P. 1968. $C_{12}H_{22}CaO_{14}$,H_2O. The most widely used of the salts of calcium for conditions in which there is a deficiency or lack of calcium. **Calcium gluconate injection,** B.P. 1968, a sterile solution containing 10 per cent of calcium gluconate, for intravenous administration.

Calcium hydroxide. B.P. 1968. $Ca(OH)_2$. An antacid and astringent. **Calcium hydroxide solution,** B.P. 1968, also known as lime water, a solution containing not less than 0·15 per cent w/v calcium hydroxide.

Calcium lactate. B.P. 1968. $C_6H_{10}CaO_6$, 5H_2O. A soluble calcium salt with the same action as calcium gluconate. **Calcium lactate tablets,** B.P. 1968, each contains 300 mg. of calcium lactate.

Calcium phosphate. B.P.C. 1968. A non-hygroscopic diluent for powders.

Calcium sodium lactate. B.P.C. 1968. $C_{12}H_{20}CaNa_2O_{12}$,4H_2O. A soluble salt with the same action as calcium gluconate.

Calcium sulphate, dried. B.P.C. 1968. $CaSO_4,\frac{1}{2}H_2O$. The salt used for the preparation of plaster of Paris.

Calcium trisodium pentetate. The B.P. Commission approved name for the calcium chelate of the trisodium salt of diethylenetriamine-NNN′N″N‴-penta-acetic acid. A chelating agent.

Calciuria. The presence of calcium in the urine.

Calculosis. The condition characterized by, or the tendency to, the deposition of calculi in the body.

Calculus. A concretion, or stone, composed predominantly, or entirely, of mineral salts, and found mainly in ducts or hollow organs, such as the gall-bladder, bile ducts, bladder, and ureter. (*Plural:* calculi.)

Calf. The fleshy part of the back of the leg, formed mainly of the gastrocnemius muscles.

Calix. A cup-shaped cavity. (*Plural:* calices.) **Renal calices,** the primary divisions of the renal pelvis.

Calliper. A two-pronged instrument with pointed ends, for the measurement of diameters, such as the pelvic diameter in obstetrics. **Calliper splint,** a splint made of two iron rods secured to a padded ring, and used in the treatment of a fractured femur.

Callisthenics. Gymnastics aimed at producing beauty and grace of movement.

Callosity. A circumscribed thickening of the skin. (*Plural:* callosities.)

Callus. Callosity. The unorganized bony tissue formed between the two ends of a fractured bone. (*Plural:* calluses.)

Calomel. Mercurous chloride. A one-time popular powerful purgative.

Calor. Heat.

Calorie. A unit of heat. The **small calorie** (cal.) is the amount of heat required to raise the temperature of 1 gramme of water from 14·5° to 15·5°C. The **large calorie** (Cal., kcal.), the one used in nutritional studies, is 1000 times the small calorie.

Calorimeter. An instrument for measuring heat production.

Calorimetry. Measurement of heat production or absorption.

Calvaria. The vault of the skull.

Calvities. Baldness, especially of the upper part of the head.

Calx. Lime or chalk.

Camphor. B.P. 1968. $C_{10}H_{16}O$. A crystalline substance obtained from the wood of *Cinnamonum camphora* (L.). It is a carminative and has also a mild expectorant action. Applied externally it is a mild analgesic and rubefacient. **Camphor liniment,** B.P. 1968, 20 per cent w/w of camphor in arachis oil. Camphorated oil.

Campimetry. A specialized form of perimetry.

Camptodactylia. A state of permanent flexion of one or more interphalangeal joints.

Canal. A duct or channel. **Adductor (subsartorial) canal,** an aponeurotic tunnel in the middle third of the thigh, which contains the femoral artery and vein and the saphenous nerve. **Alimentary canal,** the digestive tract from the mouth to the anus. **Alveolar canals,** the canals that transmit the posterior alveolar vessels and nerves to the molar teeth. **Anal canal,** the terminal section of the alimentary canal, stretching from the lower end of the ampulla of the rectum to the anus, and measuring about 3·8cm. in the adult. **Carotid canal,** the canal in the petrous part of the temporal bone, that transmits the internal carotid artery. **Central canal of the cochlea,** the small canal in the cochlea that transmits the cochlear nerve. **Central canal of the spinal cord,** the canal that traverses the entire length of the spinal cord, is continued through the medulla oblongata and opens into the fourth ventricle of the brain. **Cervical canal,** the canal of the cervix uteri. **Canal of the epididymis,** the first part of the efferent duct of the testis. **Ethmoidal canals (anterior and posterior),** canals in the ethmoid bone that transmit the anterior and posterior ethmoidal nerves and vessels. **Facial canal,** the canal that transmits the facial nerve through the petrous temporal to the stylomastoid foramen. **Femoral canal,** the medial compartment of the femoral sheath. **Haversian canals,** the minute canals in compact bone that transmit the arteries and veins. **Hyaloid canal,** a narrow canal that runs from the optic disc to the centre of the posterior surface of the lens. **Hypoglossal canal,** the canal in the base of the skull that transmits the hypoglossal nerve. **Infra-orbital canal,** the canal in the floor of the orbit that transmits the infra-orbital nerve. **Inguinal canal,** an oblique canal, about

4cm. long, extending from the deep to the superficial inguinal ring. It contains the spermatic cord in the male and the round ligament of the uterus in the female. **Mandibular canal,** the canal in the mandible that transmits the inferior alveolar nerve and vessels. It divides into **mental** and **incisive canals. Nasolacrimal canal,** the canal, about 1cm. long, that transmits the nasolacrimal duct. **Optic canal,** the canal in the posterior wall of the orbit that transmits the optic nerve and the ophthalmic artery. **Greater palatine canal,** the canal in the lateral wall of the nasal cavity that transmits the greater palatine nerves and arteries. **Palatinovaginal canal,** the canal between the vaginal process of the medial pterygoid plate and the palatine bone. **Portal canals,** the canals surrounding the hepatic lobules. Each contains a branch of the portal vein, a branch of the hepatic artery and an interlobular bile ductule. **Pterygoid canal,** the canal piercing the root of the pterygoid process of the sphenoid. **Pudendal canal,** the canal in the lateral wall of the ischiorectal fossa that carries the internal pudendal vessels and accompanying nerves. **Sacral canal,** the canal in the sacrum that contains the cauda equina. **Semicircular canals,** three in number, superior, posterior and lateral, in the bony labyrinth. **Vertebral canal,** the canal in the vertebral column that contains the spinal cord.

Canaliculus. A small channel or canal. (*Plural:* canaliculi.) **Bile canaliculi,** minute bile capillaries in the hepatic lobules. **Cochlear canaliculus,** the small canal in the petrous bone that transmits the aqueduct of the cochlea. **Dental canaliculi,** the minute tubules in the dentine, each of which contains a dentinal fibre, which is believed to be concerned with the nourishment of the avascular dentine. **Innominate canaliculus,** a canal on the medial side of the foramen spinosum that transmits the lesser petrosal nerve. **Lacrimal canaliculi,** the ducts, one in each eyelid, that lead from the lacrimal puncta to the lacrimal sac. **Mastoid canaliculus,** a minute canal that transmits the auricular branch of the vagus nerve.

Cancellous. Spongy or reticular in appearance. A term usually applied to bony tissue.

Cancer. A term used rather loosely, usually as an alternative to carcinoma, but it is also used to denote any malignant new growth.

Cancerophobia. A morbid fear of developing a malignant growth.

Cancrum. A gangrenous, ulcerative lesion. Canker. **Cancrum oris,** a gangrenous ulcer in the mouth, liable to recur in debilitated children. Noma. Gangrenous stomatitis.

Candela. The basic unit of luminous intensity, being the luminous intensity, in the perpendicular direction, of a surface of 1/600,000 square metre of a black body at the temperature of freezing platinum under a pressure of 101,325 newtons per square metre.

Candicidin. The B.P. Commission approved name for one or more of a mixture of heptaenes with antifungal activity produced by *Streptomyces griseus* and other Streptomyces species.

Candida. A genus of yeast-like fungi. *Candida albicans*, the only important pathogenic species in the genus.

Candidiasis. Disease caused by fungi of the genus Candida.

Candle. Unit of intensity of light.

Canine. Relating to a dog. **Canine tooth,** the pointed tooth next to the incisor.

Canities. Greyness or whiteness of the hair.

Canker. A sloughing ulcer.

Cannabinol. The active principle of cannabis.

Cannabione. The resin in cannabis that contains the active principle.

Cannabis. The dried flowering or fruiting tops of the pistillate plant of *Cannabis sativa*. Synonyms are cannabis indica, Indian hemp, ganja, guaza, marihuana. **Bhang** consists of specially dried leaves and flowering shoots. **Charas** is the resinous matter collected from the leaves and flowering tops of the plants and constitutes the active principle. **Hashish** is a powdered and sifted form of charas.

Cannula. A tube, designed to fit over a trocar, for insertion into a body cavity.

Canthariasis. Infestation of the body with beetles, their larvae or eggs.

Cantharides. Spanish fly. A powder made from the dried beetle *Cantharis vesicatoria*, and at one time widely used as a vesicant and counter-irritant.

Canthus. The corner at either end of the aperture between the two eyelids. (*Plural:* canthi.)

Cap. A covering. **Duodenal cap,** the superior part of the duodenum as outlined by a radio-opaque meal.

Capacity. Power or ability to hold or contain. Volume. **Forced vital capacity,** the maximum volume of air which can be expired following a maximum inspiration, the expiratory phase being accomplished as rapidly and forcibly as possible. **Functional residual capacity,** the volume of air remaining in the lungs at the end of a normal expiration. **Inspiratory capacity,** maximal volume of air that can be inspired from the resting expiratory level. **Maximum breathing capacity,** the maximum volume of air that can be breathed per minute. **Testamentary capacity,** an individual's mental fitness to make a valid will, defined legally as 'a sound disposing mind'. **Total lung capacity,** the volume of air in the lungs at the end of maximal inspiration. **Vital capacity,** the volume of air that can be expelled during a maximum expiration following a maximum inspiration.

Capillary. One of the hair-like blood vessels in which the arterial tree terminates. (*Plural:* capillaries.)

Capitate. The largest of the carpal bones, lying in the distal row opposite the base of the third metacarpal bone.

Capitulum. A small knob or eminence on a bone. **Capitulum of the humerus,** the lateral convex surface of the lower end of the humerus that articulates with the radius.

Capreomycin. The B.P. Commission approved name for an antibiotic produced by *Streptomyces capreolus*, which is active against *Myco. tuberculosis*.

Capsicum. B.P.C. 1968. The dried ripe fruits of *Capsicum minimum* and small-fruited varieties of *C. frutescens* (L.), which is used internally as a carminative, and externally as a counter-irritant.

Capsule. A sheath around an organ or structure. A medicament enclosed in a shell of methylcellulose or prepared from a gelatin base containing glycerin. **Articular capsule,** the sheath, consisting of a fibrous capsule lined with a synovial membrane, that surrounds a synovial joint. **External capsule of the cerebrum,** a thin layer of white matter interposed between the lateral aspect of the lentiform nucleus and the claustrum. **Internal capsule of the cerebrum,** a broad band of white fibres in the medial surface of the lentiform nucleus. **Perivascular fibrous capsule,** the capsule, formed by the two layers of the lesser omentum that surrounds the hepatic artery, portal vein and the bile duct, is continuous with the fibrous capsule of the liver, and surrounds these structures in their course through the liver.

Capsulitis. Inflammation of a capsule.

Captation. The first stage of hypnotism.

Captodiamine. The B.P. Commission approved name for 4-butylthiobenzhydryl 2-dimethylaminoethyl sulphide. A tranquillizer.

Caput. A head. **Caput medusae,** the whorl of dilated veins around the umbilicus in the late stages of cirrhosis of the liver. **Caput succedanum,** the temporary swelling on the head of the new-born infant.

Caramel. Burnt sugar. B.P.C. 1968.

Caramiphen hydrochloride. B.P. 1968. $C_{18}H_{28}ClNO_2$. A drug used in the treatment of parkinsonism.

Caraway. B.P. 1968. The dried ripe fruits of *Carum carvi* (L.). Used as a carminative. **Caraway oil,** B.P.C. 1968, a distillate obtained from fresh caraway, and used as a carminative.

Carbachol. B.P. 1968. $C_6H_{15}ClN_2O_2$. A drug that has the muscarine and nicotinic actions of acetylcholine, and therefore used as a parasympathetic stimulant.

Carbamazepine. B.P.C. Supplement 1971. $C_{15}H_{12}N_2O$. A drug that is proving of value in the treatment of trigeminal neuralgia and epilepsy.

Carbenicillin sodium. B.P. Addendum 1969. A bactericidal semi-synthetic penicillin that is active against *Pseudomonas pyocyanea* and against enterobacteria. It is inactive orally.

Carbenoxolone. The B.P. Commission approved name for 3β-(3-carboxypropionyloxy)-11-oxo-olean-12-en-30-oic acid. A drug used in the treatment of peptic ulcer.

Carbimazole. B.P. 1968. $C_7H_{10}N_2O_2S$. An antithyroid substance.

Carbinoxamine. The B.P. Commission approved name for 4-chloro-α-2-pyridylbenzyl 2-dimethylaminoethyl ether. An antihistamine drug.

Carbiphene. The B.P. Commission approved name for α-ethoxy-N-methyl-N-[2-(N-methylphenethylamino)ethyl] diphenylacetamide. An analgesic.

Carbocloral. The B.P. Commission approved name for ethyl (2,2,2-trichloro-1-hydroxyethyl)carbamate. A hypnotic.

Carbohydrate. A substance containing carbon, hydrogen and oxygen, the hydrogen and oxygen usually being present in the same ratio as in water. It is either a hydroxy-aldehyde or a hydroxy-ketone. The simpler carbohydrates are known as sugars.

Carbolic acid. Phenol.

Carbolonium bromide. The B.P. Commission approved name for hexamethylenedi(carbamoyl choline bromide). A muscle relaxant.

Carbon. A non-metallic element. Symbol C. Atomic weight 12·01. Atomic number 6.

Carbon dioxide. CO_2. A gas which dissolves readily in water to form carbonic acid. One of the end-products of tissue oxidation of carbohydrate and fat. A respiratory stimulant. **Carbon dioxide snow,** a form of solid carbon dioxide used to remove warts and naevi by freezing.

Carbon monoxide. CO. A colourless, odourless gas which is highly toxic because of the facility with which it combines with haemoglobin to form the stable and asphyxiating carboxyhaemoglobin.

Carboxyhaemoglobin. The cherry-coloured compound of carbon monoxide and haemoglobin.

Carbromal. B.P. 1968. $C_7H_{13}BrN_2O_2$. A quick-acting sedative.

Carbuncle. An acute circumscribed inflammation of the skin and subcutaneous tissues, comparable to, but more extensive than, a boil. Usually due to infection with *Staphylococcus aureus*.

Carbutamide. The B.P. Commission approved name for N-butyl-N'-sulphanilylurea. A hypoglycaemic agent.

Carcin-, Carcino- (Gk *karkinos:* crab). Prefixes denoting cancer.

Carcinogen. A cancer-producing agent or factor.

Carcinogenesis. The production of carcinoma in the living tissues.

Carcinoid. Argentaffin carcinoma.

Carcinoma. A malignant tumour of epithelial cells which spreads locally and metastasizes in a completely uncontrolled manner. **Adenocarcinoma,** a columnar-cell carcinoma with formation of glandular spaces. **Anaplastic carcinoma,** a carcinoma composed of undifferentiated primitive cells. **Basal-cell carcinoma,** a carcinoma arising from the cutaneous epithelium, usually of the face, and sometimes known as a rodent ulcer. **Bronchogenic carcinoma,** a carcinoma of a bronchus. **Carcinoma-in-situ,** a precursor of squamous-cell carcinoma, found in the stratified epithelium of the skin, mouth, and cervix uteri. **Chorioncarcinoma,** a highly malignant tumour of the trophoblast. Chorionepithelioma. **Columnar-cell carcinoma,** a carcinoma derived from the columnar cells of mucous membrane. **Encephaloid carcinoma,** a soft carcinoma with a minimum of stromal tissue. **Oat-cell carcinoma,** a highly malignant form of carcinoma of the lung, so-called because the constituent cells are oat-shaped **Scirrhous carcinoma,** a hard, indurated form of carcinoma. **Squamous-cell carcinoma,** a carcinoma arising from squamous epithelium.

Carcinomatosis. Widespread dissemination of carcinoma throughout the body.

Carcinophobia. Morbid fear of cancer.

Carcinosarcoma. A mixed malignant tumour containing elements of carcinoma and sarcoma.

Cardamom fruit. B.P. 1968. The dried nearly ripe fruits of *Elettaria cardamomum* A carminative and flavouring agent.

Cardi-, Cardio- (Gk *kardia:* heart). Prefixes indicating relationship to heart.

Cardia. The upper opening of the stomach.

Cardiac. Relating to the heart.

Cardiolipin. A purified lipid extracted from bovine heart. With cholesterol and lecithin it is used as an antigen in serodiagnostic tests for syphilis.

Cardiology. The study of the heart and its diseases.

Cardiomegaly. Enlargement of the heart.

Cardiopathy. Disease of the heart.

Cardioscopy. Viewing the heart on the fluorescent screen.

Cardiospasm. Achalasia of the cardia.

Cardiovascular. Relating to the heart and the blood vessels.

Carditis. Inflammation of the heart.

Caries. A process of gradual decay of bone and teeth.

Carina. A keel-like structure.

Cariogenic. Producing caries.

Carious. Affected with caries.

Carisoprodol. The B.P. Commission approved name for 2-carbamoyl-oxymethyl-2-*N*-isopropylcarbamoyl-oxymethylpentamine. A muscle relaxant.

Carminative. A drug that facilitates eructation.

Carmine. B.P.C. 1968. The aluminium lake of the colouring matter of cochineal. Used as a colouring matter.

Carneous. Fleshy. **Carneous mole,** an impregnated ovum that has died as a result of progressive or recurrent haemorrhage, usually during the first three months of pregnancy.

Carotene. $C_{40}H_{56}$. A yellow pigment found in many foodstuffs, including carrots and egg yolk, which is a precursor of vitamin A.

Carotenoid. Lipochrome.

Carotid. The name of the principal artery in the neck.

Carotinaemia. Excess of carotene in the blood, usually due to the excessive consumption of carrots, resulting in a yellowish discoloration of the blood, skin, and mucous membrane.

Carp-, Carpo- (Gk *karpos:* wrist). Prefixes signifying relationship to the wrist.

Carpal. Pertaining to the carpus, or wrist.

Carperidine. The B.P. Commission approved name for ethyl 1-(2-carbamoylethyl)-4-phenylpiperidine-4-carboxylate. A cough suppressant.

Carphenazine. The B.P. Commission approved name for 10-{3-[4-(2-hydroxyethyl) piperazin-1-yl] propyl} 2-propionylphenothiazine. A tranquillizer.

Carpopedal. Pertaining to the wrist and foot. **Carpopedal spasm,** the painful spasms of the feet and hands that occur in tetany.

Carpus. The eight bones composing the wrist.

Carrageen. Irish moss, the dried seaweed, *Chondrus crispus,* used as an emulsifying agent for cod-liver oil and other oils, and as a substitute for gelatin in the preparation of jellies for invalids.

Carrier. A healthy or convalescent individual who is carrying, and able to convey to others, the micro-organisms responsible for one or more diseases. A healthy unaffected individual who can transmit a hereditary disease trait to his (or her) offspring.

Carrot. *Daucus carota.* A vegetable which is a relatively rich source of carotene.

Carsalam. The B.P. Commission approved name for 1,3-benzoxazine-2,4-dione. An analgesic.

Cartilage. A specialized form of connective tissue, consisting of cells, known as chondrocytes, embedded in an abundant intercellular substance or matrix. It is found in parts of the body, such as the joints and larynx, where it is necessary to have rigidity and strength combined with a modicum of elasticity. **Articular cartilage,** the cartilage that covers the articular surfaces of most synovial joints. **Arytenoid cartilages,** a pair of cartilages on the lateral aspect of the upper border of the lamina of the cricoid cartilage at the back of the larynx. **Corniculate cartilages,** two small cartilages articulating with the summits of the arytenoid cartilages. **Costal cartilages,** bars of hyaline cartilage which extend forwards from the anterior ends of the ribs. **Cricoid cartilage,** a signet-ring-shaped cartilage that forms the lower part of the anterior and lateral walls, and most of the posterior wall, of the larynx. **Cuneiform cartilages,** two small cartilages, one in each aryepiglottic fold. **Epiglottic cartilage,** the leaf-like cartilage that projects obliquely behind the tongue and the body of the hyoid bone, and in front of the entrance to the larynx. **Nasal cartilages,** the series of cartilages—septal, upper, lower, and small—that form part of the framework of the nose. **Semilunar cartilages,** or menisci, two crescentic lamellae that deepen the surfaces of the upper end of the tibia for articulation with the femoral condyles. **Thyroid cartilage,** the largest cartilage of the larynx, that forms the laryngeal prominence (or Adam's apple). **Tracheal cartilages,** 16 to 20 in number, occupying the anterior two-thirds of the circumference of the trachea.

Caruncle. A small, fleshy eminence. **Hymenal caruncles,** the remnants of the ruptured hymen. **Lacrminal caruncle,** the small reddish body in the medial angle of the eye. **Urethral caruncle,** a painful, scarlet, glistening swelling, the size of a cherry stone that may develop on the posterior wall of the female urethra.

Cascara. B.P. 1968. The dried bark of *Rhamnus purshiana,* which is a purgative.

Caseation. The precipitation of casein in the process of curdling of milk. A form of necrosis in which the tissues are converted into a cheese-like mass. This is one of the classical manifestations of chronic tuberculous degeneration.

Casein. The principal protein of milk, and the basis of curds and cheese.

Caseous. Resembling cheese or curd.

Cassava. The starch from the roots of *Manihot utilissima* and *M. aipi* from which tapioca is prepared.

Cassette. A plate-holder used in photography and radiography.

Cast. A mould formed in a tubular or hollow organ of the body, such as the renal tubules, by the extravasation of pathological material. An object formed by the solidification of a liquid poured into a mould. A stiff dressing made of bandage impregnated with plaster of Paris. A squint.

Castor oil. B.P.C. 1968. The oil obtained from *Ricinus communis* (L.). A purgative internally, and an emollient externally.

Castration. Removal of the testicles or ovaries.

Cata-, Cath- (Gk *kata:* down). Prefixes meaning down, under, lower, along. back. *See also* Kata-.

Catabolism. The breaking down of the tissues of the body for the purpose of producing energy.

Catalase. An enzyme which catalyses hydrogen peroxide to oxygen and water.

Catalepsy. The condition characterized by sudden suspension of sensation and volition, accompanied by rigidity of the limbs which remain in any posture in which they are placed.

Catalysis. Alteration in the velocity of a chemical reaction induced by a substance which remains unchanged throughout the reaction.

Catalyst. A substance that induces catalysis.

Catamenia. Menstruation.

Cataphoresis. The introduction of charged ions into the tissues by means of an electric field.

Cataplasia. A degenerative process in the tissues.

Cataplasm. A poultice.

Cataplexy. Sudden onset of weakness and tonelessness in the voluntary muscles.

Cataract. Partial or complete opacity of the lens of the eye.

Catarrh. Inflammation of a mucous membrane.

Catatonia. The phase, or type, of schizophrenia, characterized by stupor and the maintenance of a fixed posture.

Catecholamines. A generic term applied to *o*-dihydric phenols with a side chain carrying an amino group, which occur in the adrenal medulla, sympathetic nerves and the brain. They include adrenaline and noradrenaline.

Catechu. B.P.C. 1968. A dried aqueous extract prepared from the leaves and young shoots of *Uncaria gambier*. It is an astringent, used in the treatment of diarrhoea.

Catgut. Sterilized surgical catgut. B.P. 1968. Strands prepared from collagen derived from healthy mammals, purified and sterilized. It may be prepared from the washed intestines of sheep or other herbivorous animals. It is used in surgery for tying off blood vessels and for stitching wounds. **Boilable catgut,** sterilized surgical catgut B.P. which must be partly hydrated or conditioned before use. **Chromicized catgut,** catgut that has been hardened by treatment with chromium compounds. **Hardened catgut,** sterilized surgical catgut B.P. which has been treated with a suitable hardening agent designed to prolong its resistance to digestion. **Non-hardened catgut,** sterilized surgical catgut B.P. which has not been processed to reduce the rate of absorption; it is generally effective in muscle for 5 to 10 days. **Plain catgut,** a synonym for non-hardened catgut.

Catharsis. Purgation. Purification.

Cathartic. Having a purgative or purifying action. A purgative.

Catheter. A tube for passage through the urethra or other canals for purposes of drainage or withdrawing fluids.

Cathode. The negative pole or electrode of an electric current or battery.

Cation. An ion carrying a positive charge of electricity. **Cation-exchange resins,** synthetic organic polymers which bind cations at pH 5, thereby effecting changes in the electrolyte balance of the plasma. They are used in the treatment of retention oedema.

Cat-scratch fever. A disease, probably due to a virus, but not necessarily characterized by a cat scratch, in which there is general malaise and generalized enlargement of lymph glands.

Cauda. A tail or appendage. (*Plural:* caudae.) **Cauda equina,** the sheaf of nerve roots in the subarachnoid space below the termination of the spinal cord at the level of the lower border of the first lumbar vertebra.

Causalgia. Severe, insistent burning pain, usually associated with incomplete lesions of a peripheral nerve.

Caustic. Corrosive. An agent producing this effect.

Cauterize. To burn with a cautery.

Cautery. An agent used to cauterize.

Caverna. A cavity or cavern. (*Plural:* cavernae.)

Cavernitis. Inflammation of the corpus cavernosum of the penis or clitoris.

Cavernous. Relating to a cavity. **Cavernous breathing,** the characteristic form of respiration heard on auscultation over a cavity in the lungs.

Cavity. A hollow space. (*Plural:* cavities.) **Amniotic cavity,** the closed sac between the amnion and the embryo, containing the liquor amnii. **Chorionic cavity,** the general cavity of the blastocyst. **Cranial cavity,** the cavity of the skull, containing the brain, its membranes and their blood vessels. **Glenoid cavity,** the cavity in the scapula, with which the head of the humerus articulates. **Joint cavity,** the cavity in a synovial joint, surrounded by synovial membrane and containing synovial fluid. **Medullary cavity,** the cavity in long bones which is filled with bone marrow. **Nasal cavity,** the cavity of the nose, divided into two halves by the nasal septum. **Peritoneal cavity,** the potential space between the parietal and visceral layers of the peritoneum. **Pericardial cavity,** the potential space between the fibrous and serous pericardium. **Pleural cavity,** the potential space between the pulmonary and parietal pleurae. **Pulp cavity,** the cavity in a tooth. **Tympanic cavity,** the middle ear.

-cele (Gk *kēlē:* hernia). Suffix denoting a swelling of the part indicated in the first part of the word.

Cell. A mass of protoplasm containing a nucleus, which constitutes the unit of living tissue. A small cavity. In electricity a source of electrical energy. **Alpha cells,** chromophile cells in the anterior lobe of the hypophysis that contain eosinophilic granules. **Alveolar cells,** the cells lining the alveoli in the lungs. **Amacrine cells,** cells in the inner part of the inner nuclear layer of the retina. **Argentaffin (enterochromaffin) cells,** pyramidal or columnar cells in the alimentary tract that contain granules that have an affinity for silver salts which stain them black, and for chromium salts which stain them brown. **Basal cells,** the columnar cells that constitute the basal cell layer of the epidermis. **Basket cells,** large pyramidal cells in the intermediate stratum of the grey matter of the cerebellar cortex. Degenerated granulocytes. **Beta cells,** the chromophile cells of the anterior lobe of the hypophysis that contain basophilic granules. **Betz cells,** the giant pyramidal cells in the cerebral cortex. **Bipolar cells,** neurones with two processes that occur in the retina, the spiral ganglion of the cochlear nerve, and the vestibular ganglion. **Blood cells,** the cellular elements of the blood, consisting of red blood cells (erythrocytes), white blood cells (leucocytes, lymphocytes, and monocytes), and platelets. **Bone cell,** osteocyte. **Capsular cells,** cells of the spinal and sympathetic ganglia. **Cartilage cell,** chondrocyte. **Centro-acinar cells,** the cells lining the ducts of the pancreas. **Chalice cell,** goblet cell. **Chromaffin cells,** phaeochromo-cytes, cells that secrete noradrenaline and adrenaline. **Chromophile cells,** cells of the anterior lobe of the hypophysis that have an affinity for acid or basic dyes. **Chromophobe cells,** cells of the anterior lobe of the hypophysis that have little or no affinity for dyes. **Decidual cells,** connective tissue cells of the vascular endometrium of early pregnancy that contain glycogen or lipoids. **Deiter's cells,** cells in the spiral organ of the cochlea. **Dendritic cells,** epidermal melanoblasts. **Dust cells,** large cells in the lungs that are believed to be concerned with the removal of particulate matter and bacteria. **Enamel cell,** ameloblast. **End cell,** a cell incapable of further differentiation or division. **Endothelial cell,** a squamous cell lining a blood or lymph vessel, or the endocardium. **Enterochromaffin cell,** argentaffin cell. **Ependymal cells,** cells lining the central canal of the spinal cord and the cavities of the brain. **Epithelial cells,** cells constituting the epithelium of the skin, alimentary, respiratory and genito-urinary tracts. **Epithelioid cell,** a cell resembling an epithelial cell. **Fat cell,** a connective-tissue cell containing fat. **Follicular cells,** the cells that line the ovarian follicle. **Goblet cells,** modified columnar cells containing mucus, found in the nose and the alimentary tract. **Golgi cells,** nerve cells found in both the cerebrum and the cerebellum. **Granular cells,** small, round cells, with multiple dendrites, in the granular layer of the cerebellum. **Gustatory cells,** the cells of the taste buds. **Hair cells,** cells in the membranous labyrinth and the spiral organ from which project hair-like processes. **Hela cells,** the epithelial cells used in virology. **Hensen cells,** fat-containing cells in the spiral organ. **Hepatic cells,** the cells of the liver. **Interstitial cells,** large polyhedral cells lying in the connective tissue of the testes between the seminiferous tubules. **Juxta-glomerular cells,** cells around the distal convoluted tubules of the kidneys which are believed to contain renin. **Kuppfer cells,** potentially phagocytic endothelial cells lining the intralobular venous sinusoids of the liver. **Lamellar cells,** fibroblasts. **Lepra cell,** the main component of the lepromatous granuloma. **Liver cells,** the parenchymal cells of the liver. **Lutein cells,** the lutein-containing cells of the corpus luteum. **Marrow cells,** the immature red or white cells in the bone marrow. **Mast cell,** a type of connective tissue cell, surrounding blood vessels, which is believed to secrete heparin and histamine. **Mastoid air cells,** the intercommunicating cells of the mastoid antrum. **Microglial cells,** connective tissue cells of the central nervous system. **Myoepithelial cell,** a smooth muscle cell found in the lacrimal, mammary and sweat glands. **Nerve cell,** neurone. **Olfactory cells,** bipolar cells terminating in a hair-like process, lying in the olfactory mucous membrane; the receptors for smell. **Oligodendroglial cells,** oligoden-drocytes. **Oxyntic cells,** cells in the gastric mucosa that secrete hydrochloric acid. **Oxyphil cells,** eosinophilic cells in the parathyroid glands. **Paraluteal cells,** cells in the corpus luteum, derived from the cells of the tunica interna, and which produce oestradiol. **Parietal cells,** oxyntic cells. **Pigment cell,** a cell containing pigment granules. **Pineal cells,** the rounded cells of the pineal gland. **Plasma cell,** a connective tissue cell, concerned with the production of antibodies. **Prickle cell,** one of the cells of the stratum spinosum of the skin. **Purkinje cells,** the large multi-dendritic cells of the cerebellum. **Pyramidal cell,** the characteristic neurone of the cerebral cortex. **Red blood cell,** erythrocyte. **Reticular cell,** the characteristic stellate cell of reticular tissue. **Reticulo-endothelial cell,** a cell of the reticulo-endothelial system. **Satellite cell,** capsular cell. **Schwann cell,** the main constituent of the myelin sheath. **Sex cell,** spermatozoon or ovum. **Stem cell,** a cell from which other cells stem or originate. **Synovial cell,** the superficial cell of the synovial membrane. **Tactile cell,** an epithelial cell in the stratum spinosum of the epidermis. **Tendon cells,** the cells in white fibrous tissue. **Totipotent cell,** an undifferentiated embryonic cell capable of developing into any type of cell. **Wandering cells,** histiocytes. White blood cells, leucocytes. **Zymogenic cells,** the gastric cells that contain pepsinogen.

Cellacephate. B.P.C. 1968. Cellulose in which almost half of the hydroxyl groups are acetylated and about one-quarter are esterified with one of the two acid groups of phthalic acid. Used in the enteric coating of tablets and capsules.

Cellulitis. Inflammation in cellular tissue, especially subcutaneous tissue.

Cellulose. A polysaccharide that forms the basis of vegetable fibre. **Microcrystalline cellulose,** B.P.C. 1968, partially depolymerized cellulose. The non-dispersible type is used as a binder, filler, disintegrant and lubricant in tablets. The collidal type is used as a suspending agent for pharmaceutical preparations. **Oxidized cellulose,** B.P. 1968, a sterilized polyanhydroglucuronic acid, which is an absorbable haemostatic, used as such in surgery.

Cement. The substance, with a structure resembling that of bone, which forms a thin layer in teeth covering the dentine and extending from the neck to the apex of the root.

Censor. The term used in Freudian terminology to describe the mental influence, or psychic barrier, which prevents certain unnecessary wishes entering consciousness unless so disguised as to be unrecognizable.

Centi- (L *centum:* a hundred). Prefix signifying relationship to 100: usually one one-hundredth.

Centigrade. Having one hundred gradations, steps or degrees. The temperature scale, in which zero is freezing point and 100 degrees is boiling point.

Centigram. A measure of weight equal to one-hundredth part of a gramme. (*Abbreviation:* cg.)

Centimetre. A measure of length equal to one-hundredth part of a metre. (*Abbreviation:* cm.)

Centre. The mid-point of a body or surface. A collection of nerve cells. **Auditopsychic centre,** the area of the superior temporal gyrus in which auditory impressions receive their interpretation. **Auditosensory centre,** the area in the anterior transverse temporal gyrus, in which auditory impressions reach consciousness as sound. **Cardio-accelerator centre,** an

area, probably in the hypothalamic region, that controls the rate of the heart through the spinal accelerator centre. **Cardio-inhibitory centre,** an area in the dorsal nucleus of the vagus, responsible for controlling the rate of the heart. **Germinal centre,** the area in lymphoid tissue composed of lymphoblasts, the progenitors of small lymphocytes. **Motor centre,** the precentral gyrus and the adjoining part of the paracentral lobule, which control the volitional movements of the opposite side of the body. **Ossification centres,** the areas in bone, in which the process of ossification begins. **Parasympathetic centre,** the area in the hypothalamic region that controls the parasympathetic nervous system. **Respiratory centre,** the area in the medulla oblongata that controls respiration. **Sensory centre,** the lowest part of the postcentral gyrus and the adjoining part of the paracentral lobule, concerned with the conscious appreciation of sensation. **Sleep centre,** as yet ill-defined areas in the hypothalamus and thalamus concerned with the control of sleep. **Somesthetic centre,** the sensory centre. **Speech centre,** or motor speech centre, the area in the premotor cortex that controls the movements employed in speech. **Spinal cardio-accelerator centre,** cells in the lateral horns of the upper thoracic segments of the spinal cord that control the accelerator or augmentor nerves of the heart. **Sympathetic centre,** the area in the hypothalamic region that controls the sympathetic nervous system. **Visuopsychic centre,** the area in the occipital lobe concerned with the correlation of visual impressions. **Visuosensory centre,** the area in the occipital lobe that constitutes the cortical receiving centre for visual impressions.

Centri-, Centro- (L *centrum,* Gk *kentron:* centre). Prefixes meaning centre or central.

Centrifugal. Fleeing the centre.

Centrifuge. An apparatus for separating the constituents of a solution by spinning at high speeds.

Centriole. One of the granules within the centrosome.

Centripetal. Seeking, or moving to, the centre.

Centromere. The spindle attachment of the chromosome.

Centrosome. One of the inclusions in the protoplasm of the cell, that divides in the initial stage of mitosis, each part then migrating to the opposite poles of the achromatic spindle.

Centrosphere. The small area of clear cytoplasm, lying near the nucleus of the cell which contains the centrioles and with them constitutes the centrosome.

Centrum. An anatomical centre. **Centrum of vertebra,** the vertebral ossification centre.

Cephal-, Cephalo- (Gk *kephate:* head). Prefixes indicating the head.

Cephalad. Towards, or in the direction of, the head.

Cephalalgia. Headache.

Cephalexin. The B.P. Commission approved name for 7-(D-α-aminophenylacetamido)-3-methyl-3-cephem-4-carboxylic acid. An antibiotic.

Cephalhaematoma. A swelling produced by an effusion of blood below the pericranium. Caput succedanum.

Cephalic. Relating to the head.

Cephalin. A phospholipid, widely distributed throughout the body, especially in the brain and spinal cord. It has a haemostatic action.

Cephalocele. A swelling produced by extrusion of the cranial contents.

Cephaloglycin. The B.P. Commission approved name for 7-[D(−)-α-aminophenylacetamido] cephalosporanic acid. An antibiotic.

Cephaloram. The B.P. Commission approved name for 7-phenylacetamidocephaloranic acid. An antibiotic.

Cephaloridine. B.P. 1968. $C_{19}H_{17}N_3O_4S_2$. An antibiotic which is active against a range of gram-negative and gram-positive organisms, including pencillinase-producing staphylococci.

Cephalosporin C. The B.P. Commission approved name for 7-(5-amino-5-carboxyvaleramido) cephalosporanic acid. An antibiotic.

Cephalothin sodium. B.P.C. Supplement 1971. $C_{16}H_{15}N_2NaO_6S_2$. An antibiotic with an action and uses similiar to cephaloridine.

Cera. Wax.

Cerate. A medicinal preparation for external use, made with a wax basis.

Cercaria. The free-swimming larval stage of a trematode.

Cereal. An edible grain: e.g. barley, maize, millet, oats, rice, wheat.

Cerebellar. Pertaining to the cerebellum.

Cerebellum. The largest part of the hindbrain, lying behind the pons and medulla oblongata, and with an average weight of around 150 grammes

in the male. It is concerned primarily with the coordination of movement.

Cerebr-, Cerebro- (L *cerebrum:* brain). Prefixes signifying association with the brain.

Cerebral. Pertaining to the cerebrum.

Cerebration. Mental activity.

Cerebroside. A glycolipid found in the brain, adrenal gland, kidney, spleen, liver, leucocytes, thymus, lung, retina, and egg yolk.

Cerebrospinal. Pertaining to the brain and spinal cord. **Cerebrospinal fever,** meningococcal meningitis. **Cerebrospinal fluid,** the fluid that fills the ventricles of the brain and the subarachnoid spaces of the cerebrospinal axis.

Cerebrovascular. Pertaining to the arteries and veins of the brain.

Cerebrum. The largest part of the brain, consisting of the two cerebral hemipheres.

Cerium. A metallic element. Symbol Ce. Atomic weight 140·12. Atomic number 58.

Cerumen. Ear wax. The secretion of the sebaceous and ceruminous glands of the external auditory meatus.

Cervic-, Cervico- (L *cervix:* neck). Prefixes signifying relationship to the neck, whether of the body or an organ.

Cervical. Pertaining to the neck or the cervix of an organ.

Cervicitis. Inflammation of the cervix uteri.

Cervix. Neck, or constricted portion. **Cervix uteri,** neck of the uterus.

Cestode. A tapeworm.

Cetalkonium chloride. The B.P. Commission approved name for benzylhexadecylimethylammonium chloride. An anti-infective agent.

Cetomacrogol 1000. B.P.C. 1968. A non-ionic emulsifying agent.

Cetostearyl alcohol. B.P. 1968. A mixture of solid aliphatic alcohols, used to produce stable oil-in-water emulsions.

Cetoxime. The B.P. Commission approved name for *N*-benzylanilino-acetamidoxime. An antihistamine agent.

Cetrimide. B.P. 1968. A quaternary ammonium compound, which is a relatively non-toxic antiseptic with detergent properties. It is active against gram-positive organisms, less effective against gram-negative organisms, and ineffective against acid-fast bacilli.

Cetrimonium chloride. The B.P. Commission approved name for hexadecyltrimethylammonium chloride. An antiseptic detergent.

Cetylpyridinium chloride. B.P. 1968. $C_{21}H_{38}ClN,H_2O$. An antiseptic with an action similar to that of cetrimide.

Chafe. To irritate.

Chalazion. A chronic inflammatory granuloma of a meibomian gland. (*Plural*: chalazia.)

Chalicosis. A form of pneumoconiosis among stone-cutters, and due to the inhalation of fine particles of stone.

Chalk. B.P. 1968. Native calcium carbonate freed from most of its impurities. An absorbent and antacid used in mixtures and powders for the treatment of diarrhoea.

Chalone. An internal secretion with an inhibitory action.

Chalybeate. An iron-containing agent.

Chamber. An enclosed space. **Anterior chamber of the eye,** the space bounded in front by the posterior surface of the cornea, and behind by the front of the iris. **Decompression chamber,** the airtight chamber used for the decompression of patients with compressed air illness, for the routine decompression of divers, and also experimentally to investigate the effect of high and low pressures on man and animals. **Posterior chamber of the eye,** the narrow chink behind the iris and in front of the lens and its suspensory ligament.

Chancre. The primary lesion of syphilis.

Chancroid. Soft sore or chancre, induced by infection with *Haemophilus ducreyi*.

Chap. A crack or slit in the skin.

Chapped. The term applied to hands, the skin of which is cracked and fissured, usually due to exposure to damp and cold.

Charcoal. B.P.C. 1968. A fine black powder prepared from vegetable matter such as sawdust, peat, cellulose residues and coconut shells. An absorbent used in the treatment of poisoning by alkaloid drugs, and also occasionally in the treatment of intestinal flatulence.

Charcot-Leyden crystals. Sharp crystals of spermin phosphate found in the sputum in asthma.

Cheek. The side of the face.

Cheese. A rich source of nutrition derived from milk, and of which there are some 400 varieties.

Cheil-, Cheilo- (Gk *cheilos:* lip). Prefixes indicating relationship to the lips.

Cheilitis. Inflammation of the lips.

Cheilosis. The eczematous state of the lips, most marked at the corners of the mouth, induced by riboflavine deficiency.

Cheir-, Cheiro- (Gk *cheir*: hand). Prefixes meaning hand. *See also* Chir-.

Cheiropompholyx. An acute vesicular eruption of the hands and feet.

Chelation. The chemical reaction in which a complex organic molecule combines with a metal ion to form a soluble ring structure, which may bind the metal so firmly that for all practical purposes it is unionized and therefore unable to react chemically. The principle is being widely used in the treatment of metallic poisons by means of chelating agents such as sodium calciumedetate B.P.

Cheloid. Keloid.

Chemo- (Gk *chēmeia:* chemistry). Prefix signifying relationship to chemistry or a chemical.

Chemosis. Oedema of the conjunctiva.

Chemotaxis. The attraction or repulsion of living cells by chemical stimulation.

Chemotherapy. Treatment of disease by chemical agents.

Cherry bark, wild. B.P.C. 1968. The dried bark of the wild or black cherry, *Prunus serotina*, which is predominantly used as a flavouring agent. **Wild cherry syrup,** B.P.C. 1968, a preparation used for the relief of cough.

Chest. The thorax.

Chiasma. A decussation or cross-over. In meiosis the point at which two chromatids, one from each chromosome, break and join diagonally. (*Plural:* chiasmata.) **Optic chiasma,** the point of cross-over of the fibres of the optic nerves.

Chickenpox. Varicella. An acute communicable disease, with a characteristic rash, caused by the varicella-zoster virus.

Chilblain. Erythema pernio. A dusky red, circumscribed, intensely itchy swelling of the skin, usually on the fingers or toes, which occurs in susceptible individuals in cold damp weather.

Child. A human being from birth to puberty.

Childbed. The puerperium.

Childbirth. Parturition.

Chill. A sensation of cold. Feeling shivery.

Chimera. An animal whose cells are derived from two or more genetically different zygotes.

Chin. The mental protuberance of the mandible.

Chir-, Chiro- (Gk *cheir:* hand). Prefixes meaning hand.

Chiropodist. One who deals with minor diseases of the hands and feet.

Chiropody. The care of the hands and feet. The profession of a chiropodist.

Chiropractic. A system of therapeutics based on the adjustment of supposed minor displacements of the spinal cord in order to relieve presumed pressure on the nerves issuing at the intervertebral foramina.

Chiropractor. One who practises chiropractic.

Chloasma. The pigmentation of the skin which appears on the face, usually in women during pregnancy, and at the menopause.

Chlophedianol. The B.P. Commission approved name for 2-chloro-α-(2-dimethylaminoethyl)benzhydrol. A cough suppressant.

Chlor-, Chloro- (Gk *chloros:* green). Prefixes meaning green, or related to chlorine.

Chloral betaine. The B.P. Commission approved name for chloral hydrate-betaine adduct. A hypnotic.

Chloral hydrate. B.P. 1968. $C_2H_3Cl_3O_2$. A hypnotic which, when given by mouth, acts within half-an-hour, the effect lasting for around eight hours.

Chlorambucil. B.P. 1968. $C_{14}H_{19}Cl_2NO_2$. A cytotoxic agent.

Chloramine. B.P.C. 1968. C_7H_7 ClNNaO$_2$S,3H$_2$O. A bactericide.

Chloramphenicol. B.P. 1968. An antibiotic derived from *Streptomyces venezeulae*, or prepared synthetically, which has a wide range of antimicrobial activity, including *Salmonella typhi* and *S. paratyphi*. Its most serious side-effect is agranulocytosis. **Chloramphenicol cinnamate,** B.P.C. 1968, the 3-cinnamic ester of chloramphenicol, which has the same action as chloramphenicol but is tasteless. **Chloramphenicol palmitate,** B.P.C. 1968, the 3-palmitic ester of chloramphenicol which is almost tasteless. **Chloramphenicol sodium succinate,** B.P.C., 1968, the sodium salt of the 3-monosuccinic ester of chloramphenicol, suitable for intramuscular or intravenous injection.

Chlorbetamide. The B.P. Commission approved name for dichloro-*N*-(2,4-dichlorobenzyl) - *N*-(2 - hydroxyethyl)-acetamide. An amoebicide.

Chlorbutol. B.P. 1968. $C_4H_7Cl_3O$, ½H$_2$O. A mild sedative and local analgesic.

Chlorcyclizine hydrochloride. B.P. 1968. $C_{18}H_{22}Cl_2N_2$. An antihistamine with a prolonged action.

Chlordane. A chlorinated hydrocarbon insecticide.

Chlordantoin. The B.P. Commission approved name for 5-(1-ethylpentyl)-3-(trichloromethylthio) hydantoin. An antifungal agent.

Chlordiazepoxide hydrochloride. B.P. 1968. $C_{16}H_{15}Cl_2N_3O$. A tranquillizer which relieves nervous tension and anxiety states, and has a slight muscle-relaxant action.

Chlorhexadol. The B.P. Commission approved name for 2-methyl-4-(2,2,2-trichloro-1-hydroxyethoxy)-pentan-2-ol. A hypnotic.

Chlorhexidine acetate. B.P.C. 1968. $C_{26}H_{38}Cl_2N_{10}O_4$. A bactericide used as an antibacterial agent in eye-drops. **Chlorhexidine gluconate solution,** B.P. 1968, a 19 to 21 per cent w/v aqueous solution of $C_{34}H_{54}Cl_2N_{10}O_{14}$, which is a relatively non-toxic antiseptic active against gram-positive and gram-negative organisms. **Chlorhexidine hydrochloride,** B.P. 1968, $C_{22}H_{32}Cl_4N_{10}$, an antiseptic that has a more prolonged action than the gluconate and is therefore used in dusting-powders, creams and ointments.

Chloride. A salt of hydrochloric acid. A compound of chlorine with another element.

Chlorinated lime. B.P. 1968. A powerful, rapidly acting bactericide and deodorant.

Chlorine. A greenish pungent gas with an intense irritating action on mucous membranes. An element of the halogen family. Symbol Cl. Atomic weight 35·45. Atomic number 17.

Chlorisondamine chloride. The B.P. Commission approved name for 4,5,6,7-tetrachloro-2-(2-dimethylaminoethyl)-isoindoline dimethochloride. A hypotensive agent.

Chlormadinone acetate. B.P. Addendum 1969. $C_{23}H_{29}ClO_4$. A progestational steroid.

Chlormerodrin. The B.P. Commission approved name for 3-chloromercuri-2-methoxypropylurea. A diuretic. **Chlormerodrin (197Hg) injection,** B.P.C. Supplement 1971, a radioactive preparation used to locate cerebral tumours and in renal investigation.

Chlormethiazole. The B.P. Commission approved name for 5-(2-chloroethyl)-4-methylthiazole. A hypnotic.

Chlormezanone. The B.P. Commission approved name for a tranquillizer.

Chlormidazole. The B.P. Commission approved name for 1-(4-chlorobenzyl)-2-methylbenzimidazole. An antifungal agent.

Chlorocresol. B.P. 1968. C_7H_7ClO. A powerful bactericide of low toxicity.

Chloroform. B.P. 1968. $CHCl_3$. A volatile anaesthetic, which is also administered orally as a carminative, and used externally as a rubefacient.

Chloroma. A rare, greenish, nodular growth, with a predilection for the periosteum. With few exceptions the patients, often children or adolescents, have a leukaemic blood picture.

Chlorophyll. The green colouring matter of plants which has achieved a reputation as a deodorant.

Chloropsia. Green vision.

Chloropyrilene. The B.P. Commission approved name for an antihistamine agent.

Chloroquine phosphate. B.P. 1968. $C_{18}H_{32}ClN_3O_8P_2$. A potent antimalarial that is also used in the treatment of intestinal amoebiasis, systemic lupus erythematosus, and rheumatoid arthritis. **Chloroquine sulphate,** B.P. 1968, a drug with the same indications as the phosphate.

Chlorosis. A form of iron-deficiency anaemia, characterized by a greenish tint of the skin, once common in young women.

Chlorothiazide. B.P. 1968. $C_7H_6Cl N_3O_4S_2$. A non-mercurial diuretic.

Chlorotrianisene. B.P. 1968. $C_{23}H_{21}Cl O_3$. A synthetic oestrogen.

Chloroxylenol. B.P.C. 1968. C_8H_9ClO. A relatively non-toxic, non-irritant antiseptic.

Chlorphenesin. B.P. 1968. $C_9H_{11}ClO_3$. A preparation with antibacterial, antifungal and trichomonicidal properties, used in the prophylaxis and treatment of fungous infections of the skin.

Chlorpheniramine maleate. B.P. 1968. $C_{20}H_{23}ClN_2O_4$. An antihistamine drug.

Chlorphenoctium amsonate. The B.P. Commission approved name for 2,4-dichlorophenoxymethyldimethyloctyl-ammonium 4,4'-diaminostilbene-2,2'-disulphonate. An antifungal agent.

Chlorphenoxamine. The B.P. Commission approved name for N-2-(4-chloro-α-methylbenzyhydryloxy)ethyl-dimethylamine. A drug for the treatment of parkinsonism.

Chlorphentermine. The B.P. Commission approved name for 4-chloro-αα-dimethylphenethylamine. An appetite suppressant.

Chlorproguanil hydrochloride. B.P. 1968. $C_{11}H_{16}Cl_3N_5$. An antimalarial drug.

Chlorpromazine hydrochloride. B.P. 1968. $C_{17}H_{20}Cl_2N_2S$. A central nervous depressant, which inhibits autonomic activity, and is widely used in psychiatry.

Chlorpropamide. B.P. 1968. $C_{10}H_{13}Cl N_2O_3S$. A hypoglycaemic agent.

Chlorprothixene. The B.P. Commission approved name for trans-2-chloro-9-(3 - dimethylaminopropylidene) - thia-xanthen (α-form). A tranquillizer and anti-emetic.

Chlorquinaldol. The B.P. Commission approved name for 5,7-dichloro-8-hydroxy-2-methylquinoline. An antiseptic and fungicide.

Chlortetracycline hydrochloride. B.P. 1968. An antibiotic obtained from *Streptomyces aureofaciens*, which has the same range of action as tetracycline.

Chlorthalidone. B.P. 1968. $C_{14}H_{11}Cl N_2O_4S$. A non-mercurial diuretic.

Chlorthenoxazin. The B.P. Commission approved name for 2-(2-chloroethyl)-2,3-dihydro-4-oxobenz-1,3-oxazine. An analgesic and anti-inflammatory agent.

Chlorzoxazone. The B.P. Commission approved name for a muscle relaxant.

Choana. A funnel-like opening. One of the posterior nasal apertures. (*Plural:* choanae.)

Chocolate. A solid substance composed of ground cocoa-nibs to which cocoa butter, cane-sugar and vanilla (for flavouring) have been added.

Choke. Suffocate. Asphyxiate.

Choke-damp. The name given to the irrespirable gas, composed mainly of carbon dioxide, that may accumulate in coal mines or wells.

Chol-, Chole-, Cholo- (Gk *Cholē:* bile). Prefixes signifying association with bile.

Cholaemia. An excess of bile or bile constituents in the blood.

Cholagogue. A substance that stimulates the flow of bile into the intestine.

Cholangiogram. An X-ray picture of the gall-bladder.

Cholangiolitis. Inflammation of the intrahepatic bile ducts.

Cholangioma. Carcinoma of the bile ducts.

Cholangitis. Inflammation of the bile ducts.

Cholecalciferol. The B.P. Commission approved name for 9,10-secocholesta-5,7,10(19)-trien-3β-ol. Also known as vitamin D$_3$.

Cholecystectomy. Operation for removal of the gall-bladder.

Cholecystitis. Inflammation of the gall-bladder.

Cholecystogram. An X-ray picture of the gall-bladder.

Cholecystography. X-ray examination of the gall-bladder.

Cholecystostomy. Surgical drainage of the gall-bladder.

Choledochotomy. Surgical incision into the bile duct.

Choledochus. The bile duct.

Choledolithiasis. Presence of a gall-stone in the common bile duct.

Cholelithiasis. The presence of gall-stones in the gall-bladder or bile duct.

Cholelithotomy. The operation for the removal of gall-stones through an opening into the gall-bladder or bile duct.

Cholera. A serious acute intestinal disease, characterized by the sudden onset of severe diarrhoea, and due to the *Vibrio cholerae*. Endemic in the Indian sub-continent. **Cholera vaccine,** B.P. 1968, a sterile suspension of suitable strains of *Vibrio cholerae*, containing not less than 8000 million bacteria per millilitre. The immunity conferred is short lived. **Mixed cholera vaccine,** B.P. Addendum 1969, a mixture of cholera vaccine and eltor vaccine, containing not less than 4000 million bacteria (*V. cholerae*) and not less than 4000 million bacteria (*V. cholerae* biotype *el tor*) in 1ml.

Choleresis. Secretion of bile by the liver.

Choleretic. A drug that stimulates the secretion of bile.

Cholestasis. Suppression or arrest of the flow of bile.

Cholesteatoma. A rare tumour of developmental origin, occurring under the pia mater or elsewhere in the brain. A tumour of the middle ear, of debatable origin.

Cholesteatosis. Fatty degeneration due to cholesterol esters.

Cholesterol. C$_{27}$H$_{45}$OH. A steroid alcohol, normally present in the blood to the extent of 150 to 250mg. per 100ml., which is essential for the metabolism of many body processes, including the repair of cell membranes and the production of hormones.

Cholesterosis. The condition characterized by deposition of cholesterol in the wall of the gall-bladder, sometimes known as strawberry gall-bladder.

Cholestyramine. The B.P. Commission approved name for a styryl-divinylbenzene copolymer (about 2 per cent divinylbenzene) containing quaternary ammonium groups. It binds bile acids in the intestine and so prevents reabsorption of bile salts. It is therefore used in conditions characterized by retention of these products, and has been shown to relieve the associated pruritus.

Cholic acid. One of the steroid acids in bile.

Choline. One of the constituents of the vitamin B complex, which acts as a lipotropic agent and is necessary for normal growth. **Choline theophyllinate,** B.P. 1968, C$_{12}$H$_{21}$N$_5$O$_3$, a bronchodilator.

Cholinergic. Stimulated or activated by acetylcholine.

Choline salicylate. An analgesic and antipyretic.

Cholinesterase. The enzyme that inactivates acetylcholine by hydrolysis.

Choluria. The presence of bile in the urine.

Chondr-, Chondro- (Gk *chondros:* cartilage). Prefixes indicating relationship to cartilage.

Chondrectomy. Excision of a cartilage.

Chondrin. The chief constituent of cartilage matrix.

Chondritis. Inflammation of cartilage.

Chondroblast. A cell of growing cartilage tissue.

Chondroblastoma. A rare, benign tumour of the epiphysis of adolescents.

Chondrocalcinosis. A form of crystal synovitis with gout-like manifestations, due to the deposition of crystals of calcium pyrophosphate dehydrate. Pseudogout.

Chondroclast. A giant cell that absorbs cartilage.

Chondrocranium. The cartilaginous structure that is the forerunner of ossification in the development of the skull.

Chondrocyte. A mature cartilage cell.

Chondrodysplasia. Dyschondroplasia.

Chondodystrophia. Chondrodystrophy. **Chondrodystrophia foetalis,** achondroplasia.

Chondrodystrophy. A congenital defect in the formation of bone from cartilage. Chondrodystrophia.

Chondroectodermal dysplasia. A syndrome consisting of dyschondroplasia, polydactyly of the hands, congenital malformation of the heart, and ectodermal dysplasia involving the nails and teeth, and occurring as an autosomal Mendelian recessive.

Chondroitin sulphate. The chief mucopolysaccharide of cartilage, bone, heart valves, tendon and the cornea.

Chondroma. A benign tumour derived from cartilage.

Chondromalacia. The condition characterized by softening of the cartilage.

Chondro-osteodystrophy. A congenital malformation characterized by irregularity and fragmentation of the epiphyses and metaphyses of the long bones, resulting in dwarfism with deformities of the sternum, vertebrae and joints, but not the skull.

Chondrosarcoma. A highly malignant, though relatively rare, tumour derived from cartilage cells, usually at the end of long bones and in the pelvis.

Chord-, Chordo- (Gk *chordē:* cord). Prefixes signifying relationship to a cord.

Chorda. A cord-like structure. (*Plural:* chordae.) **Chorda tympani nerve,** the branch of the facial nerve that subserves taste sensation in the anterior two-thirds of the tongue, and carries secretomotor fibres to the submandibular and sublingual glands. **Chordae tendineae,** the delicate tendinous cords whereby the cusps of the mitral and tricuspid valves are attached to the papillary muscles and ventricular walls of the heart.

Chordee. A painful erection of the penis, with lateral and downward curvature.

Chorditis. Inflammation of a vocal cord.

Chordoma. A rare, slow-growing, malignant tumour derived from vestiges of the notochord, most commonly in the spheno-occipital area of the skull and the sacro-coccygeal area.

Chordotomy. Surgical division of the antero-lateral tracts of the spinal cord, for the relief of intractable pain.

Chorea. A manifestation of acute rheumatism, characterized by irregular, involuntary movements of the limbs and face. **Chorea gravidarum,** chorea occurring during pregnancy. **Huntington's chorea,** a hereditary disorder characterized by choreiform movements and progressive dementia.

Choreiform. Chorea-like.

Choreoathetosis. Abnormal movements of the body combining the features of chorea and athetosis.

Chorion. The outermost of the two foetal membranes.

Chorionepithelioma. A highly malignant tumour arising from chorionic tissue remaining in the uterus after abortion or labour, [or after incomplete evacuation or expulsion of a hydatidiform mole.

Chorionic gonadotrophin. B.P. 1968. A dry sterile preparation of the gonad-stimulating substance obtained from the urine of pregnant women.

Choroid. The thin, highly vascular membrane lining the posterior five-sixths of the eyeball. **Choroid plexus,** a highly vascular fringe of pia mater projecting into the third ventricle of the brain.

Choroiditis. Inflammation of the choroid.

Christmas disease. A disease inherited as a sex-linked recessive trait, due to deficiency of factor IX, and with the same symptoms as haemophilia.

Chrom-, Chromato-, Chromo- (Gk *chromā:* colour). Prefixes meaning colour.

Chromaffin. The term applied to certain cells with granules that stain yellowish-brown with chromic acid salts. These cells, which secrete adrenaline and noradrenaline, constitute the chromaffin system and are found in the medulla of the suprarenal glands, the paraganglia, the para-aortic nodes and elsewhere among the sympathetic plexuses.

-chromasia] (Gk *chromā:* colour). Suffix meaning condition of staining or pigmentation.

Chromatic. Pertaining to colours.

Chromatid. A daughter chromosome. One of the halves into which the chromosome divides in the prophase of mitosis.

Chromatin. The basophilic material in the nucleus, consisting of nucleoprotein.

Chromatography. The method of analysis whereby mixtures of substances are separated from each other by passage through a column of supporting medium, which may be the cellulose fibres of filter paper as in **paper chromatography,** or a stream of inert carrier gas as in **gas chromatography.**

Chromatolysis. The disappearance of the granules from a nerve cell that has been damaged or exhausted.

Chromatophore. A pigment cell in the

corium of the skin, the iris and the choroid.

Chromatopsia. Coloured vision. The condition in which all objects appear abnormally coloured.

Chromatosis. Pigmentation.

Chromidrosis. The secretion of coloured sweat.

Chromium. A metallic element. Symbol Cr. Atomic weight 51·99. Atomic number 24.

Chromium trioxide. B.P.C. 1968. CrO_3. A powerful oxidizing agent and caustic.

Chromoblastomycosis. A chronic verrucous and granulomatous infection of the skin, caused by the fungi *Hormodendrum pedrosoi*, *H. compactum* and *Phialophora verrucosa*.

Chromosome. One of the rod-shaped bodies in the nucleus of a cell that carry the genes or factors of inheritance.

Chron-, Chrono- (Gk *chronos:* time). Prefixes signifying relationship to time.

Chronaxie. A measurement of the excitability of nervous or muscular tissue.

Chrys-, Chryso- (Gk *chrysos:* gold). Prefixes meaning gold.

Chrysops. A genus of the family Tabanidae, certain African species of which transmit loiasis and an American species of which transmits tularaemia.

Chrysotherapy. Treatment of disease with gold salts.

Chyl-, Chylo- (Gk *chylos:* juice). Prefixes signifying association with chyle.

Chyle. The turbid white lymph, consisting of lymph and finely emulsified fat, in the lacteals, or lymphatic vessels draining the small intestine.

Chylomicron. One of the particles of emulsified fat, about 1 micron in diameter, found in the blood after a fatty meal and in chyle.

Chylothorax. The presence of chyle in the pleural cavity.

Chyluria. The presence of chyle in the urine.

Chyme. The partly digested food as it issues from the stomach into the intestine.

Chymotrypsin. One of the proteolytic enzymes of pancreatic juice. Its main action is on casein. It is also used in ophthalmology for the dissection of the zonule of the lens.

Chymotrypsinogen. The precursor of chymotrypsin.

Cicatrix. A scar.

Cider. An alcoholic beverage made from apples. The alcoholic content ranges from 3·7 to 10·56G./100ml.

Cilia. The plural of cilium.

Ciliary. Pertaining to cilia. **Ciliary body,** the ciliary ring, the ciliary processes and the ciliaris. **Ciliary processes,** inward foldings of the choroid that form a frill behind the iris. **Ciliary ring,** a zone, 4mm. in width, directly continuous with the anterior part of the choroid.

Cilium. One of the hair-like processes found in certain epithelial cells, such as those of the bronchi, and certain micro-organisms. An eyelash. (*Plural:* cilia.)

Cimex lectularius. The bed bug.

Cinchocaine. B.P.C. 1968. $C_{20}H_{29}N_3O_2$. A local anaesthetic. Because of its solubility in oils it is used in the preparation of ointments and oily solutions. **Cinchocaine hydrochloride,** B.P. 1968, $C_{20}H_{30}N_3O_2Cl$. A local anaesthetic.

Cinchonism. Poisoning by cinchona, quinidine or quinine.

Cineangiocardiography. A cine record of the sequence of events following the opacification of the chambers of the heart and of the heart vessels by means of a radio-opaque substance.

Cinefluorography. The cine recording of a series of successive images appearing on a fluoroscopic screen. Cineradiography.

Cineradiography. Cinefluorography.

Cingulectomy. The operation for the removal of the cingulate gyrus, used for the relief of certain psychotic disturbances.

Cingulum. A girdle or zone. A long curved bundle of association fibres, stretching from the medial surface of each central hemisphere to the temporal lobe. A v-shaped prominence on the lingual surface of the crown of the upper incisors. (*Plural:* cingula.)

Cinnamon. B.P. 1968. The dried inner bark of the shoots of coppiced trees of *Cinnamomum zeylanicum*. A carminative.

Cinnamon oil. B.P.C. 1968. An oil obtained by distillation from cinnamon. A carminative. Used largely as a flavouring agent and preservative.

Cinnarizine. The B.P. Commission approved name for 1-benzhydryl-4-cinnamylpiperazine. An antihistamine.

Circadian. Relating to biological rhythms with a circle of around 24 hours.

Circinate. Ring-shaped. Circular.

Circulation. Movement in a regular or circular course. **Collateral circulation,** the compensatory circulation that develops when a main blood vessel is blocked. **Coronary circulation,** the circulation of the blood through the coronary vessels of the heart. **Cross circulation,** perfusion of blood from one experimental animal to another. **Extracorporeal circulation,** the circulation of blood outside the body, as through a heart-lung machine. **Portal circulation.** the circulation of blood from the spleen, pancreas, stomach and intestines through the portal vein, liver and hepatic veins to the inferior vena cava. **Pulmonary circulation,** the circulation of blood from the right ventricle through the lungs to the left heart. **Systemic circulation,** the circulation of blood from the left ventricle through the body to the right side of the heart.

Ciculus. A circle. (*Plural:* circuli.) **Circulus arteriosus,** the anastomotic circle at the base of the brain formed by the two anterior cerebral arteries, the anterior communicating artery, the two internal carotid arteries, the two posterior communicating arteries and the two posterior cerebral arteries. **Circulus arteriosus iridis, major and minor,** anastomosing circles of the ciliary arteries. **Circulus vasculosus articuli,** the fringe of looped anastomoses of blood vessels around the articular margin of joints. **Circulous venosus mammae,** an anastomotic circle round the base of the nipple of the breast.

Circum- (L *circum:* around). Prefix meaning around.

Circumcision. Removal of the prepuce in the male, or the labia minora in the female.

Circumduction. Circular movement, active or passive, as of a limb.

Circumflex. Winding around.

Circumoral. Around the mouth.

Cirrhosis. Diffuse fibrosis or sclerosis of an organ. The most common form is cirrhosis of the liver, a chronic inflammatory (degenerative) lesion of mixed etiology and a multiplicity of varieties.

Cirsoid. Varicose.

Cis- (L *cis:* on this side). Prefix meaning on the same side, or following.

Cisterna. A reservoir or cistern. (*Plural:* cisternae.) **Cisterna chyli,** a sac-like dilatation, 5 to 7cm long, at the beginning of the thoracic duct to the right of the aorta in front of the 1st and 2nd lumbar vertebrae. **Subarachnoid cisternae:** *Cerebellomedullary cistern* (*cisterna magna*) in the interval between the medulla oblongata and the undersurface of the cerebellum, and continuous below with the subarachnoid space of the spinal cord. *Pontine cistern* an extensive space on the ventral surface of the pons. *Interpeduncular cistern,* the space that contains the circulus arteriosus. *Cistern of the lateral fossa,* the space that contains the middle cerebral artery *Cistern of the great cerebral vein,* between the splenium and the cerebellum.

Cistron. Gene.

Citric acid. B.P. 1968. $C_6H_8O_7,H_2O$. Used in the preparation of effervescent granules and draughts.

Citronella oil. B.P.C. 1968. Obtained by distillation from *Cymbopogon nardus* or *C. winterianus,* and used as a constituent of insect repellents, and as a perfume for soaps and brilliantine.

Citrovorum factor. Folinic acid.

Citrullinaemia. An inborn error of metabolism characterized by an inability to form uric acid from citrulin, resulting in convulsions, hepatomegaly and hypothyroidism.

Citrulline. An amino-acid formed from ornithine in the course of urea formation.

Clamidoxic acid. The B.P. Commission approved name for 2-(3,4-dichlorobenzamido)phenoxyacetic acid. An anti-rheumatic agent.

Clamp. A surgical instrument for compression.

Clasmatocyte. Histiocyte or tissue macrophage.

Claudication. Limping or lameness. **Intermittent claudication,** a condition characterized by the onset of pain in the lower limbs on walking, the result of narrowing of the arteries to the affected area with resultant ischaemia.

Claustrophobia. Abnormal dread of enclosed spaces.

Claustrum. A thin sheet of grey matter separated from the lenticular nucleus by the external capsule.

Clavicle. The collar-bone. The f-shaped bone that articulates laterally with the medial side of the acromion, and medially with the manubrium sterni.

Clavus. A corn or callous growth. A severe pain in the head described as being like that produced by driving a nail into the head.

Claw-foot. Pes cavus.

Claw-hand. A deformity of the hand, characterized by flexion and atrophy, usually due to lesions of the ulnar nerve.

Clefamide. B.P.C. 1968. $C_{17}H_{16}Cl_2N_2O_5$. An amoebicide.

Cleft. A fissure, notch, or gap. **Branchial cleft,** one of the ectodermal furrows that separate the visceral arches in the embryo. **Hypomandibular cleft,** the first visceral cleft. **Intratonsillar cleft,** a cleft in the upper part of the tonsil. **Pudendal cleft,** the cleft between the labia majora. **Visceral cleft,** branchial cleft. **Cleft palate,** a common congenital abnormality (*see* Palate).

Cleid-, Cleido- (Gk *kleis:* that which serves for closing). Prefixes indicating relationship to the clavicle.

Cleidocranial dysotosis. Craniocleidodysostosis.

Clemizole. The B.P. Commission approved name for 1-(4-chlorobenzyl)-2-pyrrolidin-1- yl-methylbenzimidazole. An antipruritic.

Clemizole pencillin. The B.P. Commission approved name for benzylpenicillin combined with clemizole. An antibiotic.

Cletoquine. The B.P. Commission approved name for 7-chloro-4-[4-(2-hydroxyethylamino)-1-methylbutyl] aminoquinoline. An anti-inflammatory agent.

Clidinium bromide. The B.P. Commission approved name for 3-benziloyloxy-1-methylquinuclidinium bromide. An anticholinergic agent.

Climacteric. The menopause.

Clindamycin. The B.P. Commission approved name for 7-chlorolincomycin, a semi-synthetic derivative of lincomycin. An antibacterial preparation active orally against a wide range of gram-positive micro-organisms.

Clinodactyly. Permanent deflexion of one or more fingers.

Clioquinol. B.P. 1968. C_9H_5ClINO. An antiseptic and amoebicide.

Clitoris. The erectile structure, partially hidden between the anterior ends of the labia minora, which is homologous with the penis.

Clivus. A sloping surface. **Clivus of the occipital bone,** a broad shallow groove that slopes upward from the foramen magnum. **Clivus of the sphenoid bone,** the sloping area behind the dorsum sellae and continuous with the clivus of the occipital bone.

Cloaca. The common urogenital and rectal chamber in the early embryo.

Clofazimine. The B.P. Commission approved name for 3-(4-chloroanilino)--10-(4-chlorophenyl)-2,10-dihydro-2-2-isopropylaminophenazine. A drug used in the treatment of leprosy.

Clofibrate. B.P. Addendum 1969. $C_{12}H_{15}ClO_3$. A drug used in the treatment of hypercholesterolaemia.

Clofluperol. The B.P. Commission approved name for 4-(4-chloro-3-trifluoromethylphenyl) - 1 - [3 - (4 - fluoro - benzoyl)propyl]piperidin-4-ol. A neuroleptic.

Clomiphene. The B.P. Commission approved name for 1-chloro-2-[4 -(2 - diethylaminoethoxy)phenyl] - 1,2 - diphenylethylene. A drug which releases endogenous pituitary gonadotrophin, and is used to induce ovulation in amenorrhoeic, infertile women.

Clomipramine. The B.P. Commission approved name for 3-chloro-5-(3-dimethylaminopropyl)-10,11-dihydrodibenz[*b,f*]azepine. An antidepressant.

Clomocycline. The B.P. Commission approved name for N^2-(hydroxymethyl) chlorotetracycline. A broadspectrum antibiotic of the tetracycline group.

Clone. The asexual progeny of a single cell.

Clonic. Relating to clonus.

Clonitazene. The B.P. Commission approved name for 2-(4-chlorobenzyl)-1-(2 -diethylaminoethyl)-5-nitrobenzimidazole. A narcotic and analgesic.

Clonorchiasis. A disease due to infestation with the liver fluke *Clonorchis sinensis*, which occurs widely in the Far East.

Clonus. The rhythmical series of contractions in response to the enhancement of tension in a muscle, such as occurs when the tendon reflexes are exaggerated after a corticospinal lesion. The two most common examples are ankle and patellar clonus.

Clopamide. The B.P. Commission approved name for 4-chloro-N-(2,6-dimethylpiperidino) - 3 - sulphamoyl - benzamide. A diuretic.

Clopenthixol. The B.P. Commission approved name for 1-[3-(2-chlorothiaxanthen-9-ylidene)propyl]-4-(2-hydroxyethyl)piperazine. A psychotropic drug.

Cloponone. The B.P. Commission approved name for β,4-dichloro-α-dichloracetamidopropiophenone. An antiseptic.

Cloquinate. The B.P. Commission approved name for chloroquine di-(8-hydroxy-7-iodoquinoline-5-sulphonate). An amoebicide.

Clorazepic acid. The B.P. Commission approved name for 7-chloro-2,3-dihydro-2,2-dihydroxy-5-phenyl-1*H*-1,4-benzodiazepine-3-carboxylic acid. A sedative.

Clorexolone. The B.P. Commission approved name for 5-chloro-2-cyclohexyl-6-sulphamcylisoindolin-1-one. A diuretic.

Clorindione. The B.P. Commission approved name for 2-(4-chlorophenyl)indane-1,3-dione. An anticoagulant.

Clorprenaline. The B.P. Commission approved name for 1-(2-chlorophenyl)-2-isopropylaminoethanol. A sympathomimetic agent.

Clostridium. A genus of gram-positive, spore-bearing, anaerobic bacilli. (*Abbreviation: Cl.*) Most species of this genus are saprophytes that grow normally in soil, water and decomposing animal and plant matter. Some are commensals in the animal and human intestine. A few produce disease, including: *Cl. welchii, Cl. septicum,* and *Cl. oedematiens,* the causes of gas gangrene; *Cl. tetani,* the cause of tetanus; and *Cl. botulinum,* the cause of botulism.

Clot. A semisolid mass of coagulated blood, lymph, or other body fluid.

Clothiapine. The B.P. Commission approved name for 2-chloro-11-(4-methylpiperazin-1-yl)dibenzo[*b, f*][1,4]thiazepine. A tranquillizer.

Clove. B.P.C. 1968. The dried flower-buds of *Eugenia caryophyllus.* A carminative. **Clove oil,** B.P. 1968, obtained by distillation from clove. Taken orally as a carminative, and applied locally as an analgesic (as in dentistry).

Cloxacillin sodium. B.P. 1968. A semi-synthetic penicillin, with an anti-bacterial spectrum similar to that of benzylpenicillin but resistant to in-activation by staphylococcal penicillinase and by gastric juice.

Clubbing. Broadening and thickening of the terminal phalanges of the fingers (or toes), such as occurs in certain forms of chronic pulmonary disease.

Club-foot. Talipes.

Clumping. Agglutination.

Cluttering. The dropping of letters and/or syllables in hurried nervous speech.

Clyster. Enema.

Coagulant. A substance that causes coagulation.

Coagulase. An enzyme that accelerates the formation of blood clots. An enzyme produced by *Staphylococcus aureus.*

Coagulate. To cause to clot.

Coagulation. The process of clot formation.

Coagulum. A clot. (*Plural:* coagula.)

Coarctation. A narrowing. **Coarctation of the aorta,** narrowing of the aortic isthmus, practically always a congenital lesion.

Coat. A covering or membrane. Tunica.

Cobalamin. One of a group of cobalt-containing enzymes which are essential for normal growth and nutrition.

Cobalt. A steel-grey metallic element, which is essential for normal haemopoiesis. Symbol Co. Atomic weight 58·93. Atomic number 27. **Cobalt-60,** a radioactive isotope widely used in the treatment of cancer.

Coca. The dried leaves of *Erythroxylum coca* or *E. truxillense,* from which cocaine is derived, and which is chewed by Peruvians as an antidote to hunger and fatigue.

Cocaine. B.P. 1968. An alkaloid in coca, which is a potent local anaesthetic but, because of its toxicity and addiction-forming propensities, its use is now almost entirely restricted to local application in ophthalmic and ear, nose and throat surgery. **Cocaine hydrochloride,** B.P. 1968, the form in which cocaine is used in aqueous solution for local application in ophthalmic and ear, nose and throat practice.

Cocainism. The mental disorder induced by addiction to cocaine.

Co-carboxylase. The B.P. Commission approved name for the pyrophosphoric ester of thiamine, which is a co-enzyme.

Co-carcinogen. A substance, or agent, that facilitates the action of a carcinogen.

Coccidioides. A genus of dimorphic fungi. *Coccidioides immitis* is the cause of coccidioidomycosis.

Coccidioidomycosis. A granulomatous disease affecting man primarily as a lung infection, and varying widely in severity. Endemic in U.S.A.

Coccus. A spherical or nearly spherical bacterium. (*Plural:* cocci.)

Coccydynia. Pain in the coccyx.

Coccyx. The triangular-shaped bone, consisting of three to five fused rudimentary vertebrae, that terminates the vertebral column.

Cochineal. B.P. 1968. The dried female insect *Dactylopius coccus.* Used as a colouring agent.

Cochlea. The anterior part of the

labyrinth of the internal ear, which resembles the shell of the common snail and contains the essential organs of hearing.

Cocillana. B.P.C. 1968. The dried bark obtained from *Guarea rusbyi.* An expectorant.

Cocoa. A preparation derived from the seeds of *Theobroma cacao*, which forms the basis of a widely used beverage. Its main constituent is theobromine.

Coconut oil, fractionated. B.P.C. 1968. The fractionated and refined oil obtained from the dried solid part of the endosperm of *Cocos nucifera*. It is used as a non-aqueous vehicle for oral preparations.

Codeine phosphate. B.P. 1968. $C_{18}H_{24}NO_7P$, $\frac{1}{2}H_2O$. A mild analgesic and antitussive.

Cod-liver oil. B.P. 1968. The fixed oil obtained from the fresh liver of the cod *Gadus morhua* and other species of Gadus. Each 1G. contains not less than 600 units of vitamin-A activity and not less than 85 units of antirachitic activity (vitamin D).

Codon. One of the groups of three bases into which the genetic code is translated along a DNA strand.

Coel-, Coelio- (Gk *koilia:* cavity). Prefixes signifying relationship to a cavity or space.

-coele (Gk *koilia:* cavity). Suffix indicating relationship to a space or cavity.

Coeliac. Relating to the abdominal cavity. **Coeliac disease,** a wasting disease of childhood, characterized by the passage of large, pale, offensive stools, due apparently to hypersensitivity to gluten in the diet.

Coelioscopy. The method of examining the peritoneal cavity by inflating it with air and then inserting a cystoscope.

Coelom. The body cavity of the embryo.

Co-enzyme. A substance associated with and activating an enzyme.

Coffee. A popular drink. **Prepared coffee,** B.P.C. 1968, the kernel of the dried ripe seed of *Coffea arabica* (L.) and other species of Coffea. It is used as a flavouring agent.

Coitophobia. Morbid fear of coitus.

Coitus. Copulation. Sexual intercourse. **Coitus interruptus,** withdrawal of the penis before ejaculation. **Coitus reservatus,** postponement or suppression of ejaculation.

Colchicine. B.P. 1968. $C_{22}H_{25}NO_6$. An alkaloid obtained from colchicum corm and seeds, used for the relief of pain in gout. It has also an anti-mitotic action and has therefore been used in the treatment of leukaemia.

Colchicum corm. B.P.C. 1968. The corm of the meadow saffron *Colchicum autumnale*. It contains 0·08 to 0·15 per cent of colchicine.

Cold. A generic name for coryza. A synonym is the common cold.

Colectomy. Surgical extirpation of the colon.

Colic. Pertaining to the colon. Spasmodic, griping pain in the abdomen.

Coliform. Resembling *Escherichia coli*.

Colistin sulphate. B.P. 1968. An antibiotic derived from a strain of *Bacillus polymyxa*, var. *colistinus*, active against a wide variety of gramnegative bacteria with the exception of strains of Proteus. **Colistin sulphomethate sodium,** B.P. 1968, a derivative of colistin sulphate that is suitable for administration by injection.

Colitis. Inflammation of the colon. **Ulcerative colitis,** a severe inflammatory disorder of the colon characterized by the passage of blood and pus, and marked systemic disturbance. Of unknown etiology.

Collagen. The major protein of connective tissue. It is converted into gelatin by boiling. **Collagen diseases,** a somewhat indeterminate group of diseases, including rheumatic fever and rheumatoid arthritis, in which the common factor is gross disturbance of connective tissue.

Collateral. Subsidiary. Secondary. **Collateral circulation,** the compensatory circulation that develops when a main blood vessel is blocked.

Colliculus. A small elevation. (*Plural:* colliculi.) **Facial colliculus,** an elongated swelling in the floor of the fourth ventricle, produced in part by the ascending portion of the root of the facial nerve. **Mid-brain colliculi,** four rounded eminences arranged in pairs: superior and inferior. The superior colliculi are concerned with visual reflexes, and the inferior colliculi with hearing. **Colliculus seminalis,** an elevation in the urethral crest, on which the orifice of the prostatic utricle is situated.

Collimation. The method of localizing brain lesions by recording the concentration of gamma rays from a previously injected radioactive substance such as ^{85}Kr or ^{133}Xe.

Collodion. A clear, syrupy fluid made from pyroxylin, and used as a protective dressing. **Flexible collodion, B.P. 1968,** a preparation containing 1·6 per cent of pyroxylin.

Colloid. Gluelike. A state of matter intermediate between true solution and suspension or emulsion. The structureless, semifluid protein which fills the vesicles of the thyroid gland and contains the active principle of the gland.

Colloidal. Relating to colloid. **Colloidal osmotic pressure,** that proportion of the total osmotic pressure of blood due to the plasma proteins. **Colloidal solution,** a solution in which a substance very finely divided into particles is suspended in another substance such as water. **Colloidal state,** the term applied to particles varying in diameter between 1 and 500 millimicrons.

Collutorium. A mouth-wash or gargyle. (*Plural:* collutoria.)

Collyrium. An eye-lotion. (*Plural:* collyria.)

Colo-, Col- (Gk *kolon:* colon). Prefixes signifying relationship to the colon.

Coloboma. A congenital abnormality, usually of the eye. It may involve the choroid, retina, iris, lens, optic disc, or eyelid.

Colomyotomy. Surgical division of the thickened circular muscle of the colon, carried out for the treatment of diverticular disease.

Colon. The large intestine from the caecum to the rectum. **Ascending colon,** about 15cm. long from the caecum to the right colic flexure below the right lobe of the liver. **Transverse colon,** 50cm. long, from the right colic flexure to the left colic flexure beneath the spleen. **Descending colon,** 25cm. long, from the left colic flexure to the inlet of the lesser pelvis. **Sigmoid colon,** 40cm. long, from the inlet of the lesser pelvis to the level of the third sacral vertebra.

Colonic. Pertaining to the colon.

Colopexy. Surgical fixation of the colon to the posterior abdominal wall.

Colophony. B.P. 1968. The residue left after distilling the volatile oil from the oleo-resin obtained from various species of Pinus. An ingredient of certain plasters and collodions.

Colorado tick fever. A tick-borne virus disease that occurs in North America.

Colorrhaphy. Suture of the colon.

Colostomy. The surgical creation of an artificial anus in the colon.

Colostrum. The first milk from the mother's breasts after the birth of her baby.

Colour. A visual sensation that varies according to which part of the spectrum is absorbed. **Colour blindness,** achromatopsia, the partial or total inability (usually the former) to appreciate colours. **Colour index,** the proportion of haemoglobin in each erythrocyte. **Complementary colours,** two colours, which blended produce white light. **Primary colours,** the colours of the spectrum: red, orange, yellow, green, blue, indigo, violet.

Colp-, Colpo- (Gk *kolpos:* a fold or hollow). Prefixes denoting the vagina.

Colpalgia. Pain in the vagina.

Colpectomy. Surgical removal of the vagina.

Colpitis. Inflammation of the vagina.

Colpocele. A hernia into the vagina.

Colpodynia. Pain in the vagina.

Colpoperineorrhaphy. A plastic operation for repair of a perineal tear.

Colpopexy. Surgical fixture of the prolapsed vagina to the abdominal wall.

Colpoplasty. A plastic operation on the vagina.

Colporrhaphy. Repair of a vaginal tear. The operation for strengthening the pelvic floor in cases of uterine prolapse.

Colposcope. An instrument for the examination of the vagina and the cervix uteri.

Colposcopy. Examination of the vagina and cervix uteri by means of the colposcope.

Colpotomy. Surgical incision of the vagina.

Column. A pillar-like, elongated structure. **Anal columns,** six to ten vertical folds of mucuous membrane in the anal canal. **Grey columns of the spinal cord,** the columns formed by the anterior, lateral, and posterior horns of grey matter. **Renal columns,** the columns of the cortex of the kidney that dip in between adjacent pyramids. **White columns of the spinal cord,** the three columns of nerve fibres—anterior, lateral, and posterior—that surround the grey matter of the spinal cord. **Vaginal columns,** two median longitudinal ridges of mucous membrane, one on the anterior and one on the posterior wall of the vagina. **Vertebral column,** the backbone, made up of seven cervical, twelve thoracic, and five lumbar vertebrae, the sacrum and the coccyx.

Coma. A state of profound uncon-sciousness, from which the patient cannot be aroused.

Comatose. In a state of coma.

Comedo. Blackhead. A hyperkeratotic plug, consisting of sebaceous material and dead cells, blocking a pilo-sebaceous orifice. One of the signs of acne vulgaris. (*Plural:* comedones.)

Commensal. Living on, or within, another organism without doing any harm to each other. A micro-organism living on or within an organism without causing any harm to the host.

Comminuted. Crushed or broken into small pieces.

Commisure. A joining. **Anterior com-misure,** a bundle of white fibres which crosses the median plane in front of the columns of the fornix in the anterior wall of the third ventricle. **Anterior white commisure,** the white matter in front of the grey commisure of the spinal cord. **Commisura bulborum,** the median band that unites the two erectile masses of the bulb of the vestibule of the vagina. **Commisure of the fornix (hippocampal commisure),** the thin sheet of trans-verse fibres that connects the medial edges of the crura of the fornix. **Grey commisure,** the grey matter sur-rounding the spinal canal. **Habenular commisure,** a band of fibres in the roof of the third ventricle, anterior to the stalk of the pineal gland, that joins the habenular ganglia of the two sides. **Labial commisure,** the junction of the upper, with the lower, lip at the corner of the mouth. **Commisures of the vulva, anterior,** the meeting of the labia major in front; **posterior,** the posterior boundary of the pudendum

Commisurotomy. The surgical division of a commisure.

Commotio. Concussion. **Commotio cerebri,** concussion of the brain. **Commotio retinae,** concussion of the retina.

Communicans. Term applied usually to a nerve or artery providing com-munication between two similar structures. (*Plural:* communicantes.)

Compatibility. The ability to coexist happily. Usually applied to: (a) drugs which can be mixed or combined without destroying each other or interfering with each other's action; (b) blood from two or more people who belong to the same blood group.

Compensation. The counterbalancing of some defect of structure or function by some other bodily development: e.g. the hypertrophy of the myocardium in cases of hypertension.

Complement. A thermolabile con-stituent of serum which acts as a catalyst for a variety of antigen-antibody reactions. **Complement-fixation,** the process that occurs when antigen and antibody unite and the union is consummated by the con-junction with it of complement. The assumption is that it is this linking up with complement that results in the lysis or destruction of the antigen.

Complex. A group of: (a) symptoms and signs producing a syndrome, or (b) [ideas as in psychology: e.g. in-feriority complex. The characteristic deviations in the record in the electro-cardiogram.

Compliance. The property of an elastic structure to comply with an imposed stretching force.

Compress. A pad of gauze or some other material folded and bandaged over an area of the body to apply com-pression. It may be either dry or damp, and applied to relieve the pain of inflammation or to control an effusion.

Compressed air illness. Caisson disease. A disease of divers and others who work under conditions of raised pressure and are decompressed too rapidly.

Con- (L *con:* with). Prefix meaning with.

Conation. The exertive power of the mind.

Concave. Hollowed.

Conception. The act of becoming pregnant. The act of forming ideas.

Conceptus. The product of conception.

Concha. A shell-shaped structure. (*Plural:* conchae.) **Concha of the auricle,** the hollow in the auricle of the ear surrounded by the antihelix and leading into the orifice of the meatus. **Nasal conchae, superior, middle and in-ferior,** three ridges of bone on the lateral wall of the nasal cavity. **Sphenoidal conchae,** the thin bones that form part of the anterior wall of the sphenoid and partially enclose the sphenoidal air sinuses.

Conchotomy. Surgical removal of a nasal concha.

Concretion. A calculus.

Concussion. A condition of widespread paralysis of the functions of the brain following a blow on the head, with a strong tendency to spontaneous re-covery.

Condom. A sheath worn over the penis during coitus to prevent conception.

Condyle. A rounded prominence at the end of a bone. Present on the femur, mandible, occiput and tibia.

Condyloma. A wart-like excrescence on the anus, penis or vulva. (*Plural:* condylomata.) **Condyloma acuminatum,** a condyloma on the genital organs or about the anus that occurs in both sexes. Venereal wart. **Condyloma latum,** a syphilitic lesion that occurs at the anal muco-cutaneous junction and sometimes on moist areas such as the female genitalia, the axillae, the under-surface of the breasts or between the toes.

Cone. A structure with a circular base and tapering to a point. **Retinal cones,** with the rods, these constitute the end-organs of vision. They play the dominant role in bright illumination (photopic vision).

Confabulation. The glib recital of fictitious tales, a manifestation of various forms of mental aberration.

Confection. A powder made into a paste with sugar or honey, of such a consistency that the powder does not separate, but the mass can be swallowed.

Confluence. A running together. **Confluence of the sinuses,** the dilated posterior extremity of the superior sagittal sinus, lodged on one side of the internal occipital protuberance. It is connected with the occipital and the transverse sinus.

Congenital. Existing at birth.

Congestion. Excessive collection of blood in a part. **Hypostatic congestion,** congestion due to gravitational accumulation of blood in a dependent part. **Passive congestion,** congestion due to deficiency in the return of venous blood. **Venous congestion,** passive congestion.

Conglutin. A protein of bovine serum which brings about agglutination of complement-coated particles.

Congo red. B.P.C. 1968. $C_{32}H_{22}N_6Na_2O_6S_2$. A dye used for the detection of amyloidosis.

Coniine. The active constituent of hemlock, an alkaloid that produces paralysis of the central nervous system and of the skeletal muscle nerve endings.

Conization. Excision of a cone of tissue, as in the treatment of chronic cervicitis.

Conjugal. Pertaining to man and wife.

Conjugate. Joined. Paired. **Conjugate deviation,** the property of binocular synkinesis, whereby, normally, abduction of one eye is accompanied by adduction of the other, and elevation or depression of one eye is always accompanied by elevation or depression, respectively, of the other. **Conjugate foci,** in refraction the positions of the object and image. **Diagonal conjugate,** in obstetrics the distance between the promontory of the sacrum and the lower margin of the symphysis pubis. **External conjugate,** in obstetrics the distance between the tip of the spine of the last lumbar vertebra and the symphysis pubis.

Conjugation. A joining together. **Conjugation of the chromosomes,** the process of coupling of genetically homologous chromosomes in the second stage (zygotene) of meiosis.

Conjunctiva. The transparent mucous membrane that lines the inner surfaces of the eyelids and is reflected over the front part of the sclera and cornea.

Conjunctivitis. Inflammation of the conjunctiva. **Angular conjunctivitis,** conjunctivitis usually due to infection with Moraxella, confined as a rule to the outer and inner canthi. **Follicular conjunctivitis,** the condition characterized by the occurrence of follicles in the conjunctiva. **Inclusion conjunctivitis,** conjunctivitis due to an organism resembling that of trachoma, and producing inclusion bodies. **Ligneous conjunctivitis,** a form of recurrent membranous conjunctivitis. **Membranous conjunctivitis,** a form of conjunctivitis in which the conjunctiva becomes covered with a fibrinous membrane. **Newcastle conjunctivitis,** conjunctivitis due to the Newcastle virus. **Phlyctenular conjunctivitis,** an allergic condition, most common in ill-nourished children. **Swimming-bath conjunctivitis,** inclusion conjunctivitis, in which the infection is transmitted through the water of swimming pools. **Vernal (spring) conjunctivitis,** a recurrent conjunctivitis in young people, with the onset of hot weather.

Connexion. A connecting structure. **Intertendinous connexions,** three bands that connect the four tendons of the extensor digitorum on the back of the hand.

Consanguinity. Blood relationship.

Consolidation. Solidification of an organ, particularly of a lung as in pneumonia.

Conspersus. A dusting-powder.

Constant. Unvarying. An invariable quantity. A number expressing a quantity or relation that, under given conditions, does not change. **Equilibrium constant,** the product of the concentrations of the products of a chemical reaction divided by the product of the concentrations of the substances entering the reaction.

Constipation. Inadequate evacuation of the bowels.

Constitution. The make-up of the individual.

Constriction. A narrowing. **Constrictions of the oesophagus,** four narrowings of the oesophagus: (a) at its beginning, (b) where it is crossed by the aortic arch, (c) where it is crossed by the left bronchus, (d) where it pierces the diaphragm. **Pyloric constriction,** the circular groove on the surface of the stomach that indicates the position of the pyloric sphincter.

Consumption. An old term applied to pulmonary tuberculosis.

Contact. A touching or connexion. An individual who has been exposed to a contagious disease. **Contact lenses,** lenses shaped to fit the eyeball.

Contagion. The principle of spread of disease by direct contact with the body of the infected individual.

Contamination. Pollution with infective material. In Freudian terminology, the running of one word into another.

Contiguous. Adjacent, or in contact.

Contra- (L *contra:* against). Prefix meaning against, opposed.

Contraception. The prevention of fertilization or conception.

Contractility. The ability to be able to contract in response to a given stimulus.

Contraction. A shortening, especially of a muscle. **Anodal closure contraction,** the muscle contraction that occurs with a constant current when the circuit is closed and the anode is the testing electrode. (*Abbreviation:* ACC.) **Anodal opening contraction,** the muscle contraction that occurs with a constant current when the circuit is opened and the anode is the testing electrode. (*Abbreviation:* AOC.) **Cathodal closure contraction,** the muscle contraction that occurs with a constant current when the circuit is closed and the cathode is the testing electrode. (*Abbreviation:* CCC.) **Cathodal opening contraction,** the muscle contraction that occurs with a constant current when the

circuit is opened and the cathode is the testing electrode. (*Abbreviation:* COC.) **Clonic contraction,** alternating contraction with partial relaxation. **Isometric contraction,** a contraction in which shortening is prevented in order to measure the tension developed. **Isotonic contraction,** a muscle contraction in which shortening is allowed but tension is controlled. **Tonic contraction,** maintained contraction.

Contracture. Permanent shortening of muscle. **Dupuytren's contracture,** progressive flexion of the fingers, usually the 4th and 5th. **Volkman's ischaemic contracture,** contracture affecting the flexor muscles of the forearm.

Contraindication. A factor which renders a given form of treatment undesirable or even bans its use.

Contralateral. Relating to the opposite side.

Contrecoup. Indicating an injury at the opposite side to which the causative blow was applied. Most commonly used in the case of the skull.

Contusion. A bruise.

Conus. A cone. An anatomical structure that is cone-like in shape. **Conus arteriosus,** the part of the right ventricle from which the pulmonary trunk arises. **Conus medullaris,** the tapering lower end of the spinal cord.

Convalescence. The period of recovery from an illness.

Convection. The transference of heat in liquids or gases by change of position of the heated particles.

Convergence. A coming together to meet at a common point, as in the case of the eyes when looking at a near object.

Conversion. Change. In psychology, transformation of emotion into physical action.

Convex. Having a rounded, bulging surface, as in the case of a lens.

Convolution. A fold or gyrus.

Convulsion. Violent, spasmodic, involuntary muscular movement. **Clonic convulsion,** one in which the contractions are intermittent. **Epileptiform convulsion,** one characterized by loss of consciousness. **Hysterical convulsion,** one produced in a dramatic fashion before an audience, and not accompanied by loss of consciousness or any harmful sequelae to the perpetrator. **Jacksonian convulsion,** one occurring in Jacksonian epilepsy and following a regular, definitive geographical course. **Tonic convulsion,** one in which there is no relaxation.

Coordination. The harmonious working together of those parts that participate mutually in a given effort or action.

Copper. A metallic element. Symbol Cu. Atomic weight 63·54. Atomic number 29.

Copper sulphate. B.P.C. 1968. $CuSO_4$, $5H_2O$. Used as an external application on account of its astringent properties. Very occasionally given internally in the treatment of microcytic anaemia. A potent fungicide and molluscicide.

Copr-, Copro- (Gk *kopros:* dung). Prefixes meaning faeces.

Copremesis. Vomiting of faecal matter.

Copro-antibody. An antibody present in faeces.

Coprolagnia. The form of sexual perversion in which sexual excitement is aroused by the thought or sight of excreta.

Coprolalia. The involuntary utterance of filthy and obscene terms.

Coprolith. A hard mass of faeces in the bowels. Faecalith.

Coprophagy. The eating of faeces.

Coproporphyrin. A porphyrin compound produced in normal haemopoiesis and excreted in the bile, faeces and urine.

Coproporphyrinuria. The presence of excess coprophyrin in the urine.

Copula. A connecting link.

Copulation. Coitus.

Cor. The heart. **Cor pulmonale,** pulmonary heart disease. **Cor triatriatum,** a congenital abnomality of the heart, in which the development of an abnormal transverse septum results in the presence of three atria. **Cor triloculare,** a congenital abnormality in which the absence of the interatrial or the interventricular septum results in a three-chambered heart.

Coracoid. Beak-like. The coracoid process.

Cord. A string-like body. **Oblique cord,** a fibrous band extending from the tuberosity of the ulna to the radius. **Spermatic cord,** the structure that suspends the testis in the scrotum, and extends from the deep inguinal ring to the posterior border of the testis. It contains the deferent duct. **Spinal cord,** the elongated part of the central nervous system which extends from the level of the upper border of the atlas vertebra to that of the lower border of the 1st lumbar vertebra. In the male its average length is 45cm., its average weight 30 grammes. **Umbilical cord,** the cord by which the foetus is connected to the placenta and

which contains the two umbilical arteries and the umbilical vein. **Vocal cords,** or vocal folds, two white folds of mucuous membrane which stretch from the middle of the angle of the thyroid cartilage to the vocal processes of the arytenoid cartilages.

Cordectomy. Surgical excision of a vocal cord.

Cordotomy. Surgical section of a column in the spinal cord.

Corectopia. Displacement of the pupil, usually to the nasal side.

Coriander. B.P. 1968. The dried ripe fruits of *Coriandrum sativum* (L.). A carminative.

Corium. The layer of skin deep to the epidermis.

Corn. A painful, localized thickening of the cuticle or epidermis.

Cornea. The anterior, projecting, transparent part of the external coat of the eye.

Corneum. The horny outer layer of the epidermis, the full name of which is the stratum corneum.

Cornu. A horn or horn-like excrescence. (*Plural:* cornua.) There are cornua on the coccyx, sacrum, hyoid bone and thyroid cartilage, and the upper and lower margins of the saphenous opening are known as cornua.

Corona. (*Plural:* coronae.) A crown or curved line. **Corona glandis,** the projecting margin of the glans penis. **Corona radiata,** the radiating mass of white fibres which pass from the internal capsule to the cerebral cortex.

Coronary. Encircling in the form of a crown. **Coronary arteries,** the arteries supplying the heart. **Coronary thrombosis,** the occlusion, partial or complete, of a coronary artery by a thrombus.

Coronoid. Shaped like a crown or a crow's beak. The coronoid process.

Corpse. A dead body.

Corpulence. Obesity.

Corpus. A body. (*Plural:* corpora.) **Corpus albicans,** the scar tissue that replaces the corpus luteum. **Corpus callosum,** the transverse commisure that connects the cerebral hemispheres, and roofs in the lateral ventricles. **Corporaca vernosa clitoridis,** the two masses of erectile tissue in the clitoris. **Corpora cavernosa penis,** the two masses of erectile tissue that constitute the bulk of the body of the penis. **Corpus cerebelli,** the anterior and middle lobes of the cerebellum. **Corpus luteum,** the mass of lutein-containing cells that develops in the site of the ruptured ovarian follicle. **Corpus quadrigemium,** colliculus of the midbrain. **Corpus spongiosum penis,** the cylindrical mass which contains the spongy part of the urethra, which is continuous proximately with the bulb of the penis and terminates in the glans penis. **Corpus striatum,** the lentiform and caudate nuclei, the amygdaloid body and the claustrum, of the cerebral hemispheres.

Corpuscle. A small mass or body. **Articular corpuscle,** a tactile end-bulb in a fibrous joint capsule. **Blood corpuscles,** the cellular contents of the blood: coloured corpuscles (erythrocytes), colourless corpuscles (leucocytes), and blood platelets. **Bulbous corpuscles,** end-organs in the skin, mucous membrane and blood vessels, which may be concerned with the recognition of cold. **Colostrum corpuscles,** fat-containing cells in colostrum. **Concentric corpuscles of the thymus,** nest-like bodies in the thymus. **Corneal corpuscle,** the cell present in each of the corneal spaces in the ground substance of the cornea. **Genital corpuscles,** end bulbs, similar to bulbous corpuscles, in the glans penis and clitoris. **Golgi-Mazzoni corpuscles,** end-organs in the conjunctiva, external genitalia, tendons and muscles. **Lamellated corpuscles,** nerve endings sensitive to pressure, found throughout the body. **Renal corpuscles,** the glomerulus and its surrounding capsule. **Tactile corpuscles,** oval bodies, particularly numerous in the corium, that subserve the sense of touch.

Cortex. The outer portion of an organ, such as the adrenal gland, the brain, and the kidney. (*Plural:* cortices.)

Cortico- (L *cortex:* bark or rind). Prefix signifying relationship with cortex.

Corticoid. Corticosteroid.

Corticosteroid. A steroid produced by the adrenal cortex.

Corticosterone. A steroid hormone in the adrenal cortex, which induces hyperglycaemia and deposition of glycogen in the liver.

Cortictrophin. B.P. 1968. Adrenocorticotrophic hormone. ACTH. The hormone which increases the rate at which corticoid hormones are secreted by the adrenal gland. **Corticotrophin gelatine injection,** B.P. 1968, a sterile solution of corticotrophin containing hydrolysed gelatin. When given intramuscularly or subcutaneously, it

gives therapeutically effective blood levels for 12 to 24 hours. **Corticotrophin zinc hydroxide injection,** B.P. 1968, a sterile aqueous suspension of corticotrophin with zinc hydroxide, which gives therapeutically effective blood levels for 48 hours after intramuscular or subcutaneous injection.

Cortisol. 17-hydroxycorticosterone. Hydrocortisone. An adrenal cortex hormone with an action comparable to that of cortisone.

Cortisone. 17-hydroxy-11-dehydrocorticosterone. A hormone secreted by the adrenal cortex, which belongs to the group of glucocorticoids. **Cortisone acetate,** B.P. 1968, the form in which cortisone is used therapeutically. It has a potent anti-inflammatory action.

Cortodoxone. The B.P. Commission approved name for 17,21-dihydroxypregn-4-ene-3,20-dione. A corticosteroid.

Coruscation. Subjective sensation of light flashes.

Corybantism. Wild, sleepless frenzy.

Corynebacteriaceae. A family of gram-positive bacteria which are rod- or club-shaped, and mostly non-motile.

Corynebacterium. A genus of micro-organisms. Gram-positive rods, arranged in pairs or palisades, some species of which produce a powerful exotoxin. *Corynebacterium acnes,* a micro-organism associated with acne. *C. diphtheriae,* the causative organism of diphtheria. *C. hofmannii,* a commensal of the throat. *C. xerosis,* a commensal in the conjunctival sac.

Coryza. A cold in the head. Rhinitis.

Costal. Relating to a rib.

Costalgia. Pain in the ribs.

Costive. Constipated.

Costo- (L *costa:* rib). Prefix indicating relationship to a rib.

Costocervical. Relating to the ribs and the neck.

Costochondral. Relating to the ribs and their cartilages.

Costophrenic. Relating to the ribs and the diaphragm.

Costosternal. Relating to the ribs and the sternum.

Costoxiphoid. Relating to the ribs and the xiphoid process.

Cotton. The hairs of the seeds of cultivated species of varieties of Gossypium. **Absorbent cotton wool,** B.P.C. 1968, a fleecy mass of soft white filaments, prepared from cotton, and consisting almost entirely of cellulose. **Capsicum cotton wool, B.P.C.**

1968, absorbent cotton wool impregnated with capsicum oleoresin and methyl salicylate. Used as a counter-irritant and to produce heat on undamaged skin. **Cotton crêpe bandage,** B.P.C. 1968, fabric of plain weave, in which the warp threads are of cotton and the weft threads of cotton or rayon or combined cotton and rayon yarn. Used in the treatment of sprains. **Cotton and rubber elastic bandage,** B.P.C. 1968, characteristic fabric of plain weave, in which the warp threads are of cotton and combined cotton and rubber yarn, and the weft threads of cotton. Used as for cotton crêpe bandage. **Cotton and rubber elastic net bandage,** B.P.C. 1968, characteristic net fabric of lace construction, in which the warp threads are of combined cotton and rubber yarn and the bobbin threads of cotton. Used as for cotton crêpe bandage. **Cotton stretch bandage,** B.P.C. 1968, characteristic fabric of plain weave, in which both warp and weft threads are of cotton. Used to protect dressings and hold them in position.

Cottonseed oil. B.P. 1968. The refined fixed oil obtained from the seeds of *Gossypium herbaceum* (L.) and other species of Gossypium. It has properties similar to those of olive oil.

Cotyledon. One of the 15 to 30 areas into which the maternal surface of the placenta is divided by a series of fissures.

Cotyloid. Cup-shaped. Pertaining to the acetabulum.

Cough. A sudden, forceful expulsion of air through the glottis.

Coulomb. The amount of electricity passed by a current of one ampere, with an electromotive force of one volt, through a resistance of one ohm in one second.

Counter. A computer. **Geiger counter,** an instrument for the detection and measuring of ionizing particles, particularly beta particles. **Scintillation counter,** an instrument for the measurement of gamma rays.

Counter-irritant. An agent that relieves pain by causing irritation of the overlying skin or of the area of skin with the same segmental nerve supply.

Counter-traction. The method used in treating fractures of the limbs, by applying traction to the limb in the opposite direction to the extension applied to bring the two parts of the limb into alignment. Counter-extension.

Cover-slip. The thin slither of glass used to cover a mounted microscopical section or culture.

Cowpox. An eruption on the teats of cows caused by a virus which is morphologically identical with the vaccinia virus.

Coxa. The hip or hip-joint. (*Plural:* coxae.) **Coxa plana,** osteochondritis deformans juvenilis. **Coxa valga,** a deformity in which the angle between the neck and the shaft of the femur is increased. The opposite of coxa vara. **Coxa vara,** a deformity characterized by a decrease in the angle between the neck and the shaft of the femur.

Coxalgia. Pain in the hip.

Coxitis. Inflammation of the hip-joint.

Coxsackie viruses. A group of viruses, 25 to 35nm in diameter, so-called because they were first isolated from two patients in the village of Coxsackie in New York State. They belong to the enterovirus family and are responsible for a range of illnesses, including aseptic meningitis, epidemic myalgia and herpangina.

Crab louse. *Phthirus pubis.*

Cradle. A frame used to keep the weight of the bedclothes off the patient. A cot.

Cramp. A painful, spasmodic, involuntary muscular contraction.

Crani-, Cranio- (Gk *kranion:* skull). Prefixes signifying relationship to the skull.

Cranial. Relating to the cranium. **Cranial nerves,** the 12 pairs of nerves arising from the brain: olfactory, optic, oculomotor, trochlear, trigeminal, abducent, facial, auditory, glossopharyngeal, vagus, accessory, hypoglossal.

Cranioclasm. The operation of avulsion of the bones of the foetal cranial vault, followed by crushing of the remaining part of the head, to allow removal of the dead foetus.

Cranioclast. Craniotomy forceps, for perforating the foetal skull and removing the dead foetus from the uterus.

Craniocleidodysotosis. A rare heredo-familial disease, characterized by defective development or absence of the clavicles, defective development of the vault and base of the skull, and often absence of the pubic ramus.

Cranio-facial dysotosis. A hereditary condition characterized by oxycephaly, atrophy of the superior maxillae, atresia of the nasal fossae, a parrot beak-shaped nose and exophthalmos.

Craniology. The scientific study of skulls.

Craniopagus. Conjoined twins with fused skulls.

Craniopharyngioma. An epidermoid, slowly growing, usually benign tumour that arises from remnants of Rathke's pouch.

Craniostenosis. A congenital abnormality of the skull due to premature synostosis of the sutures, resulting in a 'tower skull', exophthalmos and optic atrophy.

Craniosynostosis. Premature closure of the cranial sutures.

Craniotabes. Localized areas of softening of the skull.

Craniotome. An instrument for perforation and crushing of the foetal skull.

Craniotomy. Any operation on the skull: e.g. trephining. An operation to reduce the size of the foetal skull to permit the removal of a dead foetus from the uterus.

Cranium. The skull. **Cranium bifidum,** congenital gap in the skull.

Crasis. Individual temperament or constitution.

Cream. The oily or fatty part of milk from which butter is made. A viscous emulsion of semi-solid consistency, which may be of oil-in-water (aqueous cream) or water-in-oil type (oily cream), and used for external application.

Creatinase. The enzyme that converts creatine to creatinine.

Creatine. Methyl guanido-acetic acid. An amino-acid found abundantly in muscle. It is synthesized in the body and is not a necessary constituent of the diet. The urine of the healthy adult male contains no creatinine. It is present in the urine of women during menstruation and pregnancy. It occurs normally in the urine of children.

Creatine phosphate. An energy-rich compound in muscle which serves for the regeneration of adenosine triphosphate from adenosine diphosphate, an integral step in the chemical processes accompanying muscular contraction. Phosphagen. Phosphocreatine.

Creatinine. The anhydride of creatine, and an end-product of muscle metabolism. It is excreted in the urine as a waste product.

Creatinuria. An excess of creatine in the urine.

Cremation. Disposal of the dead by burning.

Crenation. The notched appearance of erythrocytes on exposure to the air or hypertonic saline.

Crepitation. A sound like that produced by rubbing hair between the fingers, and heard on auscultation over the lungs in certain diseased conditions.

Crepitus. A grating sound, as heard over a fracture when the ends rub together, and over an osteoarthritic joint.

Cresol. B.P. 1968. A mixture of cresols and other phenols obtained from coaltar. It has an action similar to that of phenol. **Cresol and soap solution,** B.P. 1968, a solution of cresol in a saponaceous solvent, containing 50 per cent v/v of cresol. Lysol.

Crest. A ridge. A narrow, elongated edge. **Ampullary crest,** a prominence on the transverse septum of the semicircular ducts of the membranous labyrinth. **Basilar crest,** the triangular prominence to which the basilar membrane of the cochlea is attached. **Conchal crest of maxilla,** the oblique ridge in the maxilla for articulation with the inferior nasal concha. **Conchal crest of palatine bone,** the horizontal ridge on the nasal surface of the palatine bone for articulation with the inferior nasal concha. **Ethmoidal crest,** the oblique ridge on the medial surface of the maxilla for articulation with the middle nasal concha. **Ethmoidal crest of the palatine bone,** the ridge on the medial surface of the palatine bone for articulation with the middle nasal concha. **Frontal crest,** the median sagittal projection on the frontal bone, to which the falx cerebri is attached. **Iliac crest,** the upper border of the ilium. **Incisor crest,** the front part of the nasal crest of the palatine bone. **Infratemporal crest,** the ridge that divides the lateral surface of the greater wing of the sphenoid bone into two. **Intertrochanteric crest,** the rounded ridge which marks the junction of the neck and the shaft of the femur. **Lacrimal bone, crest of,** the posterior border of the lacrimal groove. **Lacrimal crest, anterior, of the frontal process of the maxilla,** the ridge that gives attachment to the medial palpebral ligaments. **Lacrimal crest, posterior,** a vertical ridge dividing the lateral surface of the lacrimal bone. **Nasal crest of the maxilla,** a ridge on the medial border of the palatine process of the maxilla. **Nasal crest of the palatine bone,** part of the medial border of the horizontal plate of the palatine bone that is continuous anteriorly with the nasal crest of the maxilla. **Neural crest,** the ridge of neurectodermal cells that lies along the line of closure of the neural tube in the embryo. **Obturator crest,** the rounded ridge that bounds the pectineal surface of the superior ramus of the pubis anteriorly. **External occipital crest,** the ridge on the occipital bone that gives attachment to the ligamentum nuchae. **Internal occipital crest,** the prominent ridge on the internal surface of the occipital bone that gives attachment to the falx cerebri. **Palatine crest,** the ridge on the bony palate that gives attachment to part of the tendon of the tensor veli palatini muscle. **Pubic crest,** the rounded upper border of the body of the pubis. **Crest of head of rib,** the transverse ridge that separates the two facets of the head of the rib. **Crest of neck of rib,** the sharp upper border of the neck of the rib. **Sacral crests,** intermediate, lateral and medial, all on the dorsal surface of the sacrum. **Sphenoidal crest,** a triangular crest that forms part of the septum of the nose. **Crest of the spine of the scapula,** the subcutaneous ridge on the spine of the scapula. **Supinator crest,** the ridge on the shaft of the ulna, from which the supinator arises. **Supra-mastoid crest,** a horizontal ridge. immediately above the mastoid process. **Supraventricular crest,** the muscular ridge demarcating the infundibulum of the right ventricle. **Transverse crest of the internal acoustic meatus,** the ridge on the plate that separates the fundus of the internal acoustic meatus from the internal ear. **Urethral crest,** the longitudinal median ridge in the floor of the urethra.

Cretin. A person affected with cretinism.

Cretinism. A condition resulting from thyroid deficiency in foetal or early neonatal life, characterized by stunted physical and mental development.

Cribriform. Like a sieve. **Cribriform plate,** the perforated plate of the ethmoid bone that occupies the ethmoidal notch of the frontal bone.

Cricoid. Ringlike. The cricoid cartilage.

Crisis. The turning point in a disease. A sudden intensification of symptoms. **Dietl's crisis,** paroxysmal lumbar and abdominal pain, with vomiting and nausea, associated with kinking of the ureter in patients with a wandering kidney. **Oculogyric crisis,** involuntary fixation and deviation of the eyes, a manifestation of postencephalitic parkinsonism. **Tabetic crisis,** paroxysmal attacks of pain in tabes dorsalis. **Thyrotoxic crisis,** sudden exacerbations of symptoms and signs of thyrotoxicosis in a thyrotoxic patient following a shock or thyroidectomy.

Crista. A crest. (*Plural:* cristae.) **Crista galli,** the crestlike elevation on the upper surface of the cribriform plate.

Cromoglycic acid. The B.P. Commission approved name for 1,3-di-(2-carboxy-4-oxochromen-5-yloxy)propan-2-ol. A preparation used in the treatment of asthma.

Cropropamide. The B.P. Commission approved name for NN-dimethyl-2-(N-propylcrotonamido)butyramide. A respiratory stimulant.

Crotamiton. B.P. 1968. $C_{13}H_{17}NO$. An antipruritic. Also used in treatment of scabies.

Crotethamide. The B.P. Commission approved name for 2-(N-ethylcrotonamido)-NN-dimethylbutyr amide. A respiratory stimulant.

Croup. A generic term used to cover the manifestations of laryngeal obstruction, usually in an infant or child. The presenting symptom is usually a brassy cough, with or without symptoms and signs of respiratory distress, which may rapidly be fatal.

Crown. Corona. Crown-like. The part of a tooth projecting above the gum.

Crowning. The stage of parturition when the foetal head permanently dilates the vulval orifice.

Crural. Connected with the leg.

Crus. The leg (from knee to ankle). A leg-like or elongated structure. (*Plural:* crura.) **Crura cerebri,** two white, rope-like structures, consisting of cortico-spinal, cortinuclear and corticopontine fibres, which emerge from the cerebral hemispheres, and constitute the ventral part of the cerebral peduncles. **Crus clitoridis,** the structure that connects the corpus cavernosum of the clitoris to the pubic and ischial rami. **Crus commune,** the channel formed by the junction of the superior and posterior semicircular canals. **Crura of the diaphragm,** tendinous structures in their origin from the upper lumbar vertebrae, which meet medially to arch over the aorta. **Crus of the fornix,** the two bands of white matter that unite to form the body of the fornix. **Crura of the helix,** the two parts into which the antihelix of the external ear divides. **Crura of the superficial inguinal ring,** the margins of the ring. **Crura penis,** the masses of erectile tissue in the root of the penis, stretching from the ischial tuberosity to become continuous with the corpora cavernosa.

Crust. A covering. A scab.

Cry-, Cryo- (Gk *kryos:* cold). Prefixes meaning cold.

Crymotherapy. The treatment of disease by refrigeration.

Cryoanaesthesia. Anaesthesia by refrigeration.

Cryoglobulinaemia. The presence of cryoglobulins in the blood, as in multiple myeloma.

Cryoglobulins. Plasma proteins which precipitate spontaneously from blood serum usually only in the cold (7° to 11°C), and which usually, but not invariably, redissolve at room temperature.

Cryometer. A thermometer for measuring very low temperatures.

Cryoprecipitate. The precipitate of antihaemophilic globulin that occurs as cryoglobulin when fresh-frozen plasma thaws at 4°C.

Cryoscopy. The determination of the freezing point of a fluid.

Cryosurgery. The use of cold, destroying tissue by freezing.

Crypt. A small sac or depression. **Anal crypts,** the depressions in the lining of the anal canal, into which the anal glands open. **Tonsillar crypts,** the recesses in the tonsils.

Crypt-, Crypto- (Gk *kryptos:* hidden). Prefixes meaning hidden.

Cryptococcosis. A subacute or chronic infection of the lungs with *Cryptococcus neoformans*, which is liable to metastasize to the meninges.

Cryptococcus. A genus of *Fungi imperfecti.* A pathogenic yeast which reproduces by budding and does not give rise to a mycelium. *Cryptococcus neoformans* is the only member liable to cause infection in man.

Cryptomenorrhoea. The condition in which all the systemic manifestations of menstruation occur monthly without any external bleeding, as in cases of imperforate hymen.

Cryptophthalmos. A very rare condition in which skin passes continuously from the brow over the eye to the cheek.

Cryptorchidism. Non-descent of the testicles.

Crystalluria. The passage of crystals in the urine.

Crystal violet. B.P. 1968. $C_{25}H_{30}ClN_3$. A powerful antiseptic, with a selective action on gram-positive organisms.

Cubital. Relating to the forearm.

Cubitus. The forearm. The elbow. **Cubitus valgus,** inward deviation of the forearm on extension. **Cubitus varus,** outward deviation of the forearm on extension.

Cuboid bone. The most lateral bone of the distal row of the tarsus, situated between the calcaneus proximally and the 4th and 5th metatarsal bones distally.

Culdoscope. An instrument with a light attachment for passage through the posterior fornix of the vagina to permit visual examination of the pelvic viscera.

Culdotomy. Surgical incision of the recto-uterine pouch.

Culex. A genus of mosquitoes.

Culicidae. The family of flies, belonging to the suborder Nematorera, which is made up of three subfamilies: the only one of importance is the Culicinae (comprising all the true mosquitoes).

Culicide. An agent that kills mosquitoes.

Culicinae. The subfamily of true mosquitoes. It contains three tribes: the Anophelini, the Culicini and the Megharinini. Only the first two of these tribes are of medical importance in man.

Culicoides. A genus of biting midges of the family Ceratopogonidae.

Culmen. One of the subdivisions of the superior surface of the cerebellum.

Culture. Growth of micro-organisms or cells in an artificial medium. The medium used is known as the culture medium.

Cumetharol. The B.P. Commission approved name for 4,4′-dihydroxy-3, 3′-(2-methoxyethylidene) dicoumarin. An anticoagulant.

Cuneate. Wedge-shaped.

Cunciform bones. Three wedge-shaped bones in the tarsus that articulate with the navicular bone proximally and with the bases of the first three metatarsal bones distally.

Cuneus. A wedge-shaped area on the medial surface of the occipital lobe of the cerebral hemisphere.

Cuniculus. The burrow in the skin made by *Sarcoptes hominis.*

Cunnilingus. Licking or kissing of the vulva.

Cup. A drinking vessel. A cup-shaped depression. A cupping glass.

Cupola. A dome-shaped cup. (*Plural:* cupolae.) **Cupola of the cochlea,** the apex of the cochlea. **Cupola of the diaphragm,** the dome of the diaphragm.

Cupping. Application of a cup, or cupping glass, as a means of counter-irritation. **Dry cupping,** cupping without scarification. **Wet cupping,** cupping after scarification.

Cupula. The dome-shaped, gelatinous mass that projects from the free end of each hair cell in the semicircular canals. (*Plural:* cupulae.)

Curare. An extract derived mainly from the bark of various species of Strychnos and Chondodendron which achieved fame as the arrow poison of the South American Indians. A potent muscle relaxant.

Curd. The coagulum of milk, consisting mainly of casein.

Curettage. The scraping of the lining of a cavity with a curette for diagnostic or therapeutic purposes.

Curette. A spoon-shaped instrument used in surgery for scraping out the contents of a cavity or for scraping its wall to remove material for diagnostic or therapeutic purposes.

Curie. A unit of measure of radioactivity defined as the quantity of any radioactive nuclide in which the number of disintegrations per second is 3.70×10^{10}. (*Abbreviation:* Ci.)

Current. That which flows. A stream or flow of air, electricity or fluid. **Action current,** the electrical current accompanying activity of living tissue such as muscle or nerve. **After current,** the current occurring in muscle or nerve after cessation of the original electrical stimulus. **Alternating current,** an electric current that reverses its direction in a regular periodic manner. (*Abbreviation:* a.c.) **Anionic current,** that part of an electric current carried by the anode. **Cathodic current,** that part of an electric current carried by the cathode. **Constant current,** an uninterrupted direct current. **Direct current,** an electric current that flows continuously in one direction. **Faradic current,** an intermittent electric current derived from an induction coil. **Galvanic current,** a direct current supplied by a battery of voltaic batteries. **High-frequency current,** an alternating electric current with a frequency of 10,000 or more per second. **High-tension current,** an electric current with a high electromotive force. **Induced current,** the electric current induced in a circuit by proximity to another current. **Sinusoidal current,** an alternating current, consecutive values of which fall on a regular sine-wave curve. **Static current,** the electric current from an electrostatic machine.

Cusp. A pointed eminence. One of the prominences on the crown of a tooth. One of the segments of the heart valves.

Cutaneous. Pertaining to the skin.

Cuticle. The thin outer layer of hair. **Enamel cuticle,** the membrane covering the enamel of newly erupted teeth.

Cutis. The skin. **Cutis hyperelastica,** a congenital, hereditary disorder of connective tissue leading to hyperelasticity of the skin. **Cutis laxa,** cutis hyperelastica. **Cutis marmorata,** a reticular mottling of the skin occurring in certain subjects from exposure to cold. **Cutis rhomboidalis nuchae,** a form of chronic solar dermatitis, in which the skin of the back of the neck is red, thickened and creased.

Cyan-, Cyano- (Gk *kyanos:* blue). Prefixes meaning blue.

Cyanocobalamin. B.P. 1968. A cobalt-containing substance which may be obtained from liver or separated from the products of metabolism of various micro-organisms. The haemopoietic factor specific for the treatment of pernicious anaemia in that it represents the anti-pernicious-anaemia principle of purified liver extracts. It is also used in the treatment of other megaloblastic anaemias.

Cyanopsia. The condition in which everything appears to be coloured blue.

Cyanosis. The bluish discoloration of the skin and mucous membrane induced by deficient oxygenation of the blood. **Enterogenous cyanosis,** the condition characterized by cyanosis induced by methaemoglobin or sulphaemoglobin.

Cybernetics. The study of control and communication in man and the machine.

Cycl-, Cyclo- (Gk *kyklos:* circle). Prefixes indicating round or recurring.

Cyclamic acid. B.P. 1968. $C_6H_{13}NO_3S$. A preparation used for sweetening preparations which have an acid reaction.

Cyclandelate. The B.P. Commission approved name for 3,3,5-trimethylcyclohexl mandelate. A peripheral vasodilator.

Cyclarbamate. The B.P. Commission approved name for 1,1-di(phenyl-carbamoyloxymethyl) cyclopentane. A muscle relaxant and tranquillizer

Cycle. A recurring series of events. **Anovulatory cycle,** a sexual cycle without extrusion of an ovum. **Menstrual cycle,** the recurring series of changes in the uterus and ovaries associated with menstruation.

Cyclitis. Inflammation of the ciliary body.

Cyclizine hydrochloride. B.P. 1968. $C_{18}H_{23}ClN_2$. An antihistamine.

Cyclobarbitone calcium. B.P. 1968. $C_{24}H_{30}CaN_4O_6$. An intermediate-acting barbiturate.

Cyclocoumarol. The B.P. Commission approved name for 5',6'-dihydro-6'-methoxy-6'-methyl-4'-phenylpyrano-(3',2':3,4)coumarin. An anti-coagulant.

Cyclodialysis. The operation of opening a channel between the anterior chamber of the eye and the supra-choroidal space, for the relief of glaucoma.

Cyclodiathermy. The use of diathermy to destroy the ciliary body.

Cyclofenil. The B.P. Commission approved name for 4,4'-diacetoxy-benzyhydrylidenecyclohexane. A drug for the treatment of infertility.

Cycloguanil embonate. The B.P. Commission approved name for 4,6 - diamino- 1 -(4-chlorophenyl) - 1,2-dihydro - 2, 2 - dimethyl -1, 3, 5- triazine compound (2:1) with 4,4'-methylenedi-(3-hydroxy-2-naphthoic acid). An antimalarial drug.

Cyclomethycaine sulphate. B.P. 1968. $C_{22}H_{35}NO_7S$. A local anaesthetic.

Cyclopentamine. The B.P. Commission approved name for 1-cyclopentyl-2-methylaminopropane. A vasoconstrictor.

Cyclopenthiazide. B.P. 1968. $C_{13}H_{18}Cl$ $N_3O_4S_2$. A non-mercurial diuretic.

Cyclopentolate hydrochloride. B.P. 1968. $C_{17}H_{26}ClNO_3$. A mydriatic and cycloplegic, which acts more quickly, and for a shorter time, than atropine.

Cyclophoria. The form of heterophoria, or latent strabismus, in which the deviation of the visual axis is torsional.

Cyclophosphamide. B.P. 1968. C_7H_{15} $Cl_2N_2O_2P,H_2O$. A cytotoxic drug.

Cycloplegia. Paralysis of accommodation.

Cycloplegic. A drug that causes cycloplegia. Pertaining to cycloplegia.

Cyclopropane. B.P. 1968. C_3H_6. An inhalant anaesthetic.

Cycloserine. B.P. 1968. An antibiotic produced by *Streptomyces orchidaceus* or *S. garyphalus*, or obtained by synthesis. It is active against a wide range of gram-positive and gram-negative bacteria, including *Mycobacterium tuberculosis*.

Cyclothiazide. The B.P. Commission approved name for one of the thiazide diuretics.

Cyclothymia. The mental state characterized by swings of mood between elation and depression.

Cyclotron. The apparatus in which relatively heavy positively charged particles are accelerated by an electrical field while being kept in a spiral path by a magnetic field. Its main use is in the production of radioactive isotopes.

Cycrimine. The B.P. Commission approved name for 1-cyclopentyl-1-phenyl-3-piperidinopropan-1-ol. A drug for the treatment of parkinsonism.

Cyesis. Pregnancy.

Cymba conchae. The upper part of the concha of the external ear.

Cyn-, Cyno- (Gk *kyōn:* dog). Prefixes meaning dog-like.

Cynanche. Severe sore throat.

Cynanthropy. A delusion in which the subject believes himself to be a dog and barks like one.

Cynocephalus. A foetus with a head sloping back from the orbits and thereby resembling that of a dog.

Cynophobia. A morbid fear of dogs.

Cyprenorphine. The B.P. Commission approved name for a narcotic antagonizer.

Cyproheptadine hydrochloride. B.P. 1968. $C_{21}H_{22}ClN,1\frac{1}{2}H_2O$. An antihistamine.

Cyrtometer. An instrument for measuring the shape of the chest.

Cyst. A sac or cavity, with a definite wall. **Acquired cyst,** one produced by occlusion of a duct or obstruction to the drainage of an organ of external secretion. **Aneurysmal bone cyst,** a space occupied by thin-walled vascular channels of a cavernous nature, occurring in long bones and vertebrae. **Blood cyst,** a cavity filled with blood, usually occurring in the ovary. **Branchial cyst,** a cyst arising from epithelial cells derived from rudiments of the obliterated 2nd branchial cleft. **Chocolate cyst,** a blood cyst in the ovary in endometriosis. **Congenital cyst,** a cyst developing as a result of some fault in development. **Dental cyst,** a small cavity, containing mucoid material, attached to the root of a carious tooth. **Dentigerous cyst,** a cavity, usually in the mandible, containing the crown of an unerupted tooth. **Dermoid cyst,** a cyst due to sequestration of a piece of skin beneath one of the lines of fusion of various embryonic body processes, and containing hair follicles, sebaceous glands and sweat glands in its walls. **Distension cyst,** a cyst resulting from obstruction to the duct of a secretory gland. **Epidermal cyst,** a small encysted accumulation of horn cells in the corium. A milium. **Fimbrial cyst,** a cyst originating between the abdominal ostium of the Fallopian tube and the ovary. **Follicular cyst,** a distension cyst in an atresic ovarian follicle. **Hydatid cyst,** the cyst that occurs in the encysted stage of infestation with the tapeworm *Echinococcus granulosus.* **Implantation cyst,** a cyst formed in a misplaced portion of epithelium. **Lutein cyst,** a cyst lined with lutein cells, that arises from a corpus luteum. **Mammary cyst,** a retention cyst of one of the larger mammary ducts which becomes distended with milk during the puerperium. A galactocele. **Meibomian cyst,** a chronic inflammatory granuloma of a meibomian gland. A chalazion. **Ovarian cyst,** a cystic tumour of the ovary. **Parovarian cyst,** a cyst arising from the parovarium, which includes Gartner's ducts, Kobelt's tubules, the epoöphoron and the paroöphoron. **Placental cyst,** a small cyst in the chorionic plate of the placenta. **Sebaceous cyst,** a form of sebaceous gland naevi, found most commonly on the scalp. A wen. **Solitary bone cyst,** a cyst at or near the long bone, occurring in children and adolescents. **Synovial cyst,** multilocular cyst of the lateral meniscus of the knee. **Tarsal cyst,** meibomian cyst. **Teratoid cyst,** a dermoid cyst containing foetal remnants. **Theca-lutein cyst,** a cyst of the ovary that occurs in some cases of hydatidiform mole. **Thyroglossal cyst,** a cyst formed in the neck (occasionally the tongue) by persistence of part of the thyroglossal duct.

Cyst-, Cysto- (Gk *kystis:* a sac or bladder). Prefixes signifying association with the urinary bladder, or a cyst.

Cystadenoma. An adenoma containing cyst-like spaces, most common in the ovary.

Cystalgia. Pain in the urinary bladder.

Cystectomy. Surgical excision of the urinary bladder.

Cysteine. An amino-acid, one of the principal sources of sulphur in the diet.

Cystic. Pertaining to a cyst, the urinary bladder, or the gall-bladder. **Cystic fibrosis,** a generalized disease of mucus-secreting glands, found in children. Also known as mucoviscidosis and fibrocystic disease of the pancreas.

Cysticercosis. Infestation with *Cysticercus cellulosae.*

Cysticercus. The larval form of a tapeworm. *C. bovis,* the larva of *Taenia saginata. C. cellulosae,* the larva of *T. solium.*

Cystine. $C_6H_{12}N_2S_2O_4$. An amino-acid, one of the chief sources of sulphur in the diet.

Cystinosis. A disease due to a genetic enzyme defect resulting in the failure of the renal tubules to absorb cystine, with resulting deposition of cystine in the tissues.

Cystinuria. The excretion of cystine in the urine. Cystinosis.

Cystitis. Inflammation of the urinary bladder.

Cystitome. The knife used in opening the capsule of the lens of the eye.

Cystocele. Hernia of the urinary bladder.

Cystogram. An X-ray picture of the urinary bladder.

Cystolithiasis. Stones in the urinary bladder.

Cystometer. An instrument for measuring pressure in the urinary bladder.

Cystoplasty. A plastic operation on the urinary bladder.

Cystosarcoma phyllodes. A giant fibro-adenoma of the breast.

Cystoscope. An instrument for visual examination of the interior of the urinary bladder.

Cystostomy. The formation of a permanent or semi-permanent opening into the urinary bladder.

Cystotome. An instrument for surgical incision of the urinary bladder.

Cystotomy. A surgical incision into the urinary bladder.

Cyt-, Cyto- (Gk *kytos:* a hollow vessel). Prefixes indicating association with a cell.

Cytochrome. One of a group of iron-containing protein pigments, widely distributed in the tissues of plants and animals where they play a fundamental part in the oxidation systems of cells.

Cytodiagnosis. Diagnosis by means of examination of cells in an exudate or the like.

Cytokinesis. Division of the cell body as distinct from the nucleus.

Cytology. The study of the cell.

Cytolysis. Disintegration of cells.

Cytolysosome. The modified lysosome produced by fusion with mitochondria and other cell organelles that have become damaged.

Cytomegalic inclusion disease. Infection with cytomegalovirus, which may occur as an overwhelming neonatal infection in a child who was presumably exposed to intra-uterine infection, or in older age-groups when it may manifest itself as hepatitis, or a condition resembling infectious mononucleosis, or in patients suffering from severe debilitating disease.

Cytomegaloviruses. A group of herpesviruses, affecting man and animals. In man it causes the disease known as cytomegalic inclusion disease. Many of them have a predilection for the salivary glands.

Cytometer. An instrument for counting cells.

Cytomorphosis. The changes cells undergo during development.

Cytopenia. Reduction or lack of cells in the blood.

Cytoplasm. The protoplasm of the cell body.

Cytosis. The passage of particles or globules of liquid into cells.

Cytoskeleton. The structural framework of a cell.

Cytosome. The body of the cell exclusive of the nucleus.

Cytotoxic. Destructive of cells.

Cytotrophoblast. The inner cellular layer of the wall of the blastocyst.

Cytotropic. Having an affinity for cells.

D

Dacry-, Dacryo- (Gk *dakryon:* tear). Prefixes signifying association with tears or the lacrimal duct.

Dacryo-adenitis. Inflammation of the lacrimal gland.

Dacryocystectomy. Surgical excision of the lacrimal sac.

Dacryocystitis. Inflammation of the lacrimal sac.

Dacryocystorhinostomy. The operation of establishing drainage of the lacrimal sac into the nasal cavity.

Dacryops. A cystic swelling of the lacrimal gland due to blockage of a lacrimal duct.

Dactyl-, Dactylo- (Gk *dactylos:* finger). Prefixes indicating association with finger (or toe).

Dactylitis. Inflammation of a finger or toe.

Dactylology. The art of conversing by means of the fingers.

Dacuronium bromide. The B.P. Commission approved name for a neuromuscular blocking agent.

Damp. Moist. Foul air. **Afterdamp,** see Afterdamp. **Black damp,** the stagnant air in old workings and wells, which contains no oxygen. **Choke damp,** black damp. **Fire damp,** a gas which collects in coal mines, consisting largely of methane, which is highly explosive. **Stink damp,** an evil-smelling accumulation of gas, including sulphuretted hydrogen. **White damp,** carbon monoxide.

Dandruff. The white scales cast off from the scalp.

Danthron. The B.P. Commission approved name for 1,8-dihydroxyanthraquinone. A laxative.

Dapsone. B.P. 1968. $C_{12}H_{12}N_2O_2S$. An antibacterial drug that is the major standby in the treatment of leprosy.

Darenorubicin. The B.P. Commission approved name for an anti-tumour antibiotic produced by *Streptomyces caeruleorubidus,* which is proving of value in the treatment of leukaemia.

De- (L *de:* from, away). Prefix meaning away, from.

Dead. Lifeless. Numb.

Deaf. Unable to hear.

Deaf-mute. An individual who is deaf and dumb.

Deafness. Inability to hear. **Adhesive deafness,** deafness due to fibrosis and necrosis of the mucosa, ossicles and ligaments of the middle ear. **Central deafness,** inability to understand the meaning of sound when the external ears, auditory nerves and tracts and nuclei are normal. **Concussion deafness,** deafness caused by a blow on the head without necessarily loss of consciousness or fracture of the skull. **Conductive deafness,** deafness resulting from any interruption to the passage of sound up to and including the stapedo-vestibular joint. **Drug deafness,** deafness induced by drugs. **Industrial deafness,** deafness induced by excessive sound stimulation in any industrial process. **Perceptive deafness,** deafness due to organic lesion in the cochlea, auditory nerve and its central connexions. **Psychogenic deafness,** deafness due to emotional trauma, unaccompanied by any changes in the ears. **Senile deafness,** presbyacusis. **Sensorineural deafness,** perceptive deafness. **Toxic deafness,** deafness induced by infections or toxins.

Deamination. Removal of the amino group, NH_2, from amino-acids.

Deanol. The B.P. Commission approved name for 2-dimethylaminoethanol. A central nervous system stimulant.

Death. The cessation of life.

Debility. Lack of strength or vitality. Languor.

Débridement. Removal of devitalized tissue and accompanying foreign matter from a wound.

Debrisoquine. The B.P. Commission approved name for 2-amidino-1, 2, 3,4-tetrahydroisoquinoline. A hypotensive drug.

Deca- (Gk *deka:* ten). Prefix signifying ten.

Decagram. Ten grammes (equivalent to 154·3 grains).

Decalcification. Loss or removal of calcium salts from bone, teeth, or other calcified tissues.

Decalitre. Ten litres (equivalent to 610·3 cubic inches, or 10 quarts approximately).

Decamethonium iodide. The B.P. Commission approved name for decamethylenedi(trimethyl ammonium iodide). A muscle relaxant.

Decametre. Ten metres.

Decapitation. The process of removing a head.

Decapsulation. Surgical removal of the capsule or sheath of an organ, such as the kidney.

Decay. Decomposition. **Radioactive decay,** the decrease in activity of a radioactive substance due to nuclear disintegration.

Deceleration. Decrease in speed or rate.

Decerebration. The process of removing the brain above the red nucleus.

Deci- (L *decimus:* tenth). Prefix indicating one-tenth.

Decibel. The least intensity of sound at which a given note is heard. One-tenth of a bel. (*Abbreviation:* dB.)

Decidua. The lining membrane of the uterus during pregnancy, which is cast off at birth.

Deciduous. Cast off at maturity: e.g. the teeth of the first dentition.

Decigram. One-tenth of a gramme (equivalent to 1·54 grains).

Decilitre. One-tenth of a litre (equivalent to 0·176 pint).

Decimetre. One-tenth of a metre (equivalent to 3·9 inches). (*Abbreviation:* dm.)

Decimolar. A solution containing the tenth part of the molecular weight of a substance dissolved in one litre of solvent.

Decinormal. A standard solution one-tenth of normal strength. (*Symbol:* N/10.)

Decipara. A woman who has borne ten children.

Declive. The part of the superior surface of the vermis lying immediately behind the fissura prima.

Decoction. A liquid preparation made by boiling vegetable substances with water.

Decompensation. Failure of compensation, as in heart failure.

Decompression. Relief or removal of pressure, as in the prevention or treatment of compressed air illness in divers, and in relieving raised intracranial pressure by trephining.

Decongestive. Relieving congestion. An agent or preparation that relieves congestion.

Decontamination. The freeing of an individual or object of noxious substances such as poison gases.

Decortication. The stripping of the cortex or external layer of an organ or structure.

Decubitus. The attitude or position assumed by a patient in bed. The horizontal position. **Decubitus ulcer,** a bedsore.

Decussate. To cross or intersect.

Decussation. A crossing over, applied particularly to bands of nerve fibres in the brain.

Defaecation. Evacuation of the bowels.

Defatigation. Extreme fatigue or exhaustion.

Defeminization. Loss of the female sex characteristics.

Deferent. Carrying away.

Defervescence. The period, or process, of subsidence of fever.

Defibrillation. The arrest of cardiac fibrillation.

Defibrination. The removal of fibrin from blood.

Defloration. The act of rupturing the hymen.

Deflorescence. Disappearance of the rash in diseases characterized by a skin eruption.

Defluvium. A pulling out, as of the hair.

Degeneration. Deterioration. A retrogressive pathological change in tissues. **Amyloid degeneration,** an extracellular, mesenchymal degeneration affecting basement membranes and perivascular connective tissue. **Fatty degeneration,** deposition of fat globules in the cells. **Hepatolenticular degeneration,** a progressive disease of the nervous system accompanied by cirrhosis of the liver, and due to a disorder of copper metabolism. **Hyaline degeneration,** characterized by the presence in the tissues of hyaline, a variety of collagen. **Hyaline droplet degeneration,** a degenerative change found in the renal tubular epithelium in all conditions of gross proteinuria. **Hydropic degeneration,** cloudy swelling, characterized by vacuolation and swelling of cells due to imbibition of water. **Lardaceous degeneration,** amyloid degeneration. **Mucoid degeneration,** deposition of mucoid material in the mucopolysaccharide ground substance of connective tissue. **Red degeneration,** the red discoloration of uterine fibromas, due to rupture of the blood vessels. **Wallerian degeneration,** the degenerative changes that take place in a nerve fibre beyond its point of severance from its axon. **Waxy degeneration,** amyloid degeneration.

Deglutition. The process of swallowing.

Dehiscence. A splitting or bursting open, applied particularly to wounds.

Dehydration. Removal of water from the body, or the state produced by such removal.

Dehydrocholic acid. The B.P. Commission approved name for 3,7,12-trioxo-5β-cholanic acid. A laxative.

Dehydroemetine. The B.P. Commission approved name for an amoebicide.

Dehydrogenase. An enzyme, one of a series, that plays an essential part in biological oxidation by catalysing the transfer of hydrogen.

Dehyroretinol. Vitamin A_2.

Deliquescence. The process of liquefaction by absorption of moisture from the air.

Delirium. A state of extreme mental and motor excitement, characterized by delusions, incoherent talk and restlessness. **Delirium tremens,** the state of delirium liable to occur in chronic alcoholics (*a*) after a debauch, (*b*) in the presence of an infection, (*c*) on sudden withdrawal of alcohol.

Delouse. To free from infestation with lice.

Delusion. A belief that is not in accordance with fact, and cannot be corrected by an appeal to the reason of the person in question.

Demecarium bromide. The B.P. Commission approved name for a drug for the treatment of glaucoma.

Demecolcine. The B.P. Commission approved name for an antimitotic.

Dementia. The state of mental degeneration, due to organic causes, characterized by impairment of comprehension and memory, emotional instability, and changes in character as manifested, for instance, by indecent behaviour.

Demethychlortetracycline hydrochloride. B.P. 1968. An antibiotic produced by *Streptomyces aureofaciens*, with an antibacterial spectrum comparable with that of tetracycline, but more slowly excreted.

Demi- (L *dimidium:* half). Prefix meaning a half.

Demilune. A crescentic or semilunar body, present, for instance, in the salivary glands.

Demodex. A genus of mites. *Demodex folliculorum,* a species found in the hair follicles and sebaceous glands of man.

Demography. The study of people in relation to their grouping, environment and geographical distribution.

Demulcent. A substance that exerts a soothing influence, such as a mucilage.

Demyelination. The process of destruction of the myelin sheaths of nerves.

Denatonium benzoate. The B.P. Commission approved name for an alcohol denaturant.

Denaturation. The alteration of an organic biological substance, such as protein, resulting in a complete change in its physical properties.

Dendrite. The receptive process of the neuron, usually short and branching.

Dendritic. Relating to a dendrite. Branchlike. **Dendritic ulcer,** an ulcer in the cornea caused by the herpes virus.

Denervation. Removal of the nerves to a part.

Dengue. Breakbone fever. A disease, of the tropics and subtropics, caused by a group B arbovirus transmitted by *Aëdes aegypti,* and characterized by intense pain.

Denidation. Stripping and expulsion of the superficial layer of the uterine mucosa.

Dens. The toothlike body process that projects upwards from the body of the second cervical vertebra. **Dens serotinus,** the wisdom tooth.

Densitometer. An instrument for measuring the density of a liquid.

Density. The ratio of mass to volume.

Dent-, Denti-, Dento- (L *dens:* tooth). Prefixes signifying association with teeth.

Dentalgia. Toothache.

Dentate. Notched or toothed.

Denticle. A projecting, toothlike process. A pulp stone.

Denticulate. Provided with very small toothlike projections.

Dentifrice. A preparation for the cleaning of teeth.

Dentigerous. Containing or bearing teeth.

Dentine. The hard, elastic, yellowish-white, avascular, calcified substance surrounding the pulp and constituting the bulk of the tooth.

Dentinogenesis. The process of the development of dentine. **Dentinogenesis imperfecta,** a hereditary defect of dentine formation.

Dentition. The process of teething. The layout of the teeth in the dental arch.

Denture. A set of teeth.

Denudation. The process of laying bare.

Deodorant. A substance which removes or lessens objectionable odours.

Deontology. The study of medical ethics.

Deoxycholic acid. One of the steroid acids in bile.

Deoxycortone acetate. B.P. 1968. $C_{23}H_{32}O_4$. DOCA. A mineralocorticoid which causes sodium retention and potassium excretion. **Deoxycortone pivalate,** B.P.C. 1968, $C_{26}H_{38}O_4$, a mineralocorticoid with the same action as deoxycortone acetate.

Deoxyribonuclease. An enzyme that catalyses the hydrolysis of ribonucleic acid.

Deoxyribonucleic acid. DNA. A nucleic acid found in the cell nucleus where it forms part of the fundamental genetic material of the chromosome. It is the carrier of genetic information in living cells.

Depersonalization. The state in which a person feels unreal.

Depigmentation. Loss or removal of pigment.

Depilation. The process of destroying or removing hair.

Depressant. Any agent that reduces functional activity.

Depression. A hollow or fossa. An emotional state of dejection and unhappiness.

Depressor. A nerve or muscle that restrains or prevents.

Deprodone. The B.P. Commission approved name for a corticosteroid.

Deptropine. The B.P. Commission approved name for a bronchodilator.

Dequalinium acetate. B.P. 1968. $C_{34}H_{46}N_4O_4$. An antibacterial and antifungal preparation. **Dequalinium chloride,** B.P. 1968, $C_{30}H_{40}Cl_2N_4$, an antifungal and antibacterial agent.

Deradenitis. Inflammation of the glands of the neck.

Dereism. Mental activity when the individual is lost in fantasy.

Derm-, Derma-, Dermato- (Gk *derma, dermatos:* skin). Prefixes signifying association with the skin.

-derm (Gk *derma, dermatos:* skin). Suffix signifying association with the skin.

Dermabrasion. Skin planing. Removal of the superficial layer of the skin by abrasion, used mostly in the treatment of acne scars.

Dermacentor. A genus of ticks. Certain of them can cause tick paralysis and they may be the intermediate hosts of various rickettsial infections, relapsing fevers and viral infections. Tular-

aemia is one of the diseases in which they are vectors.

Dermal. Pertaining to the skin.

Dermanyssus. A genus of mites which afflict birds, including poultry, and cause skin eruptions in man.

Dermatitis. Inflammation of the skin.

Dermatobia. A genus of botflies. *Dermatobia hominis,* the warble fly, a common cause of deep boil-like lesions in animals and man in tropical America.

Dermatofibroma. A firm, hemispherical tumour, most commonly found in the skin of the legs.

Dermatofibrosarcoma protuberans. A locally recurrent form of fibroma of the skin.

Dermatoglyphics. The study of the patterns made by the ridges and crevices of the skin of the hands and the soles of the feet.

Dermatology. The study of the skin and its diseases.

Dermatome. The area of skin supplied by any one spinal nerve.

Dermatomyositis. A disease of unknown cause in which a specific skin eruption is associated with inflammation and atrophy of the muscles.

Dermatophagoides. A genus of mites. *Dermatophagoides pteronyssimus,* a mite living in house dust, which has recently been incriminated in the cause of house dust allergy.

Dermatophytes. The ringworm fungi.

Dermatophytosis. A fungal infection of the skin.

Dermatoplasty. A reparative operation on the skin. Skin grafting.

Dermatorrhexis. A congenital hereditary disorder of connective tissue, characterized by hyperelasticity of the skin and hypermobility of the joints.

Dermatosis. A non-specific term, usually used for groups of skin diseases.

Dermis. The corium.

Dermographia. The condition in which tracings made on the skin leave a distinct swollen reddish mark. Urticaria factitia. Dermographism.

Dermoid. Resembling the skin. **Dermoid cyst,** a developmental cyst due to the sequestration of a piece of skin beneath one of the lines of fusion of various embryonic processes, as at the outer canthus, the side of the nose, the neck and the median raphe of the perineum and scrotum.

Desalination. The removal of salt from a substance or liquid.

Desensitization. The process of removing an individual's sensitivity to a given factor, as in the treatment of allergic conditions.

Deserpidine. The B.P. Commission approved name for a tranquillizer.

Desferrioxamine mesylate. B.P. Addendum 1971. $C_{25}H_{48}N_6O_8,CH_3SO_3H$. A preparation used in the investigation and treatment of haemochromatosis.

Desipramine hydrochloride. B.P. 1968. $C_{18}H_{23}ClN_2$. An antidepressant drug which does not inhibit monoamine oxidase.

Deslanoside. The B.P. Commission approved name for a cardiac glycoside.

Desmosome. Plaque-like thickening in the cells of the stratum spinosum of the epithelium.

Desomorphine. The B.P. Commission approved name for a narcotic analgesic.

Desquamation. Scaling off of the superficial layer of the skin.

Detergent. A cleansing substance. A term which tends to be restricted to surface-active agents which carry either a negative charge (*anionic detergents*) or a positive charge (*cationic detergents*).

Detoxication. The process of removing the toxic factors from micro-organisms or poisons. The lessening of the toxicity of a micro-organism.

Detoxify. Detoxicate.

Detrition. The process of wearing away by friction.

Detritus. Broken down material.

Detrusion. A thrusting down or expulsion.

Detumescence. The subsidence of a swelling.

Deuter-, Deutero-, Deuto- (Gk *deuteros:* second). Prefixes signifying second or secondary.

Deuteranopia. The form of colour blindness in which green vision is defective.

Deutoplasm. The nutritive yolk in the ovum, consisting of fatty droplets, which nourishes the embryo in its early stages.

Deviation. A deflexion or turning away. A variation from the normal. **Angle of deviation,** in ophthalmology the angle which the line joining the object of fixation and the nodal point makes with the visual line. **Conjugate deviation,** movements of the two eyes in which the axes remain parallel. **Primary deviation,** deviation of the squinting eye when the sound eye fixates. **Secondary deviation,** deviation of the visual axis of the sound eye when the squinting eye fixates.

Dexamethasone. B.P. 1968. $C_{22}H_{29}FO_5$. A drug with the same action as cortisone, but in much lower doses.

Dexamphetamine sulphate. B.P. 1968. $C_{18}H_{28}N_2O_4S$. A sympathomimetic drug, with an action comparable with that of amphetamine.

Dextrality. Righthandedness.

Dextran. A polysaccharide used for transfusion purposes. **Dextran 40 injection,** B.P. 1968, a sterile 10 per cent w/v solution in Dextrose injection B.P. (5 per cent w/v) or in Sodium Chloride injection B.P. of dextrans, of average molecular weight—about 40,000, derived from dextrans produced by the fermentation of sucrose by means of a certain strain of *Leuconostoc mesenteroides*. It is used in a wide range of clinical conditions on account of its ability to act as a blood substitute, inhibit red-cell aggregation and lower blood viscosity. **Dextran 110 injection,** B.P. 1968, similar to Dextran 40 injection except that it is made from dextrans of molecular weight around 110,000. It is used intravenously as a blood substitute.

Dextriferron. The B.P. Commission approved name for a colloidal solution of ferric hydroxide in complex with partially hydrolysed dextrin, used in the treatment of iron-deficiency anaemia.

Dextrin. An amorphous, dextrorotatory powder produced by the incomplete hydrolysis of starch.

Dextro- (L *dexter*: right). Prefix signifying right or to the right.

Dextrocardia. Displacement of the heart to the right.

Dextromethorpan hydrobromide. B.P. 1968. $C_{18}H_{26}BrNO,H_2O$. A cough depressant.

Dextromoramide tartrate. B.P. 1968. $C_{29}H_{38}N_2O_8$. A potent analgesic.

Dextropropoxyphene hydrochloride. B.P. 1968. $C_{22}H_{30}ClNO_2$. An analgesic of potency similar to codeine, but neither antitussive nor constipating. **Dextropropoxyphene napsylate,** B.P. 1968, $C_{22}H_{29}NO_2,C_{10}H_8O_3S,H_2O$. A drug with the same action as dextropropoxyphene, but less bitter.

Dextrorphan. The B.P. Commission approved name for a narcotic analgesic.

Dextrose. Glucose. **Dextrose,** B.P. 1968, also known as anhydrous dextrose. **Dextrose injection,** B.P. 1968, a sterile solution of dextrose in Water for injection, B.P. When it is prescribed without any strength being stated, a solution containing 5 per cent w/v shall be dispensed. **Dextrose monohydrate, B.P.** 1968, medicinal glucose, $C_6H_{12}O_6,H_2O$. When glucose is prescribed, dextrose monohydrate shall be prescribed.

Dextrothyroxine. The B.P. approved name for a drug for the treatment of hypercholesterolaemia.

Di- (Gk *dis:* two). Prefix signifying two, twice or double.

Dia- (Gk *dia:* through). Prefix signifying through, across, or apart.

Diabetes insipidus. A disease characterized by polyuria and polydipsia, caused by lack of the anti-diuretic hormone.

Diabetes mellitus. A disorder of metabolism due to lack of insulin, and characterized by hyperglycaemia and usually glycosuria.

Diabetogenic. Causing diabetes mellitus.

Diacetamate. The B.P. Commission approved name for an analgesic.

Diacetylnalorphine. The B.P. Commission approved name for a narcotic analgesic.

Diachylon. Lead plaster.

Diaclasia. A fracture deliberately induced, say, for the correction of a deformity.

Diaclast. An instrument for crushing or perforating the foetal skull.

Diadochokinesia. The ability to make alternating movements, as in flexion and extension of the limbs.

Diagnosis. The art of determining the nature of disease.

Diakinesis. The final stage in the prophase of meiosis, characterized by the uncoiling and slipping apart of the chromosomes.

Dialysis. The process of separating crystalloids from colloids by means of a semipermeable membrane. **Renal dialysis,** the process whereby the functions of a failing kidney can be taken over by a dialysis machine; artificial kidney.

Diameter. The line connecting two opposite points on a circle or circular body, and passing through the centre. **Anteroposterior diameter of the inferior pelvic aperture,** from the apex of the coccyx to the lower part of the symphysis pubis. **Anteroposterior diameter of the obstetric pelvic outlet,** from the tip of the last sacral vertebra to the centre of the lower border of the symphysis pubis. **Conjugate (true conjugate; obstetric conjugate) dia-**

meter, from the lumbosacral angle to the symphysis pubis. **Oblique diameters,** from the iliopectineal eminence to the opposite sacro-iliac joint. **Transverse diameter of the inferior aperture,** the diameter of the widest part of the pelvic aperture. **Transverse diameter of the narrow pelvic plane,** as used in obstetrics, the distance between the ischial spines. **Transverse diameter of the superior pelvic aperture,** the distance between the two farthest apart points on the brim.

Diamorphine hydrochloride. B.P. 1968. $C_{21}H_{29}ClNO_5,H_2O$. Heroin. A drug with an action like morphine, but more potent.

Diampromide. The B.P. Commission approved name for an analgesic.

Diamthazole. The B.P. Commission approved name for 6-(2-diethyl-aminoethoxy)-2-dimethylaminobenzo-thiazole. An antifungal agent.

Diapedesis. Passage of blood complete with its corpuscular elements through the intact capillary wall.

Diaphoresis. Sweating.

Diaphoretic. Inducing sweating. A drug, or any other measure, that induces sweating.

Diaphragm. A disc or septum. The musculo-membranous septum separating the abdominal from the thoracic cavity.

Diaphysectomy. Surgical removal of part of the shaft of a long bone.

Diaphysis. The shaft of a long bone.

Diaphysitis. Inflammation of the shaft of a long bone.

Diarrhoea. Excessive evacuation of the bowels.

Diaschisis. The shock or disturbance that accompanies a cerebral lesion.

Diastase. The enzyme produced during the germination of barley in the process of malting, which converts starch into maltose and then dextrose.

Diastasis. Separation of an epiphysis from the shaft of a bone. The period of slower ventricular filling immediately preceding the rise in atrial pressure.

Diastole. Dilatation of the cavities of the heart.

Diathermy. The process whereby high-frequency currents are passed into the body to relieve pain, or to destroy tumours and diseased parts bloodlessly.

Diathesis. The constitution of the body.

Diatrizoic acid. The B.P. Commission

approved name for 3,5-diacetamido-2,4,6-tri-iodobenzoic acid. A radio-opaque substance.

Diazepam. B.P. Addendum 1969. $C_{16}H_{13}ClN_2O$. A tranquillizer.

Diazo- (Gk *dis:* two. Fr *azote:* nitrogen). Prefix signifying a chemical compound with two linked N atoms [$-N_2-$] united to an aromatic group and an acid radical.

Dibenzepin. The B.P. Commission approved name for 4-(2-dimethylaminoethyl)-1,4-dihydro-1-methyl-2,3: 6,7-dibenzo-1,4-diazepin-5-one. An antidepressant.

Dibromopropamidine isethionate. B.P. 1968. $C_{21}H_{30}Br_2N_4O_{10}S_2$. An antibacterial and fungistatic agent for external use.

Dibupyrone. The B.P. Commission approved name for sodium 2, 3-dimethyl -1 -phenyl -5 -pyrazolon -4 -yl - N -isobutylaminomethane sulphonate. An analgesic.

Dicephalus. A two-headed foetal monster.

Dichloralphenazone. B.P. 1968. $C_{15}H_{18}Cl_4N_2O_5$. A complex of chloral hydrate and phenazone. A sedative and hypnotic.

Dichlorodifluoromethane. B.P.C. 1968. CCl_2F_2. A refrigerant and aerosol propellent.

Dichlorophen. B.P. 1968. $C_{13}H_{10}Cl_2O_2$. A taenicide.

Dichlorophenarsine. The B.P. Commission approved name for 3-amino-4-hydroxyphenyldichloroarsine. An antifungal agent.

Dichlorotetrafluoroethane. B.P.C. 1968. $C_2Cl_2F_4$. A refrigerant and aerosol propellent.

Dichloroxylenol. The B.P. Commission approved name for 2,4-dichloro-3, 5-xylenol. A bactericide.

Dichlorphenamide. B.P. 1968. $C_6H_6Cl_2N_2O_4S_2$. A carbonic anhydrase inhibitor used in the treatment of glaucoma.

Dichromium trioxide. The B.P. Commission approved name for a diagnostic marker used in metabolic studies.

Dicophane. B.P. 1968. $C_{14}H_9Cl_5$. DDT. An insecticide and larvicide.

Dicrotism. The condition in which there are two waves to each beat of the pulse.

Dictyoma. A potentially malignant tumour originating from the pars cilaris retina.

Dicyclomine hydrochloride. B.P. 1968. $C_{19}H_{36}ClNO_2$. A drug with a peripheral action similar to, but weaker than, that of atropine.

Didactylism. The congenital condition in which there are only two digits on a hand or foot.

Dieldrin. The B.P. Commission approved name for a widely used chlorinated insecticide.

Diencephalon. The part of the brain consisting of the thalamus, metathalamus, epithalamus and hypothalamus.

Dienoestrol. B.P. 1968. $C_{18}H_{18}O_2$. An oestrogen, whose activity is weaker than that of stilboestrol.

Diet. The food and drink consumed, either naturally, under duress, or under supervision (medical or otherwise).

Dietetics. The study of diets.

Diethadione. The B.P. Commission approved name for 5,5-diethyloxazine-2,4-dione. An analeptic agent.

Diethanolamine fusidate. B.P.C. 1968. The diethanolamine salt of fusidic acid, an antibiotic obtained from *Fusidium coccineum*, and active against gram-positive organisms.

Diethazine. The B.P. Commission approved name for 10-(2-diethylaminoethyl)phenothiazine. An antiparkinsonian drug.

Diethylcarbamazine citrate. B.P. 1968. $C_{16}H_{29}N_3O_8$. A filaricide.

Diethyl phthalate. B.P.C. 1968. $C_{12}H_{14}O_4$. A solvent and plasticizer for cellulose acetate, nitrocellulose and rubber, and a denaturant of alcohol.

Diethylpropion. The B.P. Commission approved name for α-diethylaminopropiophenone. An appetite suppressant.

Diethylthiambutene. The B.P. Comission approved name for a narcotic analgesic.

Diethyltoluamide. The B.P. Commission approved name for NN-diethyl-m-toluamide. An insect repellent.

Diffraction. The bending of a ray of light and breaking it up into its components.

Diffusing. Dispersing. **Diffusing capacity,** the number of millilitres of a gas that can traverse the alveolar membrane of the lungs per minute per millilitre of mercury gradient of pressure across the membrane.

Diffusion. Spreading or dispersion. **Diffusion coefficient,** the volume in millilitres of a gas which will diffuse 0·001mm. distance over a square cm.

of surface per minute at a pressure of 1 atmosphere.

Digestion. The process of breaking down, particularly applied to the process of preparing food for absorption in the alimentary tract.

Digit. A finger or toe.

Digitalis. The dried leaf of *Digitalis purpurea*, the common foxglove. The major drug in the treatment of congestive heart failure and in the control of atrial fibrillation. **Digitalis lanata leaf,** B.P.C. 1968, the dried leaves of *Digitalis lanata*. Used as a source of digoxin and certain other glycosides. **Digitalis leaf,** B.P. 1968, the dried leaves of *Digitalis purpurea* (L.). **Prepared digitalis,** B.P. 1968, digitalis leaf reduced to a powder.

Digitoxin. B.P. 1968. A crystalline glycoside obtained from suitable species of Digitalis. It is the most potent and most cumulative of the digitalis glycosides.

Diglossia. Double or bifid tongue.

Dignathus. A foetal monster with two lower jaws.

Digoxin. B.P. 1968. A crystalline glycoside obtained from the leaves of *Digitalis lanata*. It can be given intravenously or intramuscularly as well as orally.

Dihydrallazine. The B.P. Commission approved name for 1,4-dihydrazinophthalazine. A hypotensive agent.

Dihydrocodeine tartrate. B.P. Addendum 1969. $C_{18}H_{23}NO_3,C_4H_6O_6$. An analgesic and antitussive.

Dihydrostreptomycin. An antibiotic obtained by the hydrogenation of streptomycin, with the properties of streptomycin, but less likely to cause vestibular disturbance and more likely to cause deafness.

Dihydrotachysterol. B.P. 1968. $C_{28}H_{46}O$. A drug with an action comparable with that of calciferol and vitamin D_3.

Di-iodohydroxyquinoline. B.P. 1968. $C_9H_5I_2NO$. An amoebicide.

Di-iodotyrosine. One of the precursors in the thyroid gland of tri-iodothyroxine and thyroxine.

Dilatation. Enlargement or increase in volume of a hollow organ, cavity or tube.

Dilator. An instrument for dilating or stretching an orifice.

Dill oil. B.P.C. 1968. Obtained by distillation from the dried ripe fruits of *Anethum graveolens*(L.). A carminative.

Diloxanide fuorate. B.P. 1968. $C_{14}H_{11}Cl_2NO_4$. An amoebicide.

Diluent. An agent that dilutes or renders less potent.

Dimefline. The B.P. Commission approved name for 8-dimethylaminomethyl-7-methoxy-3-methylflavone. A respiratory stimulant.

Dimenhydrinate. B.P. 1968. $C_{17}H_{21}NO,C_7H_7ClN_4O_2$. An antihistamine.

Dimenoxadole. The B.P. Commission approved name for 2-dimethylaminoethyl 2-ethoxy-2,2-diphenylacetate. A narcotic analgesic.

Dimepheptanol. The B.P. Commission approved name for 6-dimethylamino-4-4,diphenylheptan-3-ol. A narcotic analgesic.

Dimercaprol. B.P. 1968.. $C_3H_8OS_2$ B.A.L. A preparation used in the treatment of acute poisoning by certain metals, including arsenic, gold, and mercury.

Dimethicone. B.P.C. 1968. A water-repellent liquid with low surface tension used in industrial barrier creams.

Dimethindene. The B.P. Commission approved name for 2-{ 1-[2-(2-dimethylaminoethyl)inden-3-yl]ethyl }pyridine. An antihistamine.

Dimethisterone. B.P. 1968. $C_{23}H_{32}O_2$, H_2O. A synthetic progestogen.

Dimethothiazine. The B.P. Commission approved name for 10-(2-dimethylaminopropyl) -2- dimethylsulphamoylphenothiazine. A drug used in the treatment of migraine.

Dimethoxanate. The B.P. Commission approved name for 2-(2-dimethylaminoethoxy) ethyl phenothiazine-10-carboxylate. A cough suppressant.

Dimethyl phthalate. B.P. 1968. $C_{10}H_{10}O_4$. An insect repellent.

Dimethyl sulphoxide. The B.P. Commission approved name for a topical anti-inflammatory agent.

Dimethylthiambutene. The B.P. Commission approved name for 3-dimethylamino-1,1-di- (2-thienyl) but-1-ene. A narcotic analgesic.

Dimethyltubocurarine. The B.P. Commission approved name for a neuromuscular blocking agent.

Dimetria. Double uterus.

Dimorphism. Existing in two different forms.

Dinitro-orthocresol. 2-Methyl-4,6-dinitrophenol. DNOC. A herbicide and insecticide.

Dioctyl sodium sulphosuccinate. B.P.C. 1968. $C_{20}H_{37}NaO_7S$. An anionic surface-active agent used as a laxative.

Diodone injection. B.P. 1968. A contrast medium for use in intravenous and retrograde pyelography and in arteriography.

Dioestrus. The time between two periods of oestrus.

Dioptre. The unit of refractive power of a lens. One dioptre is the refractive power of a lens with a focal distance of one metre.

Dioxamate. The B.P. Commission approved name for 4-carbamoyl-oxymethyl-2-methyl-2-nonyl-1,3-dioxolan. An anti-parkinsonism drug.

Dioxaphetyl butyrate. The B.P. Commission approved name for ethyl 4-morpholino-2,2-diphenylbutyrate. A narcotic analgesic.

Dioxide. A molecule with two oxide atoms.

Dipenine bromide. The B.P. Commission approved name for 2-dicyclopentylacetoxyethyltriethyl ammonium bromide. An antispasmodic.

Dipeptidase. An enzyme in the intestinal juice that splits dipeptides to amino-acids.

Dipeptide. A compound consisting of two amino-acids with a peptide link.

Diperodon. The B.P. Commission approved name for 1,2-di(phenylcarbamoyloxy)-3-piperidinopropane. A local anæsthetic.

Diphemanil methylsulphate. The B.P. Commission approved name for 4-benzhydrylidene-1, 1-dimethylpiperidinium methylsulphate. A parasympitholytic.

Diphenadione. The B.P. Commission approved name for 2-diphenylacetylindane-1,3-dione. An anticoagulant.

Diphenhydramine hydrochloride. B.P. 1968. $C_{17}H_{22}ClNO$. An antihistamine.

Diphenidol. The B.P. Commission approved name for 1, 1-diphenyl-4-piperidinobutan-1-ol. An anti-emetic.

Diphenoxylate hydrochloride. B.P. Addendum 1971. $C_{30}H_{32}N_2O_2HCl$. A drug used in the treatment of diarrhoea.

Diphenylpyraline. The B.P. Commission approved name for 4-benzhydryloxy-1-methylpiperidine. An antihistamine.

Diphtheria. An acute infective disease caused by *Corynebacterium diphtheriae*, and characterized by a membranus exudate, usually in the tonsillar region, and systemic toxic effects. **Diphtheria antitoxin,** B.P. 1968, a preparation containing the antitoxic globulins or their derivatives that have the specific power of neutralizing *C. diphtheriae* toxin, and used for the treatment of, or inducing

passive immunity against, the disease. **Diphtheria vaccine,** B.P. 1968, available in various forms for active immunization against the disease: *Formol Toxoid (F, T)*; *Alum Precipitated Toxoid (A P T)*; *Purified Toxoid Aluminium Phosphate (PTAP)*; *Purified Toxoid Aluminium Hydroxide (PTAH)*; *Toxoid-Antitoxin Floccules (TAF)*. **Diphtheria and pertussis vaccine,** B.P. 1968, used for simultaneous immunization against diphtheria and pertussis or cases in which simultaneous immunization against tetanus is contraindicated. **Diphtheria and tetanus vaccine,** B.P. 1968, used for reinforcing doses for 5-year-old children or for children on school entry. **Diphtheria, tetanus and pertussis vaccine,** B.P. 1968, vaccine of choice for primary immunization. **Diphtheria, tetanus, pertussis and poliomyelitis vaccine,** B.P. 1968, used for active immunization of infants against these four diseases. **Diphtheria, tetanus, and poliomyelitis vaccine,** B.P. 1968, used to reinforce immunization against these three diseases.

Diphtheroid. Resembling diphtheria. **Diphtheroid bacilli,** non-toxigenic corynebacteria.

Diphyllobothrium. A genus of tapeworms. *Diphyllobothrium latum,* the fish tapeworm which infects man and may cause a megaloblastic anaemia.

Dipipanone hydrochloride. B.P. 1968. $C_{24}H_{32}ClNO,H_2O$. A potent analgesic, given intramuscularly.

Diplacusis. Difference of perception of sound in the two ears.

Diplegia. Bilateral paralysis.

Diplo- (Gk *diploos:* double). Prefix signifying double or twofold.

Diplobacillus. A bacillus occurring in pairs.

Diplococcus. A paired coccus. *Diplococcus pneumoniae,* the causative organism of lobar pneumonia. The pneumococcus.

Diploë. The spongy bone between the outer and inner tables of the skull.

Diploid. Having two sets of chromosomes.

Diplopia. Double vision.

Diplotene. The fourth stage of the prophase of the first meiotic division of the sex cells during maturation, in which the homologous chromosomes move apart except at certain points termed the chiasmata.

Diprenorphine. The B.P. Commission approved name for a narcotic analgesic.

Diprophylline. The B.P. Commission approved name for 7-(2,3-dihydroxypropyl)theophylline. A bronchodilator.

Diprosopus. A foetal monster with two faces.

Dipsomania. A morbid craving for alcohol.

Diptera. The order of insects which includes mosquitoes, flies and midges.

Dipygus. A foetal monster with a double pelvis.

Dipyridamole. The B.P. Commission approved name for a coronary vasodilator.

Dipyrone. The B.P. Commission approved name for sodium 2,3-dimethyl-1-phenyl-5-pyrazolon-4-yl-*N* methylaminomethanesulphonate. An analgesic.

Director. A device or instrument that guides.

Dis- (Gk *dis:* two. L *dis:* apart, asunder). Prefix signifying either (*a*) double, or (*b*) reversal or separation.

Disarticulation. Amputation or separation at a joint.

Disc. A flat circular structure. **Articular disc,** a disc of fibrocartilage found in synovial joints. **Intervertebral discs,** the discs interposed between the adjacent surfaces of the bodies of the vertebrae, from the axis to the sacrum, which form the chief bonds of connexion between the vertebrae. **Optic disc,** the area, 1·5mm. in diameter, of the retina pierced by the optic nerve. The centre of the disc is occupied by the central artery and vein of the retina.

Disc-, Disco- (Gk *diskos:* a disc). Prefixes meaning disc-like.

Disciform. Disc-like.

Discission. Tearing apart. Usually used in reference to the operation of removing a cataract by needling.

Discoid. Disc-shaped.

Discus. A disc.

Disease. Illness. A departure from the recognized norm of health. An illness of a specific, defined type, recognizable by its characteristic features. **Addison's disease,** chronic adrenal insufficiency. **Amyloid disease,** amyloidosis. **Banti's disease,** splenic anaemia. **Bornholm disease,** epidemic myalgia. **Caisson disease,** compressed air illness. **Coeliac disease,** a wasting disease of childhood, due to inability to absorb fat from the intestine. **Collagen diseases,** a group of diseases, including rheumatoid arthritis, characterized by changes in the collagen of the tissues. **Communicable disease,** an illness due to a specific infectious agent or its toxic products, which arises through transmission of that agent or its products from a reservoir to a susceptible host, either directly as from an infected person or animal, or indirectly through the agency of an intermediate plant or animal host, a vector, or the inanimate environment. **Fibrocystic disease of the pancreas,** cystic fibrosis; mucoviscidosis. **Foot and mouth disease,** a virus disease of cattle, very occasionally transmitted to man. **Hand, foot and mouth disease,** a mild vesicular skin eruption. **Hartnup disease,** a rare congenital disorder associated with disturbed tryptophane metabolism and characterized by aminoaciduria, pellagra and cerebellar ataxia. **Hodgkin's disease,** lymphadenoma. **Hookworm disease,** ancylostomiasis. **Hydatid disease,** infection with the cyst of *Echinococcus granulosus*. **Menière's disease,** a disease characterized by paroxysmal attacks of labyrinthine vertigo. **Maple syrup urine disease,** an inborn error of metabolism due to disordered metabolism of isoleucine, leucine and valine, and so named because of the characteristic odour of the urine. **Pink disease,** erythroedema. A wasting disease of infants accompanied by a skin rash and photophobia, which has almost disappeared since mercury was withdrawn from so-called teething powders. **Peyronie's disease,** plastic induration of the penis. **Woolsorter's disease,** anthrax. **Veno-occlusive disease of the liver,** an acute type of hepatic vein occlusion due to drinking certain bush teas.

Disinfect. To free from, or destroy, pathogenic micro-organisms.

Disinfectant. An agent capable of destroying pathogenic micro-organisms.

Disinfection. The process of destroying pathogenic micro-organisms.

Disinfestation. The process of destroying insects, parasites, rodents and other forms of vermin that transmit disease.

Dislocation. Displacement of an organ, or part of it. Applied particularly to joints.

Dismemberment. Amputation of an extremity, or part of it.

Disodium edetate. B.P. 1968. $C_{10}H_{14}N_2Na_2O_8,2H_2O$. A chelating agent, used as a decalcifying agent.

Disoma. A double-bodied foetal monster.

Disorientation. The mental state in which the individual is confused as to place, time and identity.

Disparate. Unequal. Not alike.

Dispense. To prepare and distribute medicine.

Dispersion. The act of dissemination of finely divided particles. A colloidal solution.

Displacement. Removal from the normal position. The mental process of attaching to one object painful emotions associated with another object.

Disproportion. A lack of correlation between two associated objects.

Dissect. To separate or cut apart.

Disseminated. Scattered about. **Disseminated sclerosis,** *see* Multiple sclerosis.

Dissociation. Separation. The mental disturbance in which one or more normally associated mental processes become separated from each other.

Dissolution. Disintegration. Breaking up. Death.

Dissolve. To enter into the state of solution.

Distal. Peripheral. Farthest from the centre or mid-line.

Distemper. Indisposition. A name applied to several infectious diseases in animals, particularly the virus infection in dogs known as **canine distemper.**

Distensibility. The capacity for being distended or stretched.

Distension. The act, or state, of being dilated or stretched.

Distichiasis. The state of having a double row of eyelashes.

Distigmine bromide. The B.P. Commission approved name for *NN'*-hexamethylenedi-[1-methyl-3-(methylcarbamoyloxy) pyridinium bromide]. An anticholinesterase.

Distillation. The process of vaporization and subsequent condensation.

Districhiasis. Two hairs growing from a single follicle.

Distrix. Splitting of the distal ends of the hairs.

Disulfiram. The B.P. Commission approved name for tetraethylthiuram disulphide. A drug used in the treatment of alcoholism. It acts by producing a physical aversion to alcohol.

Disulphamide. B.P.C. 1968. $C_7H_9ClN_2O_4S_2$. An oral non-mercurial diuretic.

Dithiazanine. The B.P. Commission approved name for 3,3'-diethylthiadicarbocyanine. An anthelmintic.

Dithranol. B.P. 1968. $C_{14}H_{10}O_3$. A fungicide used in the treatment of ringworm and also psoriasis. **Dithranol ointment,** B.P. 1968, 0·1 per cent of dithranol in yellow soft paraffin. **Dithranol ointment, strong,** B.P. 1968, 1 per cent of dithranol in yellow soft paraffin.

Ditophal. The B.P. Commission approved name for *SS'*-diethyl dithioisophthalate. A drug used in the treatment of leprosy.

Diuresis. The passing of increased amounts of urine.

Diuretic. Inducing diuresis. A drug that produces increased secretion of urine.

Diuria. Frequency of micturition during the day.

Diurnal. Occurring during the day.

Divagation. Incoherence of thought and speech.

Divarication. Separation.

Divergence. A spreading apart.

Diverticular. Relating to a diverticulum.

Diverticulectomy. Surgical removal of a diverticulum.

Diverticulitis. Inflammation of diverticula in the colon.

Diverticulosis. The presence of diverticula in the colon.

Diverticulum. A pouch or pocket leading off a hollow organ. (*Plural:* diverticula.) **Diverticulum ilei (Meckel's diverticulum),** a pouch which projects from the lower part of the ileum in about 2 per cent of people.

Divulsion. The act of rending or pulling apart.

Dizygotic. A twin birth from two separate zygotes.

Dizziness. The sensation resulting from a disturbed relationship of the body to space. Giddiness.

Dodecyl gallate. B.P. 1968. $C_{19}H_{30}O_5$. An antoxidant for preserving oils and fats.

Dodicin. The B.P. Commission approved name for 3,6,9-triazaheneicosanoic acid. A surface active agent.

Dofamium chloride. The B.P. [Commission approved name for an antiseptic.

Dolicho- (Gk *dolichos*: long). Prefix meaning long.

Dolichocephalic. Longheaded, the transverse diameter of the head being less than 75 per cent of the anteroposterior diameter.

Dolichostenomelia. An inherited mesenchymal disorder characterized by disorders of the skeleton, eyes and cardiovascular system.

Dolor. Pain. Anguish.

Dolorimetry. The measurement of pain.

Domiphen bromide. B.P. 1968. A mixture of alkyldimethyl-2-phenoxyethylammonium bromides. An antiseptic with antifungal activity.

Dopa. Dihydroxyphenylalanine, an amino-acid in the adrenal medulla which is decarboxylated by the enzyme, dopa decarboxylase, to dopamine which is a precursor of noradrenaline, adrenaline and melanin.

Dopamine. The B.P. Commission approved name for 2-(3,4-dihydroxyphenyl)ethylamine. A sympathomimetic.

Doraphobia. A morbid fear of touching animal skin or fur.

Dorsi-, Dorso- (L *dorsum:* back). Prefixes indicating relationship to the back or dorsum.

Dorsiflexion. Bending the foot upwards, or extending the toes.

Dorsolateral. Relating to the back and the side.

Dorsum. The back, or the back of any part. (*Plural:* dorsa.) Dorsum linguae, the upper surface of the tongue. Dorsum nasi, the ridge formed by the union of the two lateral surfaces of the nose. Dorsum sellae, the plate of bone forming the posterior boundary of the sella turcica.

Dose. The quantity of a given medicament to be given at one time. **Median effective dose,** the dose calculated to produce a given effect in 50 per cent of the test subjects. (*Abreviation:* ED_{50}.) **Median lethal dose,** the dose relative to weight that will kill 50 per cent of the animals to which it is administered. (*Abbreviation:* LD_{50}.)

Dosimetry. The accurate determination of doses, used particularly in deep X-ray therapy.

Douche. An application of water to the body.

Dowel. A metal pin inserted into a dental root cavity to fix an artificial crown.

Down's syndrome. Mongolism.

Doxapram. The B.P. Commission approved name for 1-ethyl-4-(2-morpholinoethyl) -3,3- diphenyl-2-pyrrolidone. A respiratory stimulant.

Doxycycline hydrochloride, B.P. Addendum 1971. $C_{22}H_{24}N_2O_8$, HCl, $\frac{1}{2}C_2H_5OH,\frac{1}{2}$ H_2O. An antimicrobial substance obtained from oxytetracycline or methacycline. An antibiotic with an action comparable with that of tetracycline.

Doxylamine. The B.P. Commission approved name for 2-[1-(2-dimethylaminoethoxy)-1-phenylethyl]pyridine. An antihistamine.

Drachm. An archaic apothecaries' weight, equivalent to 60 grains. **Fluid drachm,** the comparable liquid measure, equivalent to 60 minims, or one-eighth of a fluid ounce.

Dracontiasis. The disease caused by infection with *Dracunculus medinensis,* the guinea worm found in Africa, Asia, Central and South America.

Dracunculus. A genus of Nematodes belonging to the superfamily Dracunculoidea.

Dragée. A sugar-coated pill.

Drain. An appliance or material to effect drainage from a cavity.

Drastic. A violent purgative.

Draught. A volume of liquid medicine taken in one dose.

Draw-sheet. A narrow sheet placed below a patient's buttocks and covering a rubber sheet.

Drench. A draught of medicine. Usually restricted now to veterinary medicine.

Drepanocyte. A sickle-shaped erythrocyte.

Drepanocytosis. Sickle-cell anaemia.

Dressing. A covering applied to a wound.

Drill. A rotating instrument for making a hole in bone or teeth.

Drip. The continuous slow introduction of a fluid.

Dromo- (Gk *dromos:* a course). Prefix indicating association with conduction or running.

Dromograph. An instrument for recording the velocity of the blood.

Dromomania. An obsession for wandering.

Dromophobia. A morbid fear of running.

Dromotropic. Affecting the conductivity of a nerve fibre.

Droperidol. The B.P. Commission approved name for a neuroleptic.

Dropper. A bottle or teat for the dispensing of a liquid drop by drop.

Dropsy. An abnormal accumulation of fluid beneath the skin or in a body cavity.

Drosophila. A species of Diptera, including the fruit fly, widely used for genetic research.

Drostanolone. The B.P. Commission approved name for an anabolic steroid.

Droxypropine. The B.P. Commission approved name for 1-[2-(2-hydroxyethoxy)ethyl]-4-phenyl - 4 - propionylpiperidine. A cough suppressant.

Drug. A substance used as a medicine.
Duct. A passage or channel. **Alveolar ducts,** the ducts (two to eleven in number) into which each bronchiole divides. **Bellini ducts,** the collecting portion of the renal tubules. **Bile duct,** the duct formed by the junction of the cystic and common hepatic ducts. It is 7·5cm. long and 6mm. wide and terminates in the hepatopancreatic ampulla. **Cochlear duct,** a spirally arranged tube within the bony wall of the cochlea. **Cystic duct,** the duct, 3 to 4cm. long, that links the gall-bladder with the common hepatic duct. **Deferent duct,** the continuation of the duct of the epididymis. **Ejaculatory ducts,** one on each side, formed by the union of the duct of the seminal vesicle with the terminal part of the deferent duct. They are 2cm. long. **Duct of the epididymis,** the duct into which the efferent ductules open; it constitutes the body and tail of the epididymis. **Frontonasal duct,** the duct leading from the frontal sinuses into the nose. **Hepatic ducts,** two ducts which issue from the liver and unite to form the **common hepatic duct** which, 3cm. in length, is joined by the cystic duct to form the bile duct. **Intercalary ducts of the pancreas,** the fine ramifications of the pancreatic duct. **Lacrimal ducts,** the ducts, about twelve in number, that open into the superior conjunctival fornix. **Lactiferous ducts,** the ducts, fifteen to twenty in number, that drain each lobe of the mammary glands. **Lymphatic duct, right,** the duct, about 1cm. in length, that receives the lymph from the right side of the head and neck, the right upper limb, the right side of the thorax, the right lung, the right side of the heart, and part of the convex surface of the liver, and opens into the junction of the right subclavian and right internal jugular veins. **Nasolacrimal duct,** the membranous canal, 18mm. long, which extends from the lacrimal sac to the inferior meatus of the nose. **Pancreatic duct,** the duct that traverses the pancreas and unites with the bile duct to form the hepatopancreatic ampulla and then drains into the duodenum. **Para-urethral ducts,** the two ducts that drain the urethral glands in the wall of the female urethra. **Parotid duct,** the duct, 5cm. long, that drains the parotid gland and enters the mouth opposite the crown of the second upper molar tooth. **Prostatic ducts,** the ducts, twelve to twenty in number, that drain the prostate and open into the prostatic sinus in the floor of the prostatic portion of the urethra. **Semicircular ducts,** the membranous tubes lining the semicircular canals. **Sublingual ducts,** the excretory ducts, eight to twenty in number, that open into the floor of the mouth. **Submandibular duct,** the excretory duct, 5cm. long, of the submandibular gland that opens into the mouth at the side of the frenulum of the tongue. **Thoracic duct,** the duct, 38 to 45cm. long, that drains the greater part of the lymph into the blood stream at the junction of the left subclavian vein with the left internal jugular vein. It begins at the upper end of the cisterna chyli, near the lower border of the twelfth thoracic vertebra. **Thyroglossal duct,** the embryonic connexion between the thyroid gland and the floor of the mouth.

Ductule. A small duct. **Aberrant ductules,** two small tubes sometimes found in the epididymis. **Bile ductules,** the tubules in the liver into which the bile canaliculi flow. **Efferent ductules,** twelve to twenty tubes in the testes, in which the seminiferous tubules terminate. **Transverse ductules of the epoöphoron,** ten to fifteen tubules which constitutes the epoöphoron.

Ductus. Duct. **Ductus arteriosus,** the channel connecting the left pulmonary artery to the aortic arch. **Ductus endolymphaticus,** the duct given off from the posterior part of the saccule, and joined by the ductus utriculosaccularis, which ends in the saccus endolymphaticus. **Ductus reuniens,** the channel through which the cochlear duct communicates with the saccule. **Ductus venosus,** the embryonic vein connecting the umbilical vein and the inferior vena cava.

Dumb. Deprived of the faculty of speech.

Duo- (L *duo:* two). Prefix meaning two.

Duodenectomy. Partial or complete surgical excision of the duodenum.

Duodenitis. Inflammation of the duodenum.

Duodenum. The first part of the small intestine, 25cm. long, stretching from the pylorus to the jejunum.

Duralumin. An alloy of aluminium and copper used in making surgical instruments.

Dura mater. The outer of the three meninges of the brain.

Dusting-powder, absorbable. B.P. 1968. An absorbable powder prepared by treating maize starch and containing up to 2·2 per cent of magnesium oxide. It is used as a lubricant for surgeons' gloves as it is not affected by autoclaving.

Dwarf. An individual of abnormally short stature.

Dwarfism. Abnormal shortness of stature.

Dyad. A pair.

Dydrogesterone, B.P. Addendum 1971. $C_{21}H_{28}O_2$. A progestational steroid.

Dyflos. B.P.C. 1968. $C_6H_{14}FO_3P$. Di-isoprophylfluorophosphonate. DFP. A powerful inhibitor of cholinesterase.

Dynamometer. An instrument for measuring the power of muscular contraction.

Dyne. The force that will accelerate a mass of 1 gramme 1 centimetre per second. (*Abbreviation:* dyn.)

-dynia. (Gk *odynē:* pain). Suffix indicating pain.

Dys- (Gk *dys:* hard, unlucky). Prefix indicating difficult or painful.

Dysacousia. Discomfort or pain in hearing loud or moderately loud sounds.

Dysarthria. Difficulty in articulation.

Dysbasia. Difficulty in walking.

Dysboulia. Impairment of will power.

Dyschezia. Pain or difficulty in passing faeces.

Dyscrasia. An abnormal or diseased constitution.

Dysdiadokokinesia. The inability to perform rapid alternating movements, such as winding a watch.

Dysdipsia. Difficulty in drinking.

Dysenteric. Pertaining to dysentery.

Dysentery. Inflammation of the colon, resulting in the passage of frequent, watery, sometimes bloodstained stools. **Amoebic dysentery,** infection of the colon with *Entamoeba histolytica.* **Bacillary dysentery,** infection of the colon with Shigella. **Ciliate dysentery,** infection of the colon with *Balantidium coli.*

Dysergia. Muscular incoordination due to defective efferent nerve impulses.

Dysgenesis. Defective development.

Dysgeusia. Perverted sense of taste.

Dysgraphia. Inability to write properly. Writer's cramp.

Dyshaemopoiesis. Imperfect formation of blood.

Dysidrosis. A disturbance of sweat secretion. Pompophylx.

Dyskinesia. Impairment of voluntary movement.

Dyslalia. Impairment of speech due to defects in the organs of speech.

Dyslexia. Difficulty in reading or learning to read.

Dyslogia. Impairment of the power of reasoning.

Dysmelia. Malformation of the limbs.

Dysmenorrhoea. Painful menstruation.

Dysorexia. Perverted appetite.

Dysosmia. Defective sense of smell.

Dysotosis. Defective formation of bone. **Craniocleidodystosis,** a rare heredofamilial disorder, characterized by defective development or absence of the clavicles, defective development of the vault and base of the skull, and often absence of the pubic ramus. **Cranio-facial dysotosis,** a heredofamilial condition characterized by deformity of the skull due to absence of one or more of the normal cranial sutures, hypoplasia of the maxilla, a beaked nose and projecting jaw. **Dysotosis multiplex,** an inherited disorder characterized by skeletal deformity, enlargement of liver and spleen, corneal opacity, deafness, mental deficiency and heart disease. **Mandibulo-facial dysotosis,** a congenital condition due to maldevelopment of the first visceral arch and characterized by various abnormalities of the face and jaw.

Dyspareunia. Difficult or painful coitus.

Dyspepsia. Indigestion.

Dysphagia. Difficulty in swallowing.

Dysphasia. Difficulty in speaking due to a central lesion.

Dysphemia. Stammering.

Dysphonia. Impairment of the voice.

Dyspituitarism. Disordered function of the pituitary body.

Dysplasia. Abnormal development of tissue. **Fibrous dysplasia,** an abnormality of body growth accompanied by abnormal proliferation of fibrous tissue.

Dyspnoea. Shortness of breath.

Dyspraxia. Inability to perform co-ordinated movements.

Dysprosium. A rare metallic element. Symbol Dy. Atomic weight 162·50. Atomic number 66.

Dysrythmia. Disordered rhythm.

Dysstasia. Difficulty in standing.

Dystocia. Abnormal labour.

Dystonia. Lack of tone. **Torsion dystonia,** a rare syndrome characterized by involuntary movements producing twisting of the limbs and vertebral column.

Dystrophia.—Dystrophy. Dystrophia adiposogenitalis, a rare condition in children characterized by hypogonadism, obesity, skeletal abnormality and diabetes insipidus, due to dyspituitarism. **Dystrophia myotonica,** a familial disorder characterized by muscular atrophy, and often accompanied by cataract, premature baldness and testicular atrophy.

Dystrophy. Defective nutrition. **Mus-**

cular dystrophy, a genetically determined, primary, degenerative myopathy, which takes various forms: facio-scapulo-humeral type; juvenile scapulo-humeral type; femoral type; pseudohypertrophic type.

Dysuria. Difficulty or pain in micturition.

E

Ear. The organ of hearing. **Cauliflower ear,** the distorted ear resulting from repeated trauma in boxing. **External ear,** the auricle and external acoustic meatus. **Internal ear,** the bony labyrinth and the membranous labyrinth. **Middle ear,** the tympanic cavity, which stretches from the tympanic membrane to the inner ear, and contains the three ossicles.

Earache. Pain in the ear.

Ear-drops. Solutions or suspensions of medicaments in water, glycerin, diluted alcohol, propylene glycol, or other suitable solvent, intended for instillation into the ear.

Ear-drum. Tympanic membrane.

Ear-plug. A device for insertion into the external ear to protect the eardrum from sudden excessive changes of pressure.

Eburnation. Conversion of bone, or dentine, into a hard ivory-like mass.

Ec- (Gk *ek:* from, out of). Prefix meaning out of.

Ecbolic. Producing contraction of the uterus. A drug that acts in this way.

Ecchordoses. Gelatinous nodules, consisting of heterotopic chordal tissue, found projecting from the clivus or dorsum sellae.

Ecchymosis. The discoloured patch produced by extravasation of blood into the subcutaneous tissues. (*Plural:* ecchymoses.)

Eccrine. Excretory. Exocrine.

Eccyesis. Ectopic gestation.

Ecdemic. Neither endemic nor epidemic. Brought in from without.

Ecdemomania. An irrational impulse to wander.

Ecdysiasm. A morbid impulse to undress.

Ecdysis. Desquamation. Moulting.

Echidnin. Snake poison.

Echidnotoxin. A poisonous principle in snake venom.

Echino- (Gk *echinos:* hedgehog). Prefix meaning prickly or spiny.

Echinococcus. A genus of tapeworms. *Echinococcus granulosus,* the parasite of hydatid disease, transmitted to man by the dog, jackal and cat. *Echinococcus multilocularis,* a parasite of hydatid disease transmitted by the fox and tundra mouse.

Echo-acousia. The subjective sensation of hearing a sound repeated as if it were an echo.

Echo-encephalography. A method of neuroradiological examination, using ultrasonic waves.

Echographia. A form of aphasia, in which the individual can write to dictation or can copy writing but cannot express his own thoughts in writing.

Echokinesis. The involuntary repetition of gestures made by another person.

Echolalia. The meaningless repetition of words or phrases spoken by another person.

Echoviruses. A group of around 30 viruses, the name being based on the first letters of their full name: *E*nteric *C*ytopathogenic *H*uman *O*rphan. They are responsible for a range of diseases, including meningitis, respiratory infections and gastro-intestinal infections.

Eclabium. Eversion of the lip.

Eclampsia. The complication of pregnancy characterized by convulsions, proteinuria and hypertension.

Ecmnesia. Loss of memory for recent events.

Ecology. The study of the mutual relationships of living organisms to the environment and to one another.

Ecothiopate iodide. B.P. Addendum 1969. $C_9H_{23}INO_3PS$. An anticholinesterase used in the treatment of glaucoma.

Ecstasy. A morbid condition in which the mind is entirely absorbed in contemplation of one dominant idea or object.

Ectasia. Dilatation of a tubular structure.

Ecthyma. A pustular eruption accompanied by surrounding inflammation.

Ecto- (Gk *ektos:* outside). Prefix indicating on the outside.

Ectocyst. The outer layer of a cyst.

Ectodactylism. Lacking fingers or toes.

Ectoderm. The outer germinal layer of the embryo, from which arise the epidermis and epidermal appendages, the nervous system, the external sense organs, and the mucous membrane of the mouth and anus.

Ectomorphy. The type of body build in which tissues derived from the ectoderm predominate: i.e. linearity and fragility, with relative predominance of skin surface in relation to body mass.

-ectomy (Gk *ektomé:* excision). Suffix indicating surgical removal.

Ectoparasite. A parasite that lives on the surface of its host: e.g. lice.

Ectopia. Congenital displacement of an organ of the body. **Ectopia cordis,** displacement of the heart outside the thoracic cavity. **Ectopia lentis,** congenital dislocation of the lens. **Ectopia testis,** abnormal siting of the testis. **Ectopia vesicae,** extroversion of the bladder.

Ectoplasm. The outer condensation of protoplasm surrounding a cell.

-ectro (Gk *ektrosis:* miscarriage). Prefix denoting congenital absence.

Ectrodactyly. Congenital absence of one or more fingers or toes.

Ectromelia. Congenital absence of a limb or limbs.

Ectropion. Eversion of the eyelid.

Ectylurea. The B.P. Commission approved name for a sedative.

Eczema. The changes induced in the epidermis when some external agent inflames the skin. Starting with erythema this develops into vesication, the cardinal sign of eczema.

Edentia. Absence of teeth.

Edentulous. Toothless.

Edetic acid. The B.P. Commission approved name for ethylenediamine-*NNN′N′*-tetra-acetic acid. A chelating agent.

Edogestrone. The {B.P. Commission approved name for a progestational steroid.

Edrophonium chloride. B.P. 1968. $C_{10}H_{16}ClNO$. An anticholinesterase drug, with an action similar to that of neostigmine methylsulphate.

Effector. A nerve ending which transmits nerve impulses to a muscle or gland.

Efferent. Carrying away. Centrifugal.

Effervescent. Bubbling.

Effleurage. A gentle, stroking movement in massage.

Effluent. A fluid discharge.

Effluvium. An outflowing or shedding.

Effusion. A pouring out of fluid, as into a joint or serous cavity.

Egg. Ovum. The female sexual cell.

Ego. The conscious self.

Eidetic. The power of exact visualization of anything seen or imagined previously. An individual with such ability.

Eikonometer. An instrument for measuring the disparity in size of the retinal image in aniseikonia.

Ejaculation. The sudden ejection or emission of semen. **Premature ejaculation,** emission of semen at the beginning, instead of at the consummation, of coitus.

Elacin. Degenerated elastic tissue.

Elastase. An enzyme from the pancreas (now known as pancreatopeptidase E) that hydrolyses elastin.

Elastin. A scleroprotein, particularly abundant in elastic fibres.

Elastosis. Degeneration of elastic tissue.

Elbow. The joint formed between the humerus above and the radius and ulna below.

Electricity. A form of energy based on the movements of electrons and protons. **Faradic electricity,** that produced by induction. **Galvanic electricity,** that generated by a galvanic cell. **Static electricity,** that induced by friction as in a static machine.

Electro- (Gk *ēlektron:* amber). Prefix indicating relationship to electricity.

Electro-anaesthesia. Anaesthesia induced by electricity.

Electrocardiogram. The record of the variations in electric potential that occur in the heart as it beats. (Abbreviation ECG.)

Electrocardiograph. An instrument for recording an electrocardiogram.

Electrocautery. An instrument for cauterizing the tissues.

Electrocoagulation. The destruction of tissue, or the arrest of haemorrhage, by means of a high frequency current.

Electroconvulsant therapy. The electrical production of convulsions for the treatment of certain mental disturbances, particularly depression. (*Abbreviation:* ECT.)

Electrocution. Death by electricity.

Electrodesiccation. The destruction of small growths by diathermy.

Electroencephalogram. The graphic record of the electrical activity of the brain. (*Abbreviation:* EEG.)

Electroencepalograph. An instrument for recording the electrical activity of the brain.

Electrokymography. The recording by fluoroscopy of the movements of the heart or any other moving structure.

Electrolysis. The decomposition of a chemical compound by the passage through it of an electric current.

Electrolyte. A substance which in solution conducts an electric current and is decomposed by it.

Electromagnet. A temporary magnet with a core of soft iron made by passing an electric current through a surrounding coil of wire.

Electrometer. An instrument for measuring difference in electric potential.

Electromotive. Pertaining to electrical action. **Electromotive force,** the force measured in volts which causes the flow of electricity from one point to another.

Electromyography. The recording of the changes of electric potential in muscle.

Electron. The unit of negative electricity. **Electron capture,** the radioactive decay process whereby a nucleus captures one of its electrons, with the resultant emission of X-rays. **Electron volt,** the kinetic energy acquired by an electron when accelerated through a potential difference of 1 volt.

Electronics. The branch of physics dealing with the behaviour of electrons.

Electronystagmography. The recording of the movements of the eyeball in nystagmus induced by electrical stimulation.

Electro-oculography. A method of recording movements of the eye.

Electrophoresis. The use of electric forces for analytical purposes by means of the migration of charged particles between electrodes.

Electroretinography. A method of measuring changes induced by the stimulation of light in the resting potential of the retina.

Electrostatic. Pertaining to static electricity.

Electrotherapy. Treatment of disease by means of electricity.

Electuary. A soft paste containing drugs mixed with sugar or honey.

Eleidin. A scleroprotein present in the stratum lucidum.

Element. Matter consisting of atoms possessing the same atomic number.

Elephantiasis. A condition characterized by gross chronic enlargement of the cutaneous and subcutaneous tissues as a result of lymphatic obstruction, usually caused by filariasis.

Elevator. A surgical instrument for lifting a depressed part, as of bone.

Elixir. A clear, pleasantly flavoured liquid preparation of potent or nauseous drugs, which may contain a high proportion of alcohol or other solvent such as glycerin or propylene glycol, with sugar or other sweetening agent.

Elliptocyte. An elliptical or oval shaped erythrocyte.

Elliptocytosis. A rare hereditary disease in which the majority of the erythrocytes are elliptocytes and fragile, resulting in haemolytic anaemia.

Eltor vaccine. B.P. Addendum 1969. A sterile suspension of suitable strains of cholera vibrio (*V. cholerae* biotype *el tor*), containing not less than 8000 million bacteria (*V. cholerae* biotype *el tor*) in 1ml.

Elution. The process of separating the constituents of a mixture by means of washing with selective solvents.

Elutriation. A process of separating solids by means of water sifting.

Emaculation. The process of removing spots or blemishes from the skin.

Emanation. That which is given off. Effluvium.

Emasculation. Castration.

Embalm. To preserve a dead body from putrefaction by means of antiseptics and preservatives.

Embolectomy. Surgical removal of an embolus.

Embolism. The sudden blocking of a blood vessel by an embolus. **Air embolism,** an embolism caused by bubbles of air. **Fat embolism,** an embolism caused by globules of fat, usually following a fracture. **Paradoxical embolism,** an embolism caused by an embolus originating in a vein and reaching the systemic circulation through a patent foramen ovale. **Retrograde embolism,** an embolism in which the embolus has gone against the stream.

Embolus. A foreign body that occludes a blood vessel. (*Plural:* emboli.)

Embramine. The B.P. Commission approved name for *N*-2-(4-bromo-α-methylbenzhydryloxy)ethyldimethylamine. An antihistamine.

Embrasure. The space between the sloping proximal surfaces of the teeth.

Embrocation. Liniment.

Embryo. The product of conception up to the eighth week of intra-uterine life.

Embryology. The study of the embryo.

Embryonic. Pertaining to the embryo. Elementary or rudimentary.

Embryotomy. Mutilation of the foetus to

facilitate its removal from the uterus.

Embutramide. The B.P. Commission approved name for N-[2-ethyl-2-(3-methoxyphenyl)butyl]-4-hydroxy-butyramide. A narcotic analgesic.

Emepronium bromide. The B.P. Commission approved name for ethyl-dimethyl-1-methyl-3,3-diphenylpropyl ammonium bromide. An anticholinergic.

Emesis. Vomiting.

Emetic. A drug or other means which produces vomiting.

Emetine and bismuth iodide. B.P. 1968. A complex iodide of emetine and of bismuth, which has an action similar to emetine hydrochloride but has the advantage in oral administration of the emetine not being liberated until it reaches the small intestine.

Emetine hydrochloride. B.P. 1968. $C_{29}H_{42}Cl_2N_2O_4,7H_2O$. An alkaloid derived from ipecacuanha, which is an amoebicide.

Emictory. Diuretic.

Emissary. An outlet or duct. **Emissary veins,** veins connecting the cerebral venous sinuses with the veins of the scalp.

Emission. A discharge. **Nocturnal emission,** involuntary discharge of semen during sleep.

Emmenagogue. A drug or agent that induces menstruation.

Emmetropia. Normal vision.

Emollient. A substance or preparation that has a soothing and softening effect on the skin.

Empathy. Emotional identification with the feelings of another person.

Emphysema. Abnormal presence of air in the tissues. **Emphysema of the lungs,** the condition in which there is distension of the air spaces of the lungs distal to the terminal bronchioles. **Acute interstitial,** or **mediastinal, emphysema,** the condition in which air is present in the stroma of the lungs and in the subpleural connective tissues. **Surgical emphysema,** the condition in which air passes into the subcutaneous tissues following an operation or trauma.

Empirical. Based upon experience.

Emplastrum. A plaster.

Emprosthotonos. The spasm of abdominal muscles in tetanus, making the body arch forwards.

Empyema. The presence of pus in a body cavity, particularly the pleural cavity.

Emulsion. A preparation of two liquid phases, one of which is finely divided and dispersed in the other, the system being stabilized with an emulsifying agent. In pharmaceutical practice the term is restricted to oil-in-water preparations for internal use.

Emunctory. Excretory.

Emylcamate. The B.P. Commission approved name for 1-ethyl-1-methylpropyl carbonate. A tranquillizer and muscle relaxant.

En- (Gk en: in). Prefix meaning in or into.

Enamel. The hard white layer, the hardest tissue in the body, consisting mainly of the mineral phase of bone, that covers the teeth.

Enanthema. An eruption on a mucous membrane.

Enarthrodial. Pertaining to a ball-and-socket joint.

Encapsulated. Enclosed in a capsule.

Encephal-, Encephalo- (Gk enkephalos: brain). Prefixes signifying relationship to the brain.

Encephalalgia. Headache.

Encephalitis. Inflammation of the brain. (Plural: encephalitides). **Acuten encephalitis,** a form that tends to occur as a complication of the acute specific fevers, particularly measles and smallpox. **Encephalitis lethargica,** a form of acute encephalitis probably due to a virus, which is characterized by the lethargy it induces and by its distressing sequelae, such as parkinsonism, oculogyric crises, and mental changes. **Suppurative encephalitis,** cerebral abscess. **Viral encephalitis,** a wide range of geographically separated forms of encephalitis caused by arboviruses and transmitted from animal hosts by mosquitoes, ticks and mites. They include equine encephalitis, Japanese B encephalitis, Murray Valley encephalitis, St. Louis encephalitis, West Nile encephalitis, Russian spring-summer encephalitis, California encephalitis.

Encephalocele. Herniation of brain substance through a congenital or traumatic defect in the skull.

Encephalography. A method of X-raying the brain, using air as a contrast medium, introduced by lumbar or cisternal puncture. **Echo-encephalography,** a method of neuroradiological examination, using ultrasonic waves.

Encephaloid. Resembling brain tissue in appearance. A form of carcinoma with the macroscopic appearance of brain tissue.

Encephalomyelitis. Inflammation of the tissues of the brain and the spinal cord.

Encephalomyelopathy. Any disease of the brain and the spinal cord.

Encephalopathy. Any disease of the brain. **Hypertensive encephalopathy,** the sudden and transient symptoms and signs of cerebral disturbance that occur in some patients with high blood pressure. **Lead encephalopathy,** the manifestations of cerebral disturbance that may occur in lead poisoning. **Wernicke's encephalopathy,** a disturbance of the midbrain and hypothalamus due to deficiency of thiamine.

Enchondroma. A tumour arising from cartilage.

Encopresis. Involuntary passage of faeces.

Encysted. Enclosed in a capsule.

Endarterectomy. Surgical removal of an occluding thrombus or atheromatous plaque from an artery.

Endarteritis. Inflammation of the arterial intima. **Endarteritis obliterans,** an occlusive arterial lesion produced by reactive proliferation of the intima, whereby the lumen of the artery is narrowed by a concentric thickening of the arterial wall.

End-artery. An artery which does not anastomose with other arteries.

Endemic, Occurring in a particular region or community.

Endo- (Gk *endon*: within). Prefix indicating inner or within.

Endocarditis. Inflammation of the endocardium.

Endocardium. The inner endothelial lining of the heart.

Endocervicitis. Inflammation of the mucous membrane of the cervix uteri.

Endocervix. The lining membrane of the cervix uteri.

Endocrine. Pertaining to the internal secretion of a gland, or a gland with an internal secretion.

Endocrinology. The science dealing with endocrine glands and their internal secretions.

Endocyst. The inner layer of a cyst.

Endoderm. Entoderm.

Endogenous. Originating within the organism.

Endolymph. The fluid contained within the membranous labyrinth of the ear.

Endometriosis. The presence of ectopic endometrium in any site outside its normal location: i.e. the lining of the cavity of the uterus.

Endometritis. Inflammation of the lining membrane of the uterus.

Endometrium. The mucous membrane lining the uterus.

Endomorphy. The somatotype, or body build, in which tissue from the endoderm predominates, resulting in a spherical build, with a round head, prominent abdomen, much fat around the thighs or upper arms, but slender ankles and wrists.

Endomyocarditis. Inflammation of the endocardium and the myocardium.

Endomysium. The thin connective-tissue covering of fine collagen fibrils that surrounds individual muscle fibres.

Endoneurium. The connective-tissue covering of individual axons or dendrites.

Endophthalmitis. Inflammation of the internal tissues of the eye.

End-organ. The encapsulated termination of a sensory nerve.

Endoscope. An instrument for the examination of the interior of an organ, viscus or canal.

Endospore. The highly resistant resting phase of certain bacteria such as Clostridium, in which the organism can survive in a dormant state for long periods under most adverse conditions.

Endosteum. The membrane lining the medullary cavity of bone.

Endothelium. The layer of epithelial cells that line the heart, blood vessels and serous cavities.

Endotoxin. A product of bacteria that is injurious to the tissues, in virtue of which disease processes result from bacterial infection, but which, as opposed to an exotoxin, is retained within the bacterial cell until the latter dies and disintegrates.

Endotoxoid. An endotoxin so modified as to be deprived of its toxicity.

Enema. An injection of fluid into the rectum.

Enervation. Weakness. Languor.

Engorgement. Distension with fluid. Congestion.

Enophthalmos. Abnormal retraction of the eye within the orbit.

Enoxolone. The B.P. Commission approved name for 3β-hydroxy-11-oxo-olean-12-en-30-oic acid. An anti-inflammatory and antipruritic agent.

Ensiform. Shaped like a sword.

Entamoeba. A genus of the family, Amoebidae. *Entamoeba histolytica,* the causative organism of amoebiasis; the only pathogenic one found in the human alimentary tract. Other non-pathogenic ones are *Entamoeba coli* and *Entamoeba hartmanii. Entamoeba gingivalis* is a non-pathogenic organism found in the mouth in pathological conditions such as gingivitis and pyorrhoea.

Enter-, Entero- (Gk *enteron:* intestine). Prefixes indicating association with the intestine.

Enteral. Within, or by way of, the intestine.

Enteralgia. Abdominal pain or colic.

Enterectomy. Surgical excision of a part of the intestine.

Enteric. Relating to the intestine. **Enteric-coated,** referring to a tablet so coated that it will not begin disintegrating until it has passed through the stomach into the intestine. **Enteric fever,** typhoid fever.

Enteritis. Inflammation of the intestines.

Enterobacteriaceae. A family of rod-shaped, gram-negative bacteria, which includes Escherichia, Klebsiella, Proteus, Salmonella, and Shigella.

Enterobiasis. Infestation with *Enterobius vermicularis.*

Enterobius. A genus of roundworms. *Enterobius vermicularis,* variously known as the threadworm, pinworm or seatworm, is the commonest intestinal worm in the white races.

Enterocele. An intestinal hernia.

Enterocentesis. Surgical puncture of the intestine.

Enterocolitis. Inflammation of the small intestine and the colon. **Pseudomembranous enterocolitis,** an acute necrosis of the bowel mucosa, involving the ileum and colon.

Enterogastrone. A hormone derived from the mucosal lining of the small intestine which inhibits the movements and secretions of the stomach.

Enterogenous. Pertaining to the intestine. **Entorogenous cyanosis,** methaemoglobinaemia and sulphaemoglobinaemia.

Enterokinase. Enteropeptidase.

Enterolith. A concretion in the intestine.

Enteromycosis. Intestinal disease of fungal origin.

Enteropathy. Disease of the intestine. **Protein-losing enteropathy,** any disease of the gastro-intestinal tract characterized by severe loss of protein from the plasma into the intestine.

Enteropeptidase. The enzyme secreted by the duodenal mucosa that converts trypsinogen into trypsin.

Enteroptosis. Abnormal downward displacement of the intestine.

Enterorrhaphy. Surgical suture of a perforation of the intestine.

Enterospasm. Painful irregular contractions of the intestine.

Enterostomy. Establishment of a permanent opening in the intestine.

Enterotomy. A surgical incision into the intestine.

Enterotoxin. A toxin specific to the cells of the intestinal mucosa: such a toxin produced by *Staph. aureus* is a common cause of food poisoning.

Enteroviruses. A group of viruses which multiply within the cells of the intestinal tract. They include the poliovirus subgroup, the echoviruses and the Coxsackie viruses.

Entoderm. The innermost of the three germinal layers of the embryo.

Entomophobia. A morbid fear of insects.

Entropion. Rolling in of the eyelid.

Enucleate. To remove whole or entire, as in the case of a tumour.

Enuresis. The unconscious or involuntary passage of urine. **Nocturnal enuresis,** the passage of urine during sleep.

Enzootic. Pertaining to a disease in animals indigenous in a given area.

Enzyme. A catalyst of living cells.

Eonism. The morbid desire to wear the clothes of the opposite sex.

Eosin. The potassium or sodium salts of tetrabromofluorescein, used as a staining material in histology and haematology, and as a colouring matter in pharmacy.

Eosinopenia. A relative lack of eosinophil leucocytes in the blood.

Eosinophil. A cell, the granules of which have an affinity for eosin.

Eosinophilia. An increase in the number of eosinophils in the blood.

Epactal. Supernumerary.

Eparterial. Over or on an artery.

Ependyma. The lining membrane of the cerebral ventricles and the spinal canal.

Ependymoma. A tumour, usually found in the 4th ventricle, in which the spaces are lined by ependymal cells.

Ephebiatrics. The branch of medicine concerned with the care of the adolescent.

Ephebology. The study of puberty.

Ephelis. A freckle. (*Plural:* ephelides.)

Ephedrine. B.P.C. 1968. $C_{10}H_{15}NO$, $\frac{1}{2}H_2O$. An alkaloid obtained from species of Ephedra or prepared synthetically. It is a sympathomimetic amine which resembles adrenaline and amphetamine in its action and is active orally. It is used in the form **Ephedrine hydrochloride B.P.**

Epi- (Gk *epi:* on). Prefix meaning on or upon.

Epicanthus. The semilunar fold of skin situated above and sometimes covering the inner angle of the eye. It is normal in Mongol races.

Epicardia. The part of the oesophagus that lies between the stomach and the diaphragm.

Epicardium. The visceral layer of the pericardium.

Epicondyle. A prominence on a bone above the condyle.

Epicranium. The scalp.

Epicritic. The term applied to the sensory nerve fibres subserving the finer degrees of sensation of touch, pain, temperature and localization.

Epidemic. Attacking a large number of people in a given area at one time.

Epidemiology. The science dealing with the various factors affecting the incidence of disease.

Epidermis. The outer layer of the skin, consisting of a germinate zone and a horny zone. (*Plural:* epidermides.)

Epidermoid. Resembling, or pertaining to, the skin.

Epidermolysis. Loosening of the epidermis. **Epidermolysis bullosa,** a congenital skin disease characterized by bullous formation.

Epidermophyton. A genus of dermophytes or ringworm fungi. **Epidermophyton floccosum,** the commonest cause of ringworm of the groin and feet.

Epididymectomy. Surgical removal of the epididymis.

Epididymis. The convoluted first part of the efferent duct of the testis. (*Plural:* epididymides.)

Epididymitis. Inflammation of the epididymis.

Epidural. On, or outside, the dura mater.

Epigastric. Referring to the epigastrium.

Epigastrium. The upper middle anatomical region of the abdomen.

Epigastrocele. A hernia in the epigastrium.

Epiglottis. The thin plate of fibrocartilage, covered with mucous membrane that lies at the root of the tongue in front of the glottis.

Epiglottitis. Inflammation of the epiglottis.

Epignathus. A mal-development of the foetus in which the deformed remains of one twin are united to the upper jaw of the other.

Epilation. Removal of a hair by the root.

Epilepsy. A sudden, transient, recurring disturbance of cerebral function, usually characterized by convulsions and loss of consciousness.

Epileptiform. Resembling epilepsy.

Epileptoid. Like epilepsy.

Epileptogenic. Causing an epileptic fit.

Epiloia. Tuberose sclerosis.

Epimysium. The connective tissue sheath surrounding muscle.

Epineural. On the neural arch of a vertebra.

Epineurium. The connective tissue sheath surrounding a nerve.

Epioestriol. The B.P. Commission approved name for oestra-1, 3, 5 (10)-triene-3,16β,17β-triol. An oestrogen.

Epiphenomenon. An unusual event occurring in the course of a disease, and not necessarily associated with the cause of the disease.

Epiphora. Overflowing of tears on to the cheek, due to interference of flow into or through the lacrimal duct.

Epiphysial. To do with an epiphysis.

Epiphysiolysis. Separation of an epiphysis from the shaft of a bone, particularly liable to occur in adolescents at the head of the femur.

Epiphysis. The secondary centre of ossification at each end of a long bone, originally separated from the shaft by an epiphysial plate of cartilage, but ultimately joining up with the shaft at different ages, each of which is characteristic for the bone in question.

Epiphysitis. Inflammation of an epiphysis.

Epiplo- (Gk *epiploon:* omentum). Prefix indicating association with the omentum.

Epiplocele. A hernia containing omentum.

Epiploic. Related to the omentum.

Episcleritis. Inflammation of the deep subconjunctival connective tissue, including the superficial scleral lamellae.

Episiorraphy. Suturing or repair of lacerations of the labia majora or vulva.

Episiotomy. Lateral incision of the vulva at childbirth to prevent undue tearing.

Episo-(Gk *episeion*: region of the pubes). Prefix indicating association with the vulva or pudenda.

Epispadias. A congential deformity in which the urethra opens on the dorsum of the penis.

Epispastic. A blistering agent.

Epistasy. In genetics, the hiding of one hereditary characteristic by another imposed upon it.

Epistaxis. Bleeding from the nose.

Epithalamus. The trigonum habenulae, the pineal body and the posterior commisure.

Epithalaxia. Shedding of the epithelium, particularly that lining the intestine.

Epithelialization. The growth of, or conversion into, epithelium.

Epithelioid. Like epithelium.

Epithelioma. Squamous-cell carcinoma.

Epithelium. The cellular layer that covers the surfaces of the body: the external surface of the skin, the internal surfaces of the digestive, respiratory and urogenital systems, the closed serous cavities, the inner coats of the vessels, the acini and ducts of all excreting and secreting glands, the ventricles of the brain, and the spinal canal. **Ciliated epithelium,** columnar epithelium with hair-like processes or cilia. **Columnar epithelium,** epithelium made up of cylindrical or rod-shaped cells, resembling a palisade. **Corneal epithelium,** the epithelium, generally consisting of five layers, covering the cornea. **Cuboidal epithelium,** short columnar epithelium. **Cylindrical epithelium,** columnar epithelium. **Germinal epithelium,** the layer of cells covering the surface of the ovary. **Pavement epithelium,** epithelium composed of flattened cells of varying shape, usually polygonal. **Pigmented epithelium,** epithelial cells containing pigment granules, as in the retina. **Simple epithelium,** epithelium consisting of a single layer of cells. **Stratified columnar epithelium,** epithelium consisting of superimposed fusiform cells. **Stratified squamous epithelium,** epithelium consisting of several layers of cells. **Transitional epithelium,** epithelium in the ureters and urinary bladder consisting of a superficial layer of large flattened cells lying on a layer of pear-shaped cells.

Epithiazide. The B.P. Commission approved name for 6-chloro-3,4-dihydro - 3 - (2,2,2 - trifluoroethylthiomethyl)-1,2,4-benzothiadiazine-7-sulphonamide 1, 1-dioxide. A diuretic.

Epitope. The specific area of the molecule to which the antigenic specificity of each protein is due.

Epitrichium. The superficial layer of cells in the embryonic ectoderm.

Epituberculosis. One of the forms of primary tuberculous infection in childhood.

Epizootic. A disease affecting a large number of animals simultaneously.

Eponychium. The stratum corneum covering the nail in the embryo. The thin cuticular fold at the base of the nail.

Eponym. The name of a disease, structure, operation or the like, based upon a person's name: e.g. Addison's disease; circle of Willis.

Epulis. A granulomatous swelling of the interdental papilla.

Equi- (L *equus:* equal). Prefix meaning equal.

Equilibrium. Evenly balanced. Poised. In a state of repose.

Equimolar. Containing the same number of molecules.

Equinocavus. *See* Talipes.

Equinovarus. *See* Talipes.

Equinus. *See* Talipes.

Erbium. A rare metallic element. Symbol Er. Atomic weight 167·26. Atomic number 68.

Erectile. Capable of erection.

Erection. The state of erectile tissue when gorged with blood.

Eremophobia. Morbid fear of solitude or desolate places.

Erepsin. A mixture of enzymes, including amino-peptidases, in the intestinal juice, which remove from polypeptides the terminal amino-acid carrying the free amino group, and dipeptidases which convert dipeptides into amino-acids.

Erethism. An abnormal state of excitement or irritation.

Erg. The unit of work or energy, being the work done by a force of one dyne moving over one centimetre.

Ergo- (Gk *ergon:* work). Prefix indicating relationship to work.

Ergograph. An instrument for recording work done in muscular movement.

Ergometrine maleate. B.P. 1968. $C_{23}H_{27}N_3O_6$. A water-soluble alkaloid obtained from ergot or prepared by partial synthesis, which is responsible for the oxytocic activity of aqueous extracts of ergot.

Ergonomics. The science relating to man and his work.

Ergosterol. A sterol found in yeasts and moulds that acts as a precursor of vitamin D_2 or calciferol.

Ergot. B.P.C. 1968. The sclerotium of the fungus *Claviceps purpurea*, which is developed on the ovary of rye. It contains seven isomeric pairs of alkaloids, the important pharmacological ones being ergometrine and ergotamine. **Prepared ergot,** B.P.C. 1968, the standardized preparation of ergot, and the form in which the drug is administered.

Ergotamine tartrate. B.P. 1968. $C_{70}H_{76}N_{10}O_{16}$. One of the alkaloids in ergot. Its main use is in the treatment of migraine.

Ergotism. Poisoning induced by excessive consumption of medicinal preparations of ergot, or of grain contaminated with *Claviceps purpurea.*

Erogenous. Producing sexual excitement.

Erosion. A wearing away.

Erotic. Pertaining to lust or sexual passion.

Eroticism. A condition of sexual excitement.

Eroto- (Gk *eros:* love). Prefix denoting relationship to love or sexual desire.

Errhine. A drug or substance that causes or stimulates nasal discharge.

Eructation. Belching, or the bringing up of wind.

Eruption. A rash or lesion of the skin. A breaking out, as of a tooth.

Erysipelas. An acute infectious disease of the skin, due to *Streptococcus pyogenes.*

Erysipeloid. A disease caused by infection with *Erysipelothrix rhusiopathiae.*

Erysipelothrix. A member of the family Corynebacteriaceae. *E. rhusiopathiae,* the causative organism of swine erysipelas and of erysipeloid in man.

Erythema. Redness of the skin due to hyperaemia. **Erythema ab igne,** a pigmentary network on the legs produced by repeated, continuing exposure to warmth. **Erythema annulare centrifugum,** large annular pinkish-grey lesions that spread slowly in one direction and fade away in another. **Drug erythema,** also known as **fixed erythema,** an eruption due to a drug, particularly a barbiturate. **Erythema induratum,** a condition of dusky, painful, subcutaneous nodules occurring in young women. **Erythema infantum,** or napkin rash, erythema of the napkin area in infants due to infection and/or irritation. **Erythema marginatum,** a circinate erythema on the trunk in children with rheumatic fever. **Erythema multiforme,** a blotchy, bilateral, symmetrical eruption, usually on the back of the hands and forearms, produced by a variety of circulating toxins. **Erythema necro-**

ticans, a condition going on to ulceration or scarring that occurs in lepromatous leprosy. **Erythema nodosum,** painful, tender nodules, usually on the front of the legs, sometimes on the back of the forearms, that occur as an allergic vascular reaction to a blood-borne organism or toxin. **Erythema pernio,** chilblains. A dusky red, circumscribed, intensely itchy swelling of the skin, usually on the fingers or toes. **Rheumatic erythema,** a circinate erythema on the trunk in children with rheumatic fever. Erythema marginatum. **Erythema serpens,** erysipeloid. **Simple erythema,** a transient redness of the skin from physical causes such as heat. **Toxic erythema,** widespread reddening of the skin due to some toxic agent.

Erythematous. Relating to erythema.

Erythism. Redness of the hair accompanied by a ruddy complexion.

Erythr-, Erythro- (Gk *erythros:* red). Prefixes meaning red or redness.

Erythraemia. Polycythaemia vera.

Erythrasma. A reddish-brown macular eruption of the skin due to *Nocardia minutissima.*

Erythroblast. The nucleated precursor of the erythrocyte in the bone marrow.

Erythroblastosis. The presence of erythroblasts in the circulating blood. **Erythroblastosis foetalis,** a haemolytic anaemia in the foetus or new-born infant, due to incompatibility between the child's erythrocytes and the mother's serum. Haemolytic disease of the newborn.

Erythrochromia. Reddish coloration, usually due to blood.

Erythrocyanosis. Bluish-red swellings on the lower limbs of girls due to capillary stasis evoked by exposure to cold. The full title is erythrocyanosis crurum puellarum frigida.

Erythrocyte. The mature, non-nucleated red blood cell. A biconcave disc with an average diameter of $7 \cdot 2\mu$. In a healthy adult the red cell count varies from $4 \cdot 2$ million to $6 \cdot 4$ million per cubic millimetre. The average count is $5 \cdot 5$ million in males and $4 \cdot 8$ million in females.

Erythrocytometer. An instrument for counting erythrocytes.

Erythroderma. An eruption characterized by redness, desquamation, thickening and universal distribution that may be primary or secondary. Erythrodermia. Exfoliative dermatitis.

Erythroedema. Acrodynia. Pink disease.

Erythrogenesis. The formation of erythrocytes. **Erythrogenesis imperfecta,** a form of aplastic anaemia present from birth. Congenital hypoplastic anaemia.

Erythroid. Reddish in colour.

Erythromelalgia. A condition characterized by painful, paroxysmal throbbing and redness of the skin due to excessive dilatation of the blood vessels of the skin in response to heat.

Erythromycin. B.P. 1968. An antibiotic produced by *Streptomyces erythreus*, which has an antibacterial spectrum comparable to that of penicillin but in addition is active against penicillin-resistant staphylococci and Haemophilus species. **Erythromycin estolate,** B.P. 1968, the propionyl ester lauryl sulphate ($C_{52}H_{97}NO_{18}S$) of erythromycin, which has the same antibacterial spectrum, but is absorbed more rapidly, and has a more prolonged action than erythromycin. **Erythromycin ethyl carbonate,** B.P.C. 1968, a salt ($C_{40}H_{71}NO_{15}$) of erythromycin that has the same action and uses, but is less bitter. **Erythromycin stearate,** B.P. 1968, a salt of erythromycin, with the same properties but less bitter.

Erythron. The erythrocyte and all its precursors and the haemopoietic tissue from which they are derived.

Erythrophobia. Morbid fear of red colours, or of blushing.

Erythropoiesis. The formation of erythrocytes.

Erythropoietin. A glycoprotein produced mainly in the kidney that is mainly responsible for erythropoiesis.

Erythropsia. The condition in which objects look red but visual activity is not affected.

Eschar. The dry scab that forms on a burn.

Escharotic. Caustic or corrosive.

Escherichia. A genus of the family Enterobacteriaceae, the members of which are gram-negative motile rods normally resident in the intestine. The main member of the genus is *Escherichia coli.*

Eserine. Physostigmine.

Esophoria. Latent convergent strabismus.

Espundia. Mucocutaneous leishmaniasis as it occurs in South America.

Essence. A solution of volatile oil in rectified spirit.

Essential. Necessary. Idiopathic. **Essential oils,** volatile odorous principles that are soluble in alcohol, but only slightly soluble in water.

Ester. An organic compound from an alcohol and an acid by elimination of water.

Esterase. An enzyme that hydrolyses esters into their constituent acids and alcohols.

Etafedrine. The B.P. Commission approved name for 2-(ethylmethylamino)-1-phenylpropan-1-ol. A bronchodilator.

Ethacrynic acid. B.P. Addendum 1969. $C_{13}H_{12}Cl_2O_4$. An oral diuretic.

Ethambutol hydrochloride. B.P.C. Supplement 1971. $C_{10}H_{26}Cl_2N_2O_2$. An anti-tuberculosis drug.

Ethamivan. B.P.C. 1968. $C_{12}H_{17}NO_3$. A respiratory stimulant.

Ethamsylate. The B.P. Commission approved name for diethylammonium 2,5-dihydroxybenzenesulphonate. A haemostatic.

Ethane. A gaseous hydrocarbon present in illuminating gas.

Ethanolamine. B.P.C. 1968. C_2H_7NO. Combined with oleic acid (Ethanolamine oleate injection B.P.C. 1968), it is given intravenously as a sclerosing agent in the treatment of varicose veins.

Ethchlorvynol. B.P. 1968. C_7H_9ClO. A hypnotic.

Ethebenecid. The B.P. Commission approved name for 4-diethylsulphamoylbenzoic acid. A uricosuric agent.

Ether. An inhalational anaesthetic and a solvent. **Anaesthetic ether,** B.P. 1968, purified diethyl ether, used as a volatile anaesthetic. **Solvent ether,** B.P. 1968, diethyl ether which is used as a solvent for oils and resins, and for cleansing the skin.

Ethiazide. The B.P. Commission approved name for 6-chloro-3-ethyl-3,4-dihydro-1,2,4-benzothiadiazine-7-sulphonamide 1,1-dioxide. A diuretic.

Ethinamate. The B.P. Commission approved name for 1-ethynylcyclohexyl carbamate. A hypnotic.

Ethinyloestradiol. B.P. 1968. $C_{20}H_{24}O_2$. A synthetic oestrogen with the same action as oestradiol.

Ethionamide. B.P. 1968. $C_8H_{10}N_2S$. A tuberculostatic agent.

Ethisterone. B.P. 1968. $C_{21}H_{28}O_2$. A synthetic preparation with an action like that of progesterone.

Ethmoid. The cuboidal bone at the anterior part of the base of the cranium that forms part of the medial walls of the orbits, the nasal septum and the roof and lateral walls of the nasal cavity.

Ethnic. Pertaining to races and their customs.

Ethnology. The study of the origin, distribution and classification of mankind.

Ethoglucid. The B.P. Commission approved name for 1,2:15,16-diepoxy-4,7,10,13-tetraoxahexadecane. A cytotoxic agent.

Ethoheptazine. The B.P. Commission approved name for ethyl-methyl-4-phenylazacycloheptane-4-carboxylate ethylhexahydro-1-methyl-4-phenylazepine-4-carboxylate. An analgesic.

Ethomoxane. The B.P. Commission approved name for 2-butylaminomethyl-8-ethoxy-1,4-benzodioxan. An adrenaline antagonist.

Ethopropazine hydrochloride. B.P. 1968. $C_{19}H_{25}ClN_2S$. An antiparkinsonism drug.

Ethosalamide. The B.P. Commission approved name for 2-(2-ethoxyethoxy) benzamide. An analgesic and antipyretic.

Ethosuximide. B.P. 1968. $C_7H_{11}NO_2$. An anticonvulsant used in the treatment of petit mal.

Ethotoin. B.P. 1968. $C_{11}H_{12}N_2O_2$. An anticonvulsant drug.

Ethybenztropine. The B.P. Commission approved name for 3-benzhydryloxy-8-ethylnortropane. An anticholinergic.

Ethyl. The monovalent, organic radical, C_2H_-.

Ethyl biscoumacetate. B.P.C. 1968. $C_{22}H_{16}O_8$. An oral anticoagulant.

Ethyl chloride. B.P. 1968. C_2H_5Cl. A volatile anaesthetic, which is also used to produce local anaesthesia by virtue of the intense cold it can produce.

Ethyl dibunate. The B.P. Commission approved name for ethyl 2,7-di-t-butylnaphthalenesulphonate. A cough suppressant.

Ethylene. A colourless, inflammable gas used as an inhalation anaesthetic. **Ethylene alcohol,** ethylene glycol. **Ethylene glycol,** a plasticizer and a constituent of anti-freeze solutions. **Ethylene oxide,** a fumigant for foodstuffs and used for gaseous sterilization of dressings.

Ethylenediamine hydrate. B.P. 1968. $C_2H_8N_2,H_2O$. Used in the preparation of aminophylline injection.

Ethylmethylthiambutene. The B.P. Commission approved name for 3-ethylmethylamino-1,1-di-(2-thienyl)but-1-ene. A narcotic analgesic.

Ethylmorphine hydrochloride. B.P.C. 1968. $C_{19}H_{24}ClNO_3,2H_2O$. A preparation that has some of the actions of codeine and morphine but with less depressant action on the respiratory centre.

Ethyloestrenol. The B.P. Commission approved name for 17α-ethyloestr-4-en-17β-ol. An anabolic steroid.

Ethyl oleate. B.P. 1968. $C_{20}H_{38}O_2$. A preparation used as a vehicle in the preparation of injections.

Ethyl pyrophosphate. The B.P. Commission approved name for tetraethyl pyrophosphate. A drug used in the treatment of myasthenia gravis.

Ethynodiol diacetate. B.P. Addendum 1969. $C_{24}H_{32}O_4$. A progestational steroid.

Etiology. The study of the causes of disease.

Etonitazene. The B.P. Commission approved name for a narcotic analgesic.

Etorphine. The B.P. Commission approved name for a narcotic analgesic.

Etoxeridine. The B.P. Commission approved name for a narcotic analgesic.

Etryptamine. The B.P. Commission approved name for 3-(2-aminobutyl)indole. An antidepressant.

Eu- (Gk *eu:* well). Prefix indicating well or good.

Eubacteriales. The order of bacteria which includes most of the bacteria pathogenic to man.

Eucalyptol. B.P.C. 1968. $C_{10}H_{18}O$. A colourless liquid derived from eucalyptus oil, cajuput oil and other oils, which has the same action and uses as eucalyptus oil, but less irritating to mucous membranes.

Eucalyptus oil. B.P. 1968. An oil distilled from species of Eucalyptus. It is used as a counter-irritant, and as a constituent of inhalations and pastilles for upper respiratory throat infections.

Eucatropine. The B.P. Commission approved name for 1,2,2,6-tetramethyl-4-piperidyl mandelate. A mydriatic.

Euchromatin. That part of the interphase nucleus of the chromosome that stains lightly and is relatively rich in nucleic acid.

Eudipsia. Mild thirst.

Eugenics. The science and study of improvement of the human race or any other stock.

Eugenol. B.P. 1968. $C_{10}H_{12}O_2$. An antiseptic and antiputrescent with an action similar to clove oil.

Euglobulin. A plasma globulin which

is soluble in isotonic salt solution but insoluble at low ionic strength or in distilled water.

Eumycetes. Fungi.

Eunuch. A male who has been deprived of his testes.

Eupad. A mixture of equal parts of calcium chloride and boric acid which, when dissolved in water, produces eusol.

Eupepsia. Good digestion.

Euphoria. The state of being, and feeling, in good health.

Euphoriant. A drug or substance that produces a state of exaggerated euphoria.

Euploidy. In genetics, the state of possessing the normal full complement of chromosomes.

Eupraxia. Normal ability to perform coordinated movements.

Europium. A rare element. Symbol Eu. Atomic weight 151·96. Atomic number 63.

Eusol. An antiseptic solution containing equal parts of calcium chloride and boric acid. (*E*dinburgh *U*niversity *S*olution of *L*ime.)

Eustachian tube. The auditory tube, the channel through which the tympanic cavity communicates with the nasal part of the pharynx.

Euthanasia. A quiet, easy death. Putting to death an individual suffering from incurable and/or painful disease.

Euthyroid. Having a normally functioning thyroid gland.

Eutocia. Normal childbirth.

Evagination. An outpouching or protrusion.

Eventration. Protrusion of the abdominal viscera through the abdominal wall.

Evert. To turn out, or inside out.

Evisceration. Removal of internal organs of the body.

Evulsion. Forceful tearing away.

Ex- (Gk *ex:* out of). Prefix signifying without, outside, away from.

Exacerbation. Increase in severity.

Exaltation. An abnormal mental state of self-importance, well-being and ecstasy.

Exanthem. An eruptive fever, such as measles. (*Plural:* exanthemata.)

Excavator. A spoon for scraping out the contents of a cavity.

Excipient. An inert binding agent in a pharmaceutical preparation such as a tablet.

Excision. The surgical removal of an organ or part of it, or tissue.

Excitation. Stimulation.

Excoriation. The superficial destruction of small pieces of the skin or mucous membrane.

Excrement. Waste matter discharged from the body.

Excrescence. An outgrowth from the surface of the body.

Excreta. Waste materials excreted by the body.

Excrete. To eliminate or discharge from the body.

Exenteration. Evisceration.

Exeresis. Surgical excision or removal of an organ, structure or part of it.

Exergonic. In thermodynamics, the term applied to a reaction which proceeds with the liberation of free energy, as opposed to endergonic.

Exflagellation. The process whereby in the stomach of the mosquito the male macrogamete of the malaria parasite protrudes four to eight flagella-like structures.

Exfoliation. Separation in layers of pieces of dead skin or bone.

Exfoliative. Marked by profuse scaling or exfoliation. **Exfoliative dermatitis,** erythroderma.

Exhalation. Expiration. The giving off of gas or vapour.

Exhaustion. Loss of physical and/or mental power. **Heat exhaustion,** the condition produced in hot climates, due usually to the excessive loss of sodium chloride as a result of extreme sweating, due sometimes to defective sweating. **Nervous exhaustion,** a meaningless but useful term to describe the clinical condition induced by the psychological failure of an individual to stand up to some particular stress or strain—usually occupational.

Exhibitionism. Attracting attention to oneself. A form of sexual perversion characterized by the exhibition of the body, particularly the external genitalia in public.

Exhilarant. Mentally stimulating. Anything that produces mental exhilaration.

Exhumation. Disinternment of a body that has been buried.

Existential. Giving priority to total subjective experience, as distinct from underlying forces or causal explanations.

Exitus. Outlet. Death.

Exo- (Gk *exo:* outside). Prefix meaning outside.

Exocrine. Pertaining to a gland that secretes externally, or to the external secretion of a gland.

Exoenzyme. An enzyme that functions outside a cell.

Exoerthrocytic. External to an erythrocyte. Applied particularly to the developmental stage of the malaria parasite in man that takes place in the liver before gaining access to the erythrocytes.

Exogamy. In protozoa, fertilization by conjugation of gametes from different individuals.

Exogenous. Developing or originating from outside.

Exomphalos. Umbilical hernia.

Exonuclease. An enzyme that hydrolyses only the internucleotide bonds located at the ends of the nucleic acids.

Exopeptidase. An enzyme that splits off the terminal amino-acid in the process of protein digestion.

Exophoria. Latent strabismus, or heterophoria, in which the latent deviation is one of divergence.

Exophthalmometer. An instrument for measuring the degree of protrusion of the eye.

Exophthalmos. Abnormal protrusion of the eyeball.

Exoskeleton. In comparative anatomy the hard protecting and supporting structures that develop in association with the skin in some lower animals. In man, the nails and enamel of the teeth are regarded as rudimentary representatives of the exoskeleton.

Exosmosis. Diffusion or osmosis from within outwards.

Exospore. An exogenous spore produced by mycelial bacteria that is separate from the parent cell and is disseminated by air or other means.

Exostosis. An outgrowth from bone. (*Plural:* exostoses.)

Exothermic. A process characterized by the liberation of heat. Relating to the surface heat of the body.

Exotoxin. A toxin that diffuses readily from the living bacteria into the surrounding medium.

Expectorant. Aiding the removal of secretion from the air passage. A drug, [or other means, whereby the removal of bronchial secretions is facilitated.

Expectorate. To spit, or eject, the matter from the air passages.

Expectoration. The matter ejected from the air passages, or the process of ejecting it.

Expiration. Breathing out.

Expire. To breathe out. To die.

Explant. To remove a piece of tissue from the body to an artificial medium or another animal. The tissue so removed.

Exsanguinate. To deprive of blood.

Exsiccation. The process of drying.

Exsufflation. Forced expiration of air from the lungs.

Extension. The process of straightening or stretching, particularly a limb.

Extensor. A muscle that extends.

Exteriorization. The surgical fixation of an internal organ outside the body. Marsupialization.

External. On the outside. Away from the centre, as opposed to internal.

Exteroceptor. A receptor end-organ or a somatic afferent component of the nervous system that responds to stimuli from the external environment.

Extirpation. Total eradication.

Extra- (L *exter:* outward). Prefix denoting outside of, beyond, in addition.

Extract. A preparation containing the active principle of a crude drug, prepared by maceration or percolation with suitable solvents. **Dry extract,** an extract prepared by evaporating the extractive to dryness. **Liquid extract,** the extractive evaporated to a given strength.

Extraction. The process of drawing out. The making of an extract.

Extractor. An instrument for pulling out any foreign body or any natural part. **Vacuum extractor,** an instrument for removing the foetus from the uterus during labour by applying a vacuum to the head of the oncoming child.

Extraneous. Foreign to the body.

Extrapyramidal. The term applied to those descending cerebrospinal tracts that do not participate in the pyramidal system.

Extrasensory. Pertaining to phenomena perceived by means other than the currently recognized means of perception.

Extrasystole. A premature contraction of one or other of the heart chambers. Thus it may be atrial, nodal, or ventricular, depending upon whether it arises in an atrium, the atrioventricular node, or a ventricle. If it rises above the ventricles it may be described as supraventricular. If it occurs without a compensatory pause it is described as interpolated.

Extravasation. The escape of fluid from its containing vessel.

Extremity. A limb.

Extrinsic. Originating outside of a part or organ.

Extroversion. Congenital eversion of an organ, as of the bladder. The turning of an individual's interest to other people and outside things.

Extrovert. A person whose main interests lie outside himself. An outgoing individual.

Extrude. To thrust out.

Exuberant. Excessive proliferation.

Exudation. The process of fluid oozing into the tissues. The substance so exuded.

Eye. The peripheral organ of vision.

Eyeball. Embedded in the fat of the orbit, the eyeball consists of three coats: (i) an outer coat consisting of the sclera behind and the cornea in front, (ii) an intermediate vascular pigmented coat, comprising, from behind forwards, the choroid, ciliary body, and the iris; (iii) an inner nervous coat, the retina. The contents of the eyeball are the aqueous humour, the vitreous body and the lens.

Eyebrow. The arched eminence above the orbit.

Eye-drops. Sterile aqueous or oily solutions or suspensions for instillation into the eyes. They usually contain substances with anaesthetic, anti-inflammatory, antiseptic or mydriatic properties, or substances used for diagnostic purposes.

Eyeground. The fundus of the eye as seen through the ophthalmascope.

Eyelash. One of the short, thick, curved hairs attached to the free edges of the eyelids.

Eyelid. One of the two movable folds placed in front of the eye.

Eye lotion. A sterile aqueous solution which is used undiluted in first-aid or domiciliary treatment. Collyrium.

Eye ointment. A sterile preparation, usually containing a substance with anti-inflammatory, antimicrobial, antiseptic, or mydriatic properties.

Eyepiece. The lens, or series of lenses nearest the eye in an optical instrument such as a microscope or telescope.

Eye teeth. The upper canine teeth.

F

Face. The front of the head from the forehead to the chin.

Facet. A smooth flat surface on a bone or other firm structure.

Facial. Relating to the face. **Facial nerve,** the 7th cranial nerve.

-facient (L *facio:* to make). Suffix indicating that which brings about or makes.

Facies. Countenance, expression or appearance of the face.

Facilitation. The enhancement of excitability in nervous activity.

Factitious. Artificial. Not natural.

Factor. A contributing cause or component. A gene. **Antinuclear factor,** a gamma-globulin factor present in certain sera, particularly in some collagen diseases, whose specific reactivity with, and uptake by, somatic cell nuclei is demonstrated by a fluorescent anti-globulin reagent. (*Abbreviation:* ANF.) **Coagulation factors,** a series of factors that play a part in the coagulation process: *Factor I,* fibrinogen. *Factor II,* prothrombin. *Factor III,* tissue thromboplastin. *Factor IV,* ionized calcium. *Factor V,* proaccelerin. *Factor VII,* proconvertin. *Factor VIII,* antihaemophilic globulin (AHG), antihaemophilic factor (AHF). *Factor IX,* Christmas factor. *Factor X,* Stuart-Power factor. *Factor XI,* plasma thromboplastin antecedent (PTA). *Factor XII,* fibrin stabilizing factor (FSF). **Extrinsic factor,** vitamin B_{12} which in conjunction with the intrinsic factor produces the haemopoietic principle necessary for the maturation of erythrocytes. **Intrinsic factor,** a substance in normal gastric juice essential for the absorption of vitamine B_{12}. **P factor,** the hypothetical, metabolite, probably a polypeptide, with pharmacological properties resembling those of bradykinin, which is the pain-producing factor responsible for stimulating the pain-carrying nerves. **Rh factor,** Rh, or rhesus, antigen (or agglutinogen). **Rheumatoid factor,** a family of globulins of high molecular weight occurring in the serum of patients with rheumatoid arthritis.

Facultative. Optional. Able to live under different conditions. **Facultative anaerobe,** a micro-organism that is able to grow aerobically or anaerobically.

Faecalith. A mass of inspissated intestinal contents.

Faeces. The excretion from the bowels.

Faeculent. Of a faecal character.

Fahrenheit scale. The method of recording temperature, in which 32° corresponds to freezing point (0° Centigrade) and 212° to boiling point (100° Centigrade) at standard atmospheric pressure. (*Abbreviation:* F.)

Faint. Weak. Syncope. Temporary loss of consciousness.

Falciform. Crescentic.

Falx. A sickle-shaped structure. **Falx cerebelli,** the sickle-shaped process of dura mater below the tentorium cerebelli that projects into the posterior cerebellar notch. **Falx cerebri,** the sickle-shaped process of dura mater in the longitudinal fissure between the cerebral hemispheres.

Family. In biological classification the group between an order and a genus. The group of individuals constituted by parents and their offsprings.

Famprofazone. The B.P. Commission approved name for 4-isopropyl-2-methy-3 - [N-methyl- N- (α-methyl-phenyl)aminomethyl]-1-phenyl- 5 -pyrazolone. An analgesic and antipyretic.

Fango. Mud from the hot springs of Ballaglio, Italy, used in the treatment of rheumatic conditions.

Fanthridone. The B.P. Commission approved name for 5-(3-dimethylaminopropyl)phenanthridone. An antidepressant.

Faradism. Induced electricity.

Farcy. A form of glanders.

Farinaceous. Starchy. Derived from cereals.

Farmer's lung. A form of allergic disease of the lungs caused by the inhalation of dust from mouldy hay or straw.

Farnoquinone. The naturally occurring form of vitamin K_1 synthesized by certain micro-organisms in the gut.

Fascia. A sheet of fibro-areolar, membranous tissue, of variable thickness, investing the softer and more delicate organs. (*Plural:* fasciae.) **Anal fascia,** the fascia on the lower surface of the levator ani. **Antebrachial fascia,** the general sheath for the muscles of the forearm. **Axillary fascia,** the fascia lining the floor of the axillary space. **Brachial fascia,** the loose sheath for the muscles of the upper arm. **Buccopharyngeal fascia,** the outer layer of the pharynx. **Cervical fascia, superficial,** a thin lamina investing the platysma. **Cervical fascia, deep,** the fascia that invests the muscles of the neck. **Clavipectoral fascia,** a strong fibrous sheet situated under cover of the clavicular portion of the pectoralis major. **Cremasteric fascia,** the sac-like investment of the cremaster, spermatic cord and testis. **Cribriform fascia,** the portion of the superficial fascia of the thigh covering the saphenous opening. **Deep fascia,** the dense, inelastic membrane which forms sheaths for muscles. **Diaphragmatic fascia,** the fascia lining the under-surface of the diaphragm. **Endothoracic fascia,** the thin layer of areolar tissue outside the costal pleura. **Iliac fascia,** the fascia covering the psoas and the iliacus. **Infraspinate fascia,** the fascia covering the infraspinatus. **Lacrimal fascia,** the fascia that forms the roof and lateral wall of the sulcus containing the lacrimal sac. **Fascia lata,** the deep fascia of the thigh. **Lunate fascia,** the fascia that forms the pudendal canal. **Obturator fascia,** the parietal pelvic fascia covering the pelvic surface of the obturator internus. **Orbital fascia,** the loose lining of the orbit. **Parotid fascia,** the strong layer of fascia that covers the masseter. **Pectoral fascia,** the thin lamina covering the pectoralis major. **Pelvic fascia,** the fasciae of the pelvis which consist of the fascial sheaths of the pelvic muscles, the **parietal pelvic fascia:** and the fascial sheaths of the pelvic viscera, the **visceral pelvic fascia.** **Pharyngobasilar fascia,** the fibrous unit between the mucous and muscular layers of the laryngeal part of the pharynx. **Fascia propria,** the fibrous investment of a femoral hernia. **Rectovesical fascia,** the posterior wall of the prostatic sheath. **Renal fascia,** the fibro-areolar tissue surrounding the kidney and perirenal fat. **External spermatic fascia,** the outermost of the coverings of the spermatic cord and testis. **Internal spermatic fascia,** the prolongation of the transversalis fascia on the spermatic cord in the male and the round ligament of the uterus in the female as they pass through the deep inguinal ring. **Subscapular fascia,** a thin membrane attached to the circumference of the subscapular fossa. **Superficial fascia,** the fascia found immediately under the skin over the entire surface of the body. **Supraspinata fascia,** the lining of the case in which the supraspinatus is contained. **Temporal fascia,** the fascia covering the temporalis. **Thoracolumbar fascia,** the fascia covering the deep muscles of the back of the trunk. **Transversalis fascia,** the thin membrane that lies between the inner surface of the transversus and the extraperitoneal fat.

Fasciculation. Arranged in the form of fasciculi. Involuntary coarse twitching of the muscles.

Fasciculus. A bundle of fibres. (*Plural:* fasciculi.) **Fasciculus circumolivarus pyramidis,** afferent fibres to the corpus pontobulbare. **Fasciculus cuneatus,** afferent fibres in the lateral part of the posterior columns of the spinal cord that arise from spinal ganglia from the 6th thoracic upwards and end in the nucleus cuneatus. **Fasciculus fronto-occipital,** the bundle of arcuate, or association, fibres that runs from the frontal pole of the cerebrum to the occipital and temporal lobes. **Fasciculus gracilis,** the ascending branches of the medial bundle of fibres of the dorsal nerve roots that runs upwards in the posterior funiculus from the lowest limit of the spinal cord, to end in the nucleus gracilis. **Intrafusal fasciculus,** a tendon fasciculus, several of which are found enclosed in the capsule containing a neurotendinous ending of Golgi, found near the junction of tendons with muscles. **Fasciculus lenticularis,** a bundle of efferent nerve fibres that runs from the globus pallidus to the red nucleus. **Longitudinal fasciculus, superior,** the largest of the arcuate fibre bundles, that runs from the frontal region of the cerebrum to the occipital and temporal lobes. **Longitudinal fasciculus, inferior,** the long arcuate fibre bundle that runs from the occipital pole to the temporal lobe. **Olfactory fasciculus,** a slender bundle of fibres that run from the fornix to the parahippocampal gyrus. **Fasciculus proprius,** one of the bundles containing fibres of the intersegmental neurone. **Fasciculus retroflexus,** efferent fibres that run from the habenular nucleus to the interpeduncular nucleus. **Subcallosal fasciculus,** the afferent fibres to the caudate nucleus from the cerebral cortex. **Subthalamic fasciculus,** fibres from the globus pallidus to the subthalamus. **Thalamic fasciculus,** a bundle of nerve fibres that run from the junction of the ansa lenticularis and the fascicularis to the ventral thalamic nuclei. **Uncinate fasciculus,** a trait that connects Broca's area and the gyri on the orbital surface of the frontal lobe with the cortex of the temporal lobe.

Fasciola. A genus of Trematoda or flukes. *Fasciola gigantica*, flukes found in Africa and the Far East, and occasionally found in man. *Fasciola hepatica*, the sheep liver fluke that occasionally infects man.

Fascioliasis. Infestation with *Fasciola hepatica*.

Fasciolopsiasis. Infestation with *Fasciolopsis buskis*, a common infection of pigs and dogs in China and the Orient where it often infects man.

Fasciolopsis. A genus of liver flukes. *Fasciolopsis buski*, the most important member of the genus from the point of view of man.

Fastidium. Distaste for food.

Fastigium. The highest temperature reached in a feverish state.

Fat. Obese. A triglyceride of fatty acids. Each gramme of fat has an energy-producing equivalent of 9·3 Calories. **Brown fat,** a deposit of fat in which the cells contain separate droplets of fat, found, particularly in the interscapular region, in some mammals, particularly those that hibernate. **Fat cell,** a cell containing glycerol esters of oleic, palmitic, and stearic acids, found in some connective tissues, and specially numerous in adipose tissue.

Fatigue. Weariness of mind or body.

Fatty acid. An acid derived from the saturated series of open chain hydrocarbons. **Saturated fatty acids,** a fatty acid, the carbon chain of which

is connected by single bonds. These include palmitic, stearic, and myristic acid. **Unsaturated fatty acid,** a fatty acid, the carbon chain of which has one or more double or triple bonds. They include linoleic acid, linolenic acid, and arachnidonic acid. These three acids are known as **essential fatty acids** because they are essential for the growth of many animals. They are present in large amounts in many vegetable oils.

Fauces. The opening between the mouth and the pharynx.

Favism. An acute haemolytic anaemia due to ingestion of broad beans or contact with their pollen. It is a hereditary disease found mostly in Italy.

Favus. A form of ringworm, common in many parts of the world outside North-west Europe, due to *Tricophyton schölenii*.

Febricula. A slight fever.

Febrifuge. An antipyretic.

Febrile. Characterized by fever.

Fecundation. Impregnation.

Fecundity. Fertility.

Feeblemindedness. Mental defectiveness which, though not amounting to imbecility, is yet so pronounced that care, supervision and control are required for the protection of the affected person or for the protection of others, or, in the case of children, involves disability of mind of such a nature and extent as to render the child incapable of receiving education at school.

Feeding. The act of giving or taking food. **Artificial feeding,** the introduction of food into the body by any means other than by the mouth. The feeding of infants with milk other than that from the mother. **Breast feeding,** the feeding of an infant from the mother's breasts. **Gastrostomy feeding,** the feeding of a patient by means of a tube through a gastrostomy opening. **Infant feeding,** the feeding of an infant which may be either artificial or breast during the first six months of life. **Intragastric feeding,** feeding by means of a thin rubber tube passed through the nose and oesophagus into the stomach. **Intravenous feeding,** feeding by means of a needle or thin polythene tube inserted into a vein. **Jejunostomy feeding,** feeding through an opening in the jejunum. **Parenteral feeding,** feeding by vein or subcutaneously. **Rectal feeding,** feeding through a tube inserted into the rectum. **Subcutaneous feeding,** feeding by means of needles inserted subcutaneously.

Fellatio. The act of taking the penis of another person into the mouth.

Felo-de-se. Suicide.

Felypressin. The B.P. Commission approved name for 2-phenylalanine-8-lysinevasopressin. A vasoconstrictor.

Feminization. The acquisition of female characteristics by the male.

Femoral. Pertaining to the femur or thigh.

Femur. The thigh bone. (*Plural:* femora.)

Fencamfamin. The B.P. Commission approved name for N-ethyl-3-phenylbicyclo[2,2,1]hept-2-ylamine. A central nervous system stimulant and appetite suppressant.

Fenclozic acid. The B.P. Commission approved name for 2-(4-chlorophenyl)thiazol-4-ylacetic acid. An antiinflammatory agent.

Fenestra. A window-like opening. (*Plural:* fenestrae.) **Fenestra cochleae,** an opening in the medial wall of the tympanic cavity into the scala tympani of the cochlea. **Fenestra vestibuli,** an opening leading from the tympanic cavity into the vestibule of the internal ear.

Fenestration. Having openings or fenestrae. The operation for otosclerosis, whereby a new opening is made into the labyrinth of the ear.

Fenfluramine. The B.P. Commission approved name for 2-ethylamino-1-(3-trifluoromethylphenyl)propane. An appetite suppressant.

Fenimide. The B.P. Commission approved name for 3-ethyl-2-methyl-2-phenylsuccinimide. A tranquillizer.

Fennel. B.P.C. 1968. The dried fruits of cultivated plants of *Foeniculum vulgare*. It has a carminative action.

Fenpipramide. The B.P. Commission approved name for 2,2,-diphenyl-4-piperidinobutyramide. A spasmolytic.

Fenpiprane. The B.P. Commission approved name for 1-(3,3-diphenylpropyl)piperidine. A spasmolytic.

Fentanyl. The B.P. Commission approved name for 1-phenethyl-4-(N-propionylanilino)piperidine. A narcotic analgesic.

Fenticlor. The B.P. Commission approved name for di-(5-chloro-2-hydroxyphenyl)sulphide. An antiseptic and fungicide.

Ferment. Undergoing fermentation. An enzyme.

Fermentation. The chemical change induced in organic matter, particularly carbohydrates, by enzymes.

Ferri- (L *ferrum:* iron). Prefix indicating a compound of ferric iron (Fe^{+++}).

Ferric ammonium citrate. B.P. 1968. A complex ammonium ferric citrate, containing not less than $20·5$ per cent and not more than $22·5$ per cent of Fe. Used in the treatment of all forms of anaemia in which there is a deficiency of iron.

Ferric citrate (^{59}Fe) injection. B.P. 1968. A sterile solution containing ^{59}Fe in the ferric state. It is used in the investigation of iron metabolism.

Ferritin. An iron-protein complex consisting of apoferritin, a protein to which iron may readily be bound. It is one of the methods whereby iron is stored in the body.

Ferro- (L *ferrum:* iron). Prefix indicating a compound of ferrous iron (Fe^{++}), or the presence of metallic iron.

Ferrous fumarate. B.P. 1968. $C_4H_2FeO_4$. Used in the treatment of anaemia in which there is lack of iron.

Ferrous gluconate. B.P. 1968. $C_{12}H_{22}FeO_{14},2H_2O$. Used in the treatment of anaemia in which there is lack of iron.

Ferrous succinate. B.P.C. 1968. A basic salt that contains 34 to 36 per cent of Fe, which is said to produce a lower incidence of gastro-intestinal side-effects than other iron salts.

Ferrous sulphate. B.P. 1968. $FeSO_4$, $7H_2O$. The commonly prescribed iron preparation for the treatment of iron-deficiency anaemia. **Dried ferrous, sulphate,** B.P. 1968, ferrous sulphate deprived of part of its water of crystallization.

Fertilization. Impregnation.

Fervescence. Rise in body temperature.

Fester. Suppurate.

Festinant. Accelerating.

Festination. The involuntary quickening of gait seen in certain nervous diseases, notably parkinsonism.

Fetid. Foul smelling.

Fetish. An inanimate object endowed with human or supernatural properties.

Fetishism. The form of perversion in which sexual excitement is aroused by the sight of clothing or the like belonging to the opposite sex.

Fetor. Stench. Offensive odour. **Fetor hepatis,** the offensive odour of the breath in cirrhosis of the liver.

Fetoxylate. The B.P. Commission approved name for 2-phenoxyethyl

1-(3-cyano-3,3-diphenylpropyl)-4-phenylpiperidine-4-carboxylate. A drug for the treatment of diarrhoea.

Fever. A rise in the body temperature above 98·4°F (37°C). A disease in which the body temperature is raised above normal. **Continued fever,** a fever which persists at an approximately steady level for a more or less definite period. **Drug fever,** a fever induced by a drug, often part of a sensitization reaction. **Ephemeral fever,** a mild degree of fever persisting for only a day or two. **Hectic fever,** a wildly fluctuating fever. **Intermittent fever,** a fever which falls to or below normal between paroxysms. **Low fever,** the persisting, resistant slight degree of fever that characterizes many terminal states or states of depression or inanition. **Malignant fever,** the fever occurring in malignant or fatal forms of infection such as typhus fever or yellow fever. **Periodic fever,** a fever in which periods of fever are separated by afebrile periods. **Quartan fever,** fever that recurs every seventy-two hours. **Quotidian fever,** fever that recurs every twenty-four hours. **Rat-bite fever,** an infection with *Spirillum minus* or *Streptobacillus moniliformis*, usually conveyed by the bite of a rat. **Relapsing fever,** a form of continued fever in which after an afebrile period of around a week the temperature shoots up again for a period. **Remittent fever,** a form of fever characterized by periods when the temperature falls to near normal and then rises again. **Tertian fever,** fever that recurs every forty-eight hours. **Undulant fever,** brucellosis. **Yellow fever,** a virus disease endemic in parts of Africa and Central and South America.

Fibr-, Fibro- (L *fibra:* fibre). Prefixes indicating association with fibre.

Fibre. A threadlike structure. **A fibres,** myelinated, somatic, afferent and efferent nerve fibres. **Adrenergic fibres,** nerve fibres that operate by liberating adrenaline and/or noradrenaline. **Afferent fibre,** the fibre of a nerve that carries impulses to the centre from the periphery. **Arcuate fibres, external anterior,** nerve fibres that run from the arcuate nuclei to the inferior cerebellar peduncle. **Arcuate fibres external, posterior,** nerve fibres that run from the accessory cuneate nucleus to the cerebellum. **Arcuate fibres, internal,** nerve fibres that rise in the nucleus gracilis and nucleus cuneatus, and become the medial lemniscus. **Argyrophilic fibres,** a network of fibres in basement membrane. **Association fibres,** nerve fibres in the spinal cord, cerebellum and cerebrum that link up or synapse with neurones without crossing to the opposite side. In the cerebrum they connect gyri with one another. **Autonomic fibres,** nerve fibres of the autonomic nervous system. **B fibres,** myelinated, efferent, preganglionic axons found in autonomic nerves. **Bone fibres,** stout collagen fibres in bone. **C fibres,** unmyelinated nerve fibres, divided into two groups: *s.C group,* efferent postganglionic sympathetic axons; *d.r.C group,* the small unmyelinated afferent axons in peripheral nerve roots and dorsal roots. **Cholinergic fibres,** nerves which liberate an acetylcholine-like transmitter. **Collagen fibres,** the predominant fibres in connective tissue. **Commissural fibres,** fibres in the spinal cord, cerebellum and cerebrum that link up neurones by crossing to the opposite side. **Dentinal fibre,** the protoplasmic prolongation of an odontoblast found in each dentinal tubule. **Efferent fibre,** the fibre of a nerve that carries impulses from the centre to the periphery. **Elastic fibres,** fibres in connective tissue that are easily stretched. **Fusimotor fibres,** a specialized efferent pathway linked with the intrafusal fibres of the muscle spindle. **Intercrural fibres,** curved, tendinous fibres that arch across the lower part of the aponeurosis of the external oblique. **Intrafusal fibres,** the muscle fibres in the muscle (or neuromuscular) spindle. **Lens fibres,** the ribbon-like fibres that make up the laminae of the lens. **Medullated (myelinated) fibres,** nerve fibres with a myelin sheath. **Moss fibres,** the main afferent fibres of the cerebellum. **Muscle fibres,** the fibres of which muscles are made up. **Cardiac muscle fibres,** the fibres of the myocardium, made up of short cylindrical cells which give off side-branches connecting with adjacent fibres. They possess the special characteristic of rhythmic contractile activity. **Striped muscle fibres,** the contractile units of skeletal muscle. **Unstriped muscle fibres,** the contractile units of muscle not under voluntary control. **Nerve fibres,** the constituents of the axon of a nerve. **Neuroglial fibres,** the fibres present in astrocytes. **Non-medullated**

(unmyelinated) fibres, nerve fibres without a myelin sheath. **Perforating fibres of Sharpey,** fibres that bind together the circumferential lamellae in bone. **Postganglionic fibres,** nerve fibres of the autonomic nervous system that constitute the neurones passing from the peripheral ganglia to the effectors. **Preganglionic fibres,** the comparable nerve fibres that rise in the central nervous system and synapse with the postganglionic nerves in the ganglia. **Projection fibres,** nerve fibres that connect the cerebellum or cerebrum with other parts of the brain or spinal cord. **Purkinje fibres,** the modified cardiac muscle fibres concerned with conduction of the cardiac impulse. **Reticular fibres,** the connective tissue fibres found in reticular tissue. **Sustenacular fibres,** the fibres of the supporting framework of the retina. **Zonular fibres,** the fibres of the suspensory ligament of the lens.

Fibril. A fine fibre.

Fibrillar. Relating to fibrils or to twitchings of muscle fibres.

Fibrillation. The formation of fibrils. Rapid twitching of muscle fibrils. **Atrial fibrillation,** a wholly incoordinated state of contraction of the fibrils of the atrial myocardium which leads to a wholly irregular rate of contraction of the ventricles. **Ventricular fibrillation,** a comparable state of affairs in the ventricular myocardium, which is invariably fatal unless it is brought very rapidly under control.

Fibrin. The insoluble protein formed from fibrinogen by the action of thrombin, that forms the basis of a clot. **Fibrin foam,** a dry artificial sponge of human fibrin used as a haemostatic.

Fibrinogen. The soluble protein in the blood that is the precursor of fibrin.

Fibrinogenopenia. A condition characterized by a haemorrhagic tendency with a prolonged coagulation time, due to lack of fibrinogen, Afibrinogenaemia.

Fibrinoid. Resembling fibrin. **Fibrinoid necrosis,** a degenerative change in collagen tissue, so-called because when stained it has the tinctorial properties of fibrin.

Fibrinokinases. Activators of plasminogen, the precursor of plasmin, the enzyme responsible for the lysis of fibrin and fibrinogen. They are found in many tissues as well as the plasma.

Fibrinolysin. An enzyme produced by certain micro-organisms, particularly streptococci, that dissolves fibrin.

Fibrinolysis. The hydrolysis of fibrin by enzyme action.

Fibrinous. Having the properties, or composed, of fibrin.

Fibro-adenoma. An adenoma containing a high proportion of fibrous tissue, predominantly found in the breast.

Fibroblast. A flattened, irregular cell with branching processes concerned with the formation of fibres in connective tissue.

Fibrocartilage. One of the forms of cartilage. **White fibrocartilage,** dense white tissue arranged in bundles with small scattered groups of cartilage cells between the bundles. **Yellow (elastic) fibrocartilage,** a matrix of yellow elastic fibres containing cartilage cells.

Fibrocyst. A cystic lesion surrounded by fibrous tissue.

Fibrocystic. Pertaining to a fibrocyst. **Fibrocystic disease of the pancreas,** a generalized disease of mucus-secreting glands, involving especially the sweat and salivary glands, and the mucus-secreting glands of the lungs and small intestine. Mucoviscidosis.

Fibrocyte. Fibroblast.

Fibrodysplasia. Abnormal development accompanied by excessive development of fibrous tissue. **Fibrodysplasia ossificans progressiva,** a rare disease, characterized by progressive ossification in tendons, ligaments and aponeuroses.

Fibroelastosis. Proliferation of fibrous and elastic tissue. **Endocardial fibroelastosis,** an uncommon congenital disease, characterized by proliferation of endocardial and subendocardial fibrous and elastic tissues.

Fibroepithelial. Association with fibrous tissue and epithelium, or indicating a proliferation of these. **Fibroepithelial polyp,** a soft, fleshy, pedunculated growth found in the neck, axillae and groins of middle-aged women. Skin tag.

Fibroid. Resembling fibrous tissue. A leiomyoma of the uterus.

Fibroma. A benign tumour consisting of circumscribed collections of fibroblasts, interspersed with collagen. **Fibroma durum,** benign hemispherical tumours of the skin, more common in women than men. **Fibroma molle,** a soft pedunculated tumour found in the neck, axillae and groins of middle-aged women.

Fibroplasia. The formation of fibrous tissue.

Fibrosarcoma. An unencapsulated malignant tumour composed of undifferentiated fibroblasts, that infiltrates the surrounding tissues and metastasizes.

Fibrose. To form fibrous tissue.

Fibrosing. The forming of fibrous tissue. **Fibrosing alveolitis,** the condition characterized by thickening of the alveolar wall as a result of excessive deposition of fibrous tissue, leading to interference of oxygen exchange in the lungs.

Fibrosis. Excessive production of fibrous tissue. **Endomyocardial fibrosis,** a common form of heart disease in Central Africa, characterized by increasing fibrosis of the endocardium and myocardium. **Pulmonary fibrosis,** the formation of fibrous tissue in the lungs, whatever the cause.

Fibrositis. The common form of non-articular rheumatism, of unknown etiology and doubtful pathology.

Fibrotic. Characterized by fibrosis.

Fibrous. Composed of tissue produced by fibroblasts.

Fibula. The slender, lateral bone of the leg.

Field. A prescribed area. **Magnetic field,** the sphere of influence of a magnet. **Visual field,** the area of vision with the eye in a fixed position.

Fig. B.P.C. 1968. The dried fruit of *Ficus carica* (L.), used in the form of Compound figs syrup, B.P.C. 1968 as a mild laxative.

Figlu. Abbreviation for Form*I*mino-*GLU*tamic acid. **Figlu test,** a test for vitamin B_{12} deficiency, based upon the amount of formiminoglutamic acid excreted in the urine following a test dose of histidine by mouth.

Filament. A thread-like structure.

Filaria. A filiform nematode, or roundworm, belonging to the superfamily Filaroidea. (*Plural:* filariae.)

Filariasis. Infestation with one or other member of the superfamily Filaroidea.

Filaricide. An agent that kills filariae.

Filarioidea. A superfamily of the Phasmida class of nematodes, or roundworms. It includes the following genera and species affecting man: *Wuchereria bancrofti, Wuchereria malayi, Onchocerca volvulus, Loa loa.*

Filiform. Filamentous.

Filum. A threadlike structure. **Filum terminale,** the non-nervous terminal filament of the spinal cord, about 20 cm. long.

Fimbria. A fringe. (*Plural:* fimbriae.) **Fimbria of the hippocampus,** a flattened band of white nerve fibres which lies above the dentate nucleus and forms the lower border of the choroidal fissure. **Ovarian fimbria,** a deeply grooved process that stretches from the infundibulum of the uterine tube to the tubal end of the ovary. **Fimbriae of the uterine tube,** the series of irregular, threadlike processes in the circumference of the infundibulum of the uterine tube.

Finger. A digit of the hand. **Mallet (baseball, drop) finger,** a deformity in which the terminal phalanx of one of the fingers is fully flexed and partially or completely powerless. **Snapping finger,** stenosing tenosynovitis. **Trigger finger,** snapping finger. **Webbed (fused) finger,** syndactylism.

Finger print. The impression of the pattern on the finger tips or thumb, recorded by inking of the finger tips followed by pressure on a sheet of paper.

Finger stall. A protective covering for the finger. Finger cot.

Firedamp. An explosive mixture of methane and air.

First aid. The emergency treatment administered to tide a patient over until he can be attended to by a qualified practitioner in hospital or elsewhere.

First intention. The term applied to the healing of a wound that takes place under aseptic conditions.

Fission. Splitting or cleaving. Asexual reproduction by division of the body into two or more parts. Splitting of an atomic nucleus.

Fissure. Cleft. Groove. **Anal fissure,** a painful crack or tear of the anus. **Antitragohelicina fissure,** the groove in the auricle that separates the helix from the antihelix. **Cerebellar fissures,** the closely set fissures in the surface of the cerebellum. **Choroid fissure,** the infolding of the choroid plexus of the lateral ventricle. **Choroidal fissure,** the gap in the caudal part of the optic cup, in the embryonic eye. **Horizontal fissure,** the most extensive of the grooves on the developing cerebellum. **Longitudinal cerebral fissure,** the deep median cleft that incompletely separates the cerebral hemispheres. **Oral fissure,** the junction of the upper with the lower lip.

Orbital fissure, inferior, the fissure that separates the inferior and lateral walls of the orbit posteriorly. **Orbital fissure, superior,** the fissure that separates the superior and lateral walls of the orbit and transmits the oculomotor, trochlear and abducent nerves and the terminal branches of the ophthalmic nerve. **Palpebral fissure** the elliptical space between the open eyelids. **Petro-occipital fissure,** the fissure that separates the area of bone in front of the foramen magnum from the petrous part of the temporal bone. **Petrotympanic fissure,** the fissure that lodges the anterior process and anterior ligament of the malleolus. **Postcentral fissure,** the fissure between the alae of the central lobule of the cerebellum and the culmen. **Post-lingual fissure,** the fissure that separates the lingula from the central lobule of the cerebellum. **Postlunate fissure,** the Y-shaped fissure on the upper surface of the middle lobe of the cerebellum. **Postpyramidal fissure,** the fissure that separates the uvula from the pyramid of the cerebellum. **Prepyramidal fissure,** the fissure separating the nodule from the rest of the inferior vermis. **Prima fissure,** the V-shaped fissure on the superior surface of the cerebellum. **Pterygoid fissure,** the angular cleft that separates the two plates of the pterygoid process. **Pterygomaxillary fissure,** the fissure that separates the anterior and medial walls of the infratemporal fossa. **Retrotonsillar fissure,** the deep fissure on the inferior surface of the cerebellar hemisphere, which partially circumscribes the tonsil. **Secunda fissure,** the postpyramidal fissure. **Squamotympanic fissure,** the fissure that separates the medial part of the articular portion of the mandibular fossa from the tympanic part of the temporal bone. **Transverse fissure,** a transverse slit below the splenium of the corpus callosum. **Tympanomastoid fissure,** the fissure between the tympanic part of the temporal bone and the mastoid. **Vestibular fissure,** the narrow fissure between the spiral laminae of the cochlea.

Fistula. An abnormal channel leading from some natural cavity to the exterior or from one such cavity to another (*Plural:* fistulae.) **Anal fistula,** the sequel to an ischiorectal abscess that has burst in two directions, with an external orifice on the skin surface and an internal one in the anal canal. Fistula-in-ano. **Branchial fistula,** an abnormal communication between the tonsillar region of the pharynx and the lower part of the neck, due to failure of the normal obliteration of the cervical sinus. **Bronchial fistula,** an abnormal tract leading from a bronchus to the pleural cavity or to the exterior of the body. **Bronchopleural fistula,** a communication between a bronchus and the pleural cavity, which may occur as a complication of empyema. **Cranico-aural fistula,** a communication between the cranial cavity and the middle ear, usually the result of a head injury. **Cranionasal fistula,** a communication between the cranial cavity and the nasal cavity, usually the result of a head injury. **Duodenal fistula,** a communication between the duodenum and either the exterior (*external duodenal fistula*) or some other viscus, usually the gall-bladder (*internal duodenal fistula*). **Faecal fistula,** a communication between some part of the intestine and either the exterior (*external faecal fistula*) or another viscus (*internal faecal fistula*). **Gastrocolic fistula,** a communication between the stomach and colon, usually a sequel to a gastrojejunal ulcer. **Pancreatic fistula,** a communication between the pancreas and the exterior. **Parotid fistula,** a communication between the parotid gland and the exterior of the face, due usually to a wound or operation, **Salivary duct fistula. Rectovaginal fistula,** an opening between the rectum and the vagina. **Rectovesical fistula,** a communication between the rectum and bladder. **Thyroglossal fistula,** a communication between a cyst in a persisting thyroglossal duct and the exterior of the neck. **Tracheo-oesophageal fistula,** a congenital communication between the trachea and the oesophagus. **Umbilical fistula,** a communication between the abdominal cavity and the exterior, that may be congenital or acquired. **Vesicovaginal fistula,** a communication between either the bladder or a ureter and the vagina.

Fit. A sudden convulsive seizure.

Fixation. The act of fixing or making firm. Loss of mobility in a joint. In histology, the rapid killing of tissues so as to preserve them in as natural a state as possible. In psychiatry, arrest of psychic or emotional development at a premature stage.

Flaccid. Flabby. Soft.

Flagellation. A form of massage by tapping with the fingers. A form of sexual perversion in which erotic pleasure is aroused by being whipped or whipping someone else.

Flagellum. A long, hair-like process. (*Plural:* flagella.)

Flap. A partially detached layer of tissue.

Flare. The area of redness surrounding a point of irritation of the skin.

Flat-foot. The deformity of the foot characterized by flattening of the normal arch of the foot.

Flatulence. The presence of excessive gas in the stomach.

Flatus. Gas in the gastro-intestinal tract.

Flavo- (L *flavus:* yellow). Prefix indicating yellow.

Flavoprotein. One of a group of enzymes, so called because they contain as prosthetic groups either flavin mononucleotide or flavine adenine dinucleotide.

Flea. A member of the order Siphonaptera. *Pulex irritans*, the common flea in man. *Tunga penetrans*, the jigger flea. Xenopsylla, the genus of fleas that include the vectors of plague: e.g. *Xenopsylla cheopis. Ctenocephalides felis*, the cat flea. *Ctenocephalides canis*, the dog flea.

Flesh. The muscular tissue of the body. **Goose flesh,** the roughness of the skin caused by contraction of the arrectores pilorum, produced usually by cold or fright. **Proud flesh,** excessive granulation tissue round a wound or other lesion.

Flex. To bend.

Flexibilitas cerea. The abnormal state, a form of catalepsy, in which the limbs remain in any position into which they are moved.

Fleximeter. An instrument for measuring the degree of flexion in a joint.

Flexure. A bend. Flexion.

Floccillation. The aimless, fitful picking at the bedclothes that may occur in low delirium.

Flocculation. The coalescence and precipitation of the fine particles of the disperse phase in a colloidal system. A test used in bacteriology for the detection and measurement of antigen.

Flocculus. The small, partially detached portion of the cerebellum, lying immediately below the vestibulo-cochlear nerve.

Flooding. Profuse bleeding from the uterus, commonly due to either a miscarriage, excessive menstrual flow or following childbirth.

Florantyrone. The B.P. Commission approved name for 4-(fluoranthen-8-yl)-4-oxobutyric acid. A drug that stimulates the secretion of bile acid.

Floss. Untwisted silk threads.

Flour. The meal produced by the grinding or milling of wheat.

Flow. An issue. **Renal plasma flow,** the amount of plasma flow to the kidney as measured by clearance of certain substances. (*Abbreviation:* RPF.)

Flowmeter. An instrument for measuring the rate of flow of gases or liquids.

Fluanisone. The B.P. Commission approved name for 4-fluoro-γ-[4-(2-methoxyphenyl)piperazin-1-yl] butyrophenone. A neuroleptic.

Fluclorolone acetonide. The B.P. Commission approved name for a corticosteroid.

Flucloxacillin. The B.P. Commission approved name for a semi-synthetic penicillin derived from the 6-amino-penicillanic nucleus, which is acid stable and therefore active when given orally.

Fluctuation. The thrill or wave-like motion induced by tapping with the finger over a fluid-containing cavity with non-rigid walls.

Fludrocortisone acetate. B.P. 1968. $C_{23}H_{31}FO_6$. An orally administered cortcosteroid with powerful glucocorticoid and mineralocorticoid actions.

Flufenamic acid. The B.P. Commission approved name for N-($\alpha\alpha\alpha$-trifluoro-m-tolyl) anthranilic acid. An anti-inflammatory agent.

Flugestone. The B.P. Commission approved name for 9α-fluoro-11β, 17-dihydroxypregn-4-ene-3,20-dione. A progestational steroid.

Fluid. A liquid. Flowing. **Amniotic fluid,** the liquid (1 litre in volume at birth) in the amniotic cavity that provides buoyant support for the foetus. **Cerebrospinal fluid,** the clear, slightly alkaline fluid secreted by the choroid plexuses, which fills the cerebral ventricles and the sub-archnoid space of the cerebrospinal axis. **Synovial fluid,** the lubricating fluid in joints secreted by the synovial membrane. Synovia. **Tissue fluid,** the colourless, watery fluid that occupies the tissue space in areolar and fibro-areolar tissues and the coelomic spaces of the pericardial, pleural and peritoneal sacs.

Fluke. A trematode worm. **Intestinal**

flukes, *Fasicolopsis buski*, *Heterophyes heterophyes*. Liver flukes, *Clonorchis sinensis*, *Fasciola hepatica*, *Opisthorchis viverrini*. Lung fluke, *Paragonimus westermani*.

Flumedroxone. The B.P. Commission approved name for 17α-hydroxy-6α-trifluoromethylpregn-4-ene-3,20-dione. A drug for the treatment of migraine.

Flumethasone. The B.P. Commission approved name for a corticosteroid.

Flumethiazide. The B.P. Commission approved name for 6-trifluoromethyl-1,2,4 - benzothiadiazine - 7 - sulphonamide 1,1-dioxide. A diuretic.

Fluo- (L *fluere:* to flow). Prefix indicating flow. In chemistry, indicating presence of fluorine.

Fluocinolone acetonide. B.P. 1968. $C_{24}H_{30}F_2O_6$. A corticosteroid for topical application.

Fluocortolone hexanoate. B.P. Addendum 1969. $C_{28}H_{39}FO_5$. A corticosteroid for topical application.

Fluocortolone pivalate. B.P. Addendum, 1969. $C_{27}H_{37}FO_5$. A corticosteroid used topically in the treatment of skin diseases.

Fluopromazine. The B.P. Commission approved name for 10-(3-dimethylaminopropyl) 2-trifluoromethylphenothiazine. A tranquillizer.

Fluorescein sodium. B.P. 1968. $C_{20}H_{10}Na_2O_5$. An ophthalmic preparation used in the form of eye-drops for detecting ocular lesions and foreign bodies.

Fluorescence. The property, when illuminated, to radiate unpolarized light of a different wave-length from that of the light absorbed.

Fluoridation. The procedure of adding salts of fluoride to drinking water to bring the concentration of fluorides up to 1 part per million, as a prophylactic measure against dental caries.

Fluorine. One of the halogen series of elements, which is present in bone and teeth. Symbol F. Atomic weight 18·99. Atomic number 9.

Fluorometholone. The B.P. Commission approved name for a corticosteroid.

Fluoroscope. An instrument for rendering X-rays visible after they have passed through the body, by projecting them on a fluorescent screen of calcium tungstate.

Fluorosis. The condition resulting from the excessive intake of fluorine.

Fluorouracil. The B.P. Commission approved name for 5-fluorouracil. An antineoplastic agent.

Fluoxymesterone. B.P. 1968. $C_{20}H_{29}$

FO_3. An androgenic hormone, active by mouth, which is several times more potent than methyltestosterone.

Fluperolone. The B.P. Commission approved name for a corticosteroid.

Fluphenazine hydrochloride. B.P. Addendum 1969. $C_{22}H_{26}F_3N_3OS,2HCl$. A tranquillizer.

Fluprednisolone. The B.P. Commission approved name for a corticosteroid.

Fluprofen. The B.P. Commission approved name for 2-(2'-fluoro-4-biphenyl)propionic acid. An anti-inflammatory agent and analgesic.

Flurandrenolone. The B.P. Commission approved name for a corticosteroid.

Flurothyl. The B.P. Commission approved name for di-(2,2,2-trifluoroethyl) ether. A central nervous system stimulant.

Flush. Redness. To wash out. **Hectic flush**, the reddening of the face that accompanies a high or hectic fever. **Hot flushes**, the sensation of heat, sometimes accompanied by flushing, that occurs spasmodically during the menopause. **Malar flush**, the area of hyperaemia over the malar bone that occurs in patients with mitral stenosis.

Flutter. Rapid vibration. Agitation. **Atrial flutter**, a condition in which the atria beat rapidly and regularly at a rate of 180 to 360 a minute. **Diaphragmatic flutter**, rapid, irregular contractions of the diaphragm.

Flux. Excessive discharge from any of the orifices of the body.

Fly. A member of the order Diptera, but the term is used loosely to describe almost any two-winged insect.

Focal. Relating to a focus. **Focal distance (or length)**, the distance of the principal focus of a lens from the lens.

Focus. The point of convergence of light rays after passing through a lens. The centre of activity. **Principal focus**, the point of convergence of parallel rays refracted through a lens.

Foetus. The unborn young of a viviparous mammal in its later stages of development. In man it is usually defined as the unborn child from the 8th week of conception to birth. **Foetus compressus (or papyraceus)**, a foetus in a twin pregnancy that has died early in pregnancy and then become mummified.

Fold. A ridge or bend. Plica. **Alar folds**, two fringe-like folds of the synovial membrane that project into the knee joint. **Aryepiglottic fold**, a fold of mucous membrane that stretches on each side between the side of the epiglottis and the apex of the arytenoid cartilage. **Axillary fold, anterior,** the rounded lower border of the pectoralis major. **Axillary fold, posterior,** the fold formed by the latissimus dorsi with the underlying teres major. **Caecal folds,** the two folds that form the lateral boundaries of the retrocaecal recess. **Circular folds,** large transverse folds of mucous membrane that project into the lumen of the small intestine **Duodenal fold,** a sickle-shaped fold of peritoneum, behind which lies the superior duodenal recess. **Duodenomesocolic fold,** a triangular peritoneal fold, behind which lies the inferior duodenal recess. **Gastropancreatic folds,** two sickle-shaped folds of peritoneum that are drawn into the omental bursa by the hepatic and left gastric arteries. **Glossoepiglottic folds,** three folds (one median and two lateral) formed by mucous membrane as it is reflected from the upper part of the anterior surface of the epiglottis on to the pharyngeal part of the tongue and the lateral wall of the pharynx. **Gluteal fold,** the lower border of the gluteus maximus that demarcates the buttock from the thigh. **Ileocaecal fold,** a peritoneal fold that extends from the anterior and inferior part of the ileum to the front of the meso-appendix. **Infrapatellar fold,** the fold formed by the alar folds which reaches to the front of the intercondylar fossa of the femur. **Lacrimal fold,** a fold of mucous membrane just above the opening of the nasolacrimal duct. **Malleolar folds,** two bands (medial and lateral) that reach from the tympanic sulcus to the lateral process of the malleus. **Nail fold,** the fold of skin that overlaps the root of the nail. **Palmate folds,** the arboriform folds that line the walls of the cervix uteri. **Paraduodenal fold,** a falciform peritoneal fold, behind which lies the paraduodenal recess. **Peritoneal folds,** the series of folds which bound recesses in the peritoneal cavity. **Presplenic fold,** the fan-shaped peritoneal fold that extends from the gastrosplenic ligament to the phrenicocolic ligament. **Rectal folds,** a series of three transverse folds of the mucous membrane of the rectum. **Recto-uterine folds,** two crescentic peritoneal folds which pass backwards from the cervix uteri, one on each side of the rectum, to the posterior wall of the lesser pelvis. **Rectovaginal fold,** the peritoneal fold that is reflected from

the back of the posterior fornix of the vagina on to the front of the rectum. **Sacrogenital folds,** the peritoneal folds that extend from the sides of the bladder backwards on either side of the rectum, to the front of the sacrum. **Salpingopalatine fold,** a fold of mucous membrane that stretches from above the pharyngeal opening of the auditory tube to the soft palate. **Salpingopharyngeal fold,** the vertical fold of mucous membrane that extends from the pharyngeal opening of the auditory tube to the wall of the pharynx. **Sublingual fold,** the ridge in the floor of the mouth, produced by the underlying sublingual salivary gland. **Umbilical folds,** three folds of the peritoneum lining the lower part of the anterior abdominal wall. The *median* contains the urachus, the *medial* contains the obliterated umbilical artery, and the *lateral* contains the inferior epigastric artery. **Ureteric folds,** the folds produced in the mucous membrane of the bladder by the ureters as they run obliquely through the bladder wall. **Uterovesical fold,** the fold of peritoneum which is reflected on to the upper surface of the bladder from the front of the uterus. **Vestibular folds,** two thick, pink folds of mucous membrane, each of which contains a vestibular ligament, and extends from the angle of the thyroid cartilage to the arytenoid cartilage. The space between them is the rima vestibuli. **Vocal folds,** two sharp, white folds of mucous membrane which extend from the angle of the thyroid cartilage to the vocal processes of the arytenoid cartilages. They form the lateral boundaries of the rima glottidis.

Folic acid. B.P. 1968. Pteroylglutamic acid. Present in many foods, particularly green leafy vegetables, meat, offal and cereals, it is essential for the maturation of red blood cells and indeed for the growth of all cells. It is used in the treatment of macrocytic and megaloblastic anaemias, but not pernicious anaemia.

Folie. Mental disorder. **Folie à deux,** the simultaneous development of psychosis in two closely associated persons, when one person seems to have influenced the other.

Folinic acid. An enzymatic conversion product of folic acid that plays a part in erythropoietic metabolism, probably as a co-enzyme. Citrovorum factor.

Folium. A leaf, or leaf-like structure.

One of the leaflike subdivisions of the cerebellar cortex. (*Plural:* folia.)

Follicle. A small sac, crypt or gland. **Graafian follicle**, or **vesicular ovarian follicle**, the follicle in the ovary in which the ovum develops. **Hair follicle**, the involution of the epidermis and superficial portion of the corium that houses the root of a hair. **Lymplatic follicles**, or **nodules**, the masses of lymphocytes in the cortex of a lymph node, the small and large intestine, the stomach and the tonsils. **Splenic follicles**, or **Malpighian bodies**, the sites of lymphocyte production in the spleen. **Thyroid follicles**, the colloid-containing vesicles of the thyroid.

Follicle-stimulating hormone. The B.P. Commission approved name for an extract of human postmenopausal urine containing primarily the follicle-stimulating hormone.

Folliculitis. Inflammation of a follicle. **Folliculitis barbae**, infection of the hair follicles of the beard region with *Staphylococcus aureus*. Sycosis. **Folliculitis decalvans**, cicatricial alopecia.

Folliculosis. A disease characterized by excessive numbers of lymph follicles.

Fomentation. A warm application to the surface of the body.

Fomes. Any article or substance capable of transmitting contagious disease. (*Plural:* fomites.)

Fomites. Plural of fomes.

Fontanelle. Unossified membranous interval in the skull at birth, of which there are six: *anterior, posterior,* and two pairs, *mastoid* and *sphenoidal.*

Fonticulus. Fontanelle. (*Plural:* fonticuli.)

Food. Nourishment.

Foot. The portion of the lower limb situated below the ankle joint. **Footdrop**, drooping of the foot due to inability to dorsiflex it.

Foramen. A natural aperture or opening. (*Plural:* foramina.) **Caecum foramen of tongue**, a median pit in the sulcus terminalis. **Epiploic foramen**, a vertical slit-like passage, about 3 cm. long, that runs from the upper part of the right border of the omental bursa into the greater sac. **Ethmoidal foramina**, two foramina that lead from the orbit to the anterior cranial fossa. **Infraorbital foramen**, the foramen in the maxilla about 1cm. below the infraorbital margin, that transmits the infraorbital vessels and nerve. **Interventricular foramen**, the foramen through which the third and lateral

ventricles of the brain communicate. **Intervertebral foramen**, the opening between the pedicles of contiguous vertebrae, through which pass the spinal vessels and nerves. **Jugular foramen**, the large foramen between the occipital bone and the jugular fossa of the petrous temporal that transmits the inferior petrosal sinus, the glossopharyngeal, vagus and accessory nerves and the internal jugular vein. **Foramen magnum**, the opening in the base of the occipital bone, through which the medulla oblongata joins the spinal cord. **Mandibular foramen**, the opening on the medial surface of the ramus of the mandible, through which pass the inferior alveolar nerve and vessels. **Mastoid foramen**, the foramen above the base of the mastoid process. **Mental foramen**, the anterior opening of the mandibular canal on the body of the mandible. **Obturator foramen**, a large, oval gap in the hip bone below and in front of the acetabulum. **Foramen ovale**, the opening in the interatrial septum which normally closes at birth or soon afterwards. **Foramen ovale of the sphenoid**, an opening on the infratemporal surface of the greater wing of the sphenoid that transmits the mandibular division of the trigeminal nerve. **Foramen rotundum**, the opening in the greater wing of the sphenoid that transmits the maxillary nerve. **Sacral pelvic foramina**, four pairs of foramina in the pelvic surface of the sacrum that communicate through the intervertebral foramina with the sacral canal. **Sciatic foramina (greater and lesser)**, the two foramina into which the sciatic notch is divided by the sacrotuberous and sacrospinous ligaments. **Foramen singulare**, the opening in the floor of the internal acoustic meatus for the passage of the nerve to the posterior semicircular duct. **Foramen spinosum**, the opening on the infratemporal surface of the greater wing of the sphenoid that transmits the middle meningeal artery. **Stylomastoid foramen**, an opening behind the root of the styloid process that transmits the facial nerve. **Foramen transversarium**, the canal in the transverse process of the cervical vertebrae. **Vertebral foramen**, the foramen enclosed by the body and vertebral arch of a vertebra, which houses the spinal cord.

Forceps. A surgical instrument for holding, lifting or compressing tissue or a dressing. Bands of white tissue in the corpus callosum: *forceps major, forceps minor.*

Fore- (Old English *fore:* in front of). Prefix meaning in front, before.

Forearm. The arm between the elbow and the wrist.

Forebrain. Prosencephalon.

Foregut. The cephalic portion of the embryonic digestive tube, from which arises the pharynx, oesophagus, stomach and duodenum.

Forehead. That part of the face above the eyes.

Forensic. Relating to courts of law.

Foreskin. Prepuce.

Forewaters. The liquor amnii in the bag of membranes which forms the fluid wedge between the oncoming foetus and the cervix in the initial stages of labour.

Formaldehyde solution. B.P. 1968. An aqueous solution, stabilized with methyl alcohol, and containing not less than 34 per cent w/w, and not more than 38 per cent w/w, of formaldehyde. It is a powerful antiseptic.

Formalin. Formaldehyde solution B.P.

Formation. A structure. **Hippocampal formation,** part of the rhinencephalon. **Reticular formation,** scattered grey matter in the brain stem, intersected by nerve fibres. It plays an important part in regulating the threshold of sensory perception, as well as many autonomic functions.

Forme fruste. An incomplete or atypical form of a disease.

Formication. A form of paraesthesia characterized by a sensation as of ants crawling over the skin.

Forminitrazole. The B.P. Commission approved name for 2-formamido-5-nitrothiazole. A drug for the treatment of trichomoniasis.

Formulary. A collection of prescriptions and preparations of drugs.

Fossa. A depression. (*Plural:* fossae.) **Acetabular fossa,** a depression in the floor of the acetabulum. **Coronoid fossa,** a hollow on the humerus immediately above the trochlea on the anterior surface of the medial condyle. **Cranial fossa, anterior,** the anterior depression of the base of the skull, the floor of which consists of the orbital parts of the frontal bone, the cribriform plate of the ethmoid, and the lesser wings and anterior part of the body of the splenoid. **Cranial fossa, middle,** the middle depression of the base of the skull, which is bounded posteriorly by the superior

borders of the petrous parts of the temporal bones and the dorsum sellae of the sphenoid. **Cranial fossa, posterior,** the posterior depression of the base of the skull. **Cubital fossa,** the triangular hollow in front of the elbow. **Hypophyseal fossa,** the hollow in the middle cranial fossa that lodges the hypophysis cerebri. **Iliac fossa,** the hollow formed by the medial aspect of the ilium. **Incudis fossa,** the small depression that lodges the short process of the incus. **Infraclavicular fossa,** the hollow immediately below the clavicle. **Infraspinous fossa,** the hollow below the spine of the scapula. **Infratemporal fossa,** the space behind the maxilla. **Intercondylar fossa,** the space separating the two condyles of the femur posteriorly. **Interpeduncular fossa,** the hollow lying between the optic chiasma in front, the pons behind, and the optic tracts and cerebral peduncles laterally. **Intrabulbar fossa,** the dilatation at the commencement of the spongy portion of the male urethra. **Ischiorectal fossa,** the wedge-shaped space that lies between the sphincter ani externus medially and the tuberosity of the ischium laterally. **Lacrimal fossa,** the hollow that lodges the orbital part of the lacrimal gland. **Malleolar fossa,** the depression that lies posterior to the articular facet of the lower end of the fibula. **Mandibular fossa,** the cavity in which rests the condyle of the mandible. **Navicular fossa,** the dilatation of the spongy portion of the male urethra within the glans penis. **Olecranon fossa,** the hollow on the posterior surface of the condyle of the lower end of the humerus that lodges the tip of the olecranon. **Fossa ovalis,** the oval depression on the wall of the atrium. **Ovarian fossa,** the depression on the lateral wall of the lesser pelvis that houses the ovary. **Pararectal fossa,** the space lying on either side of the rectum. **Paravesical fossa,** the space lying on either side of the bladder. **Piriform fossa,** a small recess lying on each side of the laryngeal orifice. **Popliteal fossa,** the space at the back of the knee. **Pterygoid fossa,** the space between the lateral and medial pterygoid plates of the sphenoid. **Pterygopalatine fossa,** the small pyramidal space below the apex of the orbit. **Radial fossa,** the small depression above the capitulum. **Rhomboid fossa,** the floor of the 4th ventricle. **Scaphoid fossa of the auricle,** the depression between the helix and the antihelix. **Sublingual fossa,** the depression on the internal surface of the mandible that lodges the sublingual salivary gland. **Submandibular fossa,** the hollow on the internal surface of the mandible that lodges the submandibular salivary gland. **Supraspinous fossa,** the hollow above the spine of the scapula. **Temporal fossa,** the region bounded by the zygomatic arch, the temporal line and the frontal process of the zygomatic bone. **Triangular fossa,** the depression between the two crura of the antihelix. **Trochanteric fossa,** the depressed area on the medial aspect of the greater trochanter of the femur. **Vestibular fossa,** the depression between the frenulum of the labia minora and the vaginal orifice.

Fovea. A shallow pit or hollow. (*Plural:* foveae.) **Fovea centralis,** a pit 3mm. to the temporal side of the optic disc, which is the most sensitive part of the retina. **Foveae inferior and superior,** two dimples on the floor of the fourth ventricle. **Pterygoid fovea,** a depression on the medial side of the neck of the condylar process of the mandible.

Foveola. A small pit or depression. (*Plural:* foveolae.) **Granular foveolae,** a series of irregular depressions on each side of the sagittal sinus.

Fracture. A break, usually in the continuity of bone. **Bennett's fracture** or **fracture-dislocation,** fracture of the base of the thumb. **Closed fracture,** a fracture in which the skin is intact. **Colles' fracture,** fracture of the lower end of the radius with displacement of the hand backwards and outwards. **Comminuted fracture,** a fracture in which the bone is broken in more than one place. **Complicated fracture,** a fracture complicated by injury to a bloodvessel, nerve, joint or viscus. **Compound fracture,** a fracture communicating with the exterior. **Compression fracture,** a fracture of a vertebral body by vertical crushing. **Extracapsular fracture,** a fracture near a joint but penetrating the joint capsule. **Fissure fracture,** a crack in a bone without an actual break. **Greenstick fracture,** a fracture in which the soft bone of a child cracks and bends, but the periosteum remains intact. **Impacted fracture,** a fracture in which the end of one fragment is driven into the cancellous bone of the other. **Malunited fracture,** a fracture that

has healed with deformity and/or shortening. **March fracture,** fracture of the 2nd, 3rd and 4th metatarsals. **Pathological fracture,** a fracture of a bone weakened by disease. **Pott's fracture,** the fracture produced by forceful abduction or eversion of the ankle, usually resulting in fracture of the lower end of the fibula and the medial malleolus. **Simple fracture,** closed fracture, **Spiral fracture,** a fracture in which the break runs spirally up the bone. **Spontaneous fracture,** a pathological fracture. **Subperiosteal fracture,** a fracture without any break of the periosteum. **Ununited fracture,** a fracture in which union fails to take place.

Fracture-dislocation. A fracture of a bone involving the neighbouring joint.

Fragilitas, Fragility. **Fragilitas crinium,** a condition characterized by fragility of the hair with consequent breaking of it. **Fragilitas ossium,** osteogenesis imperfecta.

Framboesia. Yaws.

Framycetin. The B.P. Commission approved name for an antibiotic produced by *Streptomyces decaris,* which is active against a wide range of organisms.

Freckle. A small, brown, pigmented macule on the skin of fair-skinned people, which appears or increases in intensity on exposure to sunshine.

Freemartin. A masculinized female twin calf, the other twin having been a male.

Fremitus. A thrill or vibration detectable by touch. **Vocal fremitus,** the vibration in the chest caused by the voice and felt by palpation.

Frenulum. A small fold of skin or mucous membrane. (*Plural:* frenula.) **Frenulum clitoridis,** the junction of the labia minora below the clitoris. **Frenulum of the labia minora,** the fold connecting the labia minora posteriorly. **Frenulum linguae,** the crescentic fold connecting the under-surface of the tongue to the floor of the mouth. **Frenulum of the lips,** the fold of mucous membrane that connects the inner surface of the lip in the median plane to the corresponding gum. **Frenulum of the prepuce,** the fold that connects the under-surface of the prepuce with the glans penis. **Frenulum veli,** a ridge that passes from the longitudinal sulcus between the colliculi to the superior medullary velum.

Frigidity. Sexual coldness.

Frontal bone. The bone that forms the forehead as far back as the parietal bones.

Frostbite. Damage to the tissues, usually of the extremities, caused by exposure to extreme cold.

Frottage. The rubbing movement in massage. A form of sexual stimulation by rubbing against women or their clothes.

Frotteur. One who achieves sexual satisfaction from frottage.

Fructosaemia. Laevulosaemia.

Fructose. A monosaccharide which occurs naturally in fruits and honey. It is present in the free state in the seminal plasma. Laevulose.

Fructosekinase. An enzyme in the liver which with ATP (adenosine triphosphate) converts fructose to fructose-6-phosphate.

Fructosuria. The excretion of fructose in the urine.

Frusemide. B.P. 1968. $C_{12}H_{11}ClN_2O_5S$. An oral diuretic that acts by reducing the resorption of electrolytes by the proximal and distal renal tubules and the loop of Henle.

Fuchsine. A red stain used in bacteriology. Magenta, B.P.C. 1968.

-fugal, -fuge (L *fuga:* flight). Suffixes implying flying from, or that which causes flight.

Fugue. A state of prolonged amnesia, in which the individual appears to act in a conscious manner, but on recovery from which he is completely oblivious of the state.

Fulguration. Destruction of tissue by electric sparks.

Fumagillin. The B.P. Commission approved name for an antibiotic produced by certain strains of *Aspergillus fumigatus*, which has an amoebicidal action.

Fumigation. Disinfecting by exposure to the vapour of antiseptics.

Fundus. The base or bottom of an organ. (*Plural:* fundi.) **Fundus of the gall-bladder**, the expanded end of the gall-bladder that projects beyond the inferior border of the liver. **Fundus of the stomach**, the part of the stomach that lies to the left of, and above, the level of the cardiac orifice. **Fundus of the urinary bladder**, the base of the bladder which is directed backwards and downwards. In the female it is closely related to the anterior wall of the vagina. In the male it is related to the rectum. **Fundus of the uterus**, the part of the body of the uterus

that lies above a plane passing through the points of entrance of the uterine tubes.

Fungate. To grow exuberantly—like a fungus.

Fungicide. A substance that kills fungi.

Fungoid. Resembling a fungus. Exuberant in growth.

Fungous. Resembling a fungus.

Fungus. A member of a group of non-photosynthetic micro-organisms possessing relatively rigid cell walls. The class of true fungi, Eumycetes, includes four morphological groups: moulds, yeasts, yeast-like fungi, and dimorphic fungi. The infections they cause are known as mycoses. (*Plural:* fungi.)

Funiculitis. Inflammation of a funiculus, particularly the spermatic cord.

Funiculus. A cord-like structure. A small bundle of fibres. Fasciculus. (*Plural:* funiculi.) **Funiculus separans,** an oblique ridge on the floor of the fourth ventricle. **Spinal funiculi,** three bands of white matter: *anterior funiculus* lying between the anterior median fissure and the most lateral of the bundles of the ventral nerve roots that emerge on the anterolateral aspect of the spinal cord; *lateral funiculus,* lying between the ventral nerve roots and the posterolateral sulcus; *posterior funiculus* lying between the posterolateral sulcus and the posterior median septum.

Furazolidone, B.P.C. 1968. $C_8H_7N_3O_5$. A bactericide used in the treatment of gastroenteritis.

Furethidine. The B.P. Commission approved name for ethyl 4-phenyl-1-[2-(tetrahydrofurfuryloxy)ethyl] - piperidine-4-carboxylate. A narcotic analgesic.

Furfur. Epidermal scale. Dandruff. (*Plural:* furfures.)

Furfuraceous. Resembling dandruff. Scaly. Desquamating.

Furrow. A groove. **Nasolabial furrow,** the furrow that passes from the side of the nose to the upper lip.

Furuncle. A boil.

Furunculosis. The presence of repeated boils or furuncles.

Fusafungine. The B.P. Commission approved name for an antibiotic produced by *Fusarium lateritium* 437. It is largely used as a nose spray.

Fusidic acid. The B.P. Commission approved name for an antibiotic produced by a strain of Fusidium, which is proving of value in the treatment of staphylococcal infections resistant to penicillin.

Fusiform. Spindle-like.

Fusobacterium. A genus of Bacteroidacae, which has six members. Only one, *Fusobacterium fusiforme*, is of proven pathogenicity in man. It is a concomitant of *Borrelia vincenti* in Vincent's angina, gingivitis and stomatitis.

G

Gadolinium. A rare element. Symbol Gd. Atomic weight 157·25, Atomic number 64.

Gaffkya. The group of gram-positive cocci that occur mainly in groups of four, or multiples thereof. *Gaffkya-tetragena*, a commensal of the upper respiratory tract.

Gag. An instrument for holding the mouth open. To retch.

Gait. The manner of walking. **Ataxic gait**, the unsteady gait typical of a lesion involving the posterior columns of the spinal cord, such as tabes dorsalis. **Festinating gait**, a gait of short hurrying steps. **Scissor gait**, a spastic, cross-legged gait as in spastic paraplegia. **Spastic gait**, the gait in which the legs are stiff, held close together and with the toes tending to drag on the ground. **Steppage gait**, the gait in which the feet are lifted abnormally clear of the ground, as in foot-drop. **Tabetic gait**, the classical ataxic gait of tabes dorsalis.

Galact- (Gk *gala:* milk). Prefix indicating a relationship to milk.

Galactagogue. An agent that increases the flow of milk.

Galactocele. A milk-containing cyst in the breast.

Galactokinase. An enzyme that plays a part in the conversion of galactose to glactose-1-phosphate.

Galactophoritis. Inflammation of the milk ducts.

Galactorrhoea. Excessive or spontaneous secretion of milk.

Galactosaemia. An inborn error of metabolism characterized by absence of the enzyme that converts galactose to glucose.

Galactose. A monosaccharide that occurs in nature in the combined form as a constituent of lactose, in certain complex lipids and in some proteins.

Galactoside. A glycoside formed from galactose.

Galactosuria. The excretion of galactose in the urine.

Galea. A helmet-like structure. **Galea aponeurotica**, the aponeurosis covering the upper part of the cranium.

Galenical. An archaic term for a medicine prepared from plants according to official formulae as laid down, for example, in a pharmacopoeia.

Galeophobia. A morbid fear of cats.

Gall. Bile.

Gallamine triethiodide. B.P. 1968. $C_3H_{60}I_3N_3O_3$. A muscle relaxant.

Gall-bladder. The pear-shaped reservoir for the storage and concentration of bile, with a capacity of 30 to 50ml., lying on the under-surface of the right lobe of the liver.

Gallipot. A small jar for holding ointments and confections.

Gallium. A rare metallic element. Symbol Ga. Atomic weight 69·72. Atomic number 31.

Gallon. A liquid measure in the imperial system, equivalent to four quarts or 4·545 litres.

Gall-stone. A concretion in the biliary system, usually the gall-bladder.

Galvanic. Pertaining to galvanism.

Galvanism. Direct current electricity produced by chemical means.

Galvano-. The prefix from Galvani, the Italian physicist, denoting association with direct current electricity.

Galvanocautery. Cautery by a wire heated by a galvanic current.

Galvanometer. An instrument for measuring the strength of an electric current.

Gamete. A sexual or germ cell.

Gameto- (Gk *gametē:* wife; *gametēs:* husband). Prefix indicating association with a gamete.

Gametocide. An agent capable of killing gametes or gametocytes, usually referring to the malarial gametocytes.

Gametocyte. A precursor of a gamete. The sexual phase of the malaria parasite in the intermediate host.

Gametogony. The stage in the sexual cycle of the malaria parasite, in which gametocytes are produced.

Gamma. The third letter of the Greek alphabet (γ). A microgram, or one-millionth of a gramme.

Gamma benzene hexachloride. B.P. 1968. $C_6H_6Cl_6$. An acaricide, insecticide, and larvicide.

Gammexane. $C_6H_6O_6$. A powerful synthetic insecticide, active against a wide range of insects, including houseflies, fleas, mosquitoes, cockroaches and bed-bugs.

Gamo- (Gk *gamos:* marriage). Prefix indicating an association with marriage or sexual union.

Gamomania. A morbid desire to marry.

Gamophobia. A morbid fear of marriage.

Gangli-, Ganglio- (Gk *ganglion:* a knot). Prefixes signifying relationship to a knot or ganglion.

Ganglion. A knotlike mass of nerve cells. A cystic swelling in a tendon sheath. (*Plural:* ganglia.) **Aberrant ganglia,** groups of nerve cells sometimes found on the dorsal roots of the upper cervical nerves between the spinal ganglia and the spinal cord. **Aorticorenal ganglia,** the lower part of the coeliac ganglia. **Basal ganglia,** masses of grey matter embedded within the thalamus. **Cardiac ganglion,** a small ganglion in the cardiac plexus situated immediately below the arch of the aorta. **Carotid ganglion,** a small ganglion in the internal carotid plexus on the side of the internal carotid artery. **Cervical ganglia,** three ganglia in the cervical part of the sympathetic trunk. The **inferior cervical ganglion,** usually fused with the first thoracic ganglion to form the cervicothoracic ganglion, lies between the base of the transverse process of the seventh cervical vertebra and the neck of the first rib, and sends branches mainly to the heart. The **middle cervical ganglion,** sometimes absent, lies opposite the sixth cervical vertebra, may be fused with the superior cervical ganglion, and sends branches mainly to the thyroid. The **superior cervical ganglion** is placed opposite the second and third cervical vertebrae, and sends branches to the head and the heart. **Cervical ganglion of the uterus,** a ganglion near the cervix uteri. **Cervicothoracic ganglion,** a ganglion formed by the fusion of the inferior cervical ganglion and the first thoracic ganglion. **Ciliary ganglion,** a small ganglion near the apex of the orbit. **Coeliac ganglia,** two large ganglia in the coeliac plexus. **Genicular ganglion,** the sensory ganglion of the facial nerve. **Glossopharyngeal ganglia,** two ganglia, the **inferior,** situated in a notch in the lower border of the petrous portion of the temporal bone and the **superior** in the upper part of the groove in which the nerve is lodged as it passes through the jugular foramen. **Impar ganglion,** a small ganglion on the front of the coccyx. **Intermediate ganglia,** microscopic ganglia on the grey rami communicantes in the cervical and lumbar region. **Lumbar ganglia,** four ganglia on the lumbar part of the sympathetic trunk. **Mesenteric ganglia,** two ganglia, the **interior** at the origin of the inferior mesenteric artery, and the **superior** in the upper part of the superior mesenteric plexus. **Otic ganglion,** a peripheral ganglion of the parasympathetic system immediately below the foramen ovale. **Parasympathetic ganglia,** four peripheral ganglia found in connexion with the cranial part of the parasympathetic system: the ciliary, pterygopalatine, otic, and submandibular ganglia. **Phrenic ganglion,** a small ganglion at the junction of the right phrenic plexus with the phrenic nerve. **Pterygopalatine ganglion,** the largest of the peripheral ganglia of the parasympathetic system, deeply placed in the pterygopalatine fossa. **Sacral ganglia,** the four or five ganglia of the pelvic part of the sympathetic trunk. **Spinal ganglia,** collections of nerve cells on the dorsal roots of the spinal nerves. **Spiral ganglion,** the sensory ganglion of the cochlear nerve. **Splanchnic ganglion,** a ganglion on the lesser splanchnic nerve. **Stellate ganglion,** the cervicothoracic ganglia. **Submandibular ganglion,** one of the peripheral ganglia of the parasympathetic system, placed above the deep part of the submandibular gland, and connected functionally with the facial nerve and its chorda tympani branch. **Sympathetic ganglia,** the twenty-two or twenty-three ganglion, not necessarily all discrete, of the sympathetic nervous system. **Thoracic ganglia,** the twelve ganglia, not necessarily all discrete, associated with the thoracic part of the sympathetic system. **Trigeminal ganglion,** the ganglion, situated near the apex of the petrous part of the temporal bone, from which arise the fibres of the sensory root of the trigeminal nerve. **Vagus ganglia,** the two ganglia of the vagus nerve: the **inferior ganglion,** on the nerve after its exit from the jugular foramen, which is connected with the hypoglossal nerve and the superior cervical ganglion of the sympathetic trunk; the **superior ganglion**, on the nerve in the jugular foramen. **Vertebral ganglion**, a small ganglion, lying just above the subclavian artery and the beginning of the vertebral artery, which may be fused with the middle cervical ganglion. **Vestibular ganglion**, the ganglion situated in the internal acoustic meatus, from which the fibres of the vestibular nerve take origin.

Ganglionectomy. Excision of a ganglion.

Ganglioneuroma. A tumour arising from ganglionic nerve cells.

Gangosa. An ulcerated condition of the nasopharynx, occurring in the tertiary stage of yaws.

Gangrene. Mortification of the flesh. **Dry gangrene**, mummification. **Gas gangrene**, the gangrenous state occurring in a wound contaminated with Clostridia. **Moist gangrene**, gangrene in which the affected tissues are moist and putrefying.

Gap. An opening or discontinuity. **Auscultatory gap**, the silent period that sometimes occurs just below the systolic blood pressure, when this is being recorded by auscultation.

Gargle. A solution used for rinsing the throat. The process of using such a solution.

Gargoylism. A genetically determined hereditary disorder characterized by skeletal deformity, including a large head with coarse features (hence the name), hepatomegaly, splenomegaly, corneal opacity, deafness, heart disease and mental subnormality.

Gas. A physical state in which the molecules are free to move in all directions. **Coal gas,** a mixture of methane, carbon monoxide and hydrogen, produced by the distillation of coal, and used for heating and lighting purposes. **Laughing gas,** nitrous oxide. **Marsh gas,** methane. **Mustard gas,** mustine. **Tear gas,** any gas that is used by the police or military to control mobs by producing harmless lacrimation.

Gas gangrene. Infection with certain clostridia: *Clostridium welchii, Cl. oedematiens,* and *Cl. septicum.* The *British Pharmacopoeia* contains a **Gas-Gangrene Antitoxin** against each, as well as a mixed antitoxin containing antitoxin against all three.

Gasterophilus. A species of warble or bot flies which infest horses, and the larvae of which may cause a creeping skin eruption in man.

Gastr-, Gastro- (Gk *gastrer:* stomach). Prefixes indicating association with the stomach.

Gastralgia. Pain in the stomach.

Gastrectasia. Dilatation of the stomach.

Gastrectomy. Surgical excision of part of, or the whole of, the stomach.

Gastric. To do with the stomach.

Gastrin. A hormone liberated from the mucosa of the pyloric antrum, which stimulates gastric secretion and increases the tone of the musculature of the stomach and small intestine.

Gastritis. Inflammation of the stomach.

Gastrocolic. Pertaining to the stomach and colon.

Gastroduodenal. Pertaining to the stomach and duodenum.

Gastroduodenostomy. Surgical establishment of an anastomosis between the stomach and duodenum.

Gastrodynia. Pain in the stomach.

Gastroenteritis. Inflammation of the stomach and intestine.

Gastroenterostomy. A surgical anastomosis between the stomach and intestine.

Gastroepiploic. Pertaining to the stomach and the greater omentum.

Gastrogenous. Arising from the stomach.

Gastro-intestinal. Pertaining to the stomach and intestine.

Gastrojejunostomy. The surgical creation of an anastomosis between the stomach and jejunum.

Gastrolith. A concretion in the stomach.

Gastrology. The study of the stomach.

Gastro-oesophageal. Pertaining to the stomach and oesophagus.

Gastro-oesophagostomy. A surgical anastomosis between the stomach and oesophagus.

Gastropexy. Surgical fixation of the stomach to the abdominal wall.

Gastroptosis. Downward displacement of the stomach.

Gastrorrhoea. Excessive secretion of gastric juice.

Gastroscope. An instrument for inspecting the interior of the stomach.

Gastrostaxis. Oozing of blood from the gastric mucosa.

Gastrostomy. The establishment of an artificial opening in the stomach.

Gastrotomy. A surgical incision into the stomach.

Gastrula. The early stage of embryonic development following the blastula.

Gatophobia. Morbid fear of cats.

Gaucher's disease. A hereditary disease

characterized by the abnormal storage of cerebroside, particularly in the bone marrow, liver and spleen.

Gaultheria. A species of evergreen plant, from which oil of wintergreen is obtained.

Gauss. The unit of magnetic induction. (*Symbol: G.*)

Gauze. A thin, open-web tissue used for surgical dressings.

Gavage. Feeding by stomach tube.

Gefarnate. The B.P. Commission approved name for a mixture of isomers of 3,7-dimethylocta-2,6-dienyl 5,9,13-trimethyltetradeca-4,8,12-trienoate. It is used in the treatment of peptic ulcer by virtue of its regenerative and protective action on the gastric and duodenal mucosa.

Gel. A colloid which is firm in consistence but contains much water.

Gelatin. A protein derived from collagen by boiling. It dissolves in boiling water and on cooling sets as a jelly. It is of poor nutritive value as it is lacking in several essential amino-acids. **Absorbable gelatin sponge,** B.P. 1968, a sterile, absorbable, water-insoluble gelatin used as a haemostatic.

Gelotherapy. Treatment by the induction of hilarity.

Gelsemium. B.P.C. 1968. The dried rhizome and roots of *Gelsemium sempervirens* (L.), which depresses the central nervous system, and in the form of the tincture is used in the treatment of migraine and trigeminal neuralgia.

Gemmule. A small bud. A term usually ascribed to the small buds that appear on dendrites.

Gene. The biological unit of heredity. **Dominant gene,** a gene which produces its characteristic in the individual. **Recessive gene,** a gene that only produces its characteristic if carried by both parents. **Sex-linked gene,** a gene located on a sex chromosome.

Generate. To produce or procreate.

Generation. Procreation. The period of time lapsing from the birth of an individual to the birth of his offspring.

Generic. Relating to a genus or group.

Genesiology. The science of reproduction or heredity.

Genetic. Relating to reproduction. Inherited.

Genetics. The study of heredity.

Genial. Relating to the chin.

-genic (Gk *gennan:* to produce). Suffix indicating productive of, or producing.

Genicular. Pertaining to the knee.

Geniculum. A sharp bend. (*Plural:* genicula.) **Geniculum of the facial nerve,** the sharp backward bend of the facial nerve in the facial canal.

Genio- (Gk *geneion:* chin). Prefix indicating association with the chin.

Genion. The chin. The tip of the mental protuberance.

Genioplasty. Plastic surgery on the chin.

Genital. Relating to the reproductive tract or to reproduction.

Genitalia. The organs of reproduction.

Genito- (L *genitalis:* genital). Prefix indicating relationship to the organs of reproduction (or birth).

Genito-urinary. Relating to the genital and urinary organs.

Geno- (Gk *genos:* offspring). Prefix indicating relationship to reproduction or sex.

Genome. A complete set of chromosomes derived from one parent.

Genotype. The genetic constitution of an individual.

Gentamicin sulphate. B.P. Supplement 1971. A mixture of the sulphates of the antimicrobial substances produced by *Micromonospora purpurea.* A broad-spectrum antibiotic active against a wide range of gram-positive and gram-negative organisms.

Gentian. B.P. 1968. The dried fermented rhizome and root of *Gentiana lutea* (L). It is used, usually in the form of **Compound gentian tincture,** B.P. 1968, or **Compound gentian infusion,** B.P. 1968, as a bitter to stimulate the appetite.

Genu. The knee. (*Plural:* genua.) **Genu of the corpus callosum,** the anterior end of the corpus callosum. **Genu of the facial nerve,** the loop of the facial nerve round the nucleus of the abducent nerve. **Genu of the internal capsule,** the junction of the anterior and posterior limbs of the internal capsule. **Genu valgum,** knock-knee. **Genu varum,** bow-leg.

Genus. A taxonomic group intermediate between family and species. (*Plural:* genera.)

Geo- (Gk *gē:* earth). Prefix meaning earth or soil.

Geophagia. The practice of eating earth.

Geotropism. The influence of gravity on growth.

Ger-, Gerat- (Gk *gēras:* old age). Prefixes indicating relationship to old age.

Geriatrician. A specialist in the care of old people.

Geriatrics. The branch of medicine

concerned with the care of the elderly.
Germ. A microbe. An egg, seed, or spore. **Germ cell,** the ovum or spermatozoon. **Germ disc,** the thick plate of large irregularly ranged cells in the formative mass of the early embryo. **Dental germ,** the rudiments of a tooth.

Germanium. A rare metallic element. Symbol Ge. Atomic weight 72·59. Atomic number 32.

Germicide. A substance that kills micro-organisms.

Germinal. Pertaining to a germ. **Germinal centre,** the central core of a lymph follicle. **Germinal spot,** the nucleolus of the ovum. **Germinal vesicle,** a large spherical body in the yolk of the ovum which contains a well-defined nucleolus.

Germination. The beginning of growth in an egg, ovum, seed, or spore.

Gero-, Geronto- (Gk *gēron:* old man). Prefixes indicating relationship to old age.

Gerontology. The study of old age and the ageing process.

Gerontophilia. Love for old people.

Gestagen. A hormone with progestational activity.

Gestaltism. The psychological theory that the objects of mind come as complete forms which cannot be subdivided.

Gestation. Pregnancy. **Ectopic gestation,** development of the impregnated ovum outwith the uterus.

Gestronol. The B.P. Commission approved name for 17-hydroxy-19-norpregn-4-ene-3,20-dione. A progestational steroid.

Giardia. A genus of flagellate protozoa. *Giardia intestinalis* a flagellate protozoon that inhabits the duodenum and jejunum.

Giardiasis. Diarrhoea induced by *Giardia intestinalis.*

Gibbous. Humped or hump-backed.

Giddiness. Dizziness.

Gigantism. The state of abnormal overgrowth induced by excessive secretion of the growth hormone before fusion of the epiphyses.

Ginger. B.P. 1968. The rhizome of *Zingiber officinale.* It is used as a carminative or a flavouring agent.

Gingiva. The gum. (*Plural:* gingivae.)

Gingivectomy. Surgical excision of gingival tissue.

Gingivitis. Inflammation of the gums.

Gingivo- (L *gingiva:* gum). Prefix indicating association with the gums.

Ginglymus. A hinge joint in which there is movement in one plane only,

and the bones are connected together by strong collateral ligaments: e.g. the interphalangeal joints.

Girdle. A belt or binder. A circular arrangement of bone. **Pelvic girdle,** the bony ring formed by the hip bones, sacrum and coccyx. **Shoulder girdle,** the arch formed by the scapulae and clavicles.

Gitalin. One of the glycosides in *Digitalis purpurea.*

Gizzard. The second, muscular stomach of birds, in which the food is ground up.

Glabella. The median elevation on the frontal bone where the two superciliary arches meet.

Glabrous. Hairless. Smooth.

Gland. An accumulation of cells which perform some excretory or secretory function. **Anal glands,** a series of secretory glands, containing mucin, in the anal canal, which are liable to become infected and lead to abscess or fistula formation. **Apocrine glands,** glands, the secretion of which contains part of the secreting cells. **Areolar glands,** sebaceous glands in the areola of the breast which become enlarged during pregnancy and lactation. **Arytenoid glands,** mucous glands in the aryepiglottic fold. **Body glands,** the gastric glands in the body and fundus of the stomach. They consist of *oxyntic* (or *parietal*) cells that secrete hydrochloric acid, and *zymogenic* cells that contain pepsinogen, the precursor of pepsin. **Bronchial glands,** seromucous glands in the mucous membrane of the bronchi. **Buccal glands,** mucous glands in the cheeks. **Bulbo-urethral glands,** two small, rounded glands, about the size of a pea, situated lateral to the membranous urethra, deep to the perineal membrane. **Cardiac glands,** the gastric glands, few in number, near the cardiac orifice, which are mainly mucus secreting. **Ceruminous glands,** the glands in the external acoustic meatus that secrete wax. **Ciliary glands,** the glands in the eyelids, arranged in several rows close to the free margin of the eyelid. **Ductless gland,** a gland without a duct, whose secretion passes straight into the blood; an endocrine gland. **Duodenal glands,** mucoid-secreting glands in the duodenum. **Endocrine gland,** a ductless gland in which the secretion is passed direct into the bloodstream. **Exocrine gland,** a gland whose secretion is voided via a duct. **Gastric glands,** the glands in the stomach which comprise the *cardiac glands*, the *body glands*, and the *pyloric glands*. **Genital glands**, ovary, and testis. **Holocrine glands**, glands whose function is entirely secretory, and whose cells disintegrate to produce the secretion: e.g., sebaceous glands. **Intestinal glands**, glands in the small and large intestine, containing many goblet cells. **Labial glands**, glands in the lips, resembling the mucous salivary glands. **Lacrimal gland**, the gland in the upper, outer part of each orbit that secretes tears. **Laryngeal glands**, mucus-secreting glands in the larynx that lubricate the vocal cords. **Lingual glands**, serous and mucous glands in the tongue. **Lymph glands**, lymph nodes. Encapsulated collections of lymphoid tissue. **Mammary gland**, the milk-secreting gland of the female; rudimentary in the male. **Merocrine glands**, glands the secretion of which contains no part of the secreting cells. **Molar glands**, four or five of the larger buccal glands situated around the terminal part of the parotid duct. **Mucous glands**, glands that secrete mucus. **Nasal glands**, serous glands in the nasal mucous membrane, rich in enzymes. **Oesophageal glands**, mucous glands in the oesophagus. **Palatine glands**, mucous glands in the soft palate. **Parathyroid glands**, four small ductless glands lying on the back of the thyroid gland that secrete the hormone controlling the metabolism of calcium and phosphorus. **Parotid gland**, the largest of the salivary glands weighing about 25 grammes, and lying below the external acoustic meatus between the mandible and the sternocleido-mastoid. **Preputial glands**, small glands on the corona of the glans penis and on the neck of the penis that secrete smegma. **Prostate gland**, the gland surrounding the male urethra, the acid secretion of which, with that of the seminal vesicles, provides the bulk of the seminal fluid. **Pyloric glands**, the gastric glands in the pylorus; they are predominantly mucous in type. **Salivary glands**, the parotid, sublingual and submandibular glands. **Sebaceous glands**, small, sacculated, glandular organs in the corium that secrete sebum. **Serous glands**, glands that secrete a thin, watery fluid. **Sublingual gland**, the smallest of the three main salivary glands, situated beneath the mucous membrane of the floor of the mouth

on the inner surface of the mandible close to the symphysis. **Submandibular gland**, one of the three major salivary glands, about the size of a walnut, and situated in the digastric triangle and extending up under the mandible. **Sudoriferous glands**, sweat glands. **Suprarenal glands (or adrenal glands)**, two small flattened bodies lying atop of each kidney, the cortex of which secretes the corticosteroid hormones, and the medulla of which secretes adrenaline and noradrenaline. They are ductless glands. **Sweat glands**, glands found in almost every part of the skin, that secrete sweat. **Tarsal glands**, modified sebaceous glands in the eyelids. **Thymus gland**, a ductless gland in the anterior and superior mediastina of the thorax, which plays an important part in immunogenesis. **Thyroid gland**, a ductless gland in the neck, weighing around 25 grammes, heavier in women than in men, which secretes thyroxine and triiodothyronine. **Vestibular glands**, the **lesser vestibular glands** are numerous small mucous glands in the vestibule of the vagina; the **greater vestibular glands** are two small bodies, one on each side of the vaginal orifice, which are the homologues of the bulbo-urethral glands in the male.

Glanders. A disease of horses, caused by *Loefflerella mallei*, and communicable to man.

Glandular. Pertaining to a gland or glands. **Glandular fever**, infectious mononucleosis. An acute febrile disease of infective, but unknown, origin, characterized by enlargement of lymph glands.

Glans. A glandlike body. **Glans clitoridis**, the free extremity of the clitoris. **Glans penis**, the conical end of the corpus spongiosum which constitutes the free end of the penis.

Glasses. Spectacles.

Glaucoma. A disease of the eye characterized by raised intra-ocular pressure.

Gleet. The thin sticky urethral discharge in chronic gonorrhoea.

Glenoid. Resembling a pit or cavity. **Glenoid cavity**, the socket in the scapula, into which fits the head of the humerus.

Glia. Neuroglia.

Gliadin. One of the main proteins in wheat.

Glio- (Gk *glia:* glue). Prefix signifying relationship to a gluey substance, or neuroglia.

Glioma. A tumour composed of neuroglial cells.

Gliosome. One of the small granules in neuroglia cells.

Globin. The protein of haemoglobin.

Globulin. A class of proteins insoluble in water and soluble in weak saline solution, which are found widespread in nature. They constitute one of the three main types of plasma protein. Alpha$_1$ (α_1)-globulins include a fraction which combines with bilirubin, and a fraction, α_1-lipoprotein of the plasma, which is responsible in part for the carriage of lipids and steroids. The alpha$_2$(α_2)-globulin fraction includes the mucoproteins and the haptoglobulins. The beta (β)-globulins include the β-lipoprotein responsible for the transport of lipids in blood, globulins which bind iron (transferrin) and copper (caeruloplasmin), and prothrombin. The gamma (γ)-globulins include all known antibodies. **Antihaemophilic globulin,** factor viii. A globulin in normal plasma that corrects the defect in haemophilia. Antihaemophilic factor.

Globulinuria. The presence of globulin in the urine.

Globus. A sphere or ball. (*Plural:* globi.) **Globus hystericus,** the choking sensation of a ball in the throat a not uncommon manifestation of hysteria or emotional upset. **Globus pallidus,** the medial portion of the lentiform nucleus.

Glomangioma. A glomus tumour which occurs in the skin of the extremities and causes acute paroxysmal pain.

Glomerular. Pertaining to a glomerulus.

Glomerulitis. Inflammation of a glomerulus.

Glomerulonephritis. The form of nephritis in which the primary inflammatory change (of unknown etiology) occurs in the glomeruli. A form of Bright's disease.

Glomerulosclerosis. The form of Bright's disease, or nephritis, characterized predominantly by sclerotic changes in the glomeruli.

Glomerulus. The tuft of capillaries which constitutes the beginning of the renal tubule. (*Plural:* glomeruli.)

Glomus. The arteriolar-venous anastomosis found in the nail-bed, the tips of the fingers and toes, the ears, hands and feet, which acts as a regulator in the flow of blood and thereby in the conservation of heat (*Plural:* glomerglomera.)

Gloss-, Glosso- (Gk *glōssa:* tongue). Prefixes signifying relationship to the tongue.

Glossa. The tongue.

Glossal. Pertaining to the tongue.

Glossalgia. Pain in the tongue.

Glossectomy. Surgical excision of the tongue.

Glossina. A genus of biting flies. Tsetse flies.

Glossitis. Inflammation of the tongue.

Glossodynia. Pain in the tongue.

Glossolabial. Pertaining to the tongue and the lips.

Glossolalia. Unintelligible jargon.

Glossopharyngeal. Relating to the tongue and the pharynx. **Glossopharyngeal nerve,** the 9th cranial nerve.

Glossoplasty. Plastic or reparative surgery on the tongue.

Glossopyrosis. Burning sensation in the tongue.

Glossotrichia. Hairy tongue.

Glottis. The vocal apparatus of the larynx. The triangular space between the vocal folds. Rima glottidis.

Glucagon. The hyperglycaemia-glycogenolytic factor produced by the alpha-cells of the pancreatic islets, which is a potent stimulus to insulin secretion in man.

Gluco- (Gk *gleukos:* sweetness). Prefix indicating relationship to sweetness or glucose.

Glucocorticoid. A corticoid, or corticosteroid, that affects the metabolism of glucose.

Glucokinase. The enzyme which converts glucose to glucose 6-phosphate, the first stage in glycolysis.

Gluconeogenesis. The formation of carbohydrate from non-carbohydrate precursors such as amino-acids, lactate or fat.

Glucosamine. The amino-sugar formed from glucose by the introduction of an amino group. It occurs extensively in nature in complex polysaccharides.

Glucose. $C_6H_{12}O_6$. A white, crystalline solid easily soluble in water, which has a sweet taste and is present in the blood and tisue of animals, as well as in plant and fruit juices. Dextrose. Grape sugar.

Glucoside. A glycoside formed from glucose.

Glucuronic acid. The acid formed when a carboxyl group is introduced at a carbon atom six in the glucose molecule.

Glucuronide. The form in which many drugs and some hormones are excreted in the urine, coupled with glucuronic acid.

Glutamate dehydrogenase. The enzyme which, with a co-enzyme, brings about the oxidation of glutamic acid to α-oxoglutaric acid.

Glutamic acid. $C_5H_9NO_4$. An amino-acid.

Glutamic oxaloacetic transaminase. GOT. The enzyme that catalyses the reaction between aspartic acid and α-oxoglutaric acid. The myocardium contains a higher concentration of this enzyme than any other tissue in the body. The serum transaminase (SGOT) is therefore raised following a myocardial infarction. It is also raised in disease of the liver, such as hepatitis, involving necrosis of liver cells.

Glutamic pyruvic transaminase. GPT. The enzyme that catalyses the transfer of an amine group from glutamic acid to pyruvic acid to form α-oxoglutaric acid and alanine. The serum level of the enzyme (SGPT) is raised in diseases involving necrosis of liver cells.

Glutaminase. The enzyme, found in the kidney and elsewhere in the body, that catalyses the breakdown of glutamine to ammonia and glutamic acid.

Glutamine. The amide which provides the major source of urinary ammonia. This reaction is catalysed by the enzyme glutaminase.

Glutathione. A tripeptide that plays an important part in tissue oxidations.

Gluteal. Relating to the buttocks.

Glutelin. One of a group of proteins found in the seeds of grain.

Gluten. A mixture of proteins, mainly gliadins and glutelins, present in wheat, barley and rye, which produces dough on the addition of water.

Glutethimide. B.P. 1968. $C_{13}H_{15}NO_2$. A hypnotic.

Gly-, Glyco- (Gk *glykys:* sweet). Prefixes indicating association with sweetness or sugar.

Glycalox. The B.P. Commission approved name for a polymerized complex of glycerol and aluminium hydroxide, use in the treatment of gastric hyperacidity.

Glyceraldehyde 3-phosphate. An intermediate in the glycolytic breakdown of glucose.

Glycerin. B.P. 1968. A clear, colourless, odourless, hygroscopic, syrupy liquid, with the formula propane-1,2,3-triol. It is used as a demulcent by mouth, locally with magnesium sulphate in the treatment of boils, as a suppository, and in the making of linctuses and pastilles.

Glycerite. A mixture of medicinal substances in glycerin.

Glycerol. Glycerin.

Glycerophosphate. A salt of glycerophosphoric acid. Such salts were once widely prescribed as so-called 'nerve tonics'.

Glyceryl trinitrate. $C_3H_5N_3O_9$. A substance that causes relaxation of involuntary muscle. Its main use is in the prophylaxis and relief of the pain of angina pectoris. It is also used for the relief of renal and gall-stone colic. The official *BritishPharmacopoeia* preparation is **Glyceryl trinitrate tablets**, each of which, unless otherwise specified, contains 0·5mg.

Glycine. $C_2H_5NO_2$. The simplest amino-acid. It acts as a conjugating agent combining with potentially harmful substances in the body to render them harmless.

Glycocholic acid. An acid found in bile.

Glycocyamine. Guanido-acetic acid, with which arginine and glycine react in the synthesis of creatine.

Glycogen. The form in which carbohydrate is stored in the animal body.

Glycogenesis. The process whereby glucose is converted to glycogen in the liver.

Glycogenolysis. The conversion of glycogen to glucose.

Glycol. One of a group of bivalent alcohols, widely used as plasticizers and solvents.

Glycolipid. A lipid which contains a monosaccharide in its molecule.

Glycolysis. The conversion of glucose to lactic acid, the initial series of reactions in the process of obtaining energy from glucose.

Glycoprotein. A protein-carbohydrate compound.

Glycopyrronium bromide. The B.P. Commission approved name for 3-α-cyclopentylmandeloyloxy-1,1-dimethylpyrrolidinium bromide. An anticholinergic agent.

Glycoside. A compound of a sugar and a non-sugar unit. Glycosides are widespread throughout nature and include many important pharmacological principles such as digoxin.

Glycosuria. The presence of an abnormal amount of glucose in the urine. **Renal glycosuria,** the condition in which glucose is found in the urine although the blood level is not raised.

Glycyrrhiza. A genus of perennial herbs. Liquorice B.P.

Glycyrrhizin. The principal active constituent of liquorice root.

Gnath-, Gnatho- (Gk *gnathos:* jaw). Prefixes indicating association with the jaw.

Gnathion. The lowest point on the median line of the lower jaw.

Gnathocephalus. A deformed foetus with a massive jaw as the only remnant of the skull.

Gnathodynia. Pain in the jaw.

Gnathostoma. A genus of nematode or roundworm. *Gnathostoma spinigerum,* a roundworm, infection with which is common in the East, including China, India and Thailand, and causes a wandering subcutaneous swelling.

Gnosia. The faculty of perceiving.

Goitre. An enlargement of the thyroid gland. **Colloid goitre,** a form of goitre in which the vesicles of the gland are distended with colloid. **Exophthalmic goitre,** enlargement of the thyroid gland accompanied by characteristic systemic disturbances. Thyrotoxicosis. **Lingual goitre,** a swelling at the back of the tongue due to enlargement of a thyroid gland which has not descended into its correct position during the course of development. **Nodular goitre,** nodular enlargement of the thyroid gland, which may be either simple or toxic. **Simple goitre,** enlargement of the thyroid gland without any toxic manifestations. **Substernal goitre,** enlargement of the lower end of the thyroid gland which extends behind the sternum. **Toxic goitre,** a goitre accompanied by signs and symptoms of thyrotoxicosis.

Goitrogen. A substance that induces goitre.

Gold. A precious metal, the salts of which are used in the treatment of rheumatoid arthritis. Symbol Au (L *aurum*). Atomic weight 196·97. Atomic number 79. **Gold (^{198}Au) injection,** B.P. 1968, a sterile colloidal solution of gold-168 stabilized with gelatin. Gold-168 (^{168}Au) is a radioactive isotope of gold used in the treatment of malignant effusions, and also for scanning the liver and reticulo-endothelial system.

Gomphosis. A peg-and-socket joint, as in the articulations of the roots of the teeth with the alveoli of the mandible and maxillae.

Gonad. A sexual gland, ovary or testis.

Gonadotrophin. A gonadal stimulating hormone. **Chorionic gonadotrophin,** B.P. 1968, a dry sterile preparation of the gonad-stimulating substance obtained from the urine of pregnant women. **Human chorionic gonadotrophin (HCG),** gonadrotrophin from urine from women in early pregnancy. **Human menopausal gonadotrophin (HMG),** gonadotrophin from urine from menopausal women. **Human pituitary gonadotrophin (HPG),** gonadotrophin obtained from human pituitaries at necropsy.

Gonagra. Gout in the knee.

Gonio- (Gk *gōnia:* angle). Prefix indicating relationship to an angle.

Goniometer. An instrument for measuring angles.

Gonion. The tip of the angle of the mandible.

Gonio-puncture. A surgical puncture into the subconjunctival space, carried out in certain cases of glaucoma.

Gonioscope. An instrument for the examination of the angle of the eye.

Goniotomy. An operation for relieving the pressure in certain forms of glaucoma.

Gono- (Gk *gonē:* seed). Prefix indicating association with, or pertaining to, semen.

Gonococcus. *Neisseria gonorrhoeae.* The causative organism of gonorrhoea. (*Plural:* gonococci.)

Gonocyte. The primitive germ cell of the embryo.

Gonophore. An accessory generative organ for the storage or conduction of the sexual cells, such as the oviduct or seminal vesicle.

Gonorrhoea. The inflammatory disease of the genito-urinary passages caused by *Neisseria gonorrhoeae.* A highly infectious venereal disease.

Goose flesh. The appearance of the skin produced by contraction of the arrectores pilorum, caused by some stimulus such as cold or fear. Goose skin.

Gossypium. A genus of plants from which cotton is obtained.

Goundou. An exostosis of the nasal bones, believed to be a sequel of yaws.

Gout. A constitutional disorder of purine metabolism, characterized by excess of uric acid in the blood, painful joints and systemic disturbances.

Graft. A piece of tissue removed from one part to replace missing tissue in another part.

Grain. A seed. A small particle, as of sand. A unit of weight in the imperial system: one seven-thousandth of a pound avoirdupois. Equivalent to 0·0648 gramme.

-gram (Gk *gramma*: something written). Suffix indicating that which is written or recorded.

Gramicidin. A group of polypeptide antibiotics derived from *Bacillus brevis* or by synthesis, which is active against a wide range of micro-organisms, but, because of its systemic toxicity, is used only locally.

Gramme. Gram. A unit of weight in the metric system. One-thousandth of a kilogram. The usual abbreviation is g, but the British Pharmacopoeia Commission recommends that in prescriptions the abbreviation used should be G.

Grand mal. Major epilepsy.

Granulation. Subdivision into free-flowing granules or particles. The formation of small fleshy projections on a raw surface in the process of heating.

Granule. A small particle or grain. Zymogen granule, a granule in the cells of an enzyme-producing gland, such as the pancreas and salivary glands, that is the source of zymogens.

Granulocyte. A cell containing granules. Applied particularly to the leucocytes.

Granulocytic. Pertaining to a granulocyte.

Granulocytopenia. An abnormal diminution of the number of granulocytes in the blood stream. Neutropenia.

Granuloma. A tumour composed of granulation tissue. (*Plural:* granulomas.) **Granuloma annulare,** a nodular, non-itching eruption of the skin, most common in children and young adults. **Eosinophilic granuloma of bone,** a painful bony swelling, usually of one bone, consisting of foamy macrophages, giant cells, eosinophils and polymorphs, and accompanied by eosinophilia, which occurs in older children and young adults. **Malignant granuloma,** a rare disease of unknown etiology, characterized by progressive granulomatous ulceration of the respiratory tract. **Granuloma telangietaticum,** a rapidly growing haemangioma. As it always becomes infected, it is sometimes known as *granuloma pyogenicum*. **Granuloma venereum,** an ulcerating condition of the genitals, groin and perineum,

caused by *Klebsiella granulomatis*, and found throughout the tropics. **Granuloma venereum vel inguinale,** a nodular, ulcerative condition of the anogenital region caused by *Donovania granulomatis*, which is venereally acquired. **Wegener's granuloma,** malignant granuloma in which systemic involvement has occurred; *Wegener's granulomatosis*.

Granulomatosis. A condition characterized by multiple granulomas. **Lipophagic granulomatosis,** intestinal lipodystrophy. **Progressive allergic granulomatosis,** a variant of polyarthritis nodosa, with nodular necrotic lesions in the lump, and accompanied by asthmatic attacks. **Progressive septic granulomatosis,** a condition in boys, characterized by lack of neutrophils, as a result of which they are subject to repeated infections, often staphylococcal, of the skin, lymph nodes, lungs and elsewhere. **Wegener's granulomatosis,** a form of polyarthritis nodosa affecting mainly the kidneys, lungs and upper respiratory tract.

-graph (Gk *graphos:* to write). Suffix used to denote an instrument which records.

Grapho- (Gk *graphos:* to write). Prefix indicating relationship to writing or a record.

Graphology. The science of the study of handwriting.

Graphomania. A morbid, irresistible desire to write.

Graphophobia. A morbid fear of writing.

-graphy (Gk *grophos:* to write). Suffix used to indicate the art of writing or recording.

Grattage. The removal of granulation tissue by brushing or scrubbing.

Gravel. Small, sandlike concretions in the urinary tract or biliary tract.

Gravid. Pregnant.

Gravity. Weight. The force exerted by the earth on objects. **Specific gravity,** the weight of a body compared with that of an equal volume of a standard substance.

Gripe. A sharp pain in the bowels.

Griseofulvin. B.P. 1968. $C_{17}H_{17}ClO_6$. An antifungal substance produced by the growth of certain strains of *Penicillium griseofulvum*.

Groin. The inguinal region; the depression between the abdomen and the thigh.

Grommet. A small plastic tube inserted through the tympanic membrane to allow constant aeration and drainage in cases of persistent exudative otitis media.

Groove. A hollow, long, shallow depression, or sulcus. **Anal intersphincteric groove,** the groove between the subcutaneous part of the external sphincter and the lower border of the internal sphincter. **Bicipital groove,** the *intertubercular sulcus* which lies between the two tubercles at the upper end of the humerus and lodges the tendon of the long head of the biceps. **Carotid groove,** the groove lateral to the sella turcica that houses the internal carotid artery. **Costal groove,** the groove on the lower border of the internal surface of a rib, which gives attachment to the internal intercostal membrane. **Infra-orbital groove,** the groove in the floor of the orbit that transmits the infra-orbital vessels and nerve. **Interatrial groove,** the groove that externally separates the two atria of the heart. **Interventricular grooves,** an *anterior* groove on the sternocostal surface of the heart, and a *posterior* groove on the diaphragmatic surface, that separate the two ventricles externally. **Lacrimal groove,** the groove in the medial wall of the orbit that lodges the lacrimal sac. **Mylohyoid groove,** the groove on the medial aspect of the mandibles that houses the mylohyoid nerve and vessels. **Nasolabial groove,** the groove that runs down from the side of the nose to the angle of the mouth. **Nasolacrimal groove,** a groove on the medial surface of the maxilla, lodging the nasolacrimal duct. **Neural groove,** the median groove on the dorsal surface of the embryo which is the predecessor of the neural tube. **Obturator groove,** the groove on the obturator surface of the superior ramus of the pubis, that transmits the obturator vessels and nerve. **Occipital groove,** the shallow groove on the mastoid portion of the temporal bone, that lodges the occipital artery. **Optic groove,** the *chiasmatic sulcus,* the groove in the middle cranial fossa that leads from one optic canal to the other. **Subclavian groove,** the groove on the inferior surface of the clavicle that gives insertion to the subclavius muscle. **Vertebral grooves,** the grooves on the sides of the spinous processes of the vertebrae, that lodge the deep muscles of the back.

Gruel. A semiliquid food, usually made of oatmeal or some other cereal.

Grumous. Lumpy. Clotted.

Gryposis. Abnormal curvature, usually of the nails.

Guaiphenesin. B.P.C. 1968. $C_{10}H_{14}O_4$. An expectorant which acts by reducing the tenacity of sputum.

Guamecycline. The B.P. Commission approved name for N-(4-guanidino-forminidoylpiperazin-1-ylmethyl)tetracycline. A broad-spectrum antibiotic.

Guanacline. The B.P. Commission approved name for 1-(2-guanidino-ethyl) - 1,2,3,6 - tetrahydro - 4 - picoline. A hypotensive agent.

Guanethidine sulphate. B.P. 1968. $C_{10}H_{24}N_4O_4S$. A hypotensive agent which acts by blocking transmission in post-ganglionic adrenergic nerves.

Guanoclor. The B.P. Commission approved name for [2-(2,6-dichloro-phenoxy)ethyl]aminoguanidine. A hypotensive agent.

Guanoxan. The B.P. Commission approved name for 2-guanidino-methyl-1, 4-benzodioxan. A hypotensive agent.

Gubernaculum. A guide or guiding structure. (*Plural:* gubernacula.)

Guinea-worm. The nematode worm *Dracunculus medinensis,* which causes the disease known as dracontiasis.

Gullet. Oesophagus.

Gum. Gingiva, or covering of the jaws. The mucilaginous, complex exudation of various trees or shrubs.

Gumboil. A dental abscess causing swelling of the gums.

Gumma. The granulomatous growth of tertiary syphilis. (*Plural*: gummas.)

Gustation. The sense of taste.

Gustatory. Pertaining to the sense of taste.

Gut. The intestine.

Gutta. A drop. (*Plural:* guttae.)

Gutta percha. The latex obtained from trees of the family Sapotaceae, which is used in the preparation of splints and wound dressings.

Guttate. Resembling a drop, or spotted as if by drops.

Gutter. A shallow groove. **Right lateral paracolic gutter,** the groove between the right side of the ascending colon and the posterior abdominal wall.

Gymnastics. Systematic muscular exercises.

Gyn-, Gynaec- (Gk *gynē:* woman). Prefixes indicating an association with, or pertaining to, women.

Gynaecoid. Woman-like in structure and form.

Gynaecologist. A specialist in diseases peculiar to women.

Gynaecology. The branch of medicine

concerned with diseases peculiar to women.

Gynaecomastia. Excessive development of the male breast.

Gynaephobia. Morbid fear of women.

Gynandrism. Pseudohermaphroditism in the female.

Gypsum. Calcium sulphate. When dried or calcined it becomes plaster of Paris, which is widely used in the making of plaster casts.

Gyrectomy. Surgical excision of a cerebral gyrus.

Gyro- (Gk *gyros:* ring or circle). Prefix indicating relationship to a gyrus, or meaning circular.

Gyrus. Convolution, a term applied particularly to the convolutions on the surface of the brain. (*Plural:* gyri.) **Angular gyrus,** the middle part of the inferior parietal lobule, that is concerned with the visual element in astereognosis. **Cingulate gyrus,** a gyrus on the medial surface of the cerebral hemisphere. **Cuneate gyrus,** a buried gyrus that separates the parieto-occipital sulcus and the calcarine sulcus, on the medial surface of the cerebral hemisphere. **Dentate gyrus,** a narrow gyrus on the upper surface of the parahippocampal gyrus. **Descendens gyrus,** a gyrus that lies behind the inferior and superior occipital gyri. **Frontal gyri, superior, middle, and inferior,** gyri on the superolateral surface of the cerebral hemisphere. **Interlocking gyri,** small interlocking gyri in the opposed walls of the central sulcus of the cerebral hemisphere. **Lingual gyrus,** a gyrus on the basal surface of the cerebral hemisphere, lying between the calcarine and the collateral sulci. **Long gyrus,** a gyrus on the posterior part of the insula. **Occipital gyri, superior** and **inferior,** two gyri on the lateral aspect of the occipital lobe. **Occipitotemporal gyri, medial** and **lateral,** two gyri in the basal surface of the cerebral hemisphere, the former extending from the neighbourhood of the occipital to the temporal lobe, and the latter continuous round the inferolateral margin of the hemisphere with the inferior temporal gyrus. **Orbital gyri,** four gyri on the anterior (orbital) part of the basal surface of the cerebral hemisphere. **Parahippocampal gyrus,** a gyrus on the basal surface of the cerebral hemisphere. **Paraterminal gyrus,** the strip of cortex which lies immediately in front of the lamina terminalis. **Postcentral gyrus,** the gyrus on the superolateral surface of the parietal lobe of the cerebral hemisphere, which receives somatic sensory impulses. **Precentral gyrus,** the gyrus on the superolateral surface of the cerebral hemisphere, in the frontal lobe, the cells in which give rise to some of the fibres of the pyramidal motor tracts. **Supramarginal gyrus,** the anterior part of the inferior parietal lobule, which is continuous in front with the lower part of the postcentral gyrus. **Temporal gyri, superior, middle, inferior,** and **transverse,** the first three of these, on the lateral surface of the temporal lobe, and the fourth, the transverse (of which there are four in number) forming the floor of the posterior ramus of the lateral sulcus. The higher auditory centres are situated in the anterior transverse temporal gyrus and in the contiguous portion of the superior temporal gyrus.

H

Habenula. A ribbon-like or rein-like structure. (*Plural:* habenulae.)

Hacking. The chopping stroke made with the edge of the hand in massage.

Haem. The non-protein pigment bound to globin in haemoglobin. It contains iron in the ferrous form.

Haem-, Haema-, Haemo- (Gk *haima:* blood). Prefixes indicating a relationship to blood.

Haemadsorption. The reaction in which erythrocytes are absorbed on to cells in tissue cultures on which myxoviruses are grown. It is one of the means of identifying such viruses.

Haemagglutination. The clumping together of erythrocytes as the result of the action of agglutinins.

Haemagglutinin. An antibody that causes agglutination of erythrocytes.

Haemagglutinogen. The antigen on an erythrocyte that reacts with the corresponding haemagglutinin in the blood to cause agglutination of the erythrocytes.

Haemangioblastoma. Capillary angioma.

Haemangioma. Angioma. An innocent tumour composed of dilated, tortuous blood vessels. (*Plural:* haemangiomas.)

Haemangiopericytoma. A rare vascular tumour composed of patent or collapsed capillaries surrounded by a variable number of pericytes, and of variable malignancy.

Haemaphysalis. A genus of ticks. *Haemaphysalis spinigera* is the vector of Kyasanur forest fever.

Haemarthrosis. Extravasation of blood into a joint.

Haematemesis. Vomiting of blood.

Haematin. An oxidation product of haem, which contains iron in the ferric form. It can also be obtained from myoglobin, catalase, peroxidase, and cytochrome.

Haematinic. Improving the condition of the blood. A substance which improves the blood by acting as an anti-anaemic factor.

Haematite. An iron oxide ore. **Haematite-miners' lung,** a form of pneumoconiosis in iron-ore miners caused by the inhalation of haematite dust.

Haematobium. A blood parasite. *Schistosoma haematobium,* the blood fluke that causes genito-urinary schistomiasis or bilharziasis.

Haematocele. A cyst or cavity filled with blood.

Haematocolpos. An accumulation of blood in the vagina due to some obstruction to its escape, such as an imperforate hymen.

Haematocrit. A centrifuge for separating blood cells from the plasma.

Haematocyst. A blood cyst.

Haematogenous. Blood-borne. Pertaining to blood or derived from blood.

Haematoidin. A yellow-brown crystalline substance in blood clot, which gives a bruise its yellow colour.

Haematoma. A localized collection of extravasated blood.

Haematometra. An accumulation of blood in the uterus.

Haematomyelia. Haemorrhage into the spinal cord.

Haematopoiesis. Haemopoiesis.

Haematoporphyrin. An iron-free derivative of haemoglobin, which is found in the blood and urine in sulphonal poisoning, certain cases of liver disease, and the congenital disease known as porphyria.

Haematoxylin. A widely used stain in bacteriology and histology, obtained from logwood (*Haematoxylon campechianum* (L.)).

Haematoxyphil bodies. Lilac staining foci of degraded nuclear material found in areas of filbinoid necrosis in systemic lupus erythematosus, and diagnostic of the condition.

Haematuria. The presence of blood in the urine.

Haemic. Relating to the blood.

Haemin. Haematin chloride. A dark-brown crystalline substance which forms in old blood clot and is used as a means of identifying blood.

Haemobartonella. A genus of the family Bartonellaceae, members of which are parasites of erythrocytes in lower animals, such as rats, mice and dogs.

Haemochromatosis. A rare disease in which large amounts of haemosiderin are deposited throughout the body, particularly the liver, pancreas, and skin, and characterized clinically by cirrhosis of the liver, diabetes mellitus and pigmentation. Hence the alternative name of bronzed diabetes.

Haemoconcentration. Increase in the concentration of erythrocytes in the circulating blood.

Haemocyanin. The blue, oxygen-carrying pigment in the plasma of molluscs and arthropods.

Haemocytoblast. The most primitive recognizable blood cell in the marrow which is totipotential: i.e. capable of producing red cells, white cells and platelets.

Haemocytometer. An instrument for counting cells in the blood.

Haemodialysis. The process whereby a patient's blood is passed through a cellophane tube lying in a bath of dialysing solution isotonic with blood, containing physiological concentrations of electrolytes but no urea or other nitrogenous substances. Popularly known as an artificial kidney.

Haemodilution. The state in which there is a reduced concentration of erythrocytes in the circulating blood.

Haemoglobin. An iron-containing conjugated protein consisting of globin and the iron-containing haem. It is present in the erythrocytes of vertebrates and is responsible for the transmission of oxygen from the lungs to the tissues. There are three physiological haemoglobins in man. (*Abbreviation:* Hb.) Haemoglobin A comprises about 98 per cent of adult haemoglobin. Haemoglobin A_2 normally comprises 2 per cent, but may be raised or lowered in certain abnormalities of haemoglobin formation. Haemoglobin F, or foetal haemoglobin, forms more than half the haemoglobin in the human foetus and new-born children, but is gradually replaced by haemoglobin A throughout infancy. Haemoglobin S, the abnormal haemoglobin found in sickle-cell anaemia. Other abnormal haemoglobins are Haemoglobin C, Haemoglobin D, and Haemoglobin E.

Haemoglobinaemia. The presence of free haemoglobin in the blood plasma.

Haemoglobinometer. An instrument for the determination of the amount of haemoglobin in the blood.

Haemoglobinopathy. A condition characterized by abnormality of the haemoglobin: e.g. sickle-cell anaemia.

Haemoglobinuria. The presence of haemoglobin in the urine. **Paroxysmal cold haemoglobinuria,** a disease, usually a complication of tertiary syphilis, characterized by episodes of severe haemolysis, and haemoglobinuria, due to cold haemolysins. **Paroxysmal nocturnal haemoglobinuria,** an episodic haemolytic anaemia in adults, characterized by attacks of haemoglobinuria usually occurring at night, due to a defect of the erythrocytes.

Haemogram. A written or graphic record of the blood cells and haemoglobin.

Haemohydrothorax. The presence of a blood-stained exudate in the pleural cavity.

Haemolysin. A substance that releases haemoglobin from the erythrocytes and thereby causes haemolysis.

Haemolysis. The release of haemoglobin from the erythrocytes.

Haemolytic. Causing or pertaining to haemolysis.

Haemopericardium. An effusion of blood in the pericardial sac.

Haemoperitoneum. An effusion of blood in the peritoneal cavity.

Haemophilia. A hereditary disease of males, transmitted by females, characterized by bleeding due to marked prolongation of the coagulation time.

Haemophiliac. A victim of haemophilia.

Haemophilic. Pertaining to haemophilia.

Haemophilus. A genus of bacteria belonging to the family Brucellaceae, so called in virtue of their inability to grow on culture without the addition of whole blood or certain growth-promoting substances present in blood. The important members of the genus are *H. influenzae*, *H. aegyptius*, and *H. ducreyi*.

Haemophthalmitis. The inflammatory state of the eye induced by the irritation caused by the end-products of intra-ocular haemorrhages.

Haemopneumopericardium. A combination of air and blood in the pericardial sac.

Haemopneumothorax. A combination of air and blood in the pleural cavity.

Haemopoiesis. The formation of blood.

Haemopoietic. Concerned with the formation of blood.

Haemopoietin. Intrinsic factor. The enzyme in the gastric mucosa which is responsible for the absorption of vitamin B_{12}, an essential step in normal haemopoiesis.

Haemoptysis. Spitting up of blood from the lungs.

Haemorrhage. Bleeding. The escape of blood from a blood vessel. **Accidental haemorrhage,** uterine bleeding during the last three months of pregnancy due to separation of a normally situated placenta. **Antepartum haemorrhage,** bleeding from or into the genital tract occurring either in pregnancy after the period of viability has been reached, or during labour before birth of the child. **Extradural haemorrhage,** bleeding into the extradural space, usually from the middle meningeal artery following trauma. **Internal haemorrhage,** bleeding into an organ, cavity or tissues of the body. **Petechial haemorrhage,** capillary bleeding into the skin. **Postpartum haemorrhage,** excessive bleeding, exceeding 600ml., from or into the genital tract after delivery of the child. **Primary haemorrhage,** bleeding immediately after an injury. **Secondary haemorrhage,** bleeding occurring at an interval after injury or operation or primary haemorrhage has stopped. **Splinter haemorrhage,** a linear haemorrhage under a nail, such as occurs in subacute bacterial endocarditis. **Subarachnoid haemorrhage,** bleeding into the subarachnoid space, usually from a ruptured aneurysm of the circle of Willis. **Subdural haemorrhage,** bleeding into the subdural space. **Unavoidable haemorrhage,** bleeding from placenta praevia. **Vicarious haemorrhage,** bleeding from one organ or area in place of bleeding from another site: e.g. epistazis in place of uterine bleeding in menstruation.

Haemorrhoidectomy. Surgical excision of haemorrhoids.

Haemorrhoids. Piles. A varicose state of the external haemorrhoidal veins.

Haemosialemesis. The discharge of bloodstained saliva.

Haemosiderin. An iron-containing protein complex, formed by the splitting up of haematin and stored in the body in the case of iron-overloading. It contains around 35 per cent of iron and appears as brown granules which give a Prussian-blue reaction.

Haemosiderinuria. The presence of haemosiderin in the urine.

Haemosiderosis. The accumulation of haemosiderin in the body.

Haemospermia. The presence of blood in the seminal fluid.

Haemosporidia. The order of the class Sporozoa, to which plasmodium belongs.

Haemostasis. The arrest of bleeding.

Haemostatic. A drug or procedure that arrests bleeding.

Haemothorax. Effusion of blood into a pleural cavity.

Haemozoin. The malarial pigment derived from haemoglobin which escapes from the erythrocyte when the schizont ruptures, and is finally phagocytosed by the macrophages.

Hafnia. A genus of Enterobacteriaceae which is non-pathogenic to man.

Hafnium. A rare chemical element. Symbol Hf. Atomic weight 178·49. Atomic number 72.

Hair. A slender filamentous appendage of the skin.

Halethazole. The B.P. Commission approved name for 5-chloro-2-[4-(2-diethylaminoethoxy) phenyl]-benzothiazole. An antifungal agent.

Half-life. The period during which the activity of a radioactive substance is reduced to one-half of its original value.

Halibut-liver oil. B.P. 1968. The fixed oil extracted from the fresh, or suitably preserved, livers of the halibut species belonging to the genus Hippoglossus. It contains not less than 30,000 units of vitamin A activity per gramme and usually between 2500 and 3500 units of vitamin D activity per gramme.

Halisteresis. Osteomalacia.

Halitosis. Offensive breath.

Hallucination. A mental impression of sensory vividness occurring without external stimulus.

Hallucinogen. A drug or preparation that produces distortions of perception, emotional changes, depersonalization and a variety of effects on memory, learned behaviour and other ego functions.

Hallux. The great toe. (*Plural:* halluces.) **Hallux valgus,** deviation of the great toe to the outer side of the foot. **Hallux varus,** deviation of the great toe to the inner side of the foot.

Halo. The ring of spectral colours seen round lights, as in glaucoma.

Halo- (Gk *hals:* salt). Prefix indicating relationship to a salt.

Halogen. One of the group of elements that includes bromine, chlorine, fluorine, and iodine.

Halopenium chloride. The B.P.

Commission approved name for 4-bromobenzyl-3-(4-chloro-2-isopropyl - 5 - methylphenoxy)propyldimethyl ammonium chloride. An antiseptic.

Haloperidol. B.P. Addendum 1969. $C_{21}H_{23}ClFNO_2$. A tranquillizer.

Halophilic. Requiring a salty environment. **Halophilic bacteria,** bacteria that can grow at high concentrations of sodium chloride.

Halopyramine. The B.P. Commission approved name for N-(4-chlorbenzyl)-$N'N'$-dimethyl-N-2-pyridyl-ethylene-diamine. An antihistamine.

Halothane. B.P. 1968. $C_2HBrClF_3$. A volatile anaesthetic.

Halquinol. The B.P. Commission approved name for a mixture of the chlorinated products of 8-hydroxy-quinoline compounds containing around 65 per cent of 5,7-dichloro-8-hydroxyquinoline. An anti-infective agent.

Halzoun. A form of pharyngeal fascioliasis encountered in the Middle East.

Hamamelis. B.P.C. 1968. The dried leaves of *Hamamalis virginiana* (L.). It is an astringent. **Hamamelis water,** B.P.C. 1968, prepared by macerating recently cut and partially dormant twigs of *Hamamelis virginiana* (L.) in water, distilling, and adding the requisite amount of alcohol. Distilled hazel water. Used as a cooling application to bruises and sprains, and as a haemostatic, and an eye lotion.

Hamartoma. A tumour-like malformation in which the tissues of a particular part of the body are arranged haphazardly.

Hamatum. The hamate bone, the most medial in the distal row of the carpus.

Hamstring. One of the tendons bounding the popliteal fossa.

Hamular. Hook-shaped.

Hamulus. A hook or hook-like process. (*Plural*: hamuli.) **Lacrimal hamulus,** a small hook on the crest of the lacrimal bone which articulates with the maxilla and completes the upper orifice of the bony canal for the lacrimal duct. **Pterygoid hamulus,** a slender process on the posterior border of the medial pterygoid plate, which is grooved anteriorly at its root by the tendon of the tensor veli palatini. **Spiral lamina hamulus,** a hook-shaped process in the summit of the cochlea.

Hamycin. An antibiotic derived from *Streptomyces pimprina*, which is active against *Candida albicans, Trichomonas*

vaginalis, Aspergillus niger and *Cryptococcus neoformans.*

Hand. The extremity of the upper limb, consisting of the wrist, metacarpus and fingers.

Handle. That by which something can be taken hold of. **Handle of the malleus,** that part of the malleus that is connected to the tympanic membrane.

Hangnail. A painful, loose tag of skin at the side of the nail.

Haphalgesia. Pain caused by the lightest touch.

Haplo- (Gk *haploos:* single, simple). Prefix meaning single or simple.

Haplodont. Having molar teeth without cusps or ridges.

Haploid. Having one set of chromosomes as in gametes, as opposed to the diploid state in somatic cells.

Hapt-, Hapte-, Hapto- (Gk *haptein:* to touch or hold fast). Prefixes indicating relationship to touch or to seizure.

Hapten. A non-protein substance which is not itself antigenic, but which combines with a protein to form a new antigen, which is capable of stimulating the production of specific antibodies, the specificity of which depends on the hapten fraction and not the protein fraction.

Haptoglobins. A group of α_2-globulins with the distinctive property of binding haemoglobin.

Harelip. A congenital fissure in the upper lip.

Hartnup disease. A rare congenital disorder associated with disturbed tryptophan metabolism, and characterized by aminoaciduria, pellagra and cerebellar ataxia.

Hashimoto's disease. Hashimoto's thyroiditis. A chronic inflammatory disease of the thyroid gland produced by thyroid antibodies.

Hashish. The resin of *Cannabis indica* (L.).

Haustrum. One of the sacculations of the colon. (*Plural:* haustra.)

Haustus. A draught.

Hay fever. An allergic condition of the mucous membrane of the nose, eyes and upper air passages, caused by an allergic reaction to pollen.

Head. The uppermost part of the body, containing the brain, the organs of sight, hearing, taste and smell, and the mouth. The upper part or top of any structure, including bone and muscle.

Headache. Pain in the head.

Health. The state of being free from disease mentally and physically, and the body functioning in all respects at its optimum level of efficiency.

Hearing. Perception by sound.

Hearing aid. An appliance for the amplification of sound to improve the perception of sound by a deaf person.

Heart. The hollow muscular pump, with four chambers, which maintains the circulation of the blood.

Heart block. A condition in which there is interference with the transmission of the impulse through the heart. **Arborization heart block,** interference with conduction in the finer ramifications of the Purkinje system. **Atrioventricular heart block,** interference of conduction between the atria and the ventricles, which may be complete or partial. **Bundle branch block,** interference with conduction in either the left or the right branch of the atrioventricular bundle. **Complete heart block,** complete severance of conduction between the atria and ventricles. **Sinu-atrial heart block,** interference with conduction between the sinu-atrial node and the atria.

Heartburn. A burning sensation behind the sternum. Pyrosis.

Heat. A form of kinetic energy transferred by means of conduction, or radiation. The sensation derived from exposure to hot objects. Periodic sexual excitement in animals. **Atomic heat,** the amount of heat needed to raise an atom of the substance in question from 0° to 1°C. **Conductive heat,** heat transmitted by direct contact. **Convective heat,** heat transferred or transmitted by motion from its source, as by air or water. **Latent heat,** the heat absorbed without rise of temperature in the course of conversion from solid to liquid, or from liquid to gas. **Prickly heat,** miliaria. **Radiant heat,** electromagnetic waves with a wave-length intermediate between those of red light and Hertzian waves.

Heatstroke. Heat hyperpyrexia. The condition characterized by a rise of temperature to 106°F (41·1°C) or more, induced by exposure to intense heat.

Hebephrenia. The form of schizophrenia characterized by childishness, silly giggling, grimacing, oddities of motor behaviour, lack of attention to toilet and dress, odd verbal formulations, bizarre delusions and hallucinations.

Hebetic. Pertaining to puberty.

Hebetude. Mental dullness or lethargy.

Hebiatrics. Ephebiatrics.

Hectic. The term applied to the swinging temperature in severe forms of active tuberculosis and the accompanying flush of the face. Now generally applied to such a type of pyrexia occurring in any infection.

Hecto- (Gk *hekaton:* one hundred). Prefix signifying one hundred.

Hectogram. One hundred grammes.

Hectolitre. One hundred litres.

Hectometre. One hundred metres.

Hedaquinium chloride. The B.P. Commission approved name for hexadecamethylenedi-(2-isoquinolium chloride). An antifungal agent.

Hedonia. Abnormal cheerfulness.

Hedonism. The doctrine or philosophy that inculcates that the greatest happiness [of an individual or community is the ultimate aim of life.

Hedonophobia. Morbid fear of pleasure.

Heel. The hinder part of the foot formed by the calcaneum.

Helc-, Helco- (Gk *helkos:* ulcer). Prefixes signifying association with an ulcer.

Helcoid. Resembling an ulcer.

Helcoplasty. Plastic repair of ulcers.

Helicine. Pertaining to the helix. In the form of a spiral.

Helicotrema. The small opening at the apex of the modiolus, through which the two passages in the cochlear canal of the inner ear communicate with each other.

Helio- (Gk *helios:* sun). Prefix indicating association with the sun.

Heliophobia. A morbid fear of the rays of the sun.

Heliotaxis. The reaction of a living organism whereby it grows towards (*positive heliotaxis*) or away from (*negative heliotaxis*) the sun.

Heliotherapy. Treatment of disease by exposure to the sun's rays.

Heliotropism. The property of a living organism to bend towards or away from the sun.

Helium. A gaseous element. Symbol He. Atomic weight 4·0026. Atomic number 2. **Helium,** B.P. 1968, obtained from natural petroleum gas by liquefaction and rectification at low temperature. Used as an air-helium, or oxygen-helium, mixture in easing asthmatic attacks, and as a prophylactic against caisson disease.

Helix. The convex margin of the pinna of the ear.

Helminth. A worm.

Helminthiasis. Infestation with parasitic worms.

Helminthology. The scientific study of worms.

Helo- (Gk *helos:* nail). Prefix signifying association with a nail.

Heloma. A corn or callosity.

Hemeralopia. Day blindness. The condition in which an individual can see better in dull light than in bright light.

Hemi- (Gk *hemi:* half). Prefix meaning one-half.

Hemiachromatopsia. Loss of colour vision in half of each visual field.

Hemianaesthesia. Loss of sensation on one side of the body.

Hemianalgesia. Impairment of sensation of pain on one side of the body.

Hemianopia. Loss of half the field of vision. **Altitudinal hemianopia**, loss of vision in the upper or lower visual fields. **Bilateral hemianopia**, hemianopia involving both eyes. **Bitemporal hemianopia**, loss of vision in both temporal fields. **Heteronymous hemianopia**, bilateral hemianopia in-involving either both nasal halves or both temporal halves of the field of vision. **Homonymous hemianopia**, loss of vision in the same side in each eye.

Hemiathetosis. Athetosis of one side of the body.

Hemiatrophy. Atrophy affecting one side of the body.

Hemiballism. Unilateral involuntary movements. Hemiballismus.

Hemichorea. Choreic movements restricted to one side of the body.

Hemicolectomy. Surgical removal of part of the colon.

Hemicrania. Headache limited to one side of the head.

Hemidrosis. Sweating on one side of the body.

Hemiectromelia. Defective development of the limbs on one side of the body.

Hemihyperidrosis. Excessive sweating on one side of the body.

Hemihypertrophy. Overgrowth of one side of the body.

Hemimelia. The condition characterized by imperfect development of the distal part of one or more limbs.

Hemiparaesthesia. Unilateral paraesthesia.

Hemiplegia. Paralysis of one side of the body.

Hemiptera. The order of insects, characterized by the proboscis, which is always adapted for sucking. It includes the bed bug.

Hemisacralization. Fusion of the 5th lumbar vertebra to the first segment of the sacrum on one side. A developmental abnormality.

Hemisphere. A half-sphere. **Cerebellar hemispheres**, the two hemispheres into which the cerebellum is divided. They are joined by a narrow median strip, the vermis. **Cerebral hemispheres**, the two hemispheres which form the largest part of the brain.

Hemithorax. One half of the chest.

Hemithyroidectomy. Surgical removal of one lateral lobe of the thyroid gland.

Hemlock. *Conium maculatum* (L.), a flowering plant indigenous to Britain and Central Europe, the active principle of which is coniine.

Hemp. The fibrous material obtained principally from *Cannabis sativa*, and used for the manufacture of rope. As an industrial hazard it can induce pneumoconiosis. **Indian hemp**, marihuana.

Henbane. Hyoscyamus.

Henna. An aqueous extract of the dried leaves of *Lawsonia inermis*, used as a hair dye.

Henry. The electrical inductance of a closed circuit in which an electromotive force of 1 volt is produced when the electric current in the circuit varies uniformly at the rate of 1 ampere per second.

Heparin. B.P. 1968. A sterile preparation containing the sodium salt of a complex organic acid present in mammalian tissues, and having the property, when administered parenterally (preferably intravenously) of delaying or inhibiting the clotting of blood.

Hepat-, Hepato- (Gk *hepar:* liver). Prefixes signifying association with the liver.

Hepatalgia. Pain in the liver.

Hepatectomy. Surgical removal of part of the liver in man, or the entire liver in the experimental animal.

Hepatic. Pertaining to the liver.

Hepatitis. Inflammation of the liver. **Infective (or infectious) hepatitis**, a disease caused by infection of the liver by a virus (IH) spread by faecal contamination. **Lupoid hepatitis**, a persisting, or relapsing, form of hepatitis, in which lupus erythematosus (L.E.) cells can be demonstrated in the blood. **Serum hepatitis**, a form of virus hepatitis caused by virus SH, which is transmitted parenterally, usually by the injection or transfusion of contaminated blood or blood products.

Virus hepatitis, any form of hepatitis caused by a virus.

Hepatization. The conversion of tissue into a liver-like substance, characteristically found in the lungs in lobar pneumonia. **Grey hepatization,** the stage of hepatization when the lung is packed with leucocytes and has a grey colour. **Red hepatization,** the preceding stage when the lung is red in colour because of the blood in it.

Hepatoblastoma. An embryonic malignant tumour of the liver.

Hepatocellular. Relating to the cells of the liver.

Hepatodynia. Pain in the liver.

Hepatolenticular. Pertaining to the liver and the lenticular nucleus. **Hepatolenticular degeneration,** a rare disease of the nervous system accompanied by cirrhosis of the liver, and due to a disorder of copper metabolism.

Hepatolienal. Relating to the liver and spleen.

Hepatoma. A tumour of the liver. The term is usually applied to carcinoma of the liver cells, but is also used as a synonym for a benign adenoma of the liver.

Hepatomegaly. Enlargement of the liver.

Hepatorenal. Pertaining to both liver and kidneys.

Hepatorrhaphy. Suture of a wound of the liver.

Hepatorrhexis. Rupture of the liver.

Hepatotoxic. Damaging to, or destructive of, the cells of the liver.

Hept-, Hepta- (Gk *hepta:* seven). Prefixes signifying seven.

Heptabarbitone. The B.P. Commission approved name for 5-(cylohept-1-enyl)-5-ethylbarbituric acid. A hypnotic.

Heptaminol. The B.P. Commission approved name for 6-amino-2-methyl-heptan-2-ol. A coronary vasodilator.

Herbicide. An agent that kills weeds.

Herbivorous. Living on vegetable food.

Hereditary. Transmitted from ancestors to descendants.

Heredity. The transmission of characters or traits from parents to offspring.

Heredo- (L *heres:* an heir). Prefix indicating hereditary.

Heredofamilial. Hereditary in certain families.

Hermaphrodite. An individual possessing the genital organs of both sexes.

Hermaphroditism. The condition characterized by an individual possessing the gonads of both sexes, with varying degrees of sexual ambiguity.

Hermetic. Airtight.

Hernia. Protrusion of an organ, or part of an organ, through the wall of the cavity in which it lies. **Acquired hernia,** a hernia which develops after birth and occurs through an opening which was either not present, or only partially present, at birth. **Hernia adiposa** (or **fat hernia),** protrusion of extraperitoneal fat through the abdominal wall. **Cerebellar hernia,** displacement of the cerebellum into the foramen magnum. **Cerebral hernia,** protrusion of brain tissue through a defect in the skull. **Complete hernia,** a hernia in which the hernial sac and its contents have protruded through the orifice. **Concealed hernia,** a hernia not evident on palpation. **Congenital hernia,** a hernia present at birth or through a defect present at birth. **Diaphragmatic hernia,** a hernia of abdominal contents through the diaphragm into the thoracic cavity. **Direct hernia,** an inguinal hernia in which the sac protrudes between the deep epigastric artery and the edge of the rectus muscle. **Epigastric hernia,** a hernia through the linea alba. **Femoral hernia,** a hernia through the femoral canal. **Gluteal hernia,** a hernia through the greater or lesser sciatic notch. **Hiatus hernia,** a diaphragmatic hernia through the oesophageal hiatus. **Incarcerated hernia,** an irreducible or strangulated hernia. **Incisional hernia,** a hernia through an operation scar. **Indirect hernia,** an inguinal hernia through the abdominal ring. **Inguinal hernia,** a hernia in the inguinal canal. **Internal hernia,** a hernia within the abdominal cavity. **Irreducible hernia,** a hernia that cannot be reduced except by operation. **Labial hernia,** an inguinal hernia into the labium majus. **Mesenteric hernia,** an internal hernia through a hole in the mesentery. **Oblique hernia,** an indirect hernia. **Obturator hernia,** a hernia through the obturator foramen. **Postoperative hernia,** a hernia through a surgical scar. **Reducible hernia,** a hernia that can be reduced by taxis. **Scrotal hernia,** an oblique inguinal hernia that has descended into the scrotum. **Sliding hernia,** an indirect irreducible inguinal hernia in which an extraperitoneal organ, usually the colon or caecum, descends with the sac. **Strangulated hernia,** an irreducible, incarcerated hernia to which the circulation of the blood has been arrested. **Umbilical hernia,** a hernia through the umbilicus. **Ventral hernia,**

a hernia through the anterior abdominal wall.

Herniation. The process of formation of a hernia or protrusion.

Hernio- (L *hernia:* rupture). Prefix indicating association with a hernia.

Herniorrhaphy. The radical surgical cure for a hernia.

Heroin. Diamorphine.

Herpangina. A short-term fever, with ulcers of the fauces and [pharynx, caused by a group A Coxsackie virus.

Herpes. A vesicular eruption of the skin. **Herpes gestationis,** a dermatitis-herpetiformis-like eruption that occurs, rarely, during the third trimester of pregnancy or in the puerperium. **Herpes simplex,** an acute infectious disease, caused by a virus, and characterized by a vesicular eruption. **Herpes zoster,** a virus infection of posterior root ganglia, characterized by a vesicular eruption and girdle pain. Shingles.

Herpesviruses. A group of DNA viruses. *Herpesvirus cuniculi,* virus III of rabbits; *Herpesvirus hominis,* the cause of herpes simplex in man. *Herpesvirus simiae,* virus B of monkeys. *Herpesvirus suis,* the cause of pseudo-rabies in cattle and pigs. *Herpesvirus varicellae,* the cause of chickenpox. *Cytomegaloviruses,* the cause of cytomegalic inclusion disease.

Herpetic. Relating to herpes.

Herpetiform. Resembling herpes.

Hetacillin. The B.P. Commission approved name for a semi-synthetic antibiotic derived from 6-aminopenicillanic acid, which is acid resistant and absorbed orally.

Heter-, Hetero- (Gk *heteros:* other). Prefixes indicating different, other.

Heteradenia. Abnormality in the formation or location of glandular tissue.

Heterochromatin. That part of the interphase nucleus of the chromosome that stains deeply and is considered to represent those regions of the chromosome that remain relatively inert metabolically.

Heterochromia. A difference of colour in two structures that should have the same colour. **Heterochromia iridum,** differently coloured irises or parts of the same iris.

Heterogeneous. Having dissimilar characteristics.

Heterograft. A transplant from one animal to another of a different species.

Heteronium bromide. The B.P. Commission approved name for 1,1-dimethyl-3-(α-2-thienylmandeloyloxy)

pyrrolidinium. An anticholinergic agent.

Heterophile. Having an affinity for other than the usual. **Heterophile antigen,** an antigen which appears to be specific for an antigen having no biological relationship to that constituting the immunizing stimulus.

Heterophoria. Latent squint or strabismus: i.e. a tendency to misalignment of the visual axes which is corrected by the fusional capacity.

Heterophyes. A genus of small in-intestinal flukes. *Heterophyes heterophyes,* a species found in the Middle East which infects man as a result of the eating of raw fish containing metacercariae.

Heteroplasty. The grafting of tissue from one individual to another.

Heteropsia. Inequality of vision in the two eyes.

Heterosexuality. Sexual attraction towards the opposite sex.

Heterosis. The beneficial effect of hybridization, whereby the first generation hybrid shows more vigour than either of the parent strains.

Heterotopia. A displacement of organs or tissues. Ectopia.

Heterotopic. Displaced.

Heterotrophic. Not self-sustaining. **Heterotrophic bacteria,** bacteria which obtain their carbon and energy from the dissimilation of organic compounds.

Heterotropia. Squint or strabismus.

Heterozygous. Produced by unlike genes.

Hex-, Hexa- (Gk *hex:* six). Prefixes indicating six.

Hexachlorophane. B.P. 1968. $C_{13}H_6Cl_6O_2$. A bactericide which is active against a wide variety of gram-positive organisms, and has the practical advantage of retaining its activity in the presence of soap.

Hexachromic. Capable of recognizing only six of the seven colours of the spectrum.

Hexadactylism. Possessing six digits on one or more of the extremities.

Hexadimethrine bromide. The B.P. Commission approved name for poly-(*NNN'*-*N'*-tetramethyl-*N*-trimethylenehexamethylenediammonium dibromide. A heparin antagonist.

Hexamethonium bromide. B.P.C. 1968. $C_{12}H_{30}Br_2N_2$. A ganglion-blocking hypotensive agent.

Hexamethonium iodide. The B.P. Commission approved name for hexamethylenedi(trimethylammonium iodide). A hypotensive agent.

Hexamethonium tartrate. The B.P. Commission approved name for hexamethylendi(trimethylammonium hydrogen tartrate). A hypotensive agent.

Hexamine hippurate. The B.P. Commission approved name for a 1:1 complex of hexamine and hippuric acid. An antiseptic.

Hexapropymate. The B.P. Commission approved name for 1-(prop-2-ynyl) cyclohexyl carbamate. A hypnotic.

Hexazole. The B.P. Commission approved name for a central nervous system stimulant.

Hexetidine. The B.P. Commission approved name for 5-amino-1,3,di-(2-ethylhexyl) hexahydro-5-methylpyrimidine. A bactericide and fungicide.

Hexobendine. The B.P. Commission approved name for 1,2-di-[N-methyl-3-(3,4,5-trimethoxybenzoyloxy)-propylamino]ethane. A coronary vasodilator.

Hexocyclium methylsulphate. The B.P. Commission approved name for 4-(β-cyclohexyl-β-hydroxyphenethyl)-1,1-dimethylpiperazinium methylsulphate. An anticholinergic agent.

Hexoestrol. B.P.C. 1968. $C_{18}H_{22}O_2$. An oestrogenic agent.

Hexokinase. An enzyme concerned in sugar fermentation, which catalyses the transfer of a phosphoryl group from ATP to glucose.

Hexosamine. An amino-sugar resulting from the introduction of an amino group into hexose sugars.

Hexose. A monosaccharide containing six carbon atoms in the molecule.

Hexosediphosphatase. The hydrolytic enzymes that play a part in the phosphorylation of fructose-6-phosphate.

Hexylresorcinol. B.P. 1968. $C_{12}H_{18}O_2$. An anthelminthic used for the expulsion of hookworms and dwarf tapeworms.

Hiatus. An aperture or opening. (*Plural:* hiatus or hiatuses.)

Hibernation. The dormant state in which certain animals pass the winter.

Hiccup. A clonic spasm of the diaphragm resulting in spasmodic indrawing of air to the lungs ending in a click due to sudden closure of the vocal cords.

Hidr-, Hidro- (Gk *hidrōs:* sweat). Prefixes indicating association with sweat.

Hidradenitis. Inflammation of the sweat glands. **Hydradenitis suppurativa,** an infection of the apocrine glands in the axillae or perineum.

Hidroa. Any skin condition associated with, or caused by, excessive sweating.

Hidrorrhoea. Profuse perspiration.

Hidrosis. Excessive perspiration.

Hidrotic. Related to hidrosis. An agent that causes excessive sweating.

Hierophobia. Morbid fear of sacred things or anything to do with church ritual.

Hilar. Pertaining to a hilum.

Hilum. A depression in an organ where nerves and blood vessels enter and leave.

Hindbrain. Rhombencephalon.

Hindgut. The caudal portion of the embryonic gut, from which the colon and rectum are formed.

Hip bone. A large irregular bone which consists of three parts: the ilium, the ischium, and the pubis. Between them the two hip bones form the pelvic girdles of the lower limbs.

Hippo- (Gk *hippos:* horse). Prefix indicating association with a horse.

Hippocampus. An elongated elevated structure in the medial part of the floor of the inferior horn of the lateral ventricle.

Hippus. Spasmodic alternate contraction and dilatation of the iris.

Hirsute. Hairy

Hirsuties. Excessive growth of hair.

Hirsutism. Hirsuties.

Hirudin. The anticoagulant factor in the saliva of the leech.

Hirudo. A genus of leeches.

Hist-, Histio-, Histo- (Gk *histos:* web or tissue). Prefixes indicating relationship to tissue.

Histaminase. An enzyme that inactivates histamine.

Histamine. An amine ($C_5H_9N_3$) derived from histidine, which is a powerful dilator of capillaries, stimulator of smooth muscle and stimulant of gastric secretion.

Histamine acid phosphate. B.P. 1968. $C_5H_{15}N_3O_8P_2$. A preparation used principally for diagnostic purposes in ascertaining whether an achlorhydria is histamine-resistant.

Histidine. One of the basic amino-acids, and the precursor of histamine.

Histiocyte. A cell forming part of the reticulo-endothelial system which is capable of being markedly phagocytic and is then known as a macrophage.

Histiocytoma. A small, slowly growing, benign growth of the dermis.

Histiocytosis. A condition characterized

by the appearance of histiocytes in the blood.

Histiogenic. Formed by the tissues.

Histochemistry. The study of the tissues by means of stains and dyes.

Histocompatability. The state of being immunologically identical and therefore acceptable as a homograft transplant.

Histocytic. To do with histiocytes.

Histoid. Composed of one kind of tissue. Weblike.

Histogenesis. The development of the tissues from their embryonic origins.

Histogram. A graphic representation of frequency distributions.

Histology. The study of the minute structure of the tissues.

Histones. A group of proteins, soluble in water, which includes globin, and usually occur conjugated with nucleic acid.

Histopathology. The study of the minute structure of pathological tissue.

Histoplasma. A genus of yeastlike fungi. *Histoplasma capsulatum*, a dimorphic fungus which is the cause of histoplasmosis. *Histoplasma duboisii*, the occasional causative organism of histoplasmosis in Africa.

Histoplasmin. An antigen prepared from *Histoplasma capsulatum*, and used as a skin test in the diagnosis of histoplasmosis.

Histoplasmosis. A disease of worldwide distribution, usually due to infection by *Histoplasma capsulatum*, in Africa sometimes by *H. duboisii*, and involving primarily the lungs. It may become widespread involving the reticulo-endothelial system.

Histotoxic. Poisonous to the tissues. **Histotoxic anoxia**, anoxia resulting from poisoning of the cellular respiratory enzymes.

Histotribe. Forceps for clamping tissue containing bloodvessels, to ensure haemostasis.

Hives. Urticaria.

Holism. The concept or philosophy that man is an indivisible whole.

Holmium. A rare element. Symbol Ho. Atomic weight 164·93. Atomic number 67.

Holo- (Gk *holos:* whole, complete). Prefix meaning whole, entire.

Holocrine. Signifying a gland in which the secretion includes the secreting cells, such as the sebaceous glands.

Homatropine hydrobromide. B.P. 1968. $C_{16}H_{22}BrNO_3$. A mydriatic which is often used in preference to atropine

as it acts more quickly but is less persisting.

Homaxial. Having all axes equal.

Homeo-, Homoeo- (Gk *homois:* like, unchanging). Prefixes meaning alike.

Homeostasis. The state of equilibrium in which the body is normally maintained.

Homeothermic. Having a constant body temperature, such as warm-blooded animals have.

Homo- (Gk *homos:* the same). Prefix meaning the same.

Homocentric. Having the same centre or focus.

Homochlorcyclizine. The B.P. approved name for 1-(4-chlorobenzhydryl)-4-methyl-1,4-diazacycloheptane. An antihistamine.

Homocysteine. A sulphur-containing amino-acid which is an intermediate in the biosynthesis of cysteine from methionine.

Homocytotropic. Having an affinity for cells of the same species.

Homoeopathy. The system of therapeutics instituted by Samuel Hahneman and based on the belief that like cures like (*Similia similibus curentur*) and involving the use of almost infinitesimally small doses of drugs.

Homogenate. That which has been rendered homogeneous.

Homogeneous. Constant in quality and consistency in all parts.

Homogenize. To render homogeneous or of uniform consistency.

Homogentisate oxygenase. The enzyme that metabolizes homogentisic acid, and which is absent from the body in the hereditary defect of metabolism known as alkaptonuria, and absence of which results in homogentisic acid appearing in the urine.

Homogentisic acid. An intermediary in the catabolism of tyrosine. It accumulates in the body and is therefore excreted in the urine in the hereditary metabolic defect known as alkaptonuria, as a result of the absence of homogentisate oxygenase.

Homograft. A piece of tissue transplanted from one animal to another of the same species, but not identical twins.

Homolateral. On or relating to the same side.

Homologous. Having a similar embryological orgin.

Homonymous. Having the same designation or the same relationship.

Homosexual. Pertaining to the same

sex. An individual who is sexually attracted to the same sex.

Homozygote. An individual whose somatic genes have identical genes in the same locus on one of the chromosome pairs.

Homozygous. Having both loci of a pair of chromosomes carrying identical genes.

Homunculus. A perfectly proportional dwarf. A foetus.

Honey. The secretion produced by the hive bee *Apis melliflera*, from the nectar of flowers, and which contains 75 per cent of invert sugar (a mixture of fructose and glucose) and 2 per cent sucrose. **Purified honey,** B.P.C. 1968, honey which has been melted at a temperature not exceeding 80°C and allowed to stand, after which the impurities which have floated to the surface are skimmed off, and the liquid diluted with water.

Hook. A curved instrument used for traction or for fixing a part.

Hookworm. The name given to two genera of nematodes, or roundworms: Ancylostoma and Necator. *Ancylostoma duodenale* is the cause of hookworm disease in the old world, and *Necator americanus* is the cause of hookworm disease in the new world.

Hops. The dried fruit of *Humulus lupulus*.

Hordeolum. A stye.

Hormodendrum. A species of fungi. *Hormodendrum pedrosoi* and *Hormodendrum compactum* are the causative organisms of chromoblastomycosis.

Hormone. A chemical substance which, produced in one part of the body, enters the circulation and is carried to distant organs and tissues to modify their structure and function. **Adrenocorticotrophic hormone, (ACTH)** the hormone produced by the anterior lobe of the pituitary, that controls secretions from the adrenal cortex. **Follicle stimulating hormone (FSH),** the hormone produced by the anterior lobe of the pituitary that stimulates the follicles of the ovary. **Gonadotrophic hormones,** follicle stimulating hormone, interstitial cell stimulating hormone, and luteinizing hormone. **Growth hormone,** the hormone produced by the anterior lobe of the pituitary, that affects the growth of tissue in general. **Interstitial cell stimulating hormone, (ICSH)** the hormone produced by the anterior lobe of the pituitary, that stimulates the interstitial cells of the testis to produce testosterone. **Luteinizing hormone (LH),** the hormone produced by the anterior lobe of the pituitary that brings about ovulation. **Thyrotrophic hormone,** the hormone produced by the anterior lobe of the pituitary, that controls the activity of the thyroid gland.

Horn. A protrusion or projection.

Horripilation. Erection of the hairs of the skin. Goose flesh.

Hospital. An institution or building intended for receiving the sick and injured, and in which they can receive the appropriate treatment.

Humectant. Moistening. A moistening agent.

Humeral. Relating to the humerus.

Humerus. The bone of the arm that articulates proximally with the glenoid cavity of the scapula, and distally with the radius and ulna. (*Plural:* humeri.)

Humidity. The degree of moistness or dampness, particularly of the air. **Absolute humidity,** the weight of moisture (in grains) in a cubic foot of air. **Relative humidity,** the percentage of moisture in the air, saturation being 100.

Humour. Any fluid or semi-fluid tissue of the body. **Aqueous humour,** the fluid that fills the anterior and posterior chambers of the eye. **Vitreous humour,** the fluid component of the vitreous body.

Hunger. A craving for food.

Hyal-, Hyalo- (Gk *hyalos:* glass). Prefixes meaning glass-like.

Hyalin. An acidophil, inert, refractile substance, probably a variety of collagen, that occurs in various forms of degeneration.

Hyaline. Glassy. **Hyaline degeneration,** a term used to describe a change in cells when either the whole cell or part of it becomes eosinophilic and homogeneous. **Hyaline membrane disease,** a disease found in premature infants, characterized by lining of the alveoli and bronchioles with a dense membrane. **Hyaline casts,** pale homogeneous urinary casts formed by cells showing hyaline degeneration.

Hyaloid. Having a glassy appearance. **Hyaloid membrane,** the appearance of a boundary membrane given by the concentration of the micellae on the surface of the vitreous humour.

Hyalomma. A genus of ticks.

Hyalophagia. The eating of glass.

Hyalophobia. A morbid fear of glass or of coming in contact with it.

Hyaluronidase. B.P. 1968. A mucolytic

enzyme, prepared from the testes and semen of mammals, which breaks down the hyaluronic acid of the muco-protein ground substance or tissue cement, thereby reducing its viscosity and rendering the tissues more permeable to injected fluids.

Hybrid. The offspring of parents of different species.

Hydatid. The cystic stage of *Echino-coccus granulosus.*

Hydatidiform. Having the appearance of a hydatid. **Hydatidiform mole,** a rare complication of pregnancy, character-ized by tremendous proliferation of the epithelium of the chorion.

Hydr-, Hydro- (Gk *hydōr:* water). Prefixes signifying association with water.

Hydradenoma. A benign tumour arising from sweat glands.

Hydraemia. A condition in which the blood contains an excess of water.

Hydragogue. A substance that pro-duces a watery discharge, applied to a cathartic that produces a watery stool.

Hydrallazine. The B.P. Commission approved name for 1-hydrazinoph-thalazine. A hypotensive agent.

Hydramnios. The condition character-ized by excess of fluid in the amniotic cavity.

Hydrargaphen. The B.P. Commission approved name for phenylmercury 2, 2′-dinaphthylmethane-3,3′-disulphon-ate. An anti-parasitic, anti-infective agent.

Hydrargyria. Chronic mercurial poison-ing.

Hydrargyrum. Mercury.

Hydrarthrosis. An effusion into a joint cavity. **Intermittent hydrarthrosis,** a condition characterized by recurring effusion into a joint cavity.

Hydrate. A compound containing chemically incorporated water. Hy-droxide.

Hydration. The chemical union of a substance with water.

Hydride. A chemical compound of hydrogen with one other element.

Hydroa. A bullous eruption. **Hydroa aestivale,** a bullous eruption that recurs every spring and summer, most common in boys. **Hydroa gravidarum,** dermatitis herpetiformis in pregnancy.

Hydrobromide. A salt of hydrobromic acid.

Hydrocarbon. A compound consisting of hydrogen and carbon.

Hydrocele. An encysted collection of fluid in the tunica vaginalis testis.

Hydrocephalus. The condition charac-terized by abnormal accumulation of cerebrospinal fluid within the skull. It is usually congenital, but may be acquired.

Hydrochloric acid. HCl. A pungent colourless gas that can be liquefied under pressure. **Hydrochloric acid,** B.P. 1968, an aqueous solution which contains not less than 35 per cent w/w and not more than 38 per cent w/w of HCl. **Dilute hydrochloric acid,** B.P. 1968, an aqueous solution containing 10 per cent w/w of HCl, and used as a bitter.

Hydrochloride. A compound of an alkaloid or other organic base with hydrochloric acid.

Hydrochlorothiazide. B.P. 1968. C_7H_8 $ClN_3O_4S_2$. A non-mercurial diuretic.

Hydrocolpos. A vaginal retention cyst containing a clear fluid.

Hydrocortisone. B.P. 1968. $C_{21}H_{30}O_5$. A normal secretion of the adrenal cortex in man, which has an action similar to that of cortisone. It is usually given by mouth.

Hydrocortisone acetate. B.P. 1968. $C_{23}H_{32}O_6$. A widely used preparation which has an action similar to that of cortisone.

Hydrocortisone hydrogen succinate. B.P. 1968. $C_{25}H_{34}O_8$. A preparation that has an action similar to that of cortisone, and is used in the prep-aration of hydrocortisone sodium succinate injection B.P. **Hydrocortisone sodium succinate,** B.P. 1968. $C_{25}H_{33}Na$ O_8. A preparation that has an action similar to that of cortisone. It is suitable for the preparation of intravenous or intramuscular injec-tions.

Hydrocyanic acid. HCN. One of the most potent of protoplasmic poisons. Prussic acid.

Hydroflumethiazide. B.P. 1968. $C_8H_8F_3N_3O_4S_2$. A non-mercurial diuretic.

Hydrogen. The lightest known element. Symbol H. Atomic weight 1·00797. Atomic number 1.

Hydrogenase. A bacterial enzyme which catalyses reduction by molecular hydrogen.

Hydrogenate. To add hydrogen to a compound.

Hydrogen peroxide. H_2O_2. An unstable compound readily broken down to water and oxygen. **Hydrogen peroxide solution,** B.P. 1968, an aqueous solution of hydrogen peroxide con-taining not less than 5 per cent w/v and not more than 7 per cent w/v of

H_2O_2, which is used as an antiseptic and a deodorant. **Strong hydrogen peroxide solution,** B.P. 1968, an aqueous solution of hydrogen peroxide containing not less than 26 per cent w/w and not more than 28 per cent w/w H_2O_2, corresponding to about 100 times its volume of available oxygen. It is used to prepare weaker solutions, and must never be used undiluted.

Hydrolase. One of a group of enzymes that catalyse hydrolysis of a complex molecule into two components.

Hydrolysate. The product of hydrolysis. **Protein hydrolysate,** the amino-acid mixture produced by the hydrolysis of protein and administered parenterally in certain clinical conditions.

Hydrolysis. The chemical process whereby a compound reacts with water, with the production of two or more simpler molecules with the hydroxyl atom in one and the hydrogen atom in another.

Hydrometer. An instrument for determining the specific gravity of liquids.

Hydromorphinol. The B.P. Commission approved name for 7,8-dihydro-14-hydroxymorphine. A narcotic analgesic.

Hydromorphone. The B.P. Commission approved name for 7,8-dihydromorphinone. A narcotic analgesic.

Hydromyelia. Accumulations of fluid in the distended central canal of the spinal cord.

Hydronephrosis. Distension of the pelvis and the calyces of the kidney as a result of obstruction to the outflow of urine.

Hydropericardium. A pericardial effusion.

Hydrophobia. Rabies.

Hydrophthalmos. Infantile glaucoma.

Hydropneumopericardium. The presence of gas and an effusion in the pericardial cavity.

Hydropneumoperitoneum. The presence of gas and an effusion in the peritoneal cavity.

Hydropneumothorax. The presence of gas and an effusion in the pleural cavity.

Hydrops. Dropsy. **Hydrops foetalis,** excessive accumulation of fluid in the foetus, which occurs as a feature of Rhesus incompatibility.

Hydrosalpinx. An accumulation of serous fluid in the uterine tube.

Hydrostatic. Pertaining to a liquid in equilibrium.

Hydrotherapy. The use of water as a

therapeutic measure: e.g. as baths, douches and the like.

Hydrothorax. A collection of dropsical fluid in the pleural cavity.

Hydroureter. Distension of the ureter with fluid due to some obstructive factor.

Hydrovarium. A collection of fluid in the ovary.

Hydroxamethocaine. The B.P. Commission approved name for 2-dimethylaminoethyl 4-butylaminosalicylate. A local anaesthetic.

Hydroxide. A compound that contains a hydroxyl (OH) radicle.

Hydroxocobalamin. B.P. 1968. $C_{62}H_{89}CoN_{13}O_{15}P$. A member of the group of similar compounds, including cyanocobalamin, which influence erythropoiesis and which represents the anti-pernicious-anaemia principle of purified liver extracts. Administered intramuscularly, it is therefore used in the treatment of pernicious anaemia.

Hydroxyamphetamine. The B.P. Commission approved name for 4-(2-aminoprophyl) phenol. A sympathomimetic agent and a mydriatic.

Hydroxchloroquine sulphate. B.P. 1968. $C_{18}H_{28}ClN_3O_5S$. An anti-malarial drug which is also used in the treatment of rheumatoid arthritis and lupus erythematosus.

Hydroxydione sodium succinate. The B.P. Commission approved name for sodium 21-hydroxypregnane-3,20-dione succinate. An anaesthetic.

Hydroxyglycine. One of the amino-acids only found in collagen.

Hydroxypethidine. The B.P. Commission approved name for ethyl 4-(3-hydroxyphenyl)-1-methylpiperidine-4-carboxylate. A narcotic analgesic.

Hydroxyprocaine. The B.P. Commission approved name for 2-diethylaminoethyl 4-aminosalicylate. A local anaesthetic.

Hydroxyprogesterone hexanoate. B.P. Addendum 1971. $C_{27}H_{40}O_4$. A progestational steroid.

Hydroxyproline. One of the amino-acids only found in collagen.

Hydroxystilbamidine. The B.P. Commission approved name for 4,4′-diamidino-2-hydroxystilbene. A drug used in the treatment of leishmaniasis and trypansomiasis.

Hydroxytoluic acid. The B.P. Commission approved name for 2-hydroxy-m-toluic acid. An analgesic.

Hydroxyurea. The B.P. Commission

approved name for an anti-neoplastic agent.

Hydroxyzine. The B.P. Commission approved name for 1-(4-chlorobenzhydryl) 4-[2-(2-hydroxyethoxy)-ethyl] piperazine. A tranquillizer.

Hygiene. The science of health.

Hygr-, Hygro- (Gk *hygros:* moist). Prefixes indicating moist or relationship to moisture.

Hygroma. A cystic swelling containing serous fluid.

Hygrometer. An instrument for measuring the amount of water vapour in the air.

Hygrophobia. Morbid fear of liquids, moisture, or dampness.

Hygroscope. An instrument for measuring the humidity of the atmosphere.

Hygroscopic. Capable of absorbing moisture.

Hymen. The thin fold of mucous membrane situated at the orifice of the vagina.

Hymenolepis. A genus of cestodes or tapeworms. *H. diminuta,* the rat tapeworm that sometimes infests man. *H. nana,* a dwarf tapeworm, which infests man.

Hymenoptera. The order of arthopods that includes bees, wasps and ants.

Hymenorrhaphy. Surgical suturing of the hymen or any membrane.

Hymenotomy. Surgical incision of the hymen.

Hyo- (Gk *hyoeidēs*: shaped like the letter upsilon). Prefix meaning V-shaped, and signifying association with the hyoid bone or arch.

Hyoglossal. Pertaining to the hyoid bone and the tongue.

Hyoid. The V-shaped bone suspended from the tips of the styloid processes of the temporal bones by the stylohyoid ligaments.

Hyoscine hydrobromide. B.P. 1968. $C_{17}H_{22}BrNO_4,3H_2O$. The hydrobromide of an alkaloid obtained from various solanaceous plants, which has a peripheral atropine-like action, and a central depressant action. It is widely used as a remedy for travel sickness.

Hyoscine methobromide. The B.P. approved name for a drug used in the treatment of peptic ulcer.

Hyoscyamus. B.P. 1968. The dried leaves, or leaves and flowering tops, of *Hyoscyamus niger* (L.), preparations of which are used to counteract the griping action of purgatives and to relieve spasm in the urinary tract.

Hypalgesia. Decreased sensibility to pain.

Hyper- (Gk *hyper:* above, over). Prefix signifying beyond, excessive.

Hyperacidity. An abnormal degree of acidity.

Hyperacusis. An abnormally acute sense of hearing.

Hyperaemia. Congestion due to excessive amount of blood in a part or area.

Hyperaesthesia. Excessive sensitiveness to sensory stimuli.

Hyperaldosteronism. Excessive production of aldosterone in the body. **Primary aldosteronism,** the rare condition produced by hypersecretion of aldosterone, usually by an adrenal adenoma, and characterized by hypertension, hypokalaemia and muscular wasting.

Hyperalgesia. Excessive sensitiveness to pain.

Hyperbaric. Heavier than its environment.

Hyperbilirubinaemia. The presence of excessive amounts of bilirubin in the blood.

Hypercalcaemia. Excessive calcium in the blood.

Hypercalcinuria. The presence of excessive calcium in the urine.

Hypercapnia. Excessive carbon dioxide in the blood, resulting in over-stimulation of the respiratory centre.

Hyperchloraemia. Excessive chloride in the blood.

Hyperchlorhydria. The presence of excessive hydrochloric acid in the gastric secretion.

Hypercholesterolaemia. Excessive cholesterol in the blood.

Hyperchromic. Abnormally highly coloured.

Hypercortisonism. The condition produced by excessive production of cortisone.

Hypercryaesthesia. Excessive sensitiveness to cold.

Hypercupraemia. An excessive amount of copper in the blood.

Hyperdactylism. The condition in which there is more than the normal number of fingers or toes.

Hyperemesis. Excessive vomiting. **Hyperemesis gravidarum,** the excessive vomiting that may occur during pregnancy.

Hyperendemic. Referring to an area in which a disease is highly endemic, or a disease that is highly endemic: e.g. malaria in certain parts of the tropics.

Hyperergia. Highly allergic.

Hyperextension. Forceful extension of a limb beyond the normal limits, as carried out, for instance, in certain orthopaedic procedures.

Hyperfecundation. The impregnation by separate acts of coitus of two or more ova during the same ovulation.

Hyperferraemia. Excess of iron in the serum.

Hypergammaglobulinaemia. An excess of gamma-globulin in the blood.

Hypergasia. Diminished functional activity.

Hyperglobulinaemia. Excess of globulin in the blood.

Hyperglycaemia. Excess of sugar in the blood.

Hyperidrosis. Excessive sweating.

Hyperinsulinism. The condition induced by excessive secretion of insulin.

Hyperinvolution. Excessive involution of an organ after it has undergone enlargement: e.g. the uterus after childbirth may become smaller than it was before pregnancy.

Hyperkalaemia. Excessive potassium in the blood.

Hyperkeratosis. Hypertrophy of the horny layer of the skin.

Hyperkinesia. Increased motor activity, as in muscular spasm.

Hyperlipaemia. Excess of lipids in the blood.

Hypermetamorphosis. A defect in attention whereby an individual cannot attend to anything for longer than a few seconds, with a resultant flitting of attention from one object to another.

Hypermetropia. Long sightedness, in which the rays of light are focused beyond the retina.

Hypernatraemia. Excess of sodium in the blood.

Hypernephroma. Renal carcinoma.

Hyperopia. Hypermetropia.

Hyperosmia. Abnormally sharp sense of smell.

Hyperostosis. Hypertrophy of bone. Exostosis.

Hyperparathyroidism. The condition characterized by over-activity of the parathyroid glands, marked by renal calculi, raised serum calcium and cystic formation in the bone which may lead to fractures.

Hyperperistalsis. Exaggerated peristaltic movement in the gut.

Hyperphagia. Excessive consumption of food. Gluttony.

Hyperphosphataemia. Excess of phosphates in the serum.

Hyperpiesia. The condition characterized by a raised blood pressure.

Hyperpiesis. Raised blood pressure.

Hyperplasia. Abnormal increase in the number of cells in a given tissue or organ.

Hyperploidy. The state of having more than the normal number of chromosomes.

Hyperpnoea. Breathing that is more rapid and deeper than normal.

Hyperpraxia. Excessive maniacal mental activity.

Hyperpyrexia. Excessively high body temperature: e.g., over 106°F (41°C).

Hyperreflexia. Exaggerated deep tendon reflexes.

Hyperresonance. Exaggerated resonance on percussion.

Hypersecretion. Secretion in excess of the normal.

Hypersomnia. Pathological sleepiness.

Hypersplenism. The condition characterized by enlargement of the spleen, reduction of all cellular elements in the blood and the formation of auto-antibodies.

Hypersthenia. Excessive strength or tonicity.

Hypertelorism. Abnormal distance between two paired organs.

Hypertension. Abnormally high tension, applied particularly to raised blood pressure.

Hyperthelia. The presence of supernumerary nipples.

Hyperthermia. Abnormally high body temperature. The treatment of disease by the artificial production of a high temperature.

Hyperthyroidism. The condition characterized by overactivity of the thyroid gland.

Hypertonia. Abnormally raised tone or tension, particularly of the arteries.

Hypertonic. Having excessive tension. Having an osmotic pressure greater than normal.

Hypertoxic. Excessively poisonous or toxic.

Hypertrichosis. Excessive growth of hair, or growth of hair on a part of the body not normally covered by hair.

Hypertrophy. Overgrowth. Increase in the size of a part or organ, as of the muscles in response to exercise.

Hyperuricaemia. Excess of uric acid in the blood.

Hyperuricuria. Excess of uric acid in the urine.

Hyperventilation. Increased pulmonary ventilation.

Hypervitaminosis. The abnormal state

produced by excessive consumption of one or more vitamins.

Hypervolaemia. Plethora.

Hypha. One of the filaments of the mycelium of a fungus. (*Plural:* hyphae.)

Hyphaemia. Haemorrhage into the anterior chamber of the eye.

Hyphedonia. The morbid state characterized by diminished pleasure from acts normally arousing pleasure.

Hypnagogic. Inducing sleep. Hypnotic.

Hypnagogue. Inducing sleep. Hypnotic. An agent inducing hypnosis.

Hypno- (Gk *hypnos:* sleep). Prefix indicating association with sleep.

Hypno-analysis. A form of psychotherapy, whereby a patient is psychoanalysed under the influence of hypnosis.

Hypnopaedia. Sleep learning.

Hypnosis. The artificially induced trance-like state in which an individual is in a highly suggestible state and therefore amenable to the hypnotizer's suggestions or commands.

Hypnotherapy. The use of hypnotism in therapy.

Hypnotic. Inducing sleep. A substance or procedure that induces sleep. Relating to hypnotism.

Hypnotism. The process of inducing hypnosis.

Hypo- (Gk *hypo:* under). Prefix meaning under, beneath, deficient.

Hypoacidity. Diminished acidity.

Hypoacusis. Impairment of hearing.

Hypoadrenalaemia. Abnormal diminution in the amount of suprarenal secretion in the blood.

Hypoadrenia. The state resulting from diminished activity of the adrenal glands.

Hypoaesthesia. Diminished sensibility to touch.

Hypobaric. Characterized by subnormal atmospheric pressure.

Hypobulia. Diminished will power.

Hypocalcaemia. Diminished amount of calcium in the blood.

Hypocapnia. Diminished amount of calcium dioxide in the blood.

Hypochloraemia. A diminished amount of chlorides in the blood.

Hypochlorhydria. Diminished secretion of hydrochloric acid in the stomach.

Hypochlorite. A salt of hypochlorous acid. Many hypochlorites are used as antiseptics.

Hypochlorous acid. HCO. An acid with strong bleaching, oxidizing and antiseptic propensities.

Hypocholesterolaemia. Diminished amount of cholesterol in the blood.

Hypocholia. Diminished secretion of bile.

Hypocholuria. Diminished amount of chloride in the urine.

Hypochondriac. A victim of hypochondriasis.

Hypochondriasis. A chronic mental or emotional state characterized by excessive introspection about health, with resultant exaggeration of any minor manifestation of bodily malfunctioning.

Hypochondrium. Either of the lateral regions of the upper anatomical zone of the abdomen.

Hypochromasia. The state of being deficient in colour, usually applied to the defective staining of certain blood cells in certain states of anaemia.

Hypochromatic. Deficient in colour.

Hypocoagulability. A state of diminished coagulability of the blood.

Hypocupraemia. Diminished copper in the blood.

Hypodactylia. Lack of one or more digits.

Hypoderm. The subcutaneous tissue.

Hypoderma. A genus of flies responsible for myiasis in man and cattle. Warble fly.

Hypodermic. Subcutaneous. Underneath the skin.

Hypodermoclysis. The introduction of fluids into the body by injection underneath the skin.

Hypodipsia. Diminished thirst.

Hypoferraemia. Deficiency of iron in the circulating blood.

Hypofibrogenaemia. Deficiency of fibrinogen in the circulating blood.

Hypogalactia. Inadequate secretion of milk.

Hypogammaglobulinaemia. Abnormally low amount of gamma-globulin in the circulating blood.

Hypogastric. Relating to the hypogastrium.

Hypogastrium. The median region of the lower zone of the abdomen.

Hypogeusia. Decreased taste acuity.

Hypoglossal. Beneath the tongue. **Hypoglossal nerve,** the 12th cranial nerve.

Hypoglycaemia. Deficiency of sugar in the blood.

Hypognathous. Having a protruding lower jaw or some other congenital abnormality of the lower jaw.

Hypogonadism. The condition characterized by deficient production of the hormones of the ovaries and testes.

Hypoidrosis. Diminished perspiration.

Hypoinsulinism. Diminished secretion of insulin by the pancreas.

Hypokalaemia. Diminished potassium in the blood.

Hypokinesia. Diminished power of motor function.

Hypokinetic. Marked by diminished power of movement.

Hypomania. A slight degree of mania.

Hypomenorrhoea. An abnormally small loss of blood during menstruation.

Hypomorph. An individual whose standing height is short in relationship to his sitting height.

Hyponatraemia. Diminished amount of sodium in the blood.

Hyponychium. Where the skin is attached to the under-surface of the nail just proximal to the free border of the nail.

Hypopallaesthesia. The condition characterized by diminution in the perception of vibration.

Hypoparathyroidism. The condition characterized by inadequate, or lack of, secretion of the parathyroid glands, whether induced by disease or surgical removal.

Hypophosphaturia. Diminution in the amount of phosphates excreted in the urine.

Hypophosphite. A salt of hypophosphorous acid.

Hypophrenia. Feeblemindedness.

Hypophyseal. Pertaining to the hypophysis cerebri.

Hypophysectomy. Surgical excision of the hypophysis cerebri.

Hypophysis. The hypophysis cerebri. The pituitary gland. A bi-lobed, ovoid body, 12×8mm., lying in the hypophyseal fossa of the sphenoid bone. The anterior lobe, or *adenohypophysis*, is developed from the primitive buccal cavity, the posterior lobe, or *neurohypophysis*, from the floor of the diencephalon.

Hypopiesis. Abnormally low blood pressure.

Hypopigmentation. Abnormal decrease in the amount of pigmentation.

Hypopituitarism. The condition characterized by diminished activity of the hypophysis.

Hypoplasia. Defective development of an organ or tissue.

Hypopnoea. Shallow respiration.

Hypopraxia. Listlessness.

Hypoproteinaemia. Diminution in the plasma proteins.

Hypoprothrombinaemia. Diminution of prothrombin in the blood.

Hypopyon. Accumulation of pus in the anterior chamber of the eye.

Hyposensitive. Possessing abnormally decreased sensitivity, applied particularly to the poor reaction to an allergen or antigen.

Hyposmia. Diminution of the sense of smell.

Hypospadias. A developmental abnormality in which, in the male, the urethra opens on the underside of the penis or in the perineum, whilst in the female it opens into the vagina.

Hypostasis. Accumulation of blood, usually in a dependent part, as a result of a feeble or obstructed circulation.

Hyposteatosis. Diminished secretion of sebum.

Hyposthenia. Weakness.

Hyposthenic. Debilitating.

Hyposthenuria. The condition characterized by the passage of urine of low specific gravity.

Hyposulphite. A salt of hyposulphurous acid.

Hyposynergia. A state of impaired coordination.

Hypotension. Abnormally low blood pressure.

Hypothalamus. That part of the brain consisting of the subthalamic segmental region, the structures forming the floor of the third ventricle, and the anterior part of the lateral wall of the third ventricle below and in front of the thalamus.

Hypothenar. The hypothenar eminence. The eminence on the ulnar side of the hand, or pertaining thereto.

Hypothermia. Low temperature, or the condition characterized by a low temperature, whether induced by disease or exposure, or induced artificially for therapeutic or surgical purposes.

Hypothymia. Low in spirits. Depression.

Hypothyroidism. The condition induced by under-activity of the thyroid gland. Myxoedema.

Hypotonia. Diminished tone or tension.

Hypotrichosis. Deficiency of hair.

Hypoventilation. Under-ventilation.

Hypovitaminosis. The condition induced by lack of one or more vitamins.

Hypovolaemia. Diminution in the volume of blood in the body.

Hypoxaemia. Diminution in the amount of oxygen in the blood.

Hypoxia. Oxygen want. **Anaemic hypoxia,** hypoxia where the arterial partial pressure of oxygen is normal but the oxygen-carrying capacity of the blood is reduced. **Anoxic hypoxia,**

hypoxia due to a deficient oxygen supply. **Histotoxic hypoxia,** hypoxia due to the inability of the tissues to utilize oxygen. **Stagnant hypoxia,** hypoxia due to slowing down of the local circulation.

Hypromellose. B.P.C. 1968. A mixed ether of cellulose, which has properties similar to those of methylcellulose, and is used to increase the viscosity of ophthalmic solutions, and in the preparation of anhydrous adhesive ointments for the protection of the skin.

Hypsarrhythmia. The electroencephalographic rhythm characterized by high-voltage, slow waves and spikes recurring randomly, sometimes found accompanying infantile spasms.

Hypsi- (Gk *hypsi:* high). Prefix meaning high.

Hyster-, Hystero- (Gk *hystera:* uterus). Prefixes meaning hysteria, or indicating association with the uterus.

Hysterectomy. Surgical removal of the uterus.

Hysteresis. Failure of coincidence of two associated phenomena: e.g. delayed action in the formation of gels.

Hysteria. A chronic psychoneurosis with a multiplicity of manifestations characterized by exaggerated histrionic behaviour based on conversions, with an almost infinite variety of motor, sensory or sensorial disturbances.

Hysterocele. Hernia of the uterus.

Hysterogram. An X-ray of the uterus, usually with a contrast medium. A record of the uterine contractions.

Hysteropexy. Fixation of a displaced uterus.

Hysterorrhaphy. Repair of a laceration in the uterus.

Hysterorrhexis. Rupture of the uterus.

Hysterotomy. Surgical incision of the uterus.

I

-**ia** (Gk *-ia:* a substantive-forming suffix). Suffix denoting condition and used in names of diseases.

-**iasis** (Gk *-iasis:* a suffix indicating a state or condition). Suffix used particularly to indicate a morbid condition.

Iatric. Pertaining to a physician.

Iatro- (Gk *iatros:* physician). Prefix indicating relationship to a physician or to medicine.

Iatrogenic. Doctor induced.

Ibufenac. The B.P. Commission approved name for 4-isobutylphenylacetic acid. An anti-inflammatory drug.

Ibuprofen. The B.P. Commission approved name for 2-(4-isobutylphenyl) propionic acid. An anti-inflammatory drug.

-**ic** (Gk *-ikos;* L *-icus*). Suffix signifying pertaining to. In chemistry signifying the higher of two valencies assumed by an element.

Ice. The solid produced from water by reducing its temperature to O°C.

Ichnogram. A footprint recorded when standing.

Ichor. A thin, watery discharge from an ulcer or wound.

Ichthammol. B.P. 1968. The ammonium salts of an oily substance prepared from a bituminous schist or shale. It has a slight bacteriostatic action and is used in ointments and creams in the treatment of some chronic skin diseases.

Ichthy-, Ichthyo- (Gk *ichthys:* fish). Prefixes meaning fish-like.

Ichthyoid. Fish-like.

Ichthyol. Ichthammol.

Ichthyosis. A developmental disease of the skin in which the surface is rough, dry and cracked, with a scale-like appearance.

-**icide** (L *caedere:* to kill). Suffix incating killing propensity.

Iconolagny. Sexual stimulation aroused by suggestive pictures and sculpture.

Icteric. Pertaining to jaundice.

Icterus. Jaundice.

Ictus. A stroke.

Id. The Freudian term for the unconscious reservoir of instincts, attitudes and feelings.

-**id** (Gk *eidos*: form). Suffix meaning resembling.

-**ide** (Gk *eidos:* form). Suffix indicating a binary chemical compound.

Ideation. The formation of ideas.

Ideo- (Gk *idea:* form). Prefix indicating relationship to ideas.

Idio- (Gk *idios:* one's own). Prefix indicating separate, peculiar to.

Idiocy. Profound degree of mental defect.

Idioglossia. The continued utterance of meaningless sounds.

Idiolalia. The use of language invented by oneself.

Idiopathic. Of unknown origin. Usually applied to a disease of unknown origin.

Idiopathy. A primary disease, or a disease for which there is no known cause.

Idiosyncrasy. An individual characteristic.

Idiot. An individual so mentally retarded that he is incapable of fending for himself.

Idioventricular. Pertaining to the ventricles of the heart in isolation from the atria.

Idoxuridine. B.P. Addendum 1969. $C_9H_{11}IN_2O_5$. An antiviral agent.

Ileac. Pertaining to the ileum.

Ileal. Pertaining to the ileum.

Ileectomy. Surgical excision of the ileum.

Ileitis. Inflammation of the ileum.

Ileo- (L *ileum:* intestine). Prefix indicating association with the ileum.

Ileocaecal. Pertaining to the ileum and caecum.

Ileocolic. Pertaining to the ileum and colon.

Ileocolitis. Inflammation of the ileum and colon. **Acute ileocolitis,** epidemic diarrhoea of children.

Ileostomy. A surgical opening into the ileum.

Ileum. The distal three-fifths of the small intestine beyond the duodenum, extending from the jejunum to the ileocaecal valve.

Ileus. Obstruction of the intestines.

Iliac. Pertaining to the ilium.

Ilio- (L *ilium:* flank). Prefix indicating association with the ilium.

Ilium. The uppermost of the three bones forming each side of the pelvis.

Illinition. Inunction.

Illumination. The lighting of an object. **Dark-ground illumination,** a method of illumination used in microscopy whereby most of the vertically directed rays are blocked and the object is viewed by circumferential lighting against a black background. **Focal illumination,** illumination of an object by means of light reflected from the lens of a concave mirror. **Oblique illumination,** focal illumination.

Illusion. A false interpretation of a sensory perception.

Image. A representation of an object. **Body image,** the concept of the body as represented in the cerebrum. The individual's concept of his own body. **Double image,** the two images as seen in diplopia or strabismus. **Erect image,** the image produced by rays that have not come to a focus—as in a plane mirror. **False image,** the image produced by the deviating eye in strabismus. **Inverted image,** an image which is reversed, as in the retina. **Mirror image,** the image produced by reflection from a plane mirror. **Retinal image,** the image produced by the focusing of rays on the retina. **True image,** the image seen by the undeviated eye in strabismus. **Virtual image,** erect image.

Imago. The adult stage of an insect. The psychoanalytical concept of the childhood memory of a loved person persisting into adult life.

Imbecility. A lesser degree of severe mental subnormality than idiocy.

Imbibition. The absorption of a fluid.

Imbrication. The surgical covering of a defect by means of overlapping layers.

Imfibulation. The operation of mutilating the external genitalia so as either to prevent coitus or, in the case of women, to reduce the orgasmatic pleasure of coitus to a minimum if not to abolish it altogether.

Imipramine hydrochloride. B.P. 1968. $C_{19}H_{25}ClN_2$. An antidepressant drug which does not inhibit monamine oxidase.

Immersion. Submerging in a liquid. **Immersion foot,** the condition that develops from prolonged immersion of the foot in cold, but not freezing, water.

Immune. Free from the risk of disease.

Immunity. The state of being immune, or of being protected against infection. **Acquired immunity,** immunity acquired during life as a result of exposure to infection or by the transfer of antibodies. **Active immunity,** immunity acquired by the body's own tissues as a result of stimulation by naturally or artificially acquired antigens. **Artificial immunity,** immunity induced by the administration of antigens or antibodies. **Auto-immunity,** immunity induced by the body to its own cells. **Cellular immunity,** enhanced capacity of particular cells or tissues to counteract infection. **Herd immunity,** the resistance of a group to disease. **Humoral immunity,** immunity in which the protection lies in the plasma, as in the case of antitoxin in diphtheria. **Natural immunity,** immunity acquired by exposure to, or development of, a given infection. **Non-specific immunity,** immunity acquired by one or more methods other than direct stimulation by a given antigen. **Passive immunity,** immunity imparted by direct injection, or administration, of antibodies.

Immunization. The process of inducing immunity.

Immuno- (L *immunis:* safe). Prefix indicating immune or protected.

Immunochemistry. That branch of chemistry concerned with the substances participating in the immune process.

Immunocyte. Any cell concerned with immunity.

Immunoelectrophoresis. The method of separating proteins by means of electrophoresis and then identifying them by specific immune reactions. Immunophoresis.

Immunofluorescence. The use of fluorescent dyes to stain, or label, serum antibodies, as a means of studying antigen-antibody reactions.

Immunogenesis. The process whereby immunity is developed.

Immunogenetics. The branch of genetics concerned with the inheritance of antigens and antigenic responses.

Immunoglobulin. A protein endowed with known antibody activity. Six classes of them are recognized. (*Abbreviation:* Ig.)

Immunology. The study of immunity and the immune processes.

Immunophoresis. Immunoelectrophoresis.

Immunotransfusion. Transfusion with

blood from an individual in whom the production of antibodies has been specially stimulated.

Imolamine. The B.P. Commission approved name for 4-(2-diethylamino-ethyl)-5-imino-3-phenyl-1,2,4-oxadia-zoline. A drug used in the treatment of angina pectoris.

Impaction. The condition of being firmly wedged, as may happen with the two broken ends of a fractured bone. **Dental impaction,** the state when a tooth is so firmly wedged in its socket that it cannot erupt. **Faecal impaction,** a mass of inspissated faeces wedged in the rectum.

Imperforate. Without an opening. **Imperforate anus,** a congenital condition in which a child is born without an anus. **Imperforate hymen,** a hymen without the normal opening through which the menstrual flow escapes.

Impetigo contagiosa. A highly contagious coccal, bullous disease of the skin. *Staphylococcus aureus* is the most common causative organism. **Bullous impetigo of the newborn,** pemphigus neonatorum.

Implantation. Embedding in the tissues, as of organs, or drugs, or structures, or the fertilized ovum in the uterus.

Impotence. Inability to perform the sexual act.

Impregnate. To make pregnant or fertilize. To saturate.

Impression. An indentation or shallow depression **Dental impression,** a mould of the mouth, or part of it. **Mental impression,** an effect produced upon the mind.

Impuberal. Lacking hair. Immature.

Impulse. A sudden force, physical mental or emotional.

In- (i) (L *in:* in, into). Prefix signifying in or within. (ii) (L *in:* not). Prefix meaning not, un-. (iii) (Gk *inos:* fibre). Prefix meaning fibrous.

Inanition. Physical exhaustion from lack of food.

Inappetence. Lack of appetite or desire.

Inarticulate. Unable to speak clearly. Disjointed.

In articulo mortis. At the moment of death.

Inborn. Innate. Implanted before birth.

Inbreeding. Mating by close relatives.

Incendiarism. A compulsion to set things on fire.

Incest. Sexual intercourse between persons held to be within the forbidden degrees of relationship.

Inch. One-twelfth of a foot. Equivalent to 25·399 millimetres.

Incision. A cut or wound made by a sharp instrument such as a knife or scalpel.

Incisor. One of the four front teeth on either jaw.

Incisure. A notch or incision.

Incoagulable. Incapable of coagulation or clotting.

Incompatibility. The state of being incompatible, or unable to exist together, as in the case of blood groups.

Incompetence. Inadequacy, as in the case of the heart valves when, as a result of disease, they are unable to close completely: e.g. aortic incompetence.

Incontinence. Lack of control, whether of the excretion of faeces or urine, the sexual or any other impulse.

Incoordination. Lack of the harmonious working of factors which normally are coordinated in combined operations: e.g. movements of the limbs.

Increment. Increase, enlargement or augmentation.

Incrustation. The formation of a crust.

Incubate. To maintain at the optimal temperature to allow embryos or cells to grow and develop.

Incubation. The process of incubating. The process of development of the fertilized ovum. **Incubation period,** the period elapsing between the time an individual becomes infected by a micro-organism and the first appearance of symptoms or signs of the disease.

Incubator. A chamber with controlled temperature and humidity for the growth of micro-organisms or cells, or for the treatment of premature infants.

Incubus. A heavy load on the mind. A nightmare.

Incudectomy. Surgical excision of the incus.

Incus. The anvil-shaped, movable, auditory ossicle placed between, and articulating with, the malleus and stapes.

Index. The second finger, or forefinger. The number denoting the relationship between two or more given factors. (*Plural:* indexes.) **Cephalic index,** the proportion of length to breadth of skull. **Colour index,** the mean haemoglobin content of a single erythrocyte as compared with the content of a normal erythrocyte. **Opsonic index,** a numerical expression of the opsonic power of the serum of a person for a given organism as compared with normal. **Refractive**

index, the refractive power of a substance as compared with air.

Indican. Indoxyl sulphate, which is formed from tryptopan and is excreted in the urine.

Indicanuria. The presence of an excess of indican in the urine, as occurs with excessive protein putrefaction in the gut.

Indication. A sign. A symptom or sign of disease which shows the way to, or suggests, a certain line of treatment.

Indicator. Something that shows the way. A substance used in chemistry which indicates by a colour change whether or not a given change has taken place.

Indigestion. Disturbance of the normal process of digestion.

Indigitation. Invagination. Intussusception.

Indigo carmine. B.P. 1968. $C_{16}H_8N_2Na_2O_8O_2$. Used as a test for renal function.

Indium. A metallic element. Symbol In. Atomic weight 114·82. Atomic number 49.

Indole. One of the evil-smelling compounds, helping to characterize the odour of faeces, derived from tryptophan in the gut. The bulk of it is excreted in the gut, and a small amount in the urine.

Indolent. Sluggish.

Indomethacin. B.P.C. Supplement 1971. $C_{19}H_{16}ClNO_4$. An analgesic and anti-inflammatory agent.

Indoxyl. A decomposition product of tryptophan.

Induration. Hardening.

Indusium griseum. The thin sheet of grey matter that covers the upper surface of the corpus callosum.

-ine (L inus: pertaining to). Suffix indicating an alkaloid, an organic base or a halogen.

Inebriation. The state of being intoxicated, usually applied to intoxication induced by alcohol.

Inert. Devoid of activity.

Inertia. A state of inactivity or sluggishness. Uterine inertia, absence or sluggishness of uterine contractions during labour.

In extremis. At the point of death.

Infant. A young child. Medically, usually taken to be a child under the age of 1 year. Legally, a minor or someone under the legal age of consent.

Infanticide. The murder of an infant.

Infantilism. General retardation of development. Cerebral infantilism, the infantilism seen in cases of primary mental defect, microcephaly, and the like. Coeliac infantilism, the lack of development that occurs in untreated coeliac disease. Hepatic infantilism, a rare form of infantilism occurring as a result of hepatic disease or dysfunction. Hypogonadal infantilism, lack of development due to failure of development, atrophy, or early destruction, of the gonads. Hypopituitary infantilism, lack of development due to failure of one or more of the pituitary hormones. Renal infantilism, lack of development due to early and extreme loss of renal function.

Infarct. An area, usually wedge-shaped, of necrotic tissue produced by occlusion of an end-artery.

Infarction. The process of formation of an infarct.

Infection. Invasion of the body by pathogenic micro-organisms. Airborne infection, infection transmitted by air without direct contact. Contact infection, infection transmitted by direct contact, as by kissing. Cross infection, infection transmitted from one patient to another, as in a hospital ward. Droplet infection, infection that is carried in air-borne droplets of saliva or sputum expelled by infected persons in the process of coughing, sneezing or speaking. Endogenous infection, infection in which the source is in the infected person's own body: e.g. E. coli which are harmless inhabitants of the colon but spread to the bladder and cause cystitis. Exogenous infection, infection acquired from some source outside the body. Food-borne infection, infection transmitted by food, as in food poisoning. Hand-borne infection, infection transmitted by the hands, as from the anus if the hands are not washed after defaecation. Milk-borne infection, infection transmitted by milk: e.g. brucellosis and typhoid fever. Pyogenic infection, infection due to the pus-forming bacteria: e.g. staphylococci and streptococci. Terminal infection, infection occurring immediately preceding death. Water-borne infection, infection transmitted by water: e.g. typhoid fever.

Infectious. Capable of being transmitted by infection. Infectious diseases, diseases transmitted by infection. Infectious mononucleosis, glandular fever.

Infective. Infectious.

Infecundity. Sterility or barrenness in women.

Inferior. Lower.

Infertility. Difficulty in conceiving or in inducing conception.

Infestation. Invasion of the body by animal parasites.

Inflammation. The reaction of the tissues to any insult, infection or injury short of one sufficiently severe to cause immediate death of the affected tissue. **Acute inflammation,** inflammation of rapid onset. **Catarrhal inflammation,** inflammation of mucous membrane. **Chronic inflammation,** prolonged inflammation in which destruction and inflammation are proceding at the same time as attempts at healing. **Fibrinous inflammation,** inflammation, as of serous sacs and the lungs, accompanied by marked fibrin formation. **Haemorrhagic inflammation,** inflammation accompanied by a haemorrhagic exudate, as in anthrax. **Membranous inflammation,** inflammation accompanied by membrane formation, as in membranous bronchitis. **Phlegmonous inflammation,** inflammation that goes on to a diffuse suppurative lesion. **Pseudomembranous inflammation,** inflammation accompanied by the formation of a membrane which consists of necrotic epithelium as well as fibrin and inflammatory cells, as seen in diphtheria. **Serous inflammation,** the inflammatory reaction in loose tissues, as in gas gangrene. **Suppurative inflammation,** inflammation accompanied by marked pus formation.

Influenza. An acute febrile illness caused by infection by one or more of the influenza viruses.

Influenza vaccine. B.P. 1968. An aqueous suspension of a suitable strain or strains of influenza virus, inactivated so that they are non-infective but retain their antigenic properties.

Infra- (L *infra:* beneath). Prefix meaning below, under.

Infra-red. Referring to wave-lengths beyond the red end of the spectrum: from 7700 Angstroms to 1 millimetre.

Infundibulum. A funnel or funnel-shaped passage. (*Plural:* infundibula.) **Infundibulum of the ethmoid,** the curved channel from the middle meatus of the nose that communicates with the anterior ethmoidal sinus and frontal sinus. **Infundibulum of the heart,** the section of the right ventricle from which the pulmonary artery arises. Conus arteriosus. **Infundibulum of the hypophysis,** a hollow, conical process

that projects downwards from the tuber cinereum and is continuous with the posterior lobe of the hypophysis cerebri. **Infundibulum of the lungs,** the expanded terminal portion of the embryonic lung bed. **Infundibulum of the uterine tube,** the funnel-shaped lateral end of the uterine tube.

Infusion. A preparation of a vegetable drug made by steeping it in water and then straining. Such a process, whether used for this purpose or for the extraction of the active principle from any substance. The administration of a solution parenterally.

Ingesta. Food taken into the body.

Ingestion. The taking of food into the body. The process whereby a cell takes up foreign matter.

Ingravescent. Increasing in severity or weight.

Ingredient. A component.

Inguen. The groin.

Inguinal. Pertaining to the groin.

Inhalant. A substance that is taken into the body by being breathed in.

Inhalation. The method of applying drugs in a finely divided or gaseous state so that, on being breathed in, they may come in contact with the nose, throat and lungs. A preparation used for such a purpose.

Inhaler. A device or apparatus for the administration of medicaments by inhalation.

Inheritance. That which is handed down from parent to offspring. The act of so doing.

Inhibition. The arrest or restriction of some process, whether physical, mental or emotional.

Inhibitor. That which inhibits. **Monoamine oxidase inhibitor,** a drug, or substance, that destroys, or prevents the action of, monoamine oxidase.

Inion. The external occipital protuberance.

Iniopagus. Conjoined twins fused at the occiput.

Iniops. Conjoined twins with fused thoraxes, a single head, but two faces, one of which is incomplete.

Injection. The introduction of a fluid into the body through a hollow tube. A preparation to be administered in such a way. **Hypodermic injection,** subcutaneous injection. **Intra-arterial injection,** injection direct into an artery. **Intra-articular injection,** injection into a joint cavity. **Intrabursal injection,** injection into a bursa. **Intracameral injection,** injection into the anterior chamber of the eye.

Intracardiac injection, injection into the heart. **Intracisternal injection,** injection into the cerebello-medullary cistern (cisterna magna). **Intracutaneous injection,** injection into the skin. **Intradermal injection,** injection into the skin. **Intramuscular injection,** injection into a muscle. **Intrathecal injection,** injection into the subarachnoid space. **Intravenous injection,** injection into a vein. **Intravitreous injection,** injection into the vitreous chamber. **Peridural injection,** injection around the dura mater. **Retrobulbar injection,** injection posterior to the eyeball. **Subarachnoid injection,** injection into the subarachnoid space. **Subconjunctival injection,** injection underneath the conjunctiva. **Subcutaneous injection,** injection underneath the skin.

Injury. A wound, damage, or hurt.

Inlay. That which is cut to shape and embedded, as in an external filling on a tooth, or a piece of bone fitted into a gutter to fill a gap between the two fractured sections.

Inlet. An opening or entrance. **Inlet of the larynx,** the aperture through which the laryngeal cavity opens into the pharynx. **Pelvic inlet,** the superior pelvic aperture, bounded by the brim of the pelvis. **Inlet of the thorax,** the upper bony margin of the thorax, bounded by the first thoracic vertebra behind, the superior border of the manubrium sterni in front, and the first rib on each side.

Innate. Inborn. Dependent on genetic constitution.

Innervation. The nerve supply to a part or area.

Innominate. Nameless. The hip bone.

Ino-, In- (Gk *is, inos:* fibre). Prefixes indicating relationship to a fibre or fibrous tissue.

Inoculation. The introduction into the body of micro-organisms either to stimulate the production of antibodies for the protection of the individual against a given infection, or, in the case of animals, to induce the product of antibodies for therapeutic use in medical or veterinary practice. The introduction of micro-organisms into animals for experimental purposes.

Inoculum. The material introduced in the process of inoculation.

Inorganic. Not relating to living organisms.

Inositol. One of the constituents of the vitamin B complex, deficiency of which in mice causes baldness.

Inositol nicotinate. The B.P. Commission approved name for a peripheral vasodilator.

Inotropic. Pertaining to the influences affecting muscular contractility.

Inproquone. The B.P. Commission approved name for 2,5-di-(aziridin-1-yl)-3,6-dipropoxyl-1,4-benzoquinone. An antineoplastic agent.

Inquest. An inquiry by a coroner into the cause of death.

Insalubrious. Unhealthy.

Insane. Mentally deranged.

Insanity. Mental disease. Madness.

Insect. A member of the class of Insecta of the phyllum Arthropoda.

Insecticide. A substance that destroys insects.

Insemination. The introduction of semen within the vagina. Impregnation. **Artificial semination by donor (A.I.D.),** the artificial insemination of a woman by means of semen from a male other than her husband. **Artificial insemination by husband (A.I.H.),** artificial insemination of a woman by semen from her husband.

In situ. In position.

Insolation. Treatment by exposure to the sun's rays. Sunstroke.

Insoluble. Not capable of dissolving in a liquid.

Insomnia. Inability to sleep.

Inspiration. The act of drawing air into the lungs.

Inspire. To breath in.

Inspissation. The process of hardening due to loss, or evaporation, of fluid.

Instep. The arch of the foot.

Instillation. The introduction of a fluid drop by drop.

Instinct. The inborn tendency of an individual to behave in a certain way. The basis of the inherited tendency to maintain life and to propagate the species.

Insufflation. The blowing of a powder or gas into a cavity or on to an organ of the body.

Insula. An island. An area of the cerebral cortex that lies deeply in the floor of the lateral sulcus.

Insulin. The specific antidiabetic principle. The following forms of insulin are included in the *British Pharmacopoeia* 1968. **Insulin injection,** a sterile solution of the specific antidiabetic principle of the mammalian pancreas. It contains 20, 40, or 80 units per ml. **Biphasic insulin injection,** a sterile buffered suspension of crystals containing the specific antidiabetic principle of the pancreas of the ox in a solution of the specific antidiabetic principle of the pancreas of the pig. It contains 40 or 80 units per ml. and, when given subcutaneously, produces a rapid hypoglycaemic effect within half-an-hour due to the soluble insulin fraction, while the insulin crystals, being slowly absorbed, produce a depot effect with an action beginning in about twelve hours and reaching a maximum four to twelve hours later. **Globin zinc insulin injection,** a sterile preparation of the specific anti-diabetic principle of the mammalian pancreas with a suitable globin and zinc chloride. It contains 40 or 80 units per ml. It has a delayed action intermediate in onset between that of unmodified insulin and that of protamine zinc insulin. **Isophane insulin injection,** a sterile buffered crystalline suspension of insulin, with a suitable protamine. It has a delayed action which begins about two hours after subcutaneous injection, becomes maximal after two hours, and declines after about twenty-eight hours. **Neutral insulin injection,** a sterile buffered solution of insulin from the pancreas of the ox or pig. It contains 40 or 80 units per ml. When given subcutaneously, it is slightly more rapidly absorbed than insulin injection. **Protamine zinc insulin,** a sterile suspension of insulin from mammalian pancreas, with a suitable protamine and zinc chloride. It has a delayed action which allows a slow but steady activity of insulin throughout the day. **Insulin zinc suspension,** a sterile buffered suspension of mammalian insulin with zinc chloride. It contains 40 or 80 units per ml. It has a delayed action varying in duration from twelve to thirty hours or longer. **Insulin zinc suspension (amorphous),** a sterile buffered suspension of mammalian insulin, with zinc chloride. It contains 40 to 80 units per ml. **Insulin zinc suspension (crystalline),** a sterile, buffered suspension of mammalian insulin in the form of crystals. It contains 40 to 80 units per ml.

Insulinase. A heat-labile proteolytic enzyme, particularly abundant in the liver and kidneys, that destroys insulin.

Integument. A covering.

Intelligence. The ability to comprehend. The mind.

Intention. Purpose. A process of healing. **Intention tremor,** a tremor which occurs or is accentuated on movement of the part involved, one of the

classical signs of multiple sclerosis.

Inter- (L *inter:* between). Prefix meaning between, among.

Intercalated. Interposed.

Intercostal. Between the ribs.

Intercurrent. Intervening, as applied, for example, to one disease occurring in the course of another.

Interdigitation. Interlocking of finger-like processes.

Interface. The surface forming the boundary between two phases.

Interferon. The factor responsible for the action of one virus in interfering with the growth of another, and capable of conferring on animal cells resistance to virus infection.

Intermittent. Recurrent. **Intermittent fever,** a fever which settles completely, only to recur, as in malaria. **Intermittent pulse,** a pulse in which occasional heart-beats do not get through. **Intermittent claudication,** a condition characterized by the onset of cramp-like pains in the legs in walking, due to defective blood supply to the relevant muscles.

Internal. Within. Inside.

Interneurones. Short interconnecting neurones.

Internodal. The distance between two nodes. **Internodal distance,** the distance between two nodes of Ranvier on a nerve.

Internuncial. Acting as an agent or medium between two organs or cells. **Internuncial neurones,** interneurones.

Interoceptor. A nerve-ending or receptor end-organ in the wall of the viscera and blood vessels.

Interpalpebral. Between the eyelids.

Interparietal. Intramural. Between the parietal bones. **Interparietal bone,** the squamous part of the occipital bone that may remain separate throughout life.

Interpeduncular. Between the cerebral or cerebellar peduncles.

Intersection. A division. **Tendinous intersections,** three fibrous bands that pass across the rectus muscle, one at the level of the umbilicus, one at the level of the fore end of the xiphoid process, and one midway between the xiphoid process and the umbilicus.

Intersex. The condition characterized by the presence of both male and female characteristics, as a result of a congenital developmental defect.

Interstice. A small space or gap.

Interstitial. Occurring in, or relating to, interstices. **Interstitial cells,** the cells of the connective tissue. **Interstitial**

cells of the testis, the cells lying between the seminiferous tubules that secrete testosterone. **Interstitial cell stimulating hormone (ICSH),** the hormone secreted by the anterior lobe of the hypophysis cerebri (pituitary gland) that is responsible for the appearance and development of the interstitial cells of the testis. **Interstitial fluid,** the fluid lying in the interstices of the connective tissue.

Intertrigo. The chafed or abraded condition of the skin that occurs when two surfaces of the skin rub together, as underneath the breast or between the scrotum and the thigh.

Intertrochanteric. Relating to the space between the greater and lesser trochanters of the femur.

Intestine. The alimentary tract below the stomach. **Small intestine,** this comprises the part of the intestine that extends from the stomach for 6·5 metres to the large intestine. It consists of the *duodenum,* which measures 30cm., the *jejunum* which comprises the next 2·5 metres, and the *ileum,* which comprises the next 2·5 metres and, through the ileocaecal valve leads into the large intestine. **Large intestine,** this consists of the *caecum, appendix vermiformis, ascending colon, transverse colon, descending colon, pelvic colon,* and *rectum.*

Intima. The innermost lining of a blood vessel.

Intoxication. Poisoning.

Intra- (L *intra:* within). Prefix meaning within, into.

Intra-arterial. Within or into an artery.

Intracardiac. Within or into the cavity of the heart.

Intracranial. Within or into the skull.

Intradermal. Within or into the skin.

Intramuscular. Within or into a muscle.

Intra-ocular. Within or into the eyeball.

Intrapartum. During labour.

Intraperitoneal. Within or into the peritoneal cavity.

Intrathecal. Within a sheath. Within the cerebrospinal meninges.

Intrathoracic. Within or into the thorax.

Intra-uterine. Within or into the uterus.

Intravenous. Within or into a vein.

Intravertebral. Within or into the spinal column.

Intra vitam. During life.

Intrinsic. Inherent. **Intrinsic factor,** the factor in the gastric mucosa necessary for the absorption of vitamin B_{12}, and the lack of which is the cause of pernicious anaemia.

Intro- (L *intro:* into). Prefix meaning within.

Introitus. Entrance.

Intromission. Insertion, particularly of one organ into another.

Introspection. Looking into one's mind.

Introversion. Turning outside in. A turning inward of psychic energy, and of the libido in particular.

Introvert. An individual whose libido is turned in on himself. To invaginate.

Intubation. The passage of a tube.

Intumescence. A swelling. The process of becoming swollen.

Intussusception. Invagination of a part of the intestine into the part below it, one of the important causes of intestinal obstruction in young children.

Inulin. B.P. Addendum 1969. Polysaccharide granules obtained from the tubers of *Dahlia variabilis* and other genera of the family Compositae. Used for the measurement of the glomerular filtration rate.

Inunction. The act of rubbing an ointment or some other fatty preparation into the skin.

In utero. Within the uterus. Not yet born.

In vacuo. In a vacuum.

Invagination. The process of ensheathing.

Inversion. Turning inward.

Invert. A homosexual.

Invertebrata. The division of the animal world which includes all those animals that have no spinal column.

Invertebrate. Without a vertebral column.

In vitro. In a test-tube or some comparable piece of laboratory apparatus. The opposite of *in vivo.*

In vivo. Within a living organism.

Involucrum. The sheath of new bone that grows round a piece of dead bone. A covering.

Involution. A rolling, or turning, inwards. The process of an enlarged organ returning to its original size: e.g. the uterus following parturition. Any retrograde biological change: e.g. senility.

Iobenzamic acid. The B.P. Commission approved name for N-(3-amino-2,4,6-tri-idophenzoyl)-N-β-alanine. A radio-opaque substance.

Iodate. A salt of iodic acid.

Iodide. A compound of iodine.

Iodine. A solid, non-metallic element. Symbol I. Atomic weight 126·9. Atomic number 53. It is a bactericide. Internally it is used in the preparation of the thyrotoxic patient for thyroidectomy. **Aqueous iodine solution, B.P. 1968,** also known as Lugol's solution, contains 10 per cent of potassium iodide and 5 per cent of iodine. **Weak iodine solution, B.P. 1968,** also known as iodine tincture, contains 2·5 per cent each of iodine, potassium iodide and water, in alcohol (90 per cent).

Iodipamide meglumine injection. B.P. 1968. A sterile solution of the *bis-N*-methylglucamine salt of *NN'*-di-(3-carboxy-2,4,6-tri-iodophenyl)-adipamide, a radio-opaque contrast medium used intravenously for visualization of the biliary tract.

Iodism. The morbid state induced by an overdose of, or too prolonged dosage with, iodine or iodine compounds. In some susceptible individuals it is brought on by quite small doses.

Iodized oil fluid injection. B.P. 1968. A sterile iodine-addition product of the ethyl esters of the fatty acids obtained from poppy-seed oil expressed from the ripe seeds of *Papaver somniferum* (L.). It is a contrast medium used for lymphography and sialography.

Iodothiouracil. The B.P. Commission approved name for 4-hydroxy-5-iodo-2-mercaptopyrimidine. An antithyroid agent.

Ion. An atom or group of atoms bearing an electrical charge.

Ionization. The dissociation of a substance in solution into its constituent ions.

Iontophoresis. The introduction of ions into the tissues by means of an electric current.

Iopanoic acid. B.P. 1968. $C_{11}H_{12}I_3NO_2$. A radio-opaque substance for visualization of the gall-bladder.

Iophendylate injection. B.P. 1968. Ethyl iodophenylundecanoate injection. A contrast medium for myelography.

Iopydol. The B.P. Commission approved name for *N*-(2,3-dihydroxypropyl)-3, 5-di-iodo-4-pyridone. A radio-opaque substance.

Iopydone. The B.P. Commission approved name for 3,5-di-iodo-4-pyridone. A radio-opaque substance.

Iothalamic acid. B.P. 1968. $C_{11}H_9I_3N_2O_4$. A contrast medium for diagnostic radiology.

Ipecacuanha. B.P. 1968. The dried root, or the rhizome and root, of *Cephaëlis ipecacuanha*. It contains not less than 2 per cent of alkaloids calculated as emetine. It is used in small doses as an expectorant, and in large doses as an emetic. **Ipecacuanha and opium powder,**

B.P.C. 1968, contains 100 grammes each of prepared ipecacuanha, B.P. 1968, and powdered opium, B.P. 1968, in 800 grammes of lactose. It is used as a diaphoretic. Dover's powder.

Iprindole. The B.P. Commission approved name for 5-(3-dimethylaminopropyl)-6, 7, 8, 9, 10, 11-hexahydrocylo-oct[*b*]indole. An antidepressant.

Iproclozide. The B.P. Commission approved name for *N*-4-chlorophenoxyacetyl-*N'*isopropylhydrazine. A monoamine oxidase inhibitor.

Iproniazid. The B.P. Commission approved name for *N*-isonicotinoyl-*N'*-isopropylhydrazine. A monoamine oxidase inhibitor.

Ipsilateral. Occurring on the same side.

Irid-, Irido (Gk *iris, iridos:* rainbow). Prefixes indicating relationship to the iris.

Iridectomy. Surgical removal of part of the iris.

Iridencleisis. The condition in which the iris is nipped in a small gaping wound in the cornea.

Irideremia. Congenital absence of the iris.

Iridium. A white metallic element. Symbol Ir. Atomic weight 192·2. Atomic number 77.

Iridocyclitis. Inflammation of the iris and the ciliary body.

Iridodialysis. The condition in which the iris is torn away from its ciliary attachment.

Iridodonesis. Tremulousness of the iris.

Iridoschisis. A rare condition, usually degenerative, sometimes traumatic, in origin, in which tears develop in the anterior mesodermal layer of the iris.

Iridotomy. Surgical section of the iris.

Iris. The thin, circular, contractile disc, suspended in the aqueous humour between the cornea and the lens, and perforated just to the nasal side of its centre by the circular aperture of the pupil.

Irisopsia. The appearance of rainbow colours about objects.

Iritis. Inflammation of the iris.

Iron. A malleable metal. Symbol Fe (L *ferrum*). Atomic weight 55·847. Atomic number 26. Certain of its salts are used in the treatment of irondeficiency anaemia. Others are used as styptics.

Iron dextran injection. B.P. 1968. A sterile colloidal solution containing a complex of ferric hydroxide with dextrans of average molecular weight between 5000 and 7500. It is given intramuscularly in the treatment of iron-deficiency anaemia.

Iron phosphate. B.P.C. 1968. The form of iron used principally in the form of syrups, or tablets, such as Easton's syrup or tablets.

Iron sorbitol injection. B.P. 1968. A sterile colloidal solution of a complex of ferric iron, sorbitol and citric acid, stabilized with dextrin and sorbitol. Administered intramuscularly for the treatment of iron-deficiency anaemia.

Irradiation. Treatment by some form of rays, whether X-rays, radio-isotopes, ultra-violet rays, or the like.

Irreducible. Incapable of being restored to the normal position.

Irrespirable. Unfit for respiration. Incapable of being breathed.

Irreversible. Incapable of being reversed or of cure. Permanent.

Irrigation. The method of washing out: e.g. wounds, or organs such as the bladder.

Irritability. The quality of being excitable or of responding to stimuli.

Isch-, Ischo- (Gk *ischein:* to suppress). Prefixes signifying suppression, stoppage or deficiency.

Ischaemia. Bloodlessness of a part. Local anaemia.

Ischi-, Ischio- (Gk *ischion:* hip). Prefixes signifying relationship to the hip or ischium

Ischial. Pertaining to the hip-joint.

Ischiorectal. Pertaining to the ischium and the rectum. **Ischiorectal abscess,** an abscess arising in the space between the rectum and the ischium and often resulting in a fistula.

Ischipagus. Conjoined twins united at the ischia.

Ischium. The lower and posterior part of the hip bone. (*Plural:* ischia.)

Ischuria. Suppression or retention of urine.

Island. An isolated part or structure. **Blood islands,** spherical groups of cells on the surface of the yolk sac and in the body stalk found early in the third week of embryological development, which are the precursors of the primitive blood cells. **Islands of Langerhans,** the islets of cells in the pancreas that secrete insulin. The interalveolar cell islets.

Islet. A small island. **Interalveolar cell islets,** the clusters of cells in the pancreas that secrete insulin. The islands of Langerhans.

Iso- (Gk *isos:* equal). Prefix meaning equal or alike.

Isoagglutinin. An agglutinin that acts upon the red blood cells of members of the same species.

Isoagglutinogen. An isoantigen that induces agglutination of the cells to which it is attached on exposure to the specific isoantibody.

Isoaminile. The B.P. Commission approved name for 4-dimethylamino-2-isopropyl-2-phenylvaleronitrile. A cough suppressant.

Iso-antibody. An antibody that reacts with an antigen present in another individual of the same species. Alloantibody.

Isoantigen. A substance which is present in one individual and is antigenic to some, but not all, individuals of the same species.

Isobar. Having the same atomic weight but different atomic numbers. A line drawn on a meteorological map linking up areas of equal barometric pressure.

Isobuzole. The B.P. Commission approved name for 5-isobutyl-2(4-methoxybenzene sulphonamido)-1,3,4-thiadiazole. An oral hypoglycaemic agent.

Isocarboxazid. B.P. 1968. $C_{12}H_3N_3O_2$. An antidepressant drug that inhibits monoamine oxidase.

Isochromosome. A chromosome with two equal and genetically equivalent arms.

Isodactylism. Having toes or fingers all of the same length.

Isodynamic. Of equal force or power.

Isoelectric. Of equal electric potential. **Isoelectric point,** the pH at which an amphoteric substance, such as a protein, is electrically neutral.

Isoenzyme. An enzyme that may exist in tissues in two or more components which may have the same catalytic activity but are chemically, immunologically and electrophoretically distinct.

Isoetharine. The B.P. Commission approved name for 1-(3,4-dihydroxyphenyl)-2-isopropylaminobutan-1-ol. A bronchodilator.

Isogenic. Genetically identical.

Isograft. A graft in which donor and recipient are genetically identical.

Isohaemagglutinin. Isoagglutinin.

Isohaemolysin. A haemolysin that acts on the blood of animals of the same species as that from which it is derived.

Isoimmunization. The immunization of one member of a species by an antigen lacking in himself but present naturally in other members of the species.

Isolation. The process of isolating, as, for example, the separation of an individual with an infectious disease to prevent his transmitting it to others.

Isoleucine. One of the essential amino-acids: i.e. an amino-acid that cannot be synthesized endogeneously, but is essential for growth and the maintenance of normal metabolism.

Isomer. One of two or more compounds that have the same percentage composition but differ in the relative position of the atoms within the molecule.

Isomerase. An enzyme that catalyses the internal arrangement of the component atoms of a single molecule.

Isomethadone. The B.P. Commission approved name for a narcotic analgesic.

Isometric. Of equal dimensions.

Isometropia. Equality in the refraction of the two eyes.

Isomorphous. Having the same form.

Isoniazid. B.P. 1968. $C_6H_7N_3O$. An antituberculous agent.

Isoprednidene. The B.P. Commission approved name for a corticotrophin inhibitor.

Isoprenaline sulphate. B.P. 1968. $C_{22}H_{36}N_2O_{10}S$, $2H_2O$. A sympathomimetic amine used in the treatment of asthma.

Isopropamide iodide. The B.P. Commission approved name for (3-carbamoyl-3,3-diphenylpropyl) diisopropylmethylammonium iodide. A gastro-intestinal sedative.

Isopropyl alcohol. B.P. 1968. C_3H_8O. An antibacterial agent used in the preoperative cleaning of the skin and for sterilizing instruments.

Isosthenuria. The state of fixed specific gravity of the urine that occurs in the later stages of renal failure.

Isothermal. Having the same temperature.

Isothipendyl hydrochloride. B.P.C. 1968. $C_{16}H_{20}ClN_3S$. An antihistamine.

Isotones. Atoms having the same number of nuclear neutrons but different mass numbers and different atomic numbers.

Isotonic. Of equal tension or osmotic pressure.

Isotope. Each of two or more chemical elements or atoms which have the same chemical properties but differ in atomic weight.

Isotropic. Having like properties in all respect. Equal in refracting power.

Isoxsuprine. The B.P. Commission approved name for 1-(4-hydroxyphenyl)-2-(1-methyl-2-phenoxyethyl-

amino)propan-1-ol. A peripheral vasodilator.

Isozyme. Isoenzyme.

Ispaghula. B.P.C. 1968. The dried ripe seeds of *Plantago ovata*. A laxative.

Ispaghula husk, B.P.C. 1968, the epidermis and collapsed adjacent layers removed from ispaghula.

Issue. A discharge. Offspring.

Isthmus. A narrow or constricted connecting part. **Aortic isthmus,** the slightly narrowed section of the aorta between the left subclavian artery and the attachment of the ductus arteriosus. **Isthmus of the auditory tube,** the narrow stretch of the auditory tube at the junction of the bony and cartilaginous parts. **Isthmus of the external acoustic meatus,** the constriction in the external acoustic meatus 2cm. from the bottom of the concha. **Isthmus of the fauces,** the region of the oral part of the pharynx bounded on either side by the triangular interval between the palatoglossal and palatopharyngeal arches. **Isthmus of the cingulate gyrus,** the isthmus that connects the cingulate gyrus with the parahippocampal gyrus. **Oropharyngeal isthmus,** the aperture by which the mouth communicates with the pharynx. **Pharyngeal isthmus,** the opening, between the free edge of the soft palate and the posterior wall of the pharynx, through which the nasal and oral parts of the pharynx communicate. **Isthmus of the prostate,** the band that connects the left and right lobes of the prostate. **Isthmus of the thyroid gland,** the narrow portion of the thyroid that connects together the lower parts of the two lobes. **Isthmus of the uterine tube,** the medial one-third of the tube. **Isthmus of the uterus,** the upper third of the cervix uteri.

Itch. An irritating sensation in the skin. Pruritus. Scabies.

-itis (Gk *-itis:* a feminine adjectival termination which came to denote disease). Suffix indicating an inflammatory condition.

Itramin tosylate. The B.P. Commission approved name for 2-nitratoethylamine toluene-*p*-sulphonate. A vasodilator.

Ivory. Dentine.

Ixodes. A genus of ticks of the family Ixodidae, many of which are parasitic on man.

Ixodidae. The family of hard ticks.

Ixodoidea. A superfamily of the order Acarina, the ticks.

J

Jactitation. Restless tossing about, such as may occur in grave illness.

Janiceps. A foetal monstrosity characterized by one combined head and two faces.

Jaundice. Yellow discoloration of the skin and tissues with bile pigments.

Jaws. The two bones that carry the teeth. The upper jaw is the maxilla. The lower jaw is the mandible.

Jejunal. Pertaining to the jejunum.

Jejunectomy. Surgical excision of the jejunum.

Jejunitis. Inflammation of the jejunum.

Jejuno- (L *jejunum:* empty). Prefix indicating association with the jejunum.

Jejunostomy. The establishment of an opening into the jejunum through the abdominal wall.

Jejunotomy. Surgical incision of the jejunum.

Jejunum. The stretch of the small intestine between the duodenum and the ileum.

Jelly. A colloidal semi-solid mass. (*Plural:* jellies.) **Wharton's jelly,** the mucoid connective tissue of the umbilical cord.

Jerk. A reflex or involuntary quick movement. **Ankle jerk,** the contraction of the calf muscles induced by tapping on the stretched tendo calcaneus. **Biceps jerk,** the contraction of the biceps muscles and supinator muscles induced by tapping over the lower end of the radius. **Jaw jerk,** the movement of the lower jaw induced by tapping over the tip of the mandible, with the mouth open. **Knee jerk,** the extension of the knee induced by tapping over the patellar tendon. **Triceps jerk,** the extension of the flexed elbow induced by tapping over the triceps tendon immediately above the olecranon.

Jigger. Sand-flea. *Tunga penetrans.*

Joint. A junction of two or more bones. **Acromioclavicular joint,** the plane joint between the acromial end of the clavicle and the medial margin of the acromion. **Ankle joint,** the hinge joint involving the lower end of the tibia and its malleolus, the malleolus of the fibula, and the body of the talus. The talocrural joint. **Atlanto-axial joints,** the three synovial joints whereby the atlas articulates with the axis. **Atlanto-occipital joint,** the ellipsoid joint between the superior articular facet of the atlas and the condyle of the occipital bone. **Ball-and-socket joint,** a synovial joint in which the movement is polyaxial. Spheroid joint. **Calcaneocuboid joint** the saddle-shaped joint between the calcaneus and the cuboid bone. **Carpal joints,** the intercarpal joints. **Carpometacarpal joints,** the joints between the distal row of carpal bones and the metacarpals. **Cartilaginous joint,** a joint in which the opposed bony surfaces are connected to each other by cartilage. **Compound joint,** a synovial joint with two or more articulating surfaces, sharing a common articular capsule. **Condylar joint,** a synovial joint in which the presence of two distinct pairs of articular surfaces with their long axes in parallel with each other restricts the principal movement to one plane: e.g. the knee joint. **Costochondral joints,** the joints between the lateral end of each costal cartilage and the sternal end of the rib. **Costotransverse joint,** the joint between the tubercle of a rib and the transverse process of the vertebra to which it corresponds numerically. **Costovertebral joints,** the joints between the ribs and the vertebral column. **Cricoarytenoid joint,** the synovial joint between the facet on the lateral part of the upper border of the lamina of the cricoid cartilage and the base of the arytenoid cartilage. **Cuboideonavicular joint,** a syndesmosis between the cuboid and navicular bones. **Cuneocuboid joint,** the plane joint between the cuneiform bone and the cuboid. **Cuneometatarsal joints,** the plane joints between the metatarsal and cuneiform bones. **Cuneonavicular joint,** the plane joint between the navicular and the three cuneiform bones. **Diarthrodial joint,** a synovial joint. **Digital joints,** the hinge joints between the phalanges of the fingers and toes. **Elbow joint,** the hinge joint between the trochlea of the humerus and the trochlear notch of the ulna, and between the capitulum of the humerus and the head of the radius. **Ellipsoid joint,** a joint permitting appreciable movement about two distinct axes. **Fibrous joint,** an articulation in which the surfaces of the bones are fastened together by intervening fibrous tissue, and in which there is no appreciable movement: e.g. the joints between the bones of the cranium. **Ginglymus,** a hinge joint. **Gliding joint,** a joint in which one surface glides over another without any rotary or angular movement. **Gomphosis,** articulation by insertion of a conical process into a socket, as in the articulation of the teeth with the alveoli of the jaw. Peg-and-socket joint. **Hinge joint,** a joint in which there is movement in one direction only. Ginglymus. **Hip joint,** the ball-and-socket joint formed by the reception of the head of the femur into the acetabulum. **Humero-radial joint,** that part of the elbow joint formed by the articulation between the capitulum of the humerus and the head of the radius. **Humero-ulnar joint,** that part of the elbow joint formed by the articulation between the trochlea of the humerus and the ulna. **Incudomalleolar joint,** the saddle articulation between the incus and the malleus. **Incudostapedial joint,** the ball-and-socket articulation between the incus and the stapes. **Intercarpal joints,** the joints that connect the carpal bones to one another. **Interchondral joints,** the joints between the contiguous borders of the 6th, 7th, 8th and 9th costal cartilages. **Intercuneiform joints,** the plane joints between the cuneiform bones. **Intermetacarpal joints,** the plane joints between the bases of the 2nd, 3rd, 4th and 5th metacarpal bones. **Intermetatarsal joints,** the synovial joints between the bases of the lateral four metatarsal bones. **Interphalangeal joints,** the hinge joints between the phalanges of the fingers and toes. Digital joints. **Intertarsal joints,** the subtalar (talocalcanean), talocalcaneonavicular,calcaneocuboid, cuneonavicular, cuboideonavicular, intercuneiform and cuneocuboid joints. **Intervertebral joints,** the plane joints between the articular processes

of the vertebrae. **Knee joint,** the condylar joint, composed of three articulations: two between the condyles of the femur and the menisci and condyles of the tibia, and the third between the patella and the femur. **Mandibular joint,** the condylar joint between the articular tubercle and the anterior portion of the mandibular fossa of the temporal bone above and the head of the mandible below. The temporomandibular joint. **Manubriosternal joint,** the joint between the manubrium and the body of the sternum. **Metacarpophalangeal joints,** the joints between the heads of the metacarpal bones and the proximal phalanges. **Metatarsophalangeal joints,** the ellipsoid joints between the metatarsal bones and the proximal phalanges. **Midcarpal joint,** the joint between the scaphoid, lunate and triquetral bones proximally and the second row of the carpal bones distally. **Peg-and-socket joint,** gomphosis. **Pivot joint,** a synovial joint in which the movement is limited to rotation. **Plane joint,** a synovial joint formed by the apposition of plane articular surfaces. **Radiocarpal joint,** an ellipsoid joint formed by the distal end of the radius and lower surface of the articular disc above and the scaphoid, lunate and triquetal bones below. The wrist joint. **Radio-ulnar joints,** the proximal radio-ulnar joint which is a pivot joint between the circumference of the head of the radius and osseofibrous ring formed by the radial notch of the ulna and the anular ligament; the distal radio-ulnar joint which is a pivot joint formed between the head of the ulna and the ulnar notch of the lower end of the radius. **Sacrococcygeal joint,** the symphysis between the apex of the sacrum and the base of the coccyx. **Sacro-iliac joint,** the synovial joint between the auricular surfaces of the sacrum and ilium. **Saddle joint,** a synovial joint in which the opposing surfaces are concavoconvex. **Schindylesis,** or wedge-and-groove suture, a joint where a ridge fits into a grooved surface. **Shoulder joint,** the ball-and-socket joint formed by the head of the humerus and the glenoid cavity of the scapula. **Simple joint,** a synovial joint which possesses only two articulating surfaces. **Sternal joints,** the manubriosternal and xiphisternal joints. **Sternoclavicular joint,** the modified saddle joint between the sternal end of the clavicle, the clavicular notch of the manubrium sterni, and the cartilage of the first rib. **Sternocostal joints,** the joints between the costal cartilages and the sternum. **Subtalar joint,** the joint between the calcaneus and the talus. **Symphysis pubis,** the cartilaginous joint between the pubic bones. The pubic symphysis. **Synchondrosis,** a cartilaginous joint in which the cartilage is hyaline in character and temporary in nature. **Syndesmosis,** a joint in which the opposed bony surfaces are connected by an interosseous ligament. **Synovial joint,** a joint in which the contiguous bony surfaces are covered with articular cartilage and are not attached to each other, there is a joint cavity containing synovial fluid, and the joint is completely surrounded by an articular capsule. **Talocalcanean joint,** the subtalar joint. **Talocrural joint,** the ankle joint. **Tarsometatarsal joints,** the three joints between the three cuneiform bones and cuboid bone posteriorly and the bases of the metatarsal bones anteriorly. **Temporomandibular joint,** the mandibular joint. **Tibiofibular joints,** the *tibiofibular articulation,* a plane joint between the lateral condyle of the tibia and the head of the fibula, and the *tibiofibular syndesmosis* between the lower end of the fibula and the fibular notch of the tibia. **Trochoid joint,** pivot joint.

Wrist joint, the radiocarpal joint. **Xiphisternal joint,** the joint between the xiphisternum and the body of the sternum.

Joule. The unit of work: i.e. the work done by a current of one ampere against a resistance of one ohm in one second. (*Abbreviation:* J.)

Jugular. Pertaining to the throat or neck.

Jugum. A ridge or furrow connecting two points. **Jugum sphenoidale,** the anterior portion of the upper surface of the body of the sphenoid that separates the anterior cranial fossa from the sphenoidal sinus.

Junction. A joining or meeting place. **Amelodentinal junction,** where the enamel meets the subjacent dentine in the crown of a tooth. **Anorectal junction,** where the anus and rectum joint. **Mucocutaneous junction,** the meeting between mucous membrane and skin. **Sclerocorneal junction,** the line of union between sclera and cornea.

Junket. Milk which has been acted upon by rennet.

Juxta- (L *juxta:* near). Prefix indicating nearness.

Juxta-articular. Near a joint.

Juxta-glomerular. Near to, or adjoining, a glomerulus or glomeruli.

Juxtaposition. Apposition.

Juxtapyloric. Near the pylorus.

K

Kahn reaction. A test for syphilis.

Kala-azar. Visceral leishmaniasis. A disease caused by *Leishmania donovani*, which occurs in the Mediterranean littoral, Africa and Asia, and is characterized by a chronic course, remittent fever, leucopenia, splenomegaly and hepatomegaly.

Kallidinogenase. The B.P. Commission approved name for an enzyme that splits the kinin, kallidin, from kininogen. It is a vasodilator.

Kallikrein. An enzyme that acts upon proteins in the interstitial fluid to form the vasodilator polypeptide bradykinin.

Kanamycin sulphate. B.P.C. 1968. An antimicrobial substance produced by *Streptomyces kanamyceticus*, which is active against *E. coli*, Salmonellae, Shigellae, Neisseriae, *Proteus vulgaris*, *K. pneumoniae*, *K. aerobacter*, *Myco. tuberculosis*, and many strains of staphylococci. It is active by mouth, but is liable to cause irreversible deafness.

Kaolin. A white powder consisting of aluminium silicate resulting from the decomposition of minerals containing felspar. **Heavy kaolin**, B.P. 1968, a native hydrated aluminium silicate freed from most of its impurities by elutriation and dried. It is used in the preparation of **Kaolin poultice**, B.P. 1968. **Light kaolin**, B.P. 1968, an absorbent administered orally in the treatment of diarrhoeal conditions and externally as a dusting-powder.

Kary-, Karyo- (Gk *karyon:* nucleus, nut). Prefixes indicating association with a nucleus.

Karyokinesis. Mitosis. Reproduction of cells by indirect division, the common method in higher animals.

Karyolysis. Lysis of the cell nucleus.

Karyoplasma. The protoplasm of the nucleus.

Karyorrhexis. Disintegration or rupture of the cell nucleus.

Karyotype. The systematized arrangement of the chromosomes of an individual or a cell line.

Katathermometer. A thermometer that shows the rate of loss of heat, or cooling power, of the air.

Keloid. A nodular overgrowth of skin, usually at the site of a scar: e.g. a burn or an operation scar.

Kelvin. The unit of thermodynamic temperature, being the fraction $1/273\cdot16$ of the thermodynamic temperature of the triple point of water. (*Abbreviation:* K.)

Ken-, Keno- (Gk *kenos:* empty). Prefixes meaning empty.

Kenophobia. Morbid fear of wide open spaces.

Kerat-, Kerato- (Gk *keras:* horn, cornea). Prefixes indicating relationship to the cornea or horny tissue.

Keratalgia. Pain in the cornea.

Keratectasia. Protrusion of the cornea.

Keratectomy. Surgical removal of part of, or the whole of, the cornea.

Keratic. Pertaining to the cornea. Horny.

Keratin. The scleroprotein that forms the greater part of the horny layer of the skin, as well as the nails.

Keratinization. The development of keratin or the horny layer of the skin.

Keratitis. Inflammation of the cornea.

Keratoacanthoma. A self-healing epidermal nodule, usually in the cheeks, nose, fingers and hands, in elderly people.

Keratocele. Hernia of the posterior elastic lamina through the cornea.

Keratoconjunctivitis. Inflammation of the cornea and conjunctivitis.

Keratoconus. A conical protrusion of the cornea.

Keratoderma. A local or generalized thickening of the horny layer of the skin. **Keratoderma blenorrhagica**, a condition characterized by dull-red macules, usually on the soles of the feet, that occurs in Reiter's disease.

Keratoglobus. A hemispherical protrusion of the whole cornea, occurring bilaterally as a congenital anomaly.

Keratomalacia. Softening of the cornea as a result of severe lack of vitamin A in the diet. Most common in young children.

Keratome. A knife for incising the cornea.

Keratometer. An instrument for measuring the curvature of the cornea.

Keratometry. Measurement of the curvature of the cornea.

Keratopathy. Non-inflammatory disease of the cornea.

Keratoplasty. Plastic operation on the cornea. Corneal grafting.

Keratoscope. An instrument for examining the cornea.

Keratosis. A disease of the skin characterized by overgrowth of the horny layer. It may be induced by excessive exposure to the sun or to irradiation, or by the ingestion of arsenic. **Keratosis obturans,** the condition characterized by abnormal desquamation of epithelium in the meatus of the external ear, resulting in the formation of a large ball of wax and epithelium.

Keraunophobia. A morbid fear of thunder and lightning.

Kerion. A suppurating form of ringworm.

Kernicterus. Biliary staining of the basal nuclei of the brain, with toxic degeneration of the nerve cells, that occurs in the more severe forms of icterus neonatorum.

Kerosene. The paraffin oil used in oil lamps.

Ket-, Keto- (Ger *keton:* a modification of acetone). Prefixes indicating possession of the keto, or carbonyl group.

Ketamine. The B.P. Commission approved name for 2-(2-chlorophenyl)-2-methylaminocyclohexanone. An anaesthetic.

Keto acid. An acid with the general formula of R-CO-COOH.

Ketobemidone. The B.P. Commission approved name for 4-(3-hydroxyphenyl) -1 -methyl -4 -propionylpiperidine. A narcotic analgesic.

Ketogenesis. The process whereby ketone bodies are produced.

Ketolysis. The process of breaking up of ketone bodies.

Ketonaemia. The accumulation of ketone bodies in the blood.

Ketone. An organic compound containing the carbonyl (keto) group (CO) attached to two alkyl groups.

Ketonuria. The excretion of ketone bodies in the urine.

Ketosis. The condition in which ketone bodies accumulate in the blood and appear in the urine. Most commonly encountered in starvation and diabetes mellitus.

Ketosteroid. A steroid with ketone groups on functional carbon atoms. **17-ketosteroids,** ketosteroids with a ketone group on the 17th carbon atom.

Kidney. One of the paired organs, one in each lumbar region, that secrete urine. Each is 11cm. in length, 6cm. broad and 3cm. in thickness, and weighs 150 grammes in the adult male and 135 grammes in the adult female. **Artificial kidney,** the popular name for the instrument for renal dialysis. **Double kidney,** a developmental condition in which one of the kidneys is subdivided into two. **Ectopic kidney,** a not uncommon condition in which the kidney is in an unusual site. **Floating kidney,** a kidney that is abnormally mobile. **Horseshoe kidney,** a congenital abnormality in which the upper or lower poles of opposite kidneys are fused across the midline. **Polycystic kidney,** a congenital abnormality in which, due to developmental errors, the kidney is converted into a mass of cysts. **Supernumerary kidney,** a congenital abnormality in which two kidneys develop on one side.

Kilo- (Gk *chilioi:* one thousand). Prefix meaning one thousand.

Kilocalorie. The amount of heat required to raise 1kg. of water from 15° to 16°C. (*Abbreviation:* kcal.)

Kilocycle. A measure of the frequency of electromagnetic waves: 1000 cycles per second. (*Abbreviation:* kc.)

Kilogram. The unit of mass, equal to the mass of the international prototype of the kilogram. One thousand grammes, equivalent to 2·2046 pounds. (*Abbreviation:* kg.)

Kilometre. One thousand metres, equivalent to 0·6214 mile. (*Abbreviation:* km.)

Kilovolt. One thousand volts. (*Abbreviation:* kV.)

Kilowatt. One thousand watts. (*Abbreviation:* kW.)

Kin-, Kine-, Kino- (Gk *kinesis:* to move). Prefixes signifying movement.

Kinaesthesia. The sense perception for tension and position of muscle and joints.

Kinaesthesiometer. An instrument for measuring muscular sensation.

Kinanaesthesia. Loss of deep sensibility.

Kinase. Activator of an enzyme.

Kinetic. Pertaining to motion.

Kinetics. The study of motion and acceleration under the influence of forces.

Kinins. Polypeptides that stimulate visceral smooth muscle but relax vascular smooth muscle, and increase capillary permeability. They are found in saliva, sweat and pancreatic juice, and in wasp stings.

Kink. A twist or angulation.

Klebsiella. A genus of the family Enterobacteriaceae, the members of which are gram-negative, rod-shaped, non-motile bacilli. The only two significant members are *K. pneumoniae*, which is responsible for less than 1 per cent of cases of bacterial pneumonia, and *K. aerogenes*, most of which are commensals in the intestinal tract or saprophytes in water supply.

Klepto- (Gk *kleptein:* to steal). Prefix signifying relationship to stealing.

Kleptomania. An irresistible desire to steal without necessarily having any need for the stolen property.

Kneading. Pétrissage, a movement in massage.

Knee. The condylar joint with three articulations: two between the condyles of the femur and the menisci and condyles of the tibia, and one between the patella and femur. **Beat knee,** chronic inflammation of the connective tissue over the patella, due to continuous repeated pressure and irritation, as in coal-mining. **Housemaid's knee,** prepatellar bursitis. **Knock knee,** genu valgum.

Knuckle. The prominence produced over the head of any of the metacarpal bones. **Aortic knuckle,** the radiological shadow cast by the terminal part of the arch of the aorta.

Koilo- (Gk *koilos:* hollow). Prefix indicating a hollow or concave.

Koilonychia. A spoon-shaped deformity of the nails.

Kola. The dried leaf of various species of Kola, including *Kola acuminata*, the chief constituent of which is caffeine.

Kombé. An arrow poison derived from *Strophanthus kombé.*

Koumiss. A beverage originally made by fermenting mare's milk, but may be made from other forms of milk.

Krypton. An inert gaseous chemical element present in the atmosphere. Symbol Kr. Atomic weight 83·80. Atomic number 36.

Kuru. A chronic progressive degenerative condition of the central nervous system, characterized by ataxia, dysarthria and tremor, and terminating fatally, which occurs in New Guinea. It is of unknown etiology.

Kwashiorkor. A common and severe form of malnutrition due to protein deficiency that occurs in underdeveloped countries in children when they are weaned.

Kymo- (Gk *kyma:* wave). Prefix meaning a wave or undulation.

Kymogram. The tracing made by the kymograph.

Kymograph. An instrument for recording wave-like motions.

Kypho- (Gk *kyphos:* a hump). Prefix signifying a hump or convexity.

Kyphoscoliosis. Forward and lateral curvature of the spine.

Kyphosis. Excessive forward curvature of the spine.

L

Labial. Pertaining to the lips or labium.

Labile. Unsteady, Changeable.

Labio- (L *labium:* lip). Prefix signifying association with a lip.

Labiomancy. Lip reading.

Labioplasty. Plastic surgery of the lips.

Labitome. Cutting forceps.

Labium. A lip. (*Plural:* labia.) **Labium majus,** one of the two labia majora, or prominent folds which form the lateral boundaries of the pudendal cleft. **Labium minus,** one of the two labia minora, or small cutaneous folds on each side of the vagina.

Labour. Childbirth or parturition.

Labrum. An edge or lip. (*Plural:* labra.) **Acetabular labrum,** the fibrocartilaginous rim attached to the margin of the acetabulum. **Glenoidal labrum,** the fibrocartilaginous rim attached to the margin of the glenoid cavity.

Labyrinth. An intercommunicating system of cavities. **Bony labyrinth,** cavities hollowed out of the petrous part of the temporal bone, constituting part of the internal ear, and consisting of three parts: the vestibule, the three semicircular canals, and the cochlea. **Membranous labyrinth,** a series of communicating membranous sacs and ducts contained within the bony labyrinth, consisting of the utricle and saccule within the vestibule, three semicircular ducts within the semicircular canals, and the duct of the cochlea within the cochlea.

Labyrinthitis. Inflammation of the labyrinth. Otitis interna.

Laceration. A rent or tear.

Lacertus. A fibrous band.

Lachesine chloride. B.P.C. 1968. $C_{20}H_{26}ClNO_3$. A mydriatic and cycloplegic, used as eye-drops.

Lacrimal. Pertaining to the tears.

Lacrimation. The secretion of tears.

Lacrimatory. Tear-inducing.

Lact-, Lacto- (L *lac, lactis:* milk). Prefixes signifying association with milk.

Lactalbumin. One of the three proteins in milk.

Lactase. An enzyme in the intestinal juice that hydrolyses lactose to glucose and galactose.

Lactate. A salt of lactic acid.

Lactate dehydrogenase. An isoenzyme that catalyses the oxidation of lactate to pyruvate.

Lactation. The secretion of milk. Suckling. The period during which milk is secreted.

Lacteal. One of the lymph vessels in the mesentery that convey chyle from the small intestine. Milky.

Lactic. Pertaining to milk.

Lactic acid. B.P. 1968. A mixture of lactic acid and its condensation products. It is used in the preparation of solutions containing sodium lactate, and of lactic acid milk.

Lactic dehydrogenase. The enzyme that catalyses the oxidation of lactic acid to pyruvic acid in the process of glycolysis.

Lactiferous. Secreting milk.

Lactobacillaceae. The family of micro-organisms that are gram-positive cocci or rods, mostly non-motile. It includes four genera: Diplococcus, Streptococcus, Peptostreptococcus and Lactobacillus.

Lactobacillus. The genus of acid-resistant, gram-positive, non-sporing bacilli which occur in the intestine of mammalian animals. **Lactobacillus acidophilus,** present in saliva, faeces and milk, as well as dental caries. **Lactobacillus bifidus,** found in large numbers in the faeces of breast-fed infants.

Lactogenic. Milk-producing.

Lactometer. An instrument for determining the specific gravity of milk.

Lactose. Milk sugar present in milk and synthesized in the mammary gland. On hydrolysis it yields one molecule of glucose and one of galactose. **Lactose,** B.P. 1968, obtained from the whey of milk, is used to adjust the carbohydrate content of cows' milk for infant feeding, and to give bulk to powders.

Lactosuria. The excretion of lactose in the urine.

Lactovegetarian. One subsisting on a diet of milk, eggs and vegetables.

Lacuna. A small pit or depression. (*Plural:* lacunae.) **Lacuna of bone,** one of the oblong spaces between the lamellae of bone. **Hepatic lacuna,** one of the spaces, containing the venous sinusoids, that lie between the laminae, or sheets, of liver cells. **Howship's lacuna,** one of the small pits produced in bone by osteoblasts. **Lacuna musculorum,** the lateral part of the space between the inguinal ligament and the hip bone. **Urethral lacuna,** one of the many small pit-like recesses in the urethra. **Lacuna vasorum,** the medial part of the space between the inguinal ligament and the hip bone, which transmits the femoral vessels. **Venous lacuna,** one of the small sinuses in the dura mater that communicate with the superior sagittal sinus.

Lacus lacrimalis. The triangular space separating the two eyelids at their medial angle, which contains the caruncula lacrimalis.

Laev-, Laevo- (L *laevus:* left). Prefixes meaning left, to the left. In chemistry it signifies laevorotatory.

Laevocardia. Situs inversus of the other viscera, with a normally situated heart which is almost always riddled with congenital abnormalities.

Laevophobia. Morbid dread of objects on the left side.

Laevorotatory. Rotating the plane of polarized light from right to left.

Laevulosaemia. The presence of laevulose (fructose) in the blood. An inborn error of metabolism due to lack of fructokinase.

Laevulose. $C_6H_{12}O_6$. Fructose. **Laevulose, B.P.** 1968, a preparation of laevulose also available as **Laevulose injection, B.P.** 1968, for intravenous administration.

Laevulosuria. The excretion of laevulose (fructose) in the urine.

Lagaena. The upper extremity of the duct of the cochlea.

Lageniform. Flask-shaped.

Lagnesis. Nymphomania.

Lagophthalmos. Inability to close the eye completely.

Lake. To haemolyse blood. A small collection of fluid.

Lallation. A babbling, baby-like form of speech.

Lalo- (Gk *lalein:* to babble or speak). Prefix indicating a relationship to babbling or speech.

Lambda. The point of junction of the sagittal and lambdoid sutures.

Lambliasis. Giardiasis.

Lamella. A thin plate. A small medicated disc, intended to dissolve in the lacrimal secretion. (*Plural:* lamellae.) **Articular lamella,** the compact·layer of bone on its articular surface that is firmly attached to the articular cartilage. **Lamella of bone,** one of the concentric thin plates of bone that constitute normal adult bone.

Lamina. A thin plate. (*Plural:* laminae.) **Alar lamina,** the posterolateral part of the embryonic neural tube. **Basal lamina of the choroid,** a thin structureless membrane lining the inner surface of the choroid. **Basal lamina of the neural tube,** the anterolateral part of the embryonic neural tube. **Chorocapillary lamina,** the inner layer of the choroid, consisting of an exceedingly fine capillary plexus. **Cribrosa sclerae lamina,** that part of the sclera pierced by the optic nerve. **Lamina of the cricoid cartilage,** 2 to 3cm. in height, the deep, broad posterior section of the cricoid. **External elastic lamina of arteries,** the outer layer of elastic tissue in the arterial wall. **Internal elastic lamina of arteries,** the inner layer of elastic tissue in the arterial wall. **Hepatic lamina,** one of the sheets of liver cells that form a continuous system throughout the liver. **Medullary laminae of the globus pallidus,** an *external lamina* that separates the globus pallidus from the putamen, and an *internal lamina* that subdivides it into a lateral and a medial portion. **Medullary laminae of the thalamus,** an *external lamina* of white matter that covers its lateral surface, and an *internal lamina* of white matter that divides its grey matter incompletely into three parts. **Osseous spiral lamina,** a delicate lamina in the cochlea that projects from the modiolus into the canal. **Reticular lamina of the spiral organ,** a delicate framework perforated by circular holes occupied by the free ends of the outer hair cells. **Lamina of septum pellucidum,** one of the two laminae which, separated by a narrow interval, constitute the septum pellucidum. **Suprachoroid lamina,** the delicate tissue that loosely connects the outer surface of the choroid with the sclera. **Lamina terminalis,** the anterior wall of the 3rd ventricle of the brain. **Lamina of the thyroid cartilage,** one of the two quadrilateral masses that constitute the thyroid cartilage. **Vascular lamina of the choroid,** the outer layer of the choroid. **Lamina of the vertebral arches,** one of the two broad plates directed backwards and medially from the pedicles in each vertebral arch.

Laminectomy. Surgical removal of one or more laminae of the vertebral.

Lamp. An illuminating device. **Carbon arc lamp,** a rich source of ultraviolet irradiation produced by an electric arc between carbon electrodes. **Eldridge-Green lamp,** a system of lights for testing colour vision. **Infra-red lamp** a source of infra-red heat rays produced by a surface heated to 300° to 800°C. **Kromayer lamp,** a mercury-vapour, water-cooled quartz lamp for the production of ultraviolet rays concentrated on a small area. **Mercury-vapour lamp,** a rich source of ultraviolet irradiation produced by an arc struck in mercury vaporized in a quartz lamp. **Slit lamp,** a lamp for the examination of the eye. **Sun lamp,** a lamp with an ultraviolet spectrum comparable to sunlight. **Ultraviolet lamp,** a lamp producing ultraviolet rays.

Lana. Wool.

Lanatoside C. The B.P. Commission approved name for the 3-acetyl-glucosyltridigitoxoside of dioxigenin. A drug with a digitalis-like action.

Lance. To incise or cut open.

Lanceolate. Shaped-like a lance.

Lancet. A small, double-edged pointed knife.

Lancinating. Sharp, cutting, or tearing.

Lanolin. Hydrous wool fat.

Lanthanum. A rare metallic element. Symbol La. Atomic weight 138·91. Atomic number 57.

Lanugo. The fine downy hair that covers almost the entire foetal skin around the middle of foetal life, to be shed at birth and replaced by fine hairs, termed vellus.

Lapar-, Laparo- (Gk *lapara:* flank). Prefixes signifying the loins or, less correctly, the abdomen.

Laparoscope. An endoscope for examining the peritoneal cavity.

Laparoscopy. Examination of the peritoneal cavity by means of a laparoscope.

Laparotomy. A surgical incision through the abdominal wall, usually restricted to an exploratory abdominal operation.

Lard. The purified fat of the hog.

Lardaceous. Resembling lard.

Larva. The early immature stage of life

which differs markedly from the adult, applied particularly to the first stage of insect development after leaving the egg. (*Plural:* larvae.) **Larva migrans,** creeping eruption due to larvae, often of the dog or cat hookworm, or of Hypoderma (the warble fly), burrowing under the skin.

Larvicide. An agent that kills larvae.

Laryng-, Laryngo- (Gk *larynx:* larynx). Prefixes indicating relationship to the larynx.

Laryngeal. Pertaining to the larynx.

Laryngectomy. Surgical excision of the larynx.

Laryngismus. Spasm of the larynx. **Laryngismus stridulus,** sudden spasmodic closure of the glottis which occurs in young rachitic children.

Laryngitis. Inflammation of the larynx.

Laryngocele. An air-sac communicating with the larynx.

Laryngofissure. The surgical splitting of the thyroid cartilage to gain access to the cavity of the larynx.

Laryngology. The study of the larynx and its diseases.

Laryngopharyngeal. Related to the larynx and the pharynx.

Laryngoplasty. Plastic surgery of the larynx.

Laryngoscope. An instrument for viewing the larynx.

Laryngospasm. Spasmodic closure of the glottis.

Laryngostenosis. Stricture of the larynx.

Laryngotomy. Surgical incision of the larynx through the cricoid membrane.

Laryngotracheobronchitis. An acute infection of the respiratory tract in children.

Larynx. An air passage and the organ of voice, which extends from the pharynx at the root of the tongue to the trachea. Its average length is 44mm. in the adult male and 36mm. in the adult female.

Laser. [Light Amplification by the Stimulated Emission of Radiation.] A potent form of monochromatic visible radiation, capable of engendering intense heat, that is used in surgery: e.g. in the treatment of detached retina.

Lassitude. Weakness, exhaustion.

Latah. A psychoneurosis occurring among the people of the Malay peninsula, Java and the neighbouring islands, particularly young women, characterized by a very suggestible frame of mind, whereby the individual can easily be induced into a state in which she utters strange sounds and executes imitative movements.

Latent. Concealed. Dormant.

Lateral. External, as opposed to internal (medial).

Latex. A viscid milky juice contained in the tissues of certain plants. **Latex test,** a test used in the diagnosis of rheumatoid arthritis, based upon the reaction of polystrene latex particles with rheumatoid factor, the abnormal macroglobulin present in rheumatoid arthritis.

Lathyrism. A disease characterized by acute spastic paralysis, hyperaesthesia and urinary incontinence which occurs in those who eat the lathyrus pea.

Latissimus. Broadest.

Latrine. A privy.

Laudanum. Tincture of opium.

Laudexium methylsulphate. The B.P. Commission approved name for decamethylenedi-{2-[1-(3,4-dimethoxybenzyl)-1,2,3,4-tetrahydro-6,7-dimethoxy-2-methylisoquinolinium methylsulphate] } A neuromuscular blocking agent.

Laurolinium acetate. The B.P. Commission approved name for 4-amino-1-dodecylquinaldinium acetate. A surface active agent.

Lavage. Washing out of an organ, such as the stomach.

Lavender oil. B.P.C. 1968. A preparation used largely ,in perfumery, and sometimes to disguise disagreeable odours in ointments and other preparations. It is obtained from the fresh flowering tops of *Lavandula intermedia* or *L. angustifolia*.

Laxative. A mild aperient.

Layer. A sheet or covering of more or less uniform thickness. **Basal cell layer of skin,** the layer of columnar cells in the germinative zone of the epidermis. **Clear layer of the skin,** the layer of closely packed cells in the horny zone of the epidermis. **Cuticular layer of the tympanic membrane,** the outer layer of the tympanic membrane, derived from skin and consisting of stratified epithelium, which lines the external acoustic meatus. **Endosteal layer of the dura mater,** the outer layer of the cerebral dura mater. **Ependymal layer of the neural tube,** the inner layer of the primitive, embryonic spinal cord. **Follicular layer of the ovum,** the layer of cubical cells investing the ovum. **Ganglionic layer of the cerebrum,** the layer of the cerebrum that contains the pyramidal cells.

Ganglionic layer of the retina, counting from without inwards, the sixth layer of the retina proper, consisting of a single layer of large nerve cells. **Glomerular layer of olfactory bulb,** the layer in which fibres of the olfactory nerve interlace with the terminals of descending dendrites from the mitral cells. **Granular layer of the cerebellum,** the inner layer of the cerebellar cortex. **Granular layers of the cerebrum,** an outer and an inner layer of the cerebrum, each containing granular and pyramidal cells, and constituting, from the surface inwards, the second and fourth layers, respectively, of the cerebrum. **Granular layer of the skin,** the inner layer of the horny zone of the epidermis. **Henle's layer of hair,** a single layer of cubical cells in the inner root sheath of the hair. **Horny layer of the skin,** the outer layer of the horny zone of the epidermis. **Huxley's layer of hair,** the intermediate layers of horny, nucleated cells in the inner root sheath of the hair. **Infragranular layer of cerebrum,** the deep layer of pyramidal cells in the archipallium. **Meningeal layer of the dura mater,** the inner layer of the dura mater. **Molecular layer of the cerebellum,** the outer layer of the grey matter of the cerebellum. **Molecular layer of the cerebrum,** the outer layer of the cerebral cortex. **Molecular layer of the hippocampus,** the superficial layer of the hippocampus. **Molecular layer of the olfactory bulb,** the densely packed mitral cells of the olfactory bulb. **Molecular layer of the piriform area,** the superficial layer of the piriform area. **Nerve fibre layer of the olfactory bulb,** the myelinated axons of the olfactory cells. **Nerve fibre layer of the retina,** the innermost layer of the retina proper, formed by the axons of the cells of the ganglionic layer. **Neuroglial layer of the olfactory bulb,** the mass of neuroglia in the olfactory bulb. **Nuclear layers of the retina,** from without inwards, the second and fourth layers, respectively, of the retina proper. The *outer nuclear layer* contains the cell bodies of the rod ¦and cone neurones. The *inner nuclear layer* is made up of bipolar cells, horizontal cells, and amacrine cells. **Papillary layer of the corium,** the superficial layer of the corium. **Pigmented layer of the retina,** the outer layer of the retina. **Plexiform layer of the retina,** from without inwards the third and fifth layers of the retina proper. The *outer plexiform layer* contains the rod spherules and cone footplates and the peripheral processes of cells of the inner nuclear area. The *inner plexiform layer* contains the dendrites of the ganglion cells of the ganglionic layer. **Polymorphous layer of the cerebrum,** the innermost layer of the cerebral cortex. **Prickle cell layer of the skin,** the outer layer of the germinative zone of the epidermis. **Pyramidal layer of the cerebrum,** from the surface inwards the third layer of the cerebral cortex. **Reticular layer of the corium,** the deeper layer of the corium.

Leaching. The process of washing out the soluble contents of a mixture, leaving the insoluble contents behind.

Lead. An electrocardiographic record, varying according to which part of the body the current is led off from.

Lead. A metallic element. Symbol Pb (L *plumbum*). Atomic weight 207·19. Atomic number 82.

Lead acetate. B.P.C. 1968. $C_4H_6O_4Pb$, $3H_2O$. Used in the preparation of lead lotions for the treatment of sprains.

Lead monoxide. B.P.C. 1968. PbO. Used in the preparation of **strong lead subacetate solution,** B.P.C. 1968, and of diachylon plaster-masses.

Lecithin. One of a group of phosphatidylcholines, compounds in which the phosphoric acid group of phosphatic acid is bound to choline. It is particularly abundant in nerve tissue, semen, and the yolk of egg.

Lecithinase. An enzyme that catalyses the splitting of lecithin. **Lecithinase A,** an enzyme present in the venoms of many snakes and poisonous insects, which converts lecithin into lysolecithin, a haemolytic agent.

Lectin. A substance from plants that specifically agglutinates erythrocytes of certain blood groups.

Leech. A blood-sucking annelid, *Hirudo medicinalis*, at one time widely used for drawing blood for therapeutic purposes.

Leg. The lower extremity from the knee to the ankle.

Legume. The pod or seed of a leguminous plant such as the pea.

Leio- (Gk *leios:* smooth). Prefix meaning smooth.

Leiodermia. Abnormally smooth, glossy skin.

Leiomyoma. A benign tumour composed of whorls of smooth muscle fibres, interspersed with a variable amount of fibrous tissue.

Leiomyosarcoma. A sarcoma composed of poorly differentiated smooth muscle cells.

Leishman-Donovan bodies. Another name for *Leishmania donovani*, the causative organism of leishmaniasis, or kala-azar.

Leishmania. A genus of protozoa, named after Sir William Leishman, parasitic in man, dogs and certain wild animals. *Leishmania brasiliensis*, the cause of muco-cutaneous leishmaniasis. *L. donovani*, the cause of visceral leishmaniasis (kala-azar). *L. tropica*, the cause of cutaneous leishmaniasis.

Leishmaniasis. Infection by protozoa belonging to the genus Leishmania. **Cutaneous leishmaniasis,** lesions of the skin and subcutaneous tissues caused by *Leishmania tropica. Synonyms:* Baghdad boil; Delhi boil; oriental sore. **Muco-cutaneous leishmaniasis,** chronic ulceration of exposed parts of the body, with secondary ulceration in the mucosa of the mouth and respiratory tract, caused by *Leishmania brasiliensis. Synonyms:* Bay sore; chicleros; espundia; South American leishmaniasis; uta. **Visceral leishmaniasis,** infection with *Leishmania donovani,* and resulting in remittent fever, leucopenia, splenomegaly and hepatomegaly. *Synonyms:* kala-azar, dum-dum fever, black sickness.

Lemniscus. A ribbon or band. (*Plural:* lemnisci.) **Lateral lemniscus,** nerve fibres ascending from the cochlear nuclei to the inferior quadrigeminal body and the medial geniculate body. **Medial lemniscus,** nerve fibres ascending from the cuneate and gracile nuclei of the medulla to the thalamus. **Spinal lemniscus,** the direct, upward continuation of the lateral spinothalamic tract into the brain stem. **Trigeminal lemniscus,** the secondary neurones that arise in the sensory nuclei of the trigeminal nerve and end in the ventral nucleus of the thalamus.

Lemon oil. B.P.C. 1968. The oil expressed from the outer part of the fresh pericarp of the ripe, or nearly ripe, fruit of *Citrus limon.* Used as a flavouring and perfumery agent. **Terpeneless lemon oil,** B.P.C. 1968, a preparation of lemon oil concentrated by extraction of the terpenes, and used as a flavouring agent.

Lemon peel, dried. B.P. 1968. The dried outer part of the pericarp of the ripe, or nearly ripe, fruit of *Citrus limon.* Used as a flavouring agent and a bitter.

Lens. A piece of glass, quartz or some other transparent material, with spherical surfaces, used for the refraction of light. The transparent biconvex body situated immediately behind the iris and in front of the vitreous body. (*Plural:* lenses.) **Biconcave lens,** a lens bounded by two concave surfaces. **Biconvex lens,** a lens bounded by two convex surfaces. **Bifocal lens,** a spectacle lens made of two segments, the upper for distant, and the lower for near, vision. **Contact lens,** a lens made to fit in apposition with the cornea. **Cylindrical lens,** a lens in the form of a cylinder, used to correct astigmatism. **Iseikonic lens,** a lens used to correct anisometropia.

Lenti- (L *lens, lentis:* a lentil (lens)). Prefix indicating association with a lens.

Lenticonus. Abnormal curvature of the lens of the eye, usually posterior.

Lenticular. Lens-shaped, or lentil-shaped.

Lentiform. Lens-shaped.

Lentigo. A freckle. (*Plural:* lentigines.)

Leontiasis. Leonine facies.

Lepid-, Lepido- (Gk *lepis:* flake or scale). Prefixes indicating a scale, or scaly.

Lepidic. Relating to scales. Scaly.

Lepidoptera. The order of insects that includes butterflies and moths.

Lepra. Leprosy. **Lepra reaction,** an acute allergic reaction to *Mycobacterium leprae* or its products.

Leproma. The granulomatous nodule, or macule, of leprosy.

Lepromin. The antigen prepared from bacteriologically strongly positive lepromatous tissue or its extracts.

Leprosy. The disease resulting from infection with *Mycobacterium leprae,* which tends to run a long chronic course, and to involve primarily the peripheral nerves and the skin.

Lept-, Lepto- (Gk *leptos:* slender). Prefixes indicating slender, thin, or frail.

Leptocephalous. Having an abnormally small head.

Leptocyte. An unusually thin erythrocyte. Also known as a target cell.

Leptocytosis. The presence of leptocytes in the blood, as in thalassaemia.

Leptodactyly. Abnormal slenderness of the fingers.

Leptomeninges. The pia-arachnoid.

Leptomeningitis. Inflammation of the pia-arachnoid.

Leptophonia. Weakness of the voice.

Leptosoma. A person with a thin, slender body.

Leptospira. A genus of spirochaetal organisms. *Leptospira australis,* the causal agent of 'cane fever' in North Queensland. *Leptospira autumnalis,* the causal organism of akiyami, or harvest sickness, in Japan. *Leptospira bataviae,* the causal organism of leptospirosis of rice-field workers in Italy and S.E. Asia. *Leptospira canicola,* the causal organism of canicola fever in man and of a common infection in dogs. *Leptospira grippotyphosa,* the cause of 'swamp fever'. in Europe, Asia, Africa and U.S.A. *Leptospira hebdomadis,* the causal organism of 'seven-day fever' in the East. *Leptospira icterohaemorrhagica,* the causal organism of Weil's disease (haemorrhagic jaundice). *Leptospira pomona,* the causal organism of 'seven-day fever' in Queensland and of 'swineherd's disease' in Switzerland. *Leptospira pyrogenes,* the cause of a febrile illness, with or without jaundice, in field workers in Indonesia and the Far East. *Leptospira sejroe,* the cause of a relatively mild disease in parts of Europe. *Leptospira zanoni,* one of the causal agents of 'cane fever' in Queensland.

Leptospirosis. The disease, or group of diseases, caused by Leptospira.

Leptotene. The first stage of the prophase of the first meiotic division of the sex cells during maturation, in which the as yet unsplit chromosomes become prominent.

Leresis. The garrulousness of mental, often senile, decay.

Lesbian. A female homosexual.

Lesion. A circumscribed pathological change, such as a wound, or tumour.

Lethal. Deadly.

Lethargy. Mental torpor.

Lettuce. *Lactua sativa,* a widely used green vegetable which is a relatively rich source of vitamin A. The content of vitamin C is variable.

Leuc-, Leuco- (Gk *leukos:* white). Prefixes meaning white or colourless.

Leucine. One of the amino-acids essential for growth.

Leucoagglutinin. An antibody that agglutinates white blood cells.

Leucocidin. A toxin that destroys white blood cells.

Leucocyte. A white blood cell. There are normally 4000 to 11,000 per c. mm. in the circulating blood, divided into granular cells (or polymorphonuclears), lymphocytes, and monocytes.

Leucocytosis. Any increase in the total circulating leucocytes above 11,000 per c.mm.

Leucoderma. A condition characterized by white patches of skin. Vitiligo.

Leucodystrophy. Degeneration of the white matter of the brain.

Leuco-erythroblastic. Involving both leucocytes and erythrocytes. **Leuco-erythroblastic anaemia,** a condition induced by space-occupying lesions in the bone marrow, and characterized by an anaemia with many primitive red and white blood cells in the circulation.

Leuco-erythroblastosis. Leuco-erythro-blastic anaemia.

Leucolysin. A lysin which causes disintegration of white blood cells.

Leucoma. A white scar on the cornea.

Leucon. The leucopoietic tissue and all pertaining to its products.

Leuconychia. A patchy whiteness of the nails.

Leucopenia. A decrease of the total circulating leucocytes below 4000 per c.mm.

Leucopenic. Pertaining to leucopenia.

Leucopenin. A thermolabile factor produced during pyrexia which tends to cause leucopenia.

Leucophoresis. Depletion of the white blood cells in the circulating blood, by bleeding, removing the leucocytes, and then returning the rest of the blood to the circulation.

Leucoplakia. Chronic inflammation of the mucous membrane, particularly the mouth.

Leucopoiesis. The formation of leucocytes.

Leucorrhoea. A white, or whitish, discharge from the vagina.

Leucotaxine. A polypeptide released by injured cells at the site of inflammation which causes a local increase in capillary permeability and induces migration of leucocytes through the endothelial wall.

Leucotomy. The operation of cutting the white matter of the frontal lobe of the brain, with a view to alleviating certain otherwise incurable, tense, obsessional states.

Leucotrichia. Patchy whiteness of the hair associated with leucoderma when this occurs in hair-bearing parts of the body.

Leuk- (Gk *leukos:* white). Prefix meaning white or colourless.

Leukaemia. The condition characterized by abnormal proliferation of the leucopoietic tissues, usually resulting in the appearance of large numbers of leucocytes (many immature) in the circulating blood. **Acute leukaemia,** a progressive, fatal form of the disease, which may be of the lymphatic, mono-cytic, or myeloid form. Acute lymph-atic leukaemia is the common form in childhood. **Aleukaemic leukaemia,** a type of leukaemia in which there is leukaemic infiltration of many organs, but the total white cell count of the peripheral blood is within normal limits or even leucopenic. **Atypical leukaemia,** any form of leukaemia which presents in an atypical form: e.g. without any apparent abnormality in the peripheral blood. **Basophilic leukaemia,** a form of leukaemia characterized by a high preponder-ance of basophils in the peripheral blood. **Chronic leukaemia,** the more common form of leukaemia that runs a fairly chronic course. **Eosinophilic leukaemia,** a form of chronic leu-kaemia in which there is a high pre-ponderance of eosinophils in the peripheral blood. **Lymphatic leuk-aemia,** the form of leukaemia in which the lymphocytes are involved. *Acute lymphatic leukaemia,* the commonest form of acute leukaemia, with its highest incidence in the first five years of life. Lymphocytic cells constitute 90 per cent of the total white cells and are mainly lymphoblasts. *Chronic lymphhatic leukaemia,* the most common form of leukaemia, occurring in the 35- to 80-year age-group, with a peak in the 60's. There is generalized enlargement of the lymph glands, and the small lymphocyte constitutes 85 to 99 per cent of the white blood cells. **Monocytic leukaemia,** a form of leukaemia that affects all age-groups, runs a rapidly fatal course after an insidious onset, and with monocytes constituting 50 to 90 per cent of the white blood cells. **Myeloid leukaemia,** the form of leukaemia in which the myeloid series of white blood cells predominate. *Acute myeloid leuk-aemia,* a rapidly fatal form of leukaemia, most common in children and young adults, in which myelo-blasts constitute 90 per cent of the total circulating white blood cells. *Chronic myeloid leukaemia,* a chronic form of leukaemia, most common between the ages of 35 and 65, in which there are very high white blood cell counts, with a vast preponderance of neutrophils and myelocytes.

Leukanaemia. A condition in which the blood picture resembles both leukaemia and pernicious anaemia.

Levallorphan tartrate. B.P. 1968. $C_{23}H_{31}NO_7$. An antagonist of morphine, administered intravenously.

Levamisole. The B.P. Commission approved name for $(-)$-2,3,5,6-tetrahydro-6-phenylimidazo[2,1-b]thiazole. An anthelmintic.

Levamphetamine. The B.P. Commission approved name for a sympathomimetic agent.

Levator. That which raises or elevates. Applied to certain surgical instruments and to certain muscles, which subserve this function. (*Plural:* levatores.)

Levigation. Grinding to a fine powder.

Levitation. The illusion of floating or rising on air.

Levodopa. The B.P. Commission approved name for $(-)$-3-(3,4-dihydroxyphenyl)-L-alanine. An anti-parkinsonian drug.

Levomethorpan. The B.P. Commission approved name for a cough suppressant.

Levomoramide. The B.P. Commission approved name for a narcotic analgesic.

Levophenacylmorphan. The B.P. Commission approved name for a narcotic analgesic.

Levopropoxyphene. The B.P. Commission approved name for $(-)$-4-dimethylamino-3-methyl-1,2-diphenyl-2-propionyloxybutane (α-form). A cough suppressant.

Levorphanol tartrate. B.P. 1968. $C_{21}H_{29}NO_7$, $2H_2O$. An analgesic similar to morphine in its indications, contraindications, side-effects, and habit-forming propensities, but as effective orally as parenterally.

Libido. Sexual desire.

Lice. Plural of louse.

Lichen. A group of chronic skin diseases in which the eruption consists of an aggregation of similar papules, with no tendency to suppurate. **Lichen nitidus,** an uncommon eruption of light-brown papules on the penis, flexor aspects of forearms and wrists, ankles and feet, and abdomen. **Lichen planus,** an eruption of shiny, violaceous papules, predominantly on the buccal mucosa, front of the wrists, external genitalia, back, medial aspects of thighs, shins, calves and ankles. **Lichen sclerosus et atrophicus,** a condition of lichenoid papules that in due course atrophy or become sclerosed. **Lichen scrofulosorum,** an eruption of pink-coloured papules on the trunk of children, possibly an allergic reaction to tuberculosis. **Lichen simplex,** lichenification in areas of persistent irritation or itching. **Lichen spinulosus,** an eruption of widespread horny papules, particularly on the extensor aspects of the limbs and trunk. **Lichen urticatus,** a papular urticaria of childhood.

Lichenification. Thickening and hardening of the skin, with the formation of papules.

Lichenoid. Resembling lichen.

Lidoflazine. The B.P. Commission approved name for N-{4-[4, 4-di-(4-fluorophenyl)butyl]piperazin-1-ylacetyl}-2,6-xylidine. A cardiac stimulant.

Lien. The spleen.

Lien-, Lieno- (L *lien:* spleen). Prefixes indicating association with the spleen.

Lienculus. An accessory spleen.

Lienitis. Inflammation of the spleen.

Lienorenal. Pertaining to, or in relationship to, the spleen and the kidney.

Lienteric. Related to lientery. **Lienteric diarrhoea,** a mild form of diarrhoea in which the bowels move after every meal.

Lientery. A form of diarrhoea in which undigested food is passed in the stools.

Ligament. A band of tissue that connects bones, joints or viscera. **Accessory ligament,** a joint ligament that stands clear of the fibrous capsule. **Accessory ligaments of the lateral atlanto-axial joint,** ligaments that strengthen the posterior and medial parts of the fibrous capsules of the joint, and are attached below to the body of the axis near the base of the dens, and above to the lateral mass of the atlas. **Acromioclavicular ligament,** a quadrilateral band extending between the upper part of the acromial end of the clavicle and the adjoining part of the upper surface of the acromion. **Alar ligaments of the dens,** two strong rounded cords that arise one on each side of the upper part of the dens and are inserted into the medial sides of the condyles of the occipital bone. **Anococcygeal ligament,** a mass of fibrous and muscular tissue that separates the anal canal from the coccyx. **Anular ligament of the radius,** a strong band that encircles the head of the radius. **Anular ligament of the stapes,** a ring of elastic fibres that attaches the base of the stapes to the margin of the fenestra vestibuuli. **Apical ligament of the dens,** the ligament that extends from the tip of the process of the axis to the anterior margin of the foramen magnum. **Arcuate ligament, lateral,** a thickened band in the fascia covering the quadratus lumborum, attached medially to the front of the transverse process of the first lumbar vertebra and laterally to the lower margin of the twelfth rib. **Arcuate ligament, medial,** a tendinous arch in the fascia covering the upper part of the psoas major, continuous medially with the lateral tendinous margin of the corresponding crus and attached to the body of the first or second lumbar vertebra, and laterally fixed to the transverse process of the first lumbar vertebra. **Arcuate ligament, median,** an arch across the aorta formed by the medial tendinous margins of the crura of the diaphragm. **Ligamentum arteriosum,** the impervious cord, connecting the left pulmonary artery and the arch of the aorta, which replaces the ductus arteriosus after birth. **Bifurcated ligament,** a strong band attached behind to the anterior part of the upper surface of the calcaneus, and dividing anteriorly into the calcaneonavicular ligaments. **Broad ligaments of the uterus,** two ligaments that pass from the margins of the uterus to the lateral walls of the pelvis. **Calcaneocuboid ligament, dorsal,** a thickening of the fibrous capsule over the dorsal surface of the calcaneocuboid joint. **Calcaneocuboid ligament, medial,** an extension of the bifurcated ligament, attached in front to the dorsal part of the medial side of the cuboid bone. **Calcaneocuboid ligament, plantar,** a short wide band stretching from the anterior tubercle of the calcaneus to the plantar surface of the cuboid bone. **Calcaneofibular ligament,** a long, rounded cord running backwards and downwards from the apex of the fibular malleolus to a tubercle on the lateral surface of the calcaneus. **Calcaneonavicular ligament,** an extension of the bifurcated ligament, attached in front to the navicular bone. **Calcaneonavicular ligament, plantar,** a broad, thick band connecting the sustentaculum tali of the calcaneus with the navicular bone. **Capsular ligaments,** localized thickenings in the fibrous capsules of joints. **Caroticoclinoid ligament,** a ligament connecting the anterior to the middle clinoid process of the sphenoid bone. **Carpometacarpal ligaments,** the metacarpal bone of the thumb is connected to the trapezium by *lateral, anterior* and *dorsal* ligaments as well as the capsular ligament. The second, third, fourth, and fifth metacarpal bones are connected to the carpal bones by *dorsal, palmar,* and *interosseous* ligaments. **Cervical ligament of the talus,** a ligament that stretches from the upper surface of the calcaneus to the talus. **Cervical ligament of the uterus,** a band on each side of the cervix uteri. It is attached to the side of the cervix and the vault and lateral fornix of the vagina. **Check ligaments of the eyeball,** strong, triangular extensions of the sheaths of the recti medialis et lateralis, attached to the lacrimal and zygomatic bones, respectively. **Collateral ligaments: Fibular collateral ligament,** a strong, round cord extending from the lateral epicondyle of the femur to the head of the fibula. **Metacarpophalangeal collateral ligaments,** strong rounded cords on the sides of the joints, extending from the head of the metacarpal bone to the base of the phalanx. **Metatarsophalangeal collateral ligaments,** strong, rounded cords on the sides of the joints, extending from the side of the head of the metatarsal bone to the base of the phalanx. **Radial collateral ligament of the elbow joint,** a ligament stretching from the lateral epicondyle of the humerus to the anular ligament. **Radial collateral ligament of the wrist,** a ligament that stretches from the tip of the styloid process of the radius to the scaphoid bone. **Tibial collateral ligament,** a broad, flat band attached above to the medial epicondyle of the femur and below to the medial condyle of the tibia. **Ulnar collateral ligament of the elbow joint,** a thick triangular band attached above to the medial epicondyle of the humerus and below to the coronoid process and olecranon. **Ulnar collateral ligament of the wrist joint,** a ligament extending from the styloid process of the ulna above to the triquetral and pisiform bones below. **Conoid ligament,** part of the coracoclavicular ligament. A dense band stretching from the coracoid process to the conoid process on the clavicle. **Coracoacromial ligament,** a strong, triangular band, extending between the coracoid process and the acromion. **Coraco-**

clavicular ligament, the ligament connecting the clavicle with the coracoid process of the scapula. It consists of two parts: *conoid* and *trapezoid*. Coracohumeral ligament, a broad band that extends from the root of the coracoid process to the greater tubercle of the humerus. Coronary ligament of the knee, the part of the fibrous capsule of the knee joint that connects the periphery of each meniscus to the adjacent part of the head of the tibia. Coronary ligament of the liver, the reflection of the peritoneum from the diaphragm to the superior and posterior surfaces of the right lobe. Costoclavicular ligament, the ligament extending from the upper surface of the first rib to the under-surface of the clavicle. Costocoracoid ligament, the thickened portion of the clavipectoral fascia, extending from the first rib to the coracoid process. Costotransverse ligament, the ligament connecting the neck of the rib with the transverse process of the adjacent vertebra. Costoxiphoid ligaments, the ligaments that connect the seventh costal cartilage to the xiphoid process. Cricoarytenoid ligament, posterior, the ligament that connects the cricoid cartilage with the base of the arytenoid cartilage. Cricothyroid ligament, the ligament, consisting of an anterior and a lateral part, that connects the cricoid and thyroid cartilages. The upper edge of the lateral part between its two attachments, is free and thickened slightly to form the *vocal ligament*. Cricotracheal ligament, the ligament that unites the lower border of the cricoid cartilage with the first ring of the trachea. Cruciate ligaments, an anterior and posterior, the *anterior* extending from the anterior intercondylar area of the tibia to the medial surface of the lateral condyle of the femur, and the *posterior* extending from the posterior intercondylar area of the tibia to the lateral surface of the medial condyle of the femur, Cuboideonavicular ligaments, a dorsal, a *plantar*, and an *interosseous* ligament, that connect the cuboid and navicular bones. Cuneocuboid ligaments, a *dorsal*, a *plantar*, and an *interousseous* ligament, that connect the cuneiform and cuboid bones. Cuneometatarsal ligaments, interosseous, three ligaments that connect the cuneiform with the metatarsal bones. Cuneonavicular ligaments, *dorsal* and *plantar* ligaments

that connect the navicular bone to each of the cuneiform bones. Cystoduodenal ligament, a peritoneal fold that occasionally passes from the gallbladder to the duodenum. Deltoid ligament, a strong triangular band that extends from the medial malleolus above to the talus, and the navicular bone below. Denticulatum ligament, a narrow, fibrous sheet situated on each side of the spinal cord between the ventral and dorsal nerve roots. Falciform ligament, a sickle-shaped fold, consisting of two layers of peritoneum, that connects the liver to the diaphragm and the anterior abdominal wall. Ligamenta flava, the ligaments that connect the laminae of adjacent vertebrae. Fundiform ligament, one of the two ligaments that support the weight of the body of the penis. Gastrophrenic ligament, a short peritoneal fold that passes from the diaphragm to the posterior aspect of the fundus of the stomach. Gastrosplenic ligament, a fold of peritoneum formed by the meeting of the walls of the greater sac and omental bursa between the spleen and stomach. Glenohumeral ligaments, three supplemental bands in the fibrous capsule of the shoulder joint, all attached at their scapular end to the medial margin of the glenoid cavity, whilst the other ends are attached to the lesser tubercle or anatomical neck of the humerus. Ligament of the head of the femur, a triangular band, with its apex attached to the head of the femur and its base to the acetabular notch. Hepatocolic ligament, a peritoneal fold which stretches from the under-surface of the liver to the right colic flexure. Hepatogastric ligament, the portion of the lesser omentum extending between the stomach and liver. Hepatorenal ligament, a fold of peritoneum extending from the inferior surface of the liver to the front of the right kidney. Hyoepiglottis ligament, an elastic ligament extending from the epiglottis to the hyoid bone. Iliofemoral ligament, a triangular-shaped ligament with its apex attached to the anterior inferior iliac spine, and its base attached to the trochanteric line of the femur. Iliolumbar ligament, a ligament that extends from the transverse process of the fifth lumbar vertebra to the pelvis. Inguinal ligament, the lower border of the aponeurosis of the external oblique, which stretches from the anterior superior iliac spine to the pubic tubercle. **Intercarpal ligaments,** *dorsal, palmar,* and *collateral* ligaments that connect the carpal bones. **Interchondral ligaments,** the ligaments that pass from one costal cartilage to another between the sixth and ninth cartilages. **Interclavicular ligament,** a ligament that passes from the sternal end of one clavicle to that of the other. **Interclinoid ligament,** the ligament joining the anterior to the posterior clinoid process of the sphenoid bone. **Intercornual ligaments,** ligaments that connect the cornua of the sacrum and coccyx on each side. **Intercuneiform ligaments,** *dorsal, plantar,* and *interosseous* ligaments that connect the cuneiform bones. **Intermetacarpal ligaments,** *dorsal, palmar* and *interosseous,* that connect the metacarpal bones. **Intermetatarsal ligaments,** *dorsal, plantar,* and *interosseous* ligaments that connect the metatarsal bones. **Interspinous ligaments,** thin membranous ligaments that connect adjoining spines of the vertebrae, their attachments extending from the root to the apex of each process. **Intertransverse ligaments,** ligaments between the transverse processes of the vertebrae. **Ischiofemoral ligament,** the ligament that extends from the ischium to the greater trochanter of the femur. **Lacunar ligament,** that portion of the aponeurosis of the external oblique that passes from the medial part of the inguinal ligament to the medial end of the pecten pubis. **Lateral true ligament of the bladder,** the condensation of fibro-areolar tissue that connects each side of the bladder to the tendinous arch of the pelvic fascia. **Lateral ligament of the rectum,** the fascia around the middle rectal vessels that passes from the posterolateral wall of the lesser pelvis to the rectum on each side. **Lateral ligament of the thyroid gland,** a conspicuous thickening of the pretracheal fascia that attaches the gland to the trachea and the lower part of the cricoid cartilage. **Lienorenal ligament,** the two-layered fold of peritoneum, extending from the front of the left kidney to the hilus of the spleen, which encloses the splenic vessels and the tail of the pancreas. **Longitudinal ligament, anterior,** a strong band of fibres that extends along the anterior surfaces of the vertebrae. **Longitudinal ligament, posterior,** a ligament lying within the vertebral canal on the

posterior surface of the bodies of the vertebrae and extending from the axis to the sacrum. **Lumbocostal ligament,** the band of fibres connecting the neck of the twelfth rib to the base of the first lumbar vertebra. **Nuchal ligament (ligamentum nuchae),** a fibro-elastic membrane which extends from the external protuberance and external occipital crest to the spine of the seventh cervical vertebra. **Palpebral ligament, lateral,** the band that attaches the lateral ends of the tarsi to the zygomatic bone. **Palpebral ligament, medial,** the strong tendinous band that connects the medial ends of the tarsi to the lacrimal crest and the frontal process of the maxilla. **Patellar ligament (ligamentum patellae),** the central portion of the common tendon of the quadriceps femoris, which is continued from the patella to the tuberosity of the tibia. **Pectinate ligament of the iris,** the ligament that connects the iris with the posterior elastic lamina of the cornea. **Petrosphenoidal ligament,** a fibrous band that connects the lateral margin of the dorsum sellae to the petrous part of the temporal bone. **Phrenicocolic ligament,** a peritoneal fold that attaches the left colic flexure to the diaphragm. **Pisohamate ligament,** the ligament that connects the pisiform bone to the hook of the hamate bone. **Pisometacarpal ligament,** the ligament that connects the pisiform bone to the base of the fifth metacarpal bone. **Plantar ligament, long,** a ligament attached posteriorly to the plantar surface of the calcaneus, and anteriorly to the cuboid bone. **Popliteal ligament, arcuate,** a Y-shaped system of fibres, with the stem attached to the head of the fibula, the posterior limb attached to the tibia, and the anterior limb attached to the lateral epicondyle of the femur. **Popliteal ligament, oblique,** a broad flat band derived from the tendon of the semimembranosus close to its insertion into the tibia, and passing upward to be inserted into the lateral condyle of the femur. **Pterygospinous ligament,** the ligament that stretches between the spine of the sphenoid bone and the posterior border of the lateral pterygoid plate. **Pubic ligament, arcuate,** a thick, triangular arch of fibres that connects the lower borders of the symphyseal surfaces of the two pubic bones, and forms the upper boundary of the pubic arch. **Pubic ligament,**

superior, the ligament that connects the pubic bones superiorly. **Pubofemoral ligament,** a triangular ligament with its base on the hip bone, attached to the iliopectineal eminence, the superior ramus of the os pubis, the obturator crest and obturator membrane, and blending below with the medial band of the iliofemoral ligament. **Puboprostatic ligament, lateral,** the ligament that extends from the anterior end of the tendinous arch of the pelvic fascia to blend with the upper part of the sheath of the prostate. **Puboprostatic ligament, medial,** the ligament that extends from the back of the pubic bone to the sheath of the prostate, and forms the floor of the retropubic space. **Pubovesical ligaments,** the equivalent in women of the puboprostatic ligaments in men. **Pulmonary ligament,** the double layer of mediastinal pleura that extends from the lateral edge of the oesophagus to the mediastinal surface of the lung. **Radiate carpal ligament,** the fibres of the palmar ligaments of the mid-carpal joints that radiate from the head of the capitate bone to the surrounding bones. **Radiate ligaments of the ribs,** the ligaments that connect the head of each rib with the sides of the bodies of the vertebrae and the intervertebral disc between them. **Radiate sternocostal ligaments,** broad, thin membranous bands that radiate from the sternal ends of the cartilages of the true ribs to the sternum. **Radiocarpal ligament, dorsal,** the ligament that extends from the distal end of the radius to the scaphoid, lunate and triquetral bones. **Radiocarpal ligaments, palmar,** a broad, membranous band that extends from the lower end of the radius and its styloid process to the scaphoid, lunate and triquetral bones. **Round ligaments of the uterus,** two narrow flat bands, situated between the layers of the broad ligament in front of and below the uterine tubes, which start at the lateral angle of the uterus, pass through the deep inguinal ring, down the inguinal canal to merge with the labium majus. **Sacrococcygeal ligaments,** *deep dorsal, lateral, superficial dorsal,* and *ventral,* ligaments that unite the sacrum and coccyx. **Sacroiliac ligaments,** *dorsal, interosseous,* and *ventral,* ligaments that unite the sacrum and ilium. **Sacrospinous ligament,** the thin triangular ligament, with its apex attached to the spine of

the ischium, and its base attached to the lateral margins of the sacrum and coccyx. **Sacrotuberous ligament,** a ligament attached by a broad base to the posterior iliac spines, the lower transverse tubercles of the sacrum, and the lateral margin of the lower part of the sacrum and upper part of coccyx, and extending to the ischial tuberosity and ramus of the ischium. **Sphenomandibular ligament,** a flat, thin band attached above to the spine of the sphenoid bone and below to the lingula of the mandibular foramen. **Spiral ligament of the cochlea,** a thickening of the endosteum of the outer wall of the cochlea, to which is attached the outer edge of the basilar membrane. **Sternoclavicular ligament, anterior,** a broad band attached above to the sternal end of the clavicle and below to the manubrium sterni. **Sternoclavicular ligament, posterior,** a similar, but weaker, band, covering the back of the joint. **Sternocostal ligaments, radiate,** broad, thin membranous bands radiating from the front and back of the sternal ends of the cartilages of the true ribs to the anterior and posterior surfaces of the sternum. **Sternopericardial ligaments, inferior and superior,** ligaments that attach the fibrous pericardium to the posterior surface of the sternum. **Stylohyoid ligament,** a fibrous cord that extends from the tip of the styloid process of the temporal bone to the lesser cornu of the hyoid bone. **Stylomandibular ligament,** a specialized band of the deep cervical fascia that stretches from the styloid process to the angle and posterior border of the ramus of the mandible. **Suprascapular ligament,** a thin, flat fasciculus that extends from the base of the coracoid process to the medial end of the scapular notch and thereby converts the scapular notch into a foramen. **Supraspinous ligament,** a strong fibrous cord that connects together the apexes of the spines from the seventh cervical vertebra to the sacrum. **Suspensory ligaments of the breast,** fibrous processes which pass forwards from the fascia covering the breast to the skin and nipples. **Suspensory ligament of the clitoris,** a ligament comparable to that of the suspensory ligament of the penis. **Suspensory ligament of the eye,** a thickening of the lower part of the fascial sheath of the eyeball, slung below the eyeball like a hammock. **Suspensory ligament of the lens,** a system of zonular fibres which pass from the ciliary body to the capsule of the lens and holds the lens in place. **Suspensory ligament of the ovary,** the portion of the broad ligament that extends from the infundibulum of the uterine tube and the upper pole of the ovary to the lateral wall of the lesser pelvis. **Suspensory ligament of the penis,** a triangular-shaped ligament attached above to the sympysis pubis, and blending below with the fascia penis. **Sutural ligament,** the thin layer of fibrous tissue that separates the margins of a suture. **Talocalcanean ligaments,** *interosseous, lateral,* and *medial,* that connect the talus and calcaneus. **Talofibular ligaments,** *anterior* and *posterior,* the two ligaments that connect the talus and fibula. **Talonavicular ligament,** a broad thin band connecting the neck of the talus to the dorsal surface of the navicular bone. **Temporomandibular ligament,** the ligament attached above to the root of the zygoma, and below to the neck of the mandible. **Teres ligament (ligamentum teres),** the obliterated remains of the left umbilical vein in the foetus, which begins at the umbilicus, ascends in the falciform ligament, traverses the fissure, and ends by joining the left branch of the portal vein opposite the attachment of the ligamentum venosum. **Thyroepiglottic ligament,** the elastic ligament that attaches the epiglottis to the thyroid cartilage. **Thyrohyoid ligaments,** *lateral,* round elastic cords that form the posterior borders of the thyrohyoid membrane, and connect the tips of the superior horns of the thyroid cartilage to the greater horns of the hyoid bone. **Thyrohyoid ligament, medial,** the middle, thicker part of the thyrohyoid membrane. **Tibiofibular ligaments,** *anterior, inferior, interosseous,* and *posterior,* the ligaments that connect the lower ends of the tibula and fibula, participating in the tibiofibular syndesmosis. The tibiofibular articulation between the lateral condyle of the tibia and the head of the fibula includes an anterior and a posterior ligament. **Transverse colli ligament,** a ligament that extends from the side of the cervix uteri to the vault and lateral fornix of the vagina. **Transverse ligament of the acetabulum,** strong flattened fibres that cross the acetabular notch and convert it into a foramen. **Transverse ligament of the atlas,** a thick strong band that arches across the ring of the atlas and retains the dens in contact with the anterior arch. **Deep transverse metacarpal ligaments,** three short, wide, flattened bands that connect the palmar ligaments of the second, third, fourth, and fifth metacarpophalangeal joints to one another. **Deep transverse metatarsal ligaments,** four short, wide, flattened bands that connect the palmar ligaments of adjoining metatarsophalangeal joints to one another. **Transverse humeral ligament,** a broad band passing from the lesser to the greater tubercle of the humerus. **Transverse ligament of the knee,** the ligament that connects the anterior convex margin of the lateral to the anterior end of the medial meniscus. **Superficial transverse metacarpal ligament,** a thin band stretched across the roots of the fingers and attached to the skin of the clefts and medially to the fifth metacarpal bone. **Triangular ligaments of the liver,** the *left* passes from the upper surface of the left lobe to the under-surface of the diaphragm, while the *right* connects the lateral part of the posterior aspect of the right lobe to the diaphragm. **Uterosacral ligaments,** ligaments that extend from the cervix uteri to the front of the sacrum. **Ligament of the left vena cava,** a fibrous strand, the remnant of the obliterated left common cardinal vein, which extends from the left superior intercostal vein to the back of the left atrium. **Ligamentum venosum,** the fibrous remnant of the ductus venosus, which extends from the posterior border of the left branch of the portal vein to the left hepatic vein near its point of entry into the inferior vena cava. **Vertebropelvic ligaments,** the *iliolumbar, sacrospinous,* and *sacrotuberous* ligaments. **Vestibular ligament of the larynx,** a narrow fibrous band fixed in front to the angle of the thyroid cartilage, and behind to the arytenoid cartilage. **Vocal ligament,** the free, thickened, upper edge of the lateral part of the cricothyroid ligament.

Ligase. One of a group of enzymes that catalyse the linkage of two molecules at the expense of the breakdown of a third.

Ligature. A cord, thread, or the like, for tying round a blood vessel or the like.

Light. The electromagnetic radiations that give rise to the sensation of vision when they impinge on the retina.

Lightening. The sensation of decreased abdominal pressure produced by the sinking of the gravid uterus into the pelvis in the last three weeks of pregnancy.

Ligneous. Woody. Having a wooden feeling.

Lignocaine hydrochloride. B.P. 1968. $C_{14}H_{23}ClN_2O,H_2O$. A local anaesthetic. **Lignocaine and adrenaline injection,** B.P. 1968, a sterile solution containing 2 grammes of lignocaine hydrochloride and 1ml. of adrenaline solution per 100ml.

Limb. An arm or leg

Limbus. A border or fringe. (*Plural:* limbi.) **Limbus fossae ovalis,** the prominent margin of the fossa ovalis. **Limbus laminae spiralis,** the periosteal thickening on the upper part of the osseous spiral lamina contained within the duct of the cochlea. **Limbus sclerae,** the line of union between the cornea and sclera.

Limen. Threshold. (*Plural:* limina.) **Limen insulae,** the medial part of the apex of the insula. **Limen nasi,** the curved elevation in the vestibule of the nose along which the skin of the vestibule is continuous with the mucous membrane of the nasal cavity.

Liminal. Pertaining to a threshold.

Limosis. Abnormal hunger.

Lincomycin hydrochloride. B.P. Addendum 1971. An antibiotic produced by *Streptomyces lincolnensis,* which is active against gram-positive microorganisms.

Linctus. A viscous liquid preparation, usually containing sucrose and medicinal substances, and possessing demulcent, expectorant, or sedative properties. There are thirteen linctuses in the *British Pharmaceutical Codex* 1968: codeine linctus; codeine linctus paediatric; diamorphine linctus; ipecacuanha and squill linctus, paediatric; methadone linctus; noscapine linctus; pholcodine linctus; pholcodine linctus, strong; simple linctus; simple linctus, paediatric; squill linctus, opiate (Gee's linctus); squill linctus, opiate, paediatric; tolu linctus, compound, paediatric.

Line. A streak or ridge. The connexion between two points. **Linea alba,** a tendinous raphe that extends from the xiphoid process to the symphysis pubis. **Linea aspera,** the broad rough ridge that forms the posterior border of the lateral surface of the middle third of the shaft of the femur. **Cement line,** the strongly basophilic

line that, in adult bone, demarcates each Haversian and most interstitial systems from neighbouring systems. **Cleavage lines,** the directions taken by the parallel bundles of connective tissue bands in the reticular layer of the corium. **Contour lines,** lines in the dentine which run parallel to the walls of the pulp cavity, and correspond to rest periods in the formation of the dentine. **Epiphysial line,** the peripheral margin of the epiphysial cartilage. **Flexure lines,** permanent creases in the skin, particularly evident on the palm of the hand and the flexor surfaces of the digits. **Gluteal lines,** three roughened ridges on the gluteal surface of the ilium. **Hensen's line,** the clear transverse line of low refractive index seen in the centre of the highly refractive A bands of skeletal muscle. **Intercondylar line,** the posterior border of the intercondylar fossa of the femur. **Intertrochanteric line,** the junction of the anterior surface of the neck with the shaft of the femur. **Mylohyoid line,** the oblique ridge that divides the internal surface of the mandible into two areas, running from behind the third molar tooth to the symphysis menti. **Nelaton's line,** the line joining the anterior superior iliac spine and the most prominent part of the ischial tuberosity. **Nuchal line, highest,** the higher of the two curved lines running laterally from the external occipital protuberance, and to which the galea aponeurotica is attached. **Nuchal line, inferior,** a line running laterally in the occipital bone, midway between the external occipital protuberance and the back of the foramen magnum. **Nuchal line, superior,** the lower of the two curved lines running laterally from the external occipital protuberance. **Oblique line of the mandible,** a faint ridge that runs upwards and backwards from the mental tubercle to the anterior border of the ramus. **Oblique line, anterior, of the radius,** the intermediate part of the anterior border of the radius. **Oblique line of the thyroid cartilage,** a line on the outer surface of each lamina that gives insertion to the sternothyroid muscle, and origin to the thyrohyoid muscle and the inferior constrictor of the pharynx. **Pectinate line,** the line along which the anal valves are situated. **Linea semilunaris,** the curved groove extending from the tip of the ninth costal cartilage to the pubic tubercle, and marking the lateral border of the rectus abdominis. **Soleal line**, a roughened ridge on the posterior surface of the tibia. **Spiral line of the femur**, a narrow, roughened line that bounds the posterior surface of the femur on the medial side. **Linea splendens**, a longitudinal fibrous band extending anteriorly along the median plane of the spinal pia mater. **Supracondylar lines of the femur, lateral and medial**, the two lines that bound the posterior surface of the lower third of the femur. **Sutural lines**, faint lines that radiate from the poles to the equator of the lens. **Temporal line**, a ridge which arches upwards and backwards from the zygomatic process of the frontal bone across the coronal suture to the parietal bone. **Trapezoid line**, a narrow roughened strip that runs from the conoid tubercle to the acromial end of the clavicle. **Vertical line**, a faint line on the posterior surface of the tibia. **White line**, a narrow wavy zone situated at the level of the interval between the subcutaneous part of the external sphincter and lower part of the internal sphincter of the anus. **Z line**, a line of high refractive index forming one of the transverse striations in the muscle fibril. The region between one Z line and the next is known as a sarcomere.

Linea. Line. (*Plural:* lineae.)

Lingua. Tongue. (*Plural:* linguae.) **Lingua geographica,** an idiopathic, benign form of glossitis, in which the denuded red areas of the tongue change in distribution every day. **Lingua nigra,** a blackening of the tongue. **Lingua plicata,** also known as *scrotal tongue*, a congenital condition characterized by deep sulci in the tongue.

Lingual. Pertaining to the tongue.

Linguatula. A genus of Pentastomida which occurs in the nasal cavity of carnivores and may infest man through swallowing of the eggs which develop in the liver.

Lingula. A tongue-shaped process. (*Plural:* lingulae.) **Lingula of the cerebellum,** a lamella on the superior surface of the vermis that is continuous with the superior medullary velum. **Lingula of the lung,** a small projection sometimes present at the lower part of the cardiac notch on the left lung. **Lingula of the mandible,** a thin triangular process on the medial side of the ramus of the mandible. **Lingula of the sphenoid bone,** a sharp margin on the body of the sphenoid bone.

Liniment. A liquid, or semi-liquid, preparation intended for external application. It is made with a basis of oil, alcohol, or soap solution, and may contain substances possessing analgesic, rubefacient, soothing, or stimulating properties. There are two in the *British Pharmacopoeia* 1968: camphor liniment and turpentine liniment; and seven in the *British Pharmaceutical Codex* 1968: aconite liniment; aconite, belladonna and chloroform liniment (A.B.C. Liniment); belladonna liniment; camphor liniment, ammoniated; methylsalicylate liniment; soap liniment; white liniment.

Linin. The achromatic netlike threads in the nucleus of a cell.

Linoleic acid. One of the unsaturated fatty acids referred to as essential fatty acids as they are essential for the normal growth of rats.

Linolenic acid. One of the unsaturated fatty acids referred to as essential fatty acids as they are essential for the normal growth of rats.

Linseed. The dried ripe seed of *Linum usitatissimum.*

Lint. Absorbent material used in surgical dressings. **Absorbent lint, B.P.C.** 1968, also known as lint; cotton lint; plain lint; white lint; absorbent cotton lint. Cotton cloth of plain weave, on one side of which a nap has been raised from the warp yarns. **Euflavine lint, B.P.C.** 1968, absorbent lint impregnated with euflavine.

Liothyronine sodium. B.P. 1968. $C_{15}H_{11}I_3NNaO_4$. An active principle of the thyroid gland, used in the treatment of hypothyroidism.

Lip. One of the two fleshy folds bounding the mouth. A lip-like structure bounding a cavity or groove. **Cleft lip,** harelip.

Lip-, Lipo- (Gk *lipos:* fat). Prefixes indicating association with fat.

Lipaemia. Excessive amounts of fat in the blood.

Lipase. The fat-splitting enzyme found predominantly in the pancreatic and intestinal secretions.

Lipid. One of a heterogeneous group of substances that share the property of being relatively insoluble in water and readily soluble in organic solvents such as ether, chloroform and benzene.

Lipidosis. A disorder of lipid storage. (*Plural:* lipidoses.)

Lipochondrodystrophy. An inherited disorder characterized by skeletal deformity, corneal opacity, hepatomegaly, splenomegaly, deafness, heart disease, and mental defect.

Lipochrome. One of a series of yellow pigments, soluble in fat and derived from ingested vegetables. They are responsible for the yellow colour of atheromatous plaques, fat deposits and the corpora lutea.

Lipodystrophia progressiva. A condition characterized by loss of subcutaneous fat in the upper part of the body.

Lipodystrophy. A disturbance of fat metabolism. **Intestinal dystrophy,** a disease characterized by fatty diarrhoea, multiple arthritis, loss of weight and anaemia.

Lipofucsin. One of a series of brown pigments, derived from lipids by oxidation, and present in old age and atrophic conditions.

Lipogranulomatosis. A rare condition caused by abnormal metabolism of lipids, and resulting in lipid deposits in the connective tissue and mucous membrane.

Lipoic acid. A growth factor for certain protozoa and micro-organisms, which is usually classified among the vitamins of the B group.

Lipoid. Resembling lipids or fats.

Lipolysis. The splitting or disintegration of fat.

Lipolytic. Pertaining to, or causing, lipolysis.

Lipoma. A benign tumour composed of adult adipose tissue.

Lipomatosis. An overgrowth of fatty tissue.

Lipophagic. Fat consuming. Lipolytic.

Lipopigment. A pigment that is related to fat.

Lipopolysaccharide. A toxic complex of lipid and carbohydrate in the walls of gram-negative bacteria, which possesses the antigenic specificity and toxicity of bacterial 'O' antigens.

Lipoprotein. A protein conjugated with a lipid.

Lipotropic. Increasing the metabolism of fat.

Lipping. The overgrowth of bone round a joint affected by osteoarthrosis, and visible in the X-ray film.

Lippitude, Lippitudo. Chronic blepharitis resulting in the condition known as 'blear-eyed'.

Lipsotrichia. Falling out of the hair.

Lipuria. The presence of fat in the urine.

Liquor. A solution. **Liquor amnii,** the fluid that occupies the amniotic cavity.

Liquor folliculi, the fluid that occupies the ovarian follicle.

Liquorice. B.P. 1968. The dried peeled or unpeeled root and stolon of *Glycyrrhiza glabra* and other species of Glycyrrhiza. It is a demulcent and a mild expectorant. It is also used as a flavouring agent and as an absorbent pill excipient.

Listeria. A genus of the family of Corynebacteriaceae. **Listeria monocytogenes,** a member of the genus that has been responsible for cases of meningo-encephalitis in man.

Lith-, Litho- (Gk *lithos:* stone). Prefixes indicating association with a stone or calculus.

Lithaemia. Excess of uric acid in the blood.

Lithagogue. Any agent that expels calculi from the body.

Litharge. Lead monoxide.

Lithiasis. The formation of calculi.

Lithium. An alkali metal element. Symbol Li. Atomic weight 6·939. Atomic number 3.

Lithium carbonate. B.P. Addendum, 1969. Li_2CO_3. Used in the prophylaxis and treatment of manic-depressive disorders. **Slow lithium carbonate tablets,** B.P. Addendum 1971, tablets so formulated as to release the medicament over a period of several hours.

Lithocholic acid. One of the steroid acids in bile.

Litholapaxy. The procedure of crushing a stone in the bladder preparatory to its removal in fragments.

Lithopaedion. A calcified dead foetus.

Lithotomy. Incision of the bladder for the removal of stone.

Lithotrite. An instrument for crushing a stone in the bladder.

Lithotrity. The operation of crushing a stone in the bladder.

Lithuresis. The passage of gravel in the urine.

Lithuria. Excess of uric acid or urates in the urine.

Litmus. A blue pigment derived from *Roccella tinctoria* or other species of lichens, which is reddened by acids and turned blue again by alkalis.

Litre. The volume occupied at its temperature of maximum density by a quantity of water having a mass of 1 kilogram. It is equivalent to 1000 millilitres, or 1·7598 pints. (*Abbreviation:* l.)

Littritis. Inflammation of the urethral glands.

Livedo. Bluish mottling of the skin.

Livedo reticularis, a bluish-red mottling of the skin, usually on the legs, seen particularly in children and adolescents, and most noticeable when the skin is cold.

Liver. The largest gland in the body, situated in the upper part of the abdomen, and weighing 1·4 to 1·6kg. in the male and 1·2 to 1·4kg. in the female. Its multitudinous functions include the formation of bile, a major role in the metabolism of carbohydrate, fat and protein, erythrocyte formation, the synthesis of the plasma proteins, and the processes of detoxification.

Liver fluke. *Fasicola hepatica.*

Livid. Congested and discoloured.

Lixiviation. Leaching.

Loa. A genus of filarial worms. **Loa loa,** the eyeworm. A threadlike worm (male 30 to 35mm. long; female 50 to 70mm. long); endemic in West Africa. It is transmitted by the fly, Chrysops.

Lobe. A subdivision of an organ. **Lobes of the breast,** some fifteen to twenty lobes composed of lobules. **Caudate lobe,** part of the right lobe of the liver, on the posterior surface and bounded by the tissue for the ligamentum venosum, the porta hepatis, and the inferior vena cava. **Cerebellar lobes,** an anterior, middle, and flocculonodular lobe. The *anterior lobe* comprises the lingula, central lobule, culmen, alae of the central lobules and quadrangular lobules. The *middle lobe* comprises the declive, folium vermis, tuber vermis, pyramid, uvula, lobulus simplex, biventral lobules, semilunar lobules, and tonsils. *Flocculonodular lobe,* one of the two fundamental parts into which the cerebellum is divided, consists of both flocculi, their peduncles and the |nodule. **Frontal lobe,** the anterior part of the cerebral hemisphere. **Lobes of the hypophysis cerebri,** an anterior lobe (or adenohypophysis) and a posterior lobe. **Lobes of the liver,** a left, a right, a quadrate, and a caudate lobe. **Lobes of the lungs,** the left lung has a superior and an inferior lobe; the right lung has a superior, a middle, and an inferior lobe. **Occipital lobe,** the posterior part of the cerebral hemisphere, which contains the visuosensory and visuo-psychic areas. **Parietal lobe,** that part of the cerebral hemisphere bounded in front by the central sulcus and behind by the line joining the pre-occipital notch to the superomedial margin at the point where it is cut by the parieto-occipital sulcus. **Lobes of the prostate,** a median, a left and a right lobe. **Quadrate lobe,** one of the lobes of the liver, placed on the inferior surface. **Riedel's lobe,** a broad tongue-like process of the right lobe of the liver that sometimes projects downwards to the right of the gall-bladder. **Temporal lobe,** the lobe that lies below the lateral sulcus of the cerebral hemisphere, and contains the auditory area. **Lobes of the thymus,** two unequally sized pyramidal lobes. **Lobes of the thyroid gland,** a left, and a right lobe, and sometimes a pyramidal lobe.

Lobectomy. Surgical excision of the lobe of an organ, such as the lung.

Lobelia. B.P.C. 1968. The dried aerial parts of *Lobelia inflata.* It contains 0·25 to 0·4 per cent of alkaloids, including lobeline, and is used as an antispasmodic in the treatment of asthma and chronic bronchitis.

Lobeline hydrochloride. B.P.C. 1968. $C_{22}H_{28}ClNO_2$. A respiratory stimulant.

Lobotomy. Incision into a lobe. **Frontal (prefrontal) lobotomy,** the operation for severing nerve tracts in the frontal (prefrontal) lobes of the cerebrum for the treatment of certain psychotic conditions.

Lobule. A small lobe, or a subdivision of a lobe. **Lobule of the auricle of the ear,** the soft, dependent part of the external ear. **Biventral lobule,** a lobule on the inferior surface of the cerebellum. **Central lobule,** a lobule on the superior surface of the vermis of the cerebellum. **Cortical lobules of the kidney,** the portions of the cortex that connect the renal columns with each other and intervene between the bases of the pyramids and the fibrous capsule. **Lobules of the epididymis,** the conical masses which constitute the head of the epididymis. **Lobules of the liver,** the unit of the liver, each about 1mm. in diameter and having a small central vein as its central axis, and bounded at its edge by portal canals. **Lobules of the mammary gland,** the constituents of the lobes of the gland, each consisting of a cluster of rounded alveoli which open into the branches of the lactiferous ducts. **Lobules of the pancreas,** the constituents of the pancreas, each consisting of one of the ultimate ramifications of the main duct ending in a number of alveoli. **Paracentral lobule,** the posterior portion of the anterior part of the medial surface of the cerebral hemisphere, bounded below by the cingulate sulcus. **Parietal lobule, inferior,** the part of the parietal lobe that lies below the intraparietal sulcus and behind the lower part of the postcentral sulcus. **Parietal lobule, superior,** the part of the parietal lobe lying between the superomedial margin of the cerebral hemisphere and the intraparietal sulcus. **Portal lobule,** the adjoining parts of three hepatic lobules, the bile from which drains into a bile ductule in the portal canal at the meeting place of the three hepatic lobules. **Quadrangular lobule,** the part of the superior surface of the cerebellum, lying between the postcentral fissure and the fissura prima. **Semilunar lobules, inferior,** the part of the inferior surface of the cerebellum lying between the horizontal fissure and the prepyramidal fissure. **Semilunar fissures, superior,** the posterior portion of the superior surface of the cerebellar hemispheres. **Simplex lobules,** part of the anterior portion of the superior surface of the cerebellar hemispheres. **Lobules of the testis,** the 200 to 300 cone-shaped lobules into which the testis is divided by septa given off by the tunica albuginea, each containing one to three or more convoluted tubules. **Lobules of the thymus,** the irregular lobules, each 1 to 2 mm. in diameter, into which the thymus is divided by septa from its fibrous capsule.

Lochia. The discharge of blood, mucus and tissue from the vagina following childbirth.

Lockjaw. Tetanus.

Locomotor. Pertaining to motion. **Locomotor ataxia,** tabes dorsalis.

Loculus. A small space or cavity. (*Plural:* loculi.)

Locus. A site or place. (*Plural:* loci.) **Locus coeruleus,** a bluish-grey area marking the superior part of the sulcus limitans which forms the medial eminence of the fourth ventricle.

Loefflerella. A genus of gram-negative bacilli. **Loefflerella mallei,** the causal organism of glanders. **Loefflerella pseudomallei,** the causal organism of melioidosis.

-logia, -logy- (Gk *logos:* word). Suffixes indicating the study of the subject indicated in the first part of the word.

Logo- (Gk *logos:* word). Prefix indicating association with words or speech.

Logomania. Pathological garrulity.

Logopaedics. The study of defective speech.

Logophasia. Inability to articulate correctly.

Logorrhoea. Garrulousness.

Logwood. Haematoxylin.

Loiasis. The chronic disease caused by infection with *Loa loa,* characterized by local tumours (*Calabar swellings*), eosinophilia, and varying allergic reactions.

Loin. The part of the back and the side between the ribs and the pelvis.

Longevity. Long life.

Longitudinal. In the direction of the long axis of the body.

Loop. A curve or bend. **Loop of Henle,** the bend in the renal tubule in the medullary pyramid. **Platinum loop,** a platinum wire used to transfer bacterial cultures.

Loquacity. Garrulousness.

Lorazepam. The B.P. Commission approved name for 7-chloro-5-(2-chlorophenyl)-1,3-dihydro-3-hydroxy-1,4-benzodiazepin-2-one. A tranquillizer.

Lordoscoliosis. Combined lordosis and scoliosis.

Lordosis. Forward curvature of the lumbar spine.

Lotion. A liquid preparation intended for application to the skin. There is one lotion in the *British Pharmacopoeia* 1968: calamine lotion; and ten in the *British Pharmaceutical Codex* 1968: calamine lotion, oily; copper and zinc sulphates lotion; hydrocortisone lotion; lead lotion; lead lotion, evaporating; salicylic acid lotion; salicylic acid and mercuric chloride lotion; sulphur lotion, compound; triamcinolone lotion; zinc sulphate lotion.

Loupe. A magnifying lens.

Louse. A general name for lice. (*Plural:* lice.) **Body louse,** *Pediculus vestimentorum,* or *P. corporis.* **Crab louse,** *Pediculus (Phthirus) pubis.* **Head louse,** *P. capitis.*

Loxapine. The B.P. Commission approved name for 2-chloro-11-(4-methylpiperazin-1-yl)dibenz[*b,f*] [1,4]-oxazepine. A tranquillizer.

Loxosceles. A genus of spiders found in the West Indies.

Loxoscelism. The condition induced by the bite of the Loxosceles genus of spiders. **Cutaneous loxoscelism,** the gangrenous slough that forms round the bite of a loxosceles spider.

Lozenge. A disc, in which medicaments

are incorporated in a flavoured basis and which is intended to dissolve or disintegrate slowly in the mouth. It is prepared by moulding or compression. A troche. There are eight in the *British Pharmaceutical Codex*, 1968: benzalkonium lozenges; benzocaine lozenges, compound; betamethasone lozenges; bismuth lozenges, compound; fomaldehyde lozenges; hydrocortisone lozenges; liquorice lozenges; penicillin lozenges.

Lucanthone hydrochloride. B.P. 1968. $C_{20}H_{25}ClN_2OS$. A drug used in the treatment of schistosomiasis caused by *Schistosoma haematobium*.

Lues. Syphilis.

Luetic. Syphilitic.

Lumbago. Backache.

Lumbar. Relating to the loins.

Lumbo- (L *lumbus*: loin). Prefix indicating association with the loin.

Lumbosacral. Pertaining to the lumbar spine and the sacrum.

Lumbrical. Vermiform. Resembling an earthworm. One of the four lumbrical muscles of the hands and feet.

Lumen. The channel within a tube. The unit of light flux, being the flux emitted within unit solid angle of 1 steradian by a point source having a uniform intensity of 1 candela. (*Plural:* lumina.) (*Abbreviation:* lm.)

Lunacy. Insanity.

Lunar. Pertaining to the moon.

Lunate. Moon-shaped.

Lunate bone. The crescentic-shaped bone placed between the scaphoid and triquetral bones in the middle of the proximal row of the carpus.

Lunatic. A psychotic individual.

Lungs. The essential organs of respiration, placed one on each side within the thorax, and separated from each other by the heart and the other contents of the mediastinum. The left lung has two lobes. The right lung has three lobes.

Lunula. A crescent-shaped area or organ. (*Plural:* lunulae.) Lunule. The free border of a semilunar cardiac valve on each side of the nodule. The white crescentic area at the root of a nail.

Lupoid. Resembling lupus.

Lupus. A term originally used to describe a chronic, intractable skin disease. Lupus erythematosus, an inflammatory affection of the skin, characterized by redness and scaling followed by atrophic scarring, and most common on the face. Systemic **lupus erythematosus**, a chronic in-

flammatory disease of connective tissue, probably an auto-immune process, which may affect almost any organ of the body and therefore produce protean manifestations. Lupus **verrucosus**, a warty excrescence produced by inoculation of the skin of an adult with *Mycobacterium tuberculosis*. Lupus **vulgaris**, cutaneous tuberculosis.

Luteal. Pertaining to the corpus luteum or its active principle.

Lutein. The yellow pigment of the corpus luteum.

Luteinizing. Forming luteal tissue. **Luteinizing hormone (LH)**, the hormone secreted by the anterior lobe of the pituitary gland that stimulates the formation of luteal tissue in the female, and of interstitial cells in the testes in the male.

Luteo- (L *luteus*: yellow). Prefix meaning yellow or yellowish.

Luteotrophic. Having a stimulating action on the luteal tissues of the Graafian follicle. Luteotrophic hormone (LTH), luteotrophic.

Luteotrophin. The lactogenic, or milk-stimulating, hormone secreted by the anterior lobe of the pituitary gland. Prolactin. Mammotrophin. LTH.

Lutetium. A rare element. Symbol Lu. Atomic weight 174·97. Atomic number 71.

Lux. The unit of illumination. An illumination of 1 lumen per square metre. (*Abbreviation:* lx.)

Luxation. Dislocation.

Lyase. One of a group of enzymes that catalyse the linkage of two molecules by addition at a double bond in one of them.

Lycanthropy. The delusion that one is a wolf.

Lymecycline. B.P.C. 1968. $C_{29}H_{38}N_4O_{10}$. A broad-spectrum antibiotic.

Lymph. The colourless fluid that circulates in the lymphatic vessels. It contains the same concentration of salts as plasma but a lower concentration of protein. It contains lymphocytes, and that in the thoracic duct contains a varying amount of fat globules. Lymph capillaries, the plexus of minute vessels that begin blindly in the tissue spaces and ultimately empty their contents into certain veins. Lymph duct, right, the duct about 1cm. in length, that receives the lymph from the right side of the head and neck, right upper limb, right side of the thorax, right lung, right side of the heart, and part of the liver, and opens into the angle of junction of the right subclavian and right internal jugular veins. **Lymph follicles,** dense aggregations of lymphoid tissue found in the stomach and intestine. **Lymph nodes,** small, oval or bean-shaped bodies situated in the course of lymph vessels. **Lymph nodules,** dense aggregations of lymphoid tissue in the lymph nodes. **Lymph sinuses,** the tortuous system of irregular channels within the lymphoid tissue. **Lymph trunks,** the series of lymphatic vessels, that feed into the right lymphatic duct, the thoracic duct, and the cisterna chyli. **Lymph vessels,** the vessels that carry lymph to and from the lymph nodes.

Lymph-, Lympho- (L *lympha:* water). Prefixes indicating relationship to lymph.

Lymphadenectomy. Surgical excision of a lymph node (or nodes).

Lymphadenitis. Inflammation of lymph glands.

Lymphadenography. Radiological visualization of a lymphatic node by injection of radio-opaque substances.

Lymphadenoid. Related to, or resembling, a lymph node.

Lymphadenoma. A progressive and fatal disease of lymphatic tissue characterized by enlargement of the lymph nodes. Hodgkin's disease.

Lymphadenopathy. Any morbid condition affecting the lymph nodes.

Lymphadenosis. Enlargement of lymph nodes.

Lymphadenotomy. Surgical incision of a lymph node.

Lymphagogue. Anything that stimulates the formation and flow of lymph.

Lymphangiectasis. Dilatation of the lymph vessels.

Lymphangiography. Radiological visualization of the lymphatic vessels by injection of a radio-opaque substance.

Lymphangioma. A tumour-like malformation of the lymphatic system, characterized by a dilated and cystic condition of the lymphatic vessels.

Lymphangitis. Inflammation of the lymph vessels.

Lymphatic. Pertaining to the lymph vessels and nodes. A lymph vessel.

Lymphoblast. The progenitor of a lymphocyte.

Lymphocyte. A non-granular, nucleated white blood cell which is produced in the lymphoid tissue of the body. Normal adult blood contains 1500 to 2000 lymphocytes per c.mm. **Large lymphocytes,** a young lymphocyte, 12 to 15μ in size. Large lymphocytes constitute 4 to 8 per cent of all the white blood cells in an adult, but are more numerous in the blood of infants and children. **Small lymphocyte,** a small, round cell, with a well-defined nucleus, and about the size of an erythrocyte. Small lymphocytes constitute 20 to 45 per cent of all the white blood cells in the adult.

Lymphocytic. Pertaining to lymphocytes.

Lymphocytopenia. A diminution in the number of lymphocytes in the blood.

Lymphocytopoiesis. The formation of lymphocytes.

Lymphocytosis. An increase in the number of lymphocytes.

Lymphoedema. Swelling due to lymphatic oedema.

Lymphogranuloma venereum. A venereal disease due to one of the large viruses belonging to the psittacosis group, characterized by enlargement of the inguinal glands.

Lymphoid. Resembling lymph or lymphatic tissue.

Lymphokine. A factor released from sensitized mononuclear cells in the type 4 hypersensitivity reaction, which is concerned with cell permeability and with attracting and activating macrophages and other inflammatory cells.

Lymphoma. A malignant tumour of the lymphoid tissue. **Burkitt's lymphoma,** a form of lymphoma, with a predilection for the bones of the jaw and face, which occurs predominantly in African children living below a certain altitude. **Follicular lymphoma,** a form of lymphoma with a predilection for one group of lymph glands, and which occurs in middle or later life.

Lymphopenia. A reduction in the number of lymphocytes in the circulating blood.

Lymphorrhagia. The escape of lymph from ruptured lymph vessels.

Lymphosarcoma. A malignant tumour of lymphoid tissue which is predominantly lymphocytic or lymphoblastic in structure.

Lymphuria. The presence of lymph in the urine.

Lynoestrenol. B.P. 1968. $C_{20}H_{28}O$. A progesterone-like drug that is active orally.

Lyo- (Gk *lyein:* to dissolve). Prefix meaning dissolved.

Lyophil. Water-loving. A colloid system in which the solvent and the dispersed particles mutually attract each other and is therefore stable.

Lyophilization. The process of preserving biological substances by rapid freezing and dehydration of the frozen product under high vacuum. Freeze-drying.

Lyophobe. Water-fearing. A colloid system in which there is no attraction between the solvent and the dissolved particles, and which is therefore unstable.

Lyosol. A sol in which the continuous medium is liquid.

Lyotropic. Lyophil. Readily soluble.

Lypressin. The B.P. Commission approved name for 8-lysinevasopressin. An antidiuretic hormone.

Lys-, Lysi- (Gk *lysis:* a loosening). Prefixes indicating a loosening.

Lysate. The material produced by lysis.

Lyse. To break up. To cause lysis.

Lysergic acid. A constituent of the ergot alkaloids.

Lysergic acid diethylamide. LSD. A partially synthetic ergot alkaloid which has a powerful hallucinogenic action.

Lysergide. The B.P. Commission approved name for lysergic acid diethylamide (LSD).

Lysin. An antibody that lyses cells.

Lysine. One of the essential amino-acids.

Lysis. The gradual fall in temperature, or abatement of symptoms, in an infectious disease. The solution or dissolution of cells.

-lysis (Gk *lysis:* a loosening). Suffix indicating lysis or dissolution.

Lyso- (Gk *lysis:* a loosening). Prefix indicating lysis or dissolution.

Lysogenic. Inducing lysis. Lytic.

Lysol. Cresol and soap solution, B.P.

Lysolecithin. A substance produced by the action of the enzyme lecithinase A, or lecithin, which is a surface-active agent with the ability to cause haemolysis of red blood cells.

Lysosome. A little sack of hydrolytic enzymes in the cell cytoplasm.

Lysozyme. A mucolytic enzyme, found in various body fluids, particularly human tears, and in egg white, which has a destructive lytic action on certain micro-organisms.

Lytic. Lysogenic.

M

Macaroni. Wheat paste made from a hard variety of wheat (*Triticum durum*) rich in gluten, and moulded into tubes.

Mace. The dried envelope of the seed of *Myristica fragrans*, which contains an oil closely resembling nutmeg oil, and used as a flavouring agent.

Maceration. Softening of a solid by soaking in a fluid.

Mackintosh. Waterproof sheeting.

Macr-, Macro- (Gk *makros:* large or long). Prefixes signifying enlargement.

Macrencephaly. Abnormal enlargement of the brain.

Macrobrachia. Abnormal size or length of the arms.

Macrocardius. A foetal monster with an abnormally large heart.

Macrocephaly. Excessive size of the head.

Macrocheilia. Excessively large lips.

Macrocyte. An abnormally large red blood cell.

Macrocytosis. The state distinguished by the presence of an unusually large number of macrocytes in the circulating blood.

Macrodactyly. Abnormally large fingers or toes.

Macrogamete. The female gamete.

Macrogametocyte. The female gametocyte.

Macrogenitosoma. Precocious puberty, usually the result of congenital hyperplasia or tumour of the adrenal cortex.

Macroglia. The large neuroglial cells, consisting of the astrocytes and the oligodendroglia.

Macroglobulin. A globulin with an abnormally high molecular weight of over 1,000,000.

Macroglobulinaemia. The condition characterized by the presence in the circulating blood of a macroglobulin of very high molecular weight.

Macroglossia. An abnormally large tongue.

Macrogols. Strongly hydrophilic substances which are non-irritating to the skin and are well absorbed. They are used as ingredients of water-miscible bases in preparations for external use, in which penetration of the skin is required. There are two official preparations: **Hard macrogol,** B.P.C. 1968, and **Liquid macrogol,** B.P.C. 1968. Two more have been given approved names by the British Pharmacopoeia Commission. **Macrogol 4000,** and **Macrogol 400.**

Macromastia. Abnormal enlargement of the breasts.

Macromelia. Abnormally large size of the limbs.

Macronathia. The condition characterized by an abnormally large jaw.

Macronidia. The large multicellular spore-forms produced in artificial culture by the dermatophyte fungi, according to the morphology of which the genera are distinguished.

Macronormoblast. A large normoblast.

Macronychia. Excessive length of the nails.

Macrophage. A phagocytic reticulo-endothelial cell.

Macropolycyte. A polymorphonuclear cell with a multi-segmented nucleus.

Macropsia. The condition in which objects appear to be larger than they actually are.

Macroscopic. Visible to the naked eye.

Macroscopy. Naked-eye examination.

Macrostomia. Abnormal size of the mouth.

Macula. A small spot or blemish. (*Plural:* maculae.) ¦**Macula cribrosa inferior,** holes in the lower part of the vestibule of the bony labyrinth of the internal ear, through which pass the nerves to the ampulla. **Macula cribrosa media,** holes in the medial wall of the vestibule, through which pass nerves to the saccule. **Macula cribrosa superior,** holes in the pyramid and elliptical recess of the vestibule, through which pass the nerves to the utricle and to the ampullae of the superior and lateral semicircular canals. **Macula densa,** the part of the renal tubule that lies close to the renal corpuscle in the space between the afferent and efferent arterioles. **Macula lutea,** the oval yellowish area near the centre of the posterior part of the retina, where the visual sense is most highly developed. **Macula of the saccule,** an oval thickening on the anterior wall of the saccule. **Macula of the utricle,** a thickening in the utricle which receives the utricular filaments of the vestibular nerve.

Maculae caeruliae. Bluish-grey macules sometimes present on the side of the trunk and the inner surfaces of the arms and thighs in fair-skinned people infested with *Pediculus pubis*.

Macule. Macula.

Maculo- (L *macula:* a spot). Prefix signifying relationship to a spot or macule.

Maculocerebral. Pertaining to the macula lotea and the brain. **Maculocerebral familial degeneration,** a familial disease in children, characterized by defective vision, weak intellect, convulsions and spasticity.

Maculopapular. Characterized by macules and papules—as of skin rashes.

Madarosis. Loss of the eye-lashes.

Madder. The powdered root of *Rubia tinctoria*, from which is derived the red dye known as Turkey Red.

Madura foot. Mycetoma.

Madurella. A genus of fungi, saprophytic in the soil and on vegetable matter, which can enter the tissues of man and become pathogenic, causing the condition known as maduromycosis. The genus includes *Madurella mycetomi* and *M. grisei*.

Maduromycosis. A chronic infection caused by various fungi. Madura foot.

Mafenide. The B.P. Commission approved name for *a*-aminotoluene-*p*-sulphonamide. An antibacterial agent.

Magenta. B.P.C. 1968. A mixture of the hydrochlorides of pararosaniline and rosaniline, which has antifungal and antibacterial actions. **Magenta paint,** B.P.C. 1968, also known as Castellani's paint, used in the treatment of superficial dermatophytoses.

Maggot. A fly larva, usually of the order Diptera.

Magnesia. Magnesium oxide. **Cream of magnesia,** Magnesium hydroxide Mixture B.P. **Light magnesia,** Light Magnesium oxide, B.P.

Magnesium. A mineral element. Symbol Mg. Atomic weight 24·32. Atomic number 12.

Magnesium carbonate, heavy. B.P. 1968. $3MgCO_3,Mg(OH)_2$. A hydrated basic magnesium carbonate. An antacid. **Magnesium carbonate, light,** B.P. 1968, a hydrated basic magnesium carbonate with the approximate formula, $3MgCO_3$, $Mg(OH)_2$, $3H_2O$. An antacid and laxative.

Magnesium chloride. B.P. 1968. $MgCl_2$, $6H_2O$. Used to adjust the concentration of magnesium ions in preparing solutions for haemodialysis and peritoneal dialysis.

Magnesium hydroxide. B.P.C. 1968. $Mg(OH)_2$. An antacid and mild laxative. Magnesium hydroxide mixture, B.P. 1968, cream of magnesia. An antacid and laxative containing the equivalent of 7·9 per cent w/w of $Mg(OH)_2$.

Magnesium oxide, light. B.P. 1968. MgO. An antacid and laxative. Light magnesia.

Magnesium stearate. B.P. 1968. Used as (i) a dusting powder, (ii) in creams as a barrier to chemical irritants; (iii) as a lubricant for granules in the manufacture of tablets.

Magnesium sulphate. B.P. 1968. $MgSO_4$, $7H_2O$. Epsom salts. A saline purgative. Used intravenously to lower intracranial pressure and applied as a wet compress in treatment of boils and carbuncles. **Magnesium sulphate, dried,** B.P. 1968, one of the chief ingredients of effervescent and non-effervescent aperient powders or granules.

Magnesium trisilicate. B.P. 1968. $2MgO$, $3SiO_2$. An antacid.

Magnet. Lodestone. Natural iron oxide that has the property of attracting iron. A piece of steel or iron that exhibits this property.

Maize. A cereal grain produced by *Zea mays*, the principal protein of which is zein, which lacks lysine and contains very little tryptophan.

Maize oil. B.P. 1968. The fixed oil obtained from the embryos of *Zea mays* (L.). Corn oil. Because of its high content of glycerides of unsaturated acids, it is used in diets to reduce high blood-cholesterol levels.

Mal. Disease. **Grand mal,** major epilepsy. **Petil mal,** minor epilepsy.

Mal- (L *malus:* bad). Prefix meaning bad or ill.

Malabsorption. Defective absorption.

Malacia. A softening.

Malaise. A vague and indefinite sensation of not feeling well, of uneasiness or discomfort.

Malaria. A protozoal disease of man, in which the causative organism

Plasmodium, invades certain body cells and the red blood cells, causing an infection with a characteristic periodic pyrexia.

Malassezia furfur. The yeast-like fungus that causes pityriasis versicolor.

Malate. A salt or ester of malic acid.

Male. A member of the sex that produces spermatozoa. Masculine, or belonging to the male sex.

Male fern. B.P. 1968. The rhizome, frond-bases and apical bud of *Dryopteris filix-mas*. **Male fern extract,** B.P. 1968, an extract containing 21 to 23 per cent w/w of filicin, used for the expulsion of tapeworms.

Maleic acid. B.P. 1968. $C_4H_4O_4$. Used in the preparation of ergometrine injection and methylergometrine injection.

Maleruption. Faulty eruption of a tooth.

Malethamer. The B.P. Commission approved name for maleic anhydride-ethylene polymer. An antiperistaltic agent.

Malformation. Deformity.

Malfunction. Disordered function.

Malic acid. Hydroxysuccinic acid, the acid that gives the tart taste to apples and other fruits.

Malignant. Virulent, life-threatening. **Malignant disease,** cancer. **Malignant hypertension,** a condition characterized by exceptionally high blood pressure, transient cerebral attacks and papilloedema. **Malignant pustule,** anthrax.

Malingering. Feigning disease.

Mallein. A preparation from the glanders bacillus analogous to tuberculin, and used in the diagnosis of glanders, particularly in horses.

Malleolar. Relating to a malleolus.

Malleolus. The rounded bony prominence on either side of the ankle. **Lateral malleolus,** the lower end of the fibula. **Medial malleolus,** the lower end of the tibia.

Malleus. The largest of the three auditory ossicles, so called because of its resemblance to a hammer.

Malnutrition. Faulty nutrition.

Malocclusion. Faulty occlusion or closure of the two rows of teeth.

Malpractice. Failure in the exercise of a reasonable degree of skill and care on the part of a medical practitioner in his treatment of a patient.

Malpraxis. Malpractice.

Malpresentation. Abnormal presentation of the foetus.

Malt. The substance obtained from grain, usually barley, which has been artificially germinated, and then dried and crushed. It contains dextrin, maltose and diastase. **Malt extract,** B.P.C. 1968, an extract obtained from ground malted grain of barley, or a mixture of barley and wheat. Used chiefly as a vehicle for cod-liver oil (*Malt extract with cod-liver oil, B.P.C.* 1968) and halibut-liver oil (*Malt extract with halibut-liver oil, B.P.C.*1968). It also has nutritive properties.

Maltase. An enzyme in the small intestine that converts maltose to glucose.

Maltose. A disaccharide consisting of two molecules of glucose, which occurs as an intermediate in the breakdown of starch to glucose.

Malunion. Faulty or incomplete union of a fracture.

Mamilla. Nipple. (*Plural:* mamillae.)

Mamillary. Resembling a nipple. **Mamillary bodies,** two round masses, the size of a small pea, below the grey matter of the floor of the third ventricle.

Mamma. The breast. (*Plural:* mammae.)

Mammillaria. A skin condition associated with anidrotic heat exhaustion, in which the skin is covered with pale circular elevations which bear no relation to hair follicles or openings of sweat ducts.

Mammography. X-ray examination of the breast.

Mammoplasty. A plastic operation on the breast.

Mancinism. Left handedness.

Mandible. The lower jaw.

Mandibulo-facial. Concerned with the mandible and the facial bone. **Mandibulo-facial dystrophy,** the condition characterized by a notch at the outer part of the lower eyelid, associated with maldevelopment of the first visceral arch.

Manganese. One of the trace elements of the body concerned in several enzyme systems. Symbol Mn. Atomic weight 54·938. Atomic number 25. **Manganese sulphate,** B.P.C. 1968, Mn $SO_4,4H_2O$. A preparation used occasionally for its effect in increasing the haematinic action of iron.

Mania. A form of mental disorder characterized by great excitement.

Manikin. A model of the body, or part of it, used for teaching purposes.

Manipulation. The use of forceful, passive movements in the treatment of disorders of the joints.

Mannitol. B.P. 1968. $C_6H_{14}O_6$. An

osmotic diuretic. Given intravenously as **Mannitol injection,** B.P. 1968.

Mannomustine hydrochloride. B.P.C. 1968. A cytotoxic agent.

Mannose. A monosaccharide.

Manometer. An instrument for measuring the pressure or tension of liquids or gases.

Mantoux test. One of the tuberculin tests for the diagnosis of tuberculosis, in which the tuberculin is given intracutaneously.

Manubrium. A handle-like structure. (*Plural:* manubria.) **Manubrium of the malleus,** one of the three processes of the malleus that connects it with the tympanic membrane. **Manubrium sterni,** the uppermost part of the sternum.

Maple syrup urine disease. One of the inborn errors of metabolism, in which the metabolism of isoleucine, leucine and valine is disordered, and characterized by the distinctive odour of the urine to which it owes its name.

Marasmus. Progressive wasting, especially in infants, for which there is no specific cause.

Margarine. An emulsion of animal and vegetable fats with the aqueous serum of sweet or soured milk, which contains 80 to 86 per cent fat, and is used largely as a substitute for butter.

Marihuana. Cannabis.

Marrow. The soft pulpy tissue in the hollows of the long bones and in the spaces of the spongy substance of all bones. **Red marrow,** the marrow found in adult life in the vertebrae, sternum, ribs, clavicles, scapulae, hip bones, skull bones and the upper ends of the femora and humeri. It contains a variety of blood cells and their precursors. **Yellow marrow,** the marrow found in the long bones, most of the cells in which are fat cells.

Marsupialization. Drainage of a cavity, usually a cyst, by opening it up widely and suturing the edges to the edge of the adjacent skin as to keep it open—thus forming a pouch, and hence the name.

Masculinization. The induction or development of male secondary sex characteristics in the female.

Masochism. A form of sexual perversion in which sexual excitement and pleasure are enhanced by being simultaneously beaten or humiliated.

Mass. A lump or aggregation of particles. **Formative mass,** the clump of totipotential cells, some of which are destined to form the embryo, which projects into the blastocele. **Inner cell mass,** the fomative mass. **Intermediate cell mass,** the intraembryonic mesoderm of the embryo, in the floor of the longitudinal groove that connects the paraxial portion and the lateral plate. It is also known as the nephrogenic cord. **Lateral mass of the atlas,** the two major portions of the first cervical vertebra (or atlas), connected to each in front by the anterior arch and behind by the posterior arch. **Mass number,** the total number of neutrons and protons in the nucleus of an isotope.

Massage. The method of physiotherapy characterized by a varying combination of rubbing, kneading, tapping, pinching and manipulation.

Masseur. A man who practises massage.

Masseuse. A woman who practises massage.

Mast-, Masto- (Gk *masto:* breast). Prefixes signifying relationship to the breast.

Mastalgia. Pain in the breast.

Mastectomy. Amputation of the breast.

Mastic. B.P.C. 1968. A resinous exudation from certain varieties of *Pistacia lentiscus* L. Used as a temporary filling for carious teeth, and, in the form of *Compound mastic paint,* B.P.C. 1968, as a protective covering for wounds.

Mastication. The chewing of food.

Mastigophora. The class of protozoa which possess one or more flagella. It includes the Trypanosomes.

Mastitis. Inflammation of the breast.

Mastodynia. Pain in the breast.

Mastoid. The mastoid part of the temporal bone, including the mastoid process in which it terminates behind the ear.

Mastoidectomy. The operation for drainage of the infected mastoid antrum.

Mastoiditis. Inflammation of the mastoid antrum.

Mastoplasia. Hypertrophy of the breast.

Mastoptosis. Excessive pendulousness of the breasts.

Masturbation. Production of an orgasm by self-manipulation of the genitalia.

Materia medica. The branch of medical science that deals with the sources, preparation and uses of drugs.

Matrix. The groundwork or mold on which a part is set. (*Plural:* matrices.)

Matter. Material or substance. An archaic term for pus. **Grey matter of the cerebellum, cerebrum and spinal cord,** the nerve cells and dendrites. **White matter of the cerebellum, cere-**

brum and spinal cord, the nerve fibres of the central nervous system.

Mattoid. A person, who, though passing as sane, is eccentric or mentally unbalanced in some particular respect.

Maturation. The process of maturing or ripening. The process whereby the chromosomes in the sex cells are halved in number.

Matutinal. Occurring in the morning.

Maxilla. One of the two bones that constitute the upper jaw. (*Plural:* maxillae.)

Maxillary. Pertaining to the maxillae.

Maxillofacial. Pertaining to the maxillae and the face.

Measles. An acute infectious disease, caused by a virus, and with a characteristic rash. **Measles vaccine (inactivated),** B.P. 1968, an aqueous suspension of measles virus grown in cultures of monkey kidney tissue or chick embryo cells, and inactivated. **Measles vaccine (live attenuated),** B.P. 1968, an aqueous suspension of a live attenuated strain of measles virus grown in cultures of chick embryo cells. **German measles,** rubella.

Measly. Infected with measles. Like measles. Of meat, infected with cysticerci.

Meatal. Pertaining to a meatus.

Meato- (L *meatus:* a passage). Prefix signifying meatus or opening.

Meatotomy. Surgical incision of the urinary meatus in order to enlarge it.

Meatus. A passage or opening. (*Plural:* meatus.) **External acoustic meatus,** the passage from the concha to the tympanic membrane. **Internal acoustic meatus,** the short passage in the petrous portion of the temporal bone that transmits the facial and vestibulocochlear nerves. **Inferior nasal meatus,** the space beneath the inferior concha. **Middle nasal meatus,** the space beneath the middle concha. **Superior nasal meatus,** the space beneath the superior concha.

Mebanazine. The B.P. Commission approved name for *a*-methylbenzylhydrazine. A monoamine oxidase inhibitor.

Mebeverine. The B.P. Commission approved name for an antispasmodic.

Mebezonium iodide. The B.P. Commission approved name for 4,4′-methylenedi(cyclohexyltrimethylammonium iodide). A neuromuscular blocking agent.

Mebhydrolin napadisylate. B.P.C. 1968. $C_{48}H_{48}N_4O_6S_2$. An antihistaminic.

Mebutamate. The B.P. Commission approved name for 2,2-di(carbamoyloxymethyl)-3-methylpentane. A hypotensive agent.

Mecamylamine hydrochloride. B.P. 1968. $C_{11}H_{22}ClN$. A ganglion-blocking agent.

Mechanotherapy. The provision of active physical exercise by means of mechanical contrivances.

Meclofenamic acid. The B.P. Commission approved name for *N*-(2,6-dichloro-*m*-tolyl)anthranilic acid. An anti-inflammatory agent.

Meclofenoxate. The B.P. approved name for 2-dimethylaminoethyl 4-chlorophenoxyacetate. A cerebral stimulant.

Meclozine hydrochloride. B.P. 1968. $C_{25}H_{29}Cl_3N_2$. An antihistamine, widely used in the treatment of motion sickness.

Meco- (Gk *mekos:* length). Prefix meaning length.

Meconism. Opium addiction or poisoning.

Meconium. The first faecal discharge of the new-born infant, consisting of bile, intestinal debris, and mucus.

Mecono- (Gk *mēkon:* poppy). Prefix signifying opium.

Medi-, Medio- (Gk *medius*: middle). Prefixes meaning middle, mean.

Medial. Closer to the midline.

Median. Middle. The midpoint that divides the area of a frequency curve into two halves.

Mediastinitis. Inflammation of the cellular tissue of the mediastinum.

Mediastinum. A median septum. (*Plural:* mediastina.) The interval between the two pleural sacs, extending from the sternum in front to the vertebral column behind, and from the thoracic inlet above to the diaphragm below. It is divided into two parts: an upper part known as the *superior mediastinum*, and a lower part which is subdivided into the *anterior mediastinum* in front of the pericardium, the *middle mediastinum* occupied by the pericardium and its contents, and the *posterior mediastinum* behind the pericardium. **Mediastinum testis,** an incomplete vertical septum, a projection of the tunica albuginea, that extends from the upper to near the lower end of the testis.

Medical. Pertaining to medicine.

Medicament. A medicinal substance.

Medicated. Impregnated with a medicinal substance.

Medication. Treatment by means of drugs.

Medicinal. Having healing properties.

Medicine. A drug. The healing art. The non-surgical practice of the healing art.

Medicochirurgical. Pertaining to both medicine and surgery.

Medicolegal. Pertaining to medicine and the law.

Medium. A means. A substance through which impulses are transmitted. (*Plural:* media.) **Culture medium,** the substance (or substances), solid or liquid, on which micro-organisms are grown in the laboratory.

Medroxyprogesterone. The B.P. Commission approved name for 17α-hydroxy - 6α-methylpregn-4- ene -3,20-dione. A progestational steroid.

Medulla. The inmost part. (*Plural:* medullae.) **Medulla of bone,** the bone marrow. **Medulla of hair,** the innermost part of the hair shaft. **Medulla of the kidney,** the innermost part of the kidney composed of eighteen pyramids. **Medulla of lymph node,** the innermost part of a lymph node. **Medulla oblongata,** the lowest part of the brain, continuous below with the spinal cord and above with the pons. **Medulla spinalis,** the spinal cord. **Medulla of suprarenal glands,** the inner tenth of the suprarenal gland, composed of chromaffin cells which secrete adrenaline and noradrenaline. **Medulla of thymus,** the inner part of the thymus which contains the concentric corpuscles of Hassall.

Medullated. Having a medulla, or a myelin sheath.

Medullation. The process of acquiring a myelin sheath.

Medulloblastoma. A highly malignant brain tumour found in the region of the fourth ventricle near the cerebellum, predominantly in young children.

Mefenamic acid, B.P. Addendum 1969. $C_{15}H_{15}NO_2$. An analgesic and an anti-inflammatory agent.

Mefruside. The B.P. Commission approved name for 4-chloro-N'-methyl-N'-(2-methyltetrahydrofurfuryl)-benzene-3-disulphonamide. A diuretic.

Mega- (Gk *megas:* big). Prefix meaning large. In metric system signifying one million.

Megacephaly. Unusually large size of the head.

Megacolon. Dilatation and hypertrophy of part, or the whole, of the colon.

Megacycle. One million cycles per second.

Megadactyly. Having abnormally large fingers.

Megakaryoblast. One of the primitive forms of marrow giant cells.

Megakaryocyte. The bone marrow cell from which the blood platelets are derived.

Megal-, Megalo - (Gk *megaleios:* great). Prefixes signifying great size.

Megaloblast. A nucleated red cell which is larger than a normoblast, and represents an early stage in the pathological form of erythropoiesis which results in the clinical condition known as pernicious anaemia.

Megalocyte. A large erythrocyte.

Megalomania. The condition characterized by delusions of grandeur.

Megalo-ureter. An abnormally large ureter.

-megaly (Gk *megaleios:* great). Suffix meaning great size.

Megavolt. One million volts.

Megestrol acetate, B.P. Addendum 1969, $C_{24}H_{32}O_4$. A progestational steroid.

Meglumine, B.P. 1968. $C_7H_{17}NO_5$. An organic base used in the preparation of iodinated organic acids used as contrast media. **Meglumine iothalamate injection,** B.P. 1968, a radio-opaque substance used in urography.

Megrim. Migraine.

Meio- (Gk *meion:* less). Prefix meaning less.

Meiosis. The process in the early stage of sexual reproduction, in which there are two divisions of the zygote, or fertilized ovum, but only one division of the chromosomes during the maturation of the gametes, thus ensuring that each daughter nucleus receives half the number of chromosomes characteristic of the somatic cells of the species.

Mel. Honey.

Mel-, Melo- (Gk *melos:* limb). Prefixes indicating association with a limb. (Gk *melon:* cheek). Prefixes signifying relationship with a cheek. (L *mel:* honey). Prefixes meaning honey.

Meladrazine. The B.P. Commission approved name for 2,4-di(diethyl-amino)-6-hydrazino-1,3,5-triazine. A polysynaptic inhibitor.

Melaena. The passage of dark tarry stools, containing altered blood due to bleeding in the stomach or upper part of the intestines.

Melan- (Gk *melas:* black). Prefix meaning black.

Melancholia. A mental illness characterized by extreme depression or black despair.

Melanin. The dark brown or black pigment present in the skin, the hair, the choroid coat of the eye, and the substantia nigra of the brain, as well as melanotic tumours.

Melanoblast. The precursor of the melanocyte.

Melanocyte. The cell that produces melanin.

Melanoderma. A localized increased deposition of melanin in the skin.

Melanogen. A colourless precursor of melanin.

Melanoid. Dark-coloured. Resembling melanin.

Melanoma. A tumour composed of pigmented cells. **Benign melanoma,** a mole or naevus. **Malignant melanoma,** a most malignant tumour that may arise from lentigenes, or compound or junctional naevi.

Melanonychia. Darkening of the nails by melanin.

Melanophore. A macrophage that contains melanin. **Melanophore-stimulating hormone (MSH),** the hormone secreted by the pituitary that causes darkening of the skin.

Melanoplakia. Dark pigmented patches in the mucous membrane of the mouth.

Melanosis. An abnormal deposition of melanin. **Melanosis coli,** the condition in which macrophages loaded with brown pigment are found in the mucosa of the colon.

Melanotic. Pertaining to melanosis.

Melanuria. The presence of a dark pigment in the urine.

Melarsonyl potassium. The B.P. Commission approved name for dipotassium 2-[4-(4,6-diamino-1,3,5-triazin-2-ylamino)phenyl]-1,3,2-dithiarsolan-4,5-dicarboxylate. A trypanocide.

Melarsopro. B.P. 1968. $C_{12}H_{15}AsN_6OS_2$. A trypanocide.

Melatonin. A substance isolated from the pineal gland that constructs the melanocytes in frogs, and decreases ovarian activity in rats.

Melengestrol. The B.P. Commission approved name for 17a-hydroxy-6-methyl-16-methylenepregna-4,6-diene-3,20-dione. A progestogen.

Melioidosis. A glanders-like disease, due to *Loefflerella pseudomallei,* which occurs in the Far East and U.S.A.

Melisophobia. Morbid fear of bees.

Melomania. Singing mania.

Melomelus. A foetus with rudimentary accessory limbs as well as normal limbs.

Meloplasty. Plastic surgery of the cheek.

Melorheostosis. The condition in which pathological hardening and denseness extend in a linear direction through one of the long bones of a limb, causing deformity and limitation of movement.

Melphalan. B.P. Addendum 1971. $C_{13}H_{18}Cl_2N_2O_2$. A cytotoxic agent used in the treatment of neoplastic disease.

Membrana. Membrane. (*Plural:* membranae.) **Membrana granulosa,** the cells lining the Graafian follicle.

Membrane. A thin sheet or layer. **Anal membrane,** the membrane that closes the anal end of the embryonic gut. **Atlanto-occipital membrane, anterior,** a broad dense membrane that passes between the anterior margin of the foramen magnum and the upper border of the atlas. **Atlanto-occipital membrane, posterior,** a broad thin membrane that passes between the posterior margin of the foramen magnum and the upper border of the posterior arch of the atlas. **Basement membrane,** the thin sheet of modified connective tissue underlying layers of epithelial cells, as in mucous membrane. **Basilar membrane of the cochlea,** the membrane that stretches from the tympanic lip of the osseous spiral lamina to the crista basilaris. The inner part supports the spiral organ. **Cell membrane,** the thin, elastic resilient membrane with which most cells are surrounded. **Cricovocal membrane,** the lower part of the quadrangular membrane of the larynx, which with its fellow of the opposite side connects the thyroid, cricoid and arytenoid cartilages. **Fenestrated membrane,** the yellow elastic tissue in the inner coat of the arteries, and the media of large arteries. **Fibroelastic membrane of the larynx,** the broad sheet of fibrous and elastic tissue lying beneath the mucous membrane of the larynx, and divided into the quadrangular membrane and the cricovocal membrane. **Fibrous membrane of the trachea,** the fibro-elastic membrane that encloses the cartilages of the trachea. **Hyaloid membrane,** the vitreous membrane. **Hyoglossal membrane,** the membrane that connects the root of the tongue to the hyoid bone. **Intercostal membrane, anterior,** the aponeurotic layer that extends the insertion of the external intercostal muscles to the sternum. **Intercostal membrane, posterior,** the aponeurotic continuation of the internal intercostal muscles. **Interosseous membrane, crural,** the membrane that connects the interosseous borders of the tibia and fibula and separates the muscles in the front, from those on the back, of the leg. **Interosseous membrane of the forearm,** a broad, thin sheet that stretches from the interosseous border of the radius to that of the ulna. **Krause's membrane,** the narrow dark line, the Z disc, running transversely across the middle of the I band of the striated muscle fibre. **Mucous membrane,** the membrane lining the digestive, respiratory and urogenital systems, which is kept moist by the secretion of glands **Nuclear membrane,** the outer layer of the nucleus. **Obturator membrane,** the membrane that nearly closes the obturator foramen. **Otolithic membrane,** the gelatinous mass in the utricle and saccule, which contains the otoliths, and into which the cilia project. **Perineal membrane,** a strong layer stretching horizontally across the pubic arch. **Periodontal membrane,** the membrane that covers the cement of the roots of the teeth and firmly embeds them in the alveoli of the maxilla and mandible. **Plasma membrane,** cell membrane. **Pupillary membrane,** the delicate, vascular membrane that covers the pupil in the foetus. **Quadrangular membrane,** the upper portion of the fibroelastic membrane of the larynx, which extends between the arytenoid cartilage and the cartilage of the epiglottis. **Semipermeable membrane,** a membrane that will only allow the solvent, or the solvent and the cystalloids it contains, not colloids, to pass through it. **Serous membrane,** the lining membrane of the closed cavities of the body: e.g. the peritoneal, pericardial and pleural cavities. **Suprapleural membrane,** a dome-like expansion of fascia that stretches from the first rib to the transverse process of the seventh cervical vertebra. **Synovial membrane,** the membrane that lines the fibrous capsule of joints and secretes a small amount of viscid, glairy fluid known as synovia. **Tectorial membrana** the strong fibrous band within the vertebral canal, which covers the dens, and is a continuation upwards of the posterior longitudinal ligament of the vertebral ligament. **Tectorial membrana of the cochlea,** the membrane that overlies the sulcus spiralis internus and the spiral organ of Corti **Thyrohyoid membrane,** the broad, fibroelastic layer attached below to the thyroid cartilage and above to the hyoid bone. **Tympanic membrane,** the thin, semi-transparent membrane, 8 to 10mm. in diameter, that separates the tympanic cavity from the external acoustic meatus. **Vestibular membrane,** the delicate membrane that extends from the osseous spiral lamina to the outer wall of the cochlea. **Vitelline membrane,** the innermost layer of the ovum. **Vitreous membrane,** the surface layer of the vitreous body. Hyaloid membrane.

Membranous. Resembling, or consisting of, membrane.

Memory. The knowledge of an event or fact, of which meantime we have not been thinking, with the additional consciousness that we have thought or experienced it before. (William James.)

Menadoxime. The B.P. Commission approved name for the ammonium salt of 2-methylnaphthaquinone-4-oxime-*O*-carboxymethyl ether. A drug for the treatment of hypoprothrombinaemia.

Menarche. The establishment of menstruation.

Mendelian. Pertaining to the laws of heredity laid down by G. J. Mendel.

Mendelism. The theory laid down by G. J. Mendel concerning the inheritance of certain characteristics through chromosomes, the fundamental basis of which is that the characters of sexually reproducing organisms are transmitted to the offspring in fixed ratios and without blending.

Menidrosis. Vicarious menstruation by means of bloody sweat.

Menière's disease. A disease characterised by paroxysmal attacks of labyrinthine vertigo, associated with vomiting, tinnitus and progressive deafness.

Mening-, Meningo- (Gk *meninx:* membrane). Prefixes signifying relationship with the meninges or any other membrane.

Meninges. The membranes that surround the brain and spinal cord, named from without inwards: dura mater, the arachnoid, and the pia mater.

Meningioma. A tumour of the arachnoid cells that lie on the deep surface of the dura and on the arachnoid granulations.

Meningism. The condition usually in children, characterized by the symptoms and signs of meningitis, but without any infection of the meninges.

Meningitis. Inflammation of the meninges.

Meningocele. Protrusion of the meninges of the brain or spinal cord through a defect in the skull or spinal column.

Meningococcaemia. Presence of meningococci (*Neisseria meningitidis*) in the bloodstream.

Meningococcus. *Neisseria meningitidis.*

Meningocyte. The reticulo-endothelial phagocytic cell in the meninges.

Meningo-encephalitis. Inflammation of the meninges and of the brain.

Meningo-encephalocele. Hernial protrusion of the brain and its meninges through a defect in the skull.

Meningomyelitis. Inflammation of the spinal cord and its meninges.

Meningovascular. Relating to the bloodvessels of the meninges.

Meninx primitiva. The loose mesenchyme of sclerotomic origin surrounding the spinal cord, from which the three meninges are derived.

Meniscectomy. Surgical excision of the semilunar cartilages of the knee joint.

Meniscus. A crescent-shaped structure, whether it be a lens, the upper curved surface of a column of liquid, or the semilunar cartilages of the knee joint. There are two crescentic lamellae, medial and lateral, which deepen the surfaces of the upper end of the tibia for articulation with the condyles of the femur. (*Plural:* menisci.) **Meniscus tactile,** a shallow, cup-shaped disc in hairless skin and the hair follicles.

Meno- (Gk *mēn:* month). Prefix signifying relationship with menstruation or the monthly period.

Menopause. The cessation of menstruation at the end of reproductive life. **Artificial menopause,** artificial cessation of menstruation, as by irradiation or surgery.

Menorrhagia. Excessive loss of blood during menstruation.

Menses. The monthly flow of blood at menstruation.

Mens rea. Guilty mind. Evil intent. A medico-legal concept.

Menstruation. The periodic uterine bleeding which occurs throughout the sexually active period of a woman's life—from the menarche to the menopause, unless it is interfered with by pregnancy or disease.

Menstruum. A solvent.

Mensuration. The act of measuring.

Mental. Pertaining to the mind. **Mental defect,** arrested or incomplete development of the mind Now renamed subnormality under the Mental Health Act, 1959. **Mental illness,** any disorder of the mind.

Mental. Pertaining to the chin.

Mentality. Mental power or activity.

Menthol. B.P. 1968. A natural laevo-menthol obtained from the volatile oils of various species of Mentha, or derived synthetically by the catalytic hydrogenation of thymol. Used as an inhalation or pastilles for relief of bronchitis and sinusitis.

Mento- (L *mentum:* chin). Prefix indicating association with the chin.

Mentum. The chin.

Mepacrine hydrochloride. B.P. 1968. $C_{23}H_{32}Cl_3N_3O,2H_2O$. An antimalarial drug. It is also used in the treatment of giardiasis and tapeworm infestation.

Mepenzolate bromide. The B.P. Commission approved name for 3-benziloyloxy-1,1-dimethylpiperidinium bromide. A parasympatholytic.

Mephenesin, B.P.C. 1968. $C_{10}H_{14}O_3$. A muscle relaxant.

Mephentermine sulphate. B.P. 1968. $C_{22}H_{36}N_2O_4S,2H_2O$. A sympathomimetic used in the treatment of hypotension.

Mepiprazole. The B.P. Commission approved name for 1-(3-chlorophenyl) -4 -[2 -(5 -methylpyrazol -3 -yl) ethyl] -piperazine. A psychotropic agent.

Mepivacaine. The B.P. Commission approved name for 1-methyl-2-(2,6-xylylcarbamoyl) piperidine. A local anaesthetic.

Meprobamate, B.P. 1968. $C_9H_{18}N_2O_4$. A sedative.

Meprochol. The B.P. Commission approved name for (2-methoxyprop-2-enyl)trimethylammonium bromide. A parasympathomimetic.

Mepyramine maleate. B.P. 1968. $C_{17}C_{21}H_{27}N_3O_5$. An antihistamine.

Mer-, Mero- (Gk *meros:* part). Prefix meaning part.

Meralgia. Pain in the thigh. **Meralgia paraesthetica,** pain, numbness, tingling and hyperaesthesia in the distribution of the lateral femoral cutaneous nerve.

Meralluride. The B.P. Commission approved name for a mixture of *N*-(3-hydroxymercuri-2-methoxypropyl-carbamoyl) succinamic acid and theophylline. An organic mercurial diuretic.

Mercaptomerin sodium. The B.P. Commission approved name for the disodium salt of *N*-(3-carboxymethylthiomercuri-2-methoxypropyl) camphoramic acid. An organic mercurial diuretic.

Mercaptopurine. B.P. 1968. $C_5H_4N_4S$, H_2O. A cytotoxic agent used in the treatment of acute leukaemia. It acts as an antimetabolite.

Mercurialentis. Brownish golden staining of the lens that occurs in workers exposed to elemental mercury for a year or more.

Mercuric chloride. B.P.C. 1968. $HgCl_2$. Corrosive sublimate. An antibacterial agent. Because of its toxicity, solutions for external use are coloured with indigo carmine. **Salicylic acid and mercurial chloride lotion,** B.P.C. 1968, a lotion used in the treatment of follicular infections.

Mercuric oxide, yellow. B.P.C. 1968. An antibacterial agent. In the form of **Mercuric oxide eye ointment,** B.P.C. 1968, it is used in the treatment of blepharitis and conjunctivitis.

Mercuric oxycyanide. B.P.C. 1968. An antibacterial agent.

Mercurophylline sodium. The B.P. Commission approved name for a mixture of the sodium salt of *N*-(3-hydroxymercuri-2-methoxypropyl) camphoramic acid and theophylline. An organic mercurial diuretic.

Mercury. A liquid metallic element. Quicksilver. Symbol Hg (L *hydrargum*). Atomic weight 200·59. Atomic number 80.

Mercury, ammoniated, B.P. 1968. White precipitate. A mild antiseptic.

-mere (Gk *meros:* part). Suffix meaning a part, or series of parts.

Merocrine. Pertaining to the type of secretion, or gland, in which the gland remains intact while forming its secretion.

Merozoite. The product of division of the schizont in Sporozoa, such as the Plasmodium of malaria.

Mersalyl acid. B.P. 1968. $C_{13}H_{17}HgNO_6$. An organic mercurial diuretic used in the form of **Mersalyl injection,** B.P. 1968, which contains 10 per cent of the sodium salt of mersalyl acid and 5 per cent of theophylline.

Mes-, Meso- (Gk *mesos:* middle). Prefixes meaning intermediate or middle.

Mesaortitis. Inflammation of the middle coat of the aorta.

Mesarteritis. Inflammation of the middle coat of an artery.

Mescaline. $C_{11}H_{17}NO_3$. An alkaloid isolated from the cactus, *Anhalonium lewinii,* which is a powerful hallucinogen.

Mesencephalon. The midbrain. It consists of the two *cerebral peduncles,* each of which is subdivided into the *crus cerebri* and the *tegmentum* by a barrier of pigmented grey matter, the *substantia nigra.* The tegmentum is traversed by the *cerebral aqueduct.* The portion of the tegmentum dorsal to the aqueduct is the *tectum* which comprises the four *colliculi.*

Mesenchyme. The embryonic connective tissue which gives rise to bone, cartilage, lymphatics, bloodvessels, and the connective tissues of the body.

Mesentery. A broad, fan-shaped fold of peritoneum connecting the coils of jejunum and ileum to the posterior abdominal wall.

Mesial. Median. Middle.

Mesmerism. The precursor of hypnotism.

Mesoappendix. A triangular fold of peritoneum which clothes the vermiform appendix, and is attached to the lower end of mesentery close to the ileocaecal junction.

Mesocolon. The fold of peritoneum attaching the colon to the posterior abdominal wall. **Sigmoid mesocolon,** the fold of peritoneum that attaches the sigmoid colon to the posterior abdominal wall. **Transverse mesocolon,** the broad fold of peritoneum that attaches the transverse colon to the posterior abdominal wall.

Mesoderm. The layer of the human embryo that gives origin, either directly or via the mesenchyme, to: all the connective and sclerous tissues; the teeth with the exception of the enamel; the musculature (striated and unstriated) with the exception of the musculature of the iris; the blood vascular and lymphatic systems; the urogenital system with the exception of the bladder, prostate and urethra; the cortex of the suprarenal glands, the mesothelial linings of the pericardial, pleural and peritoneal cavities.

Mesodiastole. In the middle of diastole.

Mesoduodenum. A fold of mesentery that connects the duodenum to the posterior abdominal wall in the foetus, and sometimes persists into later life.

Mesomorph. A person of medium height and stocky build.

Mesosalpinx. The part of the broad ligament encircling the uterine tube.

Mesosomes. Intracytoplasmic bodies of unknown function seen with the electron microscope in ultra-thin sections of some bacteria.

Mesotenon. The connective tissue sheath attaching a tendon to its fibrous sheath. Mesotendon. Mesotendineum.

Mesothelioma. A tumour of the pleura or peritoneum, that may be benign or malignant. The malignant form is one of the complications of asbestosis.

Mesothelium. The epithelial cells of mesodermal origin that line the serous cavities of the body.

Mesothorium. A disintegration product of thorium.

Mesovarium. The peritoneal fold that connects the anterior border of the ovary to the posterior layer of the broad ligament.

Mesterolone, The B.P. Commission approved name for 17β-hydroxy-1α-methyl-5α-ardrostan-3-one. An anabolic steroid.

Mestranol, B.P. 1968. $C_{21}H_{26}O_2$. An oestrogen.

Mesulphen, B.P.C. 1968. $C_{14}H_{12}S_{23}$. A preparation used in the treatment of scabies, pediculosis pubis, seborrhoea, and acne.

Meta- (Gk *meta:* after, between, over). Prefix indicating change, after, or next.

Metabolism. The chemical and physical changes, whereby the living lives, moves and has its being.

Metabolite. A substance produced by metabolism or by a metabolic process.

Metacarpal. Relating to the metacarpus.

Metacarpophalangeal. Pertaining to the metacarpus and the phalanges.

Metacarpus. The five bones of the hand connecting the carpus with the fingers. They are numbered from the lateral to the medial side.

Metacetamol. The B.P. Commission approved name for 3-acetamidophenol. An analgesic.

Metachromasia. The property exhibited by some tissue components of taking up certain dyes and so altering them that the colour is changed.

Metachromatic. Exhibiting metachromasia.

Metachromatin. The basophil element in chromatin.

Metagonimus. A genus of flukes. *Metagonimus yokogawai*, an intestinal parasite in the Far East acquired by eating undercooked or raw fish.

Metahexamide. The B.P. Commission approved name for *N*-(3-amino-4-methylbenzenesulphonyl)-*N'*-cyclohexylurea. A hypoglycaemic agent.

Metamere. One of the sections of paraxial mesoderm into which the vertebrate embryo is divided from the end of the third week.

Metamorphopsia. Distortion of objects seen: e.g. straight lines appear to be wavy.

Metamyelocyte. The primitive white cell intermediate between the myeloblast and the granulocyte.

Metanephros. The permanent embryonic kidney.

Metaphase. The stage of mitosis, or mitotic division, at which the chromosomes arrange themselves round the equator of the spindle.

Metaphysis. The part of the diaphysis of a long bone which lies immediately adjacent to the epiphyseal cartilage. It is the site of advancing ossification.

Metaphysitis. Inflammation of the metaphysis of a long bone.

Metaplasia. The change of one tissue into another in the adult, as, for example, occurs in certain tumours.

Metaraminol tartrate. B.P. 1968. $C_{13}H_{19}NO_8$. A sympathomimetic used in the treatment of hypotension.

Metastasis. The transfer of disease from one part of the body to another not directly connected with it, as occurs, for example, in the case of cancer. (*Plural:* metastases.)

Metatarsal. Relating to the metatarsus or a metatarsal bone.

Metatarsalgia. Pain in the foot.

Metatarsus. The five metatarsal bones in the distal part of the foot between the tarsus and the phalanges. They are numbered from the medial to the lateral side.

Metathalamus. The two geniculate bodies.

Metaxalone. The B.P. Commission approved name for 5-(3,5-xylyloxymethyl)oxazolidin-2-one. A muscle relaxant.

Metazoa. A subdivision of the animal kingdom that includes all multicellular animals whose cells become differentiated to form tissues.

Metazocine. The B.P. Commission approved name for 1,2,3,4,5,6-hexahydro-8-hydroxy-3, 6,11-trimethyl-2, 6-methano-3-benzazocine. A narcotic analgesic.

Metencephalon. The part of the hindbrain consisting of the pons, cerebellum and middle part of the fourth ventricle.

Meteorism. Distension of the gut by gas.

-meter (Gk *metron:* measure). Suffix indicating relationship to measurement, or an instrument for measurement.

Metformin hydrochloride. B.P. Addendum 1969. $C_4H_{11}N_5$, HCl. An oral hypoglycaemic agent.

Methacholine chloride, B.P.C. 1968. $C_8H_{18}ClNO_2$. A drug with the muscarinic actions of acetylcholine. It is used to terminate attacks of atrial paroxysmal tachycardia, and for the treatment of postoperative abdominal distension and urinary retention.

Methacycline hydrochloride. B.P. Addendum 1971. $C_{22}H_{22}N_2O_8$,HCl. A broad-spectrum antibiotic produced by chemical synthesis from oxytetracycline.

Methadone hydrochloride. B.P. 1968. $C_{21}H_{27}NO$,HCl. A narcotic analgesic.

Methadyl acetate. The B.P. Commission approved name for 6-dimethylamino-4, 4-diphenylheptan-3-ol. A narcotic analgesic.

Methaemalbumin. An abnormal blood pigment, in which haem is combined with plasma albumin. Its presence in the plasma may be an important sign of a haemolytic process.

Methaemoglobin. An oxidized form of haemoglobin in which the iron is in the ferric state, as opposed to the ferrous state in haemoglobin and oxyhaemoglobin.

Methaemoglobinaemia. A condition characterized by cyanosis, due to the presence of methaemoglobin in the circulating erythrocytes. The condition is usually drug induced—by one of the active derivatives, especially phenacetin.

Methaemoglobinuria. The presence of methaemoglobin in the urine.

Methallenoestril. B.P.C. 1968. $C_{18}H_{22}O_3$ A synthetic oestrogen.

Methallibure. The B.P. Commission approved name for *N*-methylthiocarbamoyl)- N´-(1-methylallylthiocarbamoyl)hydrazine. A drug that suppresses pituitary, ovarian, and adrenal function.

Methamphazone. The B.P. Commission approved name for 4-amino-6-methyl-2-phenyl-3-pyridazone. An analgesic and antirheumatic drug.

Methandienone. B.P. 1968. $C_{20}H_{28}O_2$. An anabolic steroid and weak androgen.

Methane. Marsh gas. A colourless, odourless gas that burns with a clear flame. It is produced by the decomposition of organic matter. Hence its popular name.

Methanol. Methyl alcohol.

Methanthelinium bromide. The B.P. Commission approved name for 2-diethylaminoethyl xanthen-9-carboxylate methobromide. An anticholinergic drug.

Methaphenilene. The B.P. Commission approved name for *N´N´*-dimethyl-*N*-phenyl-*N*-2-thenylethylenediamine. An antihistaminic.

Methapyrilene. The B.P. Commission approved name for *NN*-dimethyl-*N´*-(2 - pyridyl)-*N´*-(2-thenyl)ethylenediamine. An antihistaminic.

Methaqualone. B.P. Addendum 1969. $C_{16}H_{14}N_2O$. A hypnotic.

Metharbitone. The B.P. Commission approved name for 5,5-diethyl-1-methylbarbituric acid. An anticonvulsant.

Methazolamide. The B.P. Commission approved name for 5-acetylamino-4-methyl-1,3,4-thiadiazoline -2- sulphonamide. A carbonic anhydrase inhibitor.

Methdilazine. The B.P. Commission approved name for 10-1-methylpyrrolidin-3-ylmethyl) phenothiazine. An antihistaminic and an antipruritic.

Methenolone. The B.P. Commission approved name for 17β-hydroxy-1-methyl-5a-androst-1-en-3-one. An anabolic steroid.

Methicillin sodium, B.P. 1968. A semisynthetic penicillin which is not destroyed by staphylococcal penicillinase. It is, however, destroyed by acid and must therefore be given parenterally.

Methimazole. The B.P. Commission approved name for 2-mercapto-1-methylimidazole. An antithyroid drug.

Methiodal sodium. The B.P. Commission approved name for sodium iodomethanesulphonate. A radioopaque substance.

Methionine. One of the essential amino-acids.

Methisazone. The B.P. Commission approved name for 1-methylindoline-2, 3-dione 3-thiosemicarbazone. An antiviral drug.

Methixene. The B.P. Commission approved name for 9-(1-methyl-3-piperidylmethyl) thiaxanthen. An antiparkinsonian drug.

Methocarbamol. The B.P. Commission approved name for 2-hydroxy-3-(2-

methoxyphenoxy)propyl carbamate. A muscle relaxant.

Methohexitone injection. B.P. 1968. A sterile solution of a mixture of 100 parts by weight of the mono-sodium salt of methohexitone and six parts by weight of dried sodium carbonate. It is an intravenous general anaesthetic of short duration.

Methoin. B.P. 1968. $C_{12}H_{14}N_2O_2$. An anticonvulsant used in the treatment of grand mal.

Methoserpidine. B.P. 1968. $C_3H_{40}N_2O_9$. A hypotensive agent.

Methotrexate. B.P. Addendum 1969. A mixture of 4-amino-10-methylfolic acid and related substances. A cytotoxic agent used in the treatment of neoplastic disease and as an immunosuppressant.

Methotrimeprazine. The B.P. Commission approved name for 10-(3-dimethylamino-2- methylpropyl) -2 - methoxyphenothiazine. A tranquillizer.

Methoxamine hydrochloride. B.P.C. 1968. $C_{11}H_{18}ClNO_3$. A synthetic sympathomimetic amine administered intramuscularly in the treatment of hypotensive states such as postoperative shock.

Methoxyflurane. B.P. 1968. $C_3H_4Cl_2F_2O$. A volatile general anaesthetic.

Methoxyphenamine. The B.P. Commission approved name for 1-(2-methoxyphenyl)-2-methylaminopropane. A bronchodilator.

Methsuximide. The B.P. Commission approved name for N,2-dimethyl-2-phenylsuccinimide. An anticonvulsant.

Methyclothiazide. The B.P. Commission approved name for 6-chloro-3-chloromethyl-3, 4-dihydro-2-methyl-1, 2,4 - benzothiadiazine-7-sulphonamide 1,1-dioxide. A diuretic.

Methyl. The monovalent, organic radical, $CH_3—$.

Methyl alcohol. CH_3OH. A widely used industrial solvent. When ingested it is highly toxic, causing blindness. Also known as wood alcohol.

Methylamphetamine hydrochloride. B.P. 1968, $C_{10}H_{16}ClN$. A sympathomimetic used with care, as a central nervous system stimulant.

Methylated spirit, industrial. B.P.C. 1968. A mixture of 19 volumes of alcohol (95 per cent) with 1 volume of approved wood naphtha. Used externally for its astringent action.

Methylation. The process of substituting a methyl group for a hydrogen atom.

Methylbenzethonium chloride. The B.P

Commission approved name for benzyldimethyl-2-{2-[4-(1,1,3,3-tetramethylbutyl) - tolyloxy]ethoxy} ethylammonium chloride. An anti-infective agent.

Methylcellulose. B.P.C. 1968. A methyl ether of cellulose. The name, 'methylcellulose', is followed by a number indicating the approximate viscosity of a 2 per cent solution. Thus **Methylcellulose 450,** B.P. 1968, is a laxative.

Methylchromone. The B.P. Commission approved name for 2-methylchromone. A coronary vasodilator.

Methyl cysteine. The B.P. Commission approved name for methyl 2-amino-3-mercaptopropionate. A vasoconstrictor.

Methyldesorphine. The B.P. Commission approved name for 6-methyl- $\triangle^6$-deoxymorphine. A narcotic analgesic.

Methyldopa. B.P. 1968, $C_{10}H_{13}NO_4$, $1\frac{1}{2}$ H_2O. A hypotensive agent.

Methyldopate. The B.P. Commission approved name for $(-)$-3-(3, 4-dihydroxyphenyl) - 2 - methylalanine ethyl ester. A hypotensive drug.

Methylene. The radical, CH_2.

Methylene blue. B.P. 1968, $C_{16}H_{18}ClN_3S$, $2H_2O$. A weak antiseptic. Also used in the treatment of methaemoglobinaemia, and as a renal function test.

Methylergometrine maleate. B.P. 1968, $C_{24}H_{29}N_3O_6$. A uterine stimulant.

Methyl hydroxybenzoate. B.P. 1968. $C_8H_8O_3$. A preservative.

Methylpentynol. B.P.C. 1968, $C_6H_{10}O$. A short-acting hypnotic.

Methylphenidate. The B.P. Commission approved name for methyl a-phenyl-a-2-piperidylacetate. A central nervous system stimulant.

Methylprednisolone. B.P. 1968. $C_{22}H_{30}O_5$. A corticosteroid with the same action as prednisone, but at a lower dosage.

Methyl salicylate. B.P. 1968. $C_8H_8O_3$. A counter-irritant.

Methyltestosterone. B.P. 1968. $C_{20}H_{30}O_2$. An androgen which is active when taken by mouth.

Methylthiouracil. B.P. 1968. $C_5H_6N_2OS$. An antithyroid drug.

Methyprylone. B.P. 1968. $C_{10}H_{17}NO_2$. A hypnotic and sedative.

Methysergide. The B.P. Commission approved name for N-1-(hydroxymethyl)propyl - 1 - methyl - $(+)$-lysergamide. A drug used in the treatment of migraine.

Metoclopramide. The B.P. Commission approved name for 4-amino-5-chloro-N-(2-diethylaminoethyl)-2-methoxy-benzamide. An antiemetic.

Metofoline. The B.P. Commission approved name for 1-(4-chlorophenhyl)-1,2,3,4-tetrahydro-6,7-dimethoxy-2-methylisoquinoline. An analgesic.

Metolazone. The B.P. Commission approved name for 7-chloro-1,2,3,4-tetrahydro-2-methyl-4-oxo-3-o-tolyl-6-quinazolinesulphonamide. A diuretic.

Metopimazine. The B.P. Commission approved name for 10-3[3-(4-carbamoylpiperidine)propyl]-2-methanesulphonylphenothiazine. An antiemetic.

Metopon. The B.P. Commission approved name for 7,8-dihydro-5-methylmorphinone. A narcotic analgesic.

Metra-, Metro- (Gk *metra:* uterus). Prefixes meaning the uterus.

Metralgia. Pain in the uterus.

Metre. The length equal to 1,650,763·73 wave-lengths in vacuum of the radiation corresponding to the transition between the levels $2p_{10}$ and $5d_5$ of the krypton-86 atom. It is equivalent to 39·37 inches. (*Abbreviation:* m.)

Metritis. Inflammation of the uterus.

Metromalacia. Pathological softening of the uterus.

Metronidazole. B.P. 1968. $C_6H_9N_3O_3$. A trichomonacide.

Metropathia haemorrhagica. Essential uterine haemorrhage.

Metrorrhagia. Bleeding from the uterus independent of the menstrual cycle.

-metry (Gk *metrein:* to measure). Suffix indicating measurement or measuring.

Metyrapone. B.P. Addendum 1971. $C_{14}H_{14}N_2O$. An adrenocortical enzyme inhibitor.

Metyzoline. The B.P. Commission approved name for 2-(2-methylbenzo[*b*] thien-3-yl) methyl-2-imidazoline. A vasoconstrictor.

Mexenone. B.P.C. Supplement 1971. $C_{15}H_{14}O_3$. A preparation that absorbs ultraviolet radiation over a wide range, and is therefore used as a sun-screening preparation.

Miasma. A noxious effluvium.

Mica. A mineral occurring in scales, and composed of the hydrated silicate of aluminium with silicates of other minerals. Used as an insulator and lubricant.

Micelle. A multimolecular structure having the hydrophilic parts of the constituent molecules at the surface and in contact with water, while the hydrophobic parts are in the interior in a milieu of other hydrophobic groups.

Micr-, Micro- (Gk *mikros:* small). Prefixes meaning small, or one-millionth part.

Microaerophilic. Growing best in a trace only of free oxygen, as in the case of certain bacteria.

Micro-aneurysm. A small aneurysm, such as is found in vascular retinopathy.

Microangiopathy. Disease of the capillaries. **Thrombotic angiopathy**, a disease characterized by thrombocytopenia, haemolytic anaemia, transitory focal neurological symptoms, and renal involvement leading to uraemia.

Microbe. A minute, unicellular living organism.

Microbial. Pertaining to a microbe or microbes.

Microbiology. The study of microorganisms.

Microblast. A small erythroblast.

Microblepharon. The condition in which the eyelids are abnormally small.

Microcapsule. The very fine capsule surrounding some bacteria that can only be detected by electron microscopy or indirect serological means.

Microcephaly. Abnormal smallness of the head.

Microcheilia. Abnormally small lips.

Microcheiria. Abnormal smallness of the hands.

Micrococcaceae. The family of Eubacteriae that includes the Micrococcus, Staphylococcus, Gaffkya, and Sarcina. The cells are spherical and gram-positive.

Micrococcus. A genus of the family Micrococcaceae, comprising only non-pathogenic species. (*Plural:* micrococci.) *Micrococcus ureae*, a contaminant in urine that converts urea to ammonium carbonate.

Microconidium. A small unicellular spore produced by the dermatophyte fungi in artificial culture. (*Plural:* microconidia.)

Micro-culture. The method of growing micro-organisms whereby their growth can be watched under a microscope.

Microcurie. One-millionth of a curie.

Microcyte. A small red blood corpuscle.

Microcytosis. The form of anaemia characterized by an excess of microcytes in the circulating blood.

Microdactyly. Abnormally small digits.

Microdontic. Having abnormally small teeth.

Microdrepanocytic anaemia. The disease resulting from the double heterozygous inheritance of the sickle-cell and thalassaemic states.

Micro-electrode. An electrode of very fine calibre, as used in physiological investigations.

Micro-electrophoresis. Electrophoresis of very small amounts of solutions.

Microfilaria. The uncoiled embryo of a filarial worm.

Microgamete. The male gamete of the malarial plasmodium.

Microgametocyte. The male gametocyte.

Microglia. The neuroglia of mesodermal origin. **Microglial cells,** small, amoeboid, phagocytic cells scattered about the central nervous system, particularly the grey matter.

Microglossia. Smallness of the tongue.

Microgram. One-thousandth part of a milligram. (*Abbreviation:* μg; mcg. in prescriptions.)

Micrographia. Smallness of an individual's writing compared with what it used to be.

Microgyria. Abnormal smallness of the gyri of the brain.

Micro-iontophoresis. The procedure whereby the sensitivity of individual neurones to putative transmitter substances can be investigated.

Micro-lens. Contact lens.

Microlitre. One-thousandth part of a millilitre.

Micromanipulation. The investigational technique based on the use of micropipettes, micro-electrodes and the like, for the minute investigation of body function.

Micromastia. Abnormal smallness of the breasts.

Micromelia. Abnormally small arms and legs.

Micrometer. An instrument, usually in conjunction with a microscope, to measure very small objects or to measure to a fine degree.

Micrometre. One-thousandth part of a millimetre. (*Abbreviation:* μm.) Micron.

Micron. Micrometre.

Micropipette. A pipette for the measurement of very small volumes.

Micropodia. Abnormal smallness of the feet.

Micropsia. The state in which objects appear smaller than they are.

Micropuncture. The term applied to an investigational technique whereby very fine pipettes, small enough to be inserted into a glomerulus, for example, can be used to obtain samples for analysis.

Micropyle. A minute canal or pore in the ovum in certain species, through which the spermatozoa gain entry

Microscope. An instrument for magnifying objects. **Binocular microscope,** a microscope with an eyepiece for each eye but a single object. **Electron microscope,** a visual and photographic microscope, in which electrons with a wave-length of $1/20$ of an Ångström unit (100,000 times shorter than that of ordinary light) are used, thus giving a magnification of up to 100,000, which can be enlarged photographically to a magnification of 1 million. **Interference microscope,** a microscope for examining viable cells, in which the light from a single source is split, so that one part of the beam passes through the specimen and the other bypasses it. The two beams are then recombined before entering the objective lens. **Phase contrast microscope,** a microscope for the study of living cells, which alters the phase relationships of the light passing through the object and that passing round it.

Microscopy. The use of the microscope. **Dark-ground microscopy,** the method of examining delicate micro-organisms, such as spirochaetes, by oblique rays which only reach the eye of the observer when scattered by objects, such as spirochaetes of different refractive index from the medium in which they are suspended. **Fluorescence microscopy,** the method of microscopy in which a fluorescent dye is used as a stain, and examination then carried out by ultraviolet light.

Microsome. One of the fine granules in the cytoplasm of the cell.

Microsporum. A genus of *Fungi imperfecti.* One of the three genera responsible for ringworm. *Microsporum audouini,* the commonest cause of ringworm in children. *Microsporum canis,* a fungus that affects cats and dogs. *Microsporum equinium,* a fungus that affects horses. *Microsporum gypseus,* a fungus found in the soil that may infect animals and man.

Microtatobiotes. The class of micro-organisms that includes the two orders of Rickettsiales and Virales—the smallest of all living organisms.

Microthelia. Abnormal smallness of the nipples.

Microtome. An instrument for cutting sections for microscopy. **Freezing microtome,** a microtome for cutting frozen sections. **Rocking microtome,** a microtome for the cutting of serial sections.

Microtonometer. An apparatus for measuring the oxygen and carbon-dioxide tension in the blood.

Microvillus. One of the projections covered with cell membrane, and detectable by electron microscopy, which are found in certain forms of epithelium, as in the small intestine, kidneys and thyroid, as a device to increase the surface area of the cells. (*Plural:* microvilli.)

Microvolt. One-millionth of a volt.

Micturition. The act of voiding urine. Urination.

Mid- (OE *midd:* middle). Prefix meaning middle.

Midbrain. Mesencephalon.

Midge. The smallest of the blood-sucking Diptera.

Midgut. The portion of the embryonic alimentary tract that gives rise to the distal half of the duodenum, the jejunum, ileum, caecum, appendix, ascending colon and part of the transverse colon.

Midriff. The diaphragm.

Midwife. A person who is qualified to supervise women in childbirth.

Migraine. A condition characterized by recurring unilateral, frontal, or temporal headaches, accompanied by visual disturbances known as fortification figures, and nausea and/or vomiting.

Mikamycin. The B.P. Commission approved name for an antibiotic produced by *Streptomyces mitakaensis.*

Miliaria. The eruption resulting from blockage of the sweat ducts by a keratotic plug. **Miliaria crystallina,** the crop of minute glassy vericles occurring in acute febrile illnesses, and due to blockage at the orifice of the ducts. **Miliaria rubra,** the widespread, irritating, papular vesicular eruption that tends to accompany heavy sweating in Europeans in the tropics. Prickly heat.

Miliary. The size of a millet seed. **Miliary tuberculosis,** the form of acute tuberculosis in which the tubercles, the size of millet seeds, are scattered throughout the lungs and other parts of the body.

Milium. A small whitish nodule in skin, usually the face. (*Plural:* milia.)

Milk. The whitish fluid secreted by the mammary gland for the feeding of the young. **Human milk** contains 6·8g./100ml. carbohydrate, 1·5g./100ml. protein, 4g./100ml. fat, 30mg./100ml. calcium, 15mg./100ml. phosphorus, but only 0·1 to 0·2mg./100ml. iron. It also contains vitamins A, D, and C, thiamine, riboflavine and nicotinic acid. **Cow's milk** contains less carbohydrate (5g. per 100ml.), more protein (3·5g./110ml.), approximately the same amount of fat (3·5g./110ml.), more calcium (120mg./100ml.) and phosphorus (110mg./100ml.), approximately the same amount of vitamins A and D, more thiamine, and riboflavine, and less nicotinic acid and vitamin C. **Condensed milk,** milk concentrated *in vacuo* at low temperature, and then sterilized by heat at a temperature of 105°C. There are three varieties of condensed milk: whole milk unsweetened; whole milk sweetened; and skimmed milk sweetened. **Dried milk,** milk prepared by evaporating all the fluid, so that the milk is reduced to the form of a powder. **Evaporated milk,** unsweetened condensed milk. **Heat-treated milk,** the official category in England and Wales and Scotland of milk which has been pasteurized, sterilized or ultra-treated. **Homogenized milk,** milk in which the fat globules have been ruptured under high pressure so that the fat is evenly distributed throughout the milk and will not rise as cream. **Pasteurized milk,** milk that has been treated in one of two ways: (*a*) retained at a temperature of 63° to 65·5°C for at least half-an-hour and then immediately cooled to a temperature of not more than 10°C; (*b*) milk which has been retained at a temperature of not less than 71·7°C. for at least 15 seconds and then immediately cooled to a temperature of not more than 10°C. **Peptonized milk,** milk that has been treated with peptonizing powder. **Premium milk,** untreated milk in Scotland. **Roller-dried milk,** milk prepared by spreading a thin film of milk over steam-heated revolving cylinders. **Spray-dried milk,** milk powder prepared by forcing a fine spray of milk into a heated chamber where drying is almost instantaneous. **Standard milk,** untreated milk in Scotland. **Sterilized milk,** one of the official categories of heat-treated milk in England and Wales and Scotland. It is milk that has been filtered or clarified, homogenized, and then, in bottles, heated to, and maintained at, a temperature of at least 100°C. for a prescribed period. **Ultra-heat-treated milk**, one of the official categories of heat-treated milk in England and Wales and Scotland. It is milk which has been retained at a temperature of at least 132°C. for not less than one second. **Untreated milk**, one of the official categories of milk in England and Wales and Scotland. In Scotland it is also known as Premium or Standard milk.

Milli- (L *mille:* one thousand). Prefix signifying one-thousandth part.

Milliampere. One-thousandth of an ampere.

Millicurie. One-thousandth of a curie, which represents the quantity of radium emanation in equilibrium with one milligram of radium element.

Milliequivalent. The number of grammes of a substance contained in one millilitre of a normal solution. (*Abbreviation:* mEq.)

Milligram. One-thousandth of a gramme. (*Abbreviation:* mg.)

Millilitre. One-thousandth of a litre. (*Abbreviation:* ml.)

Millimetre. One-thousandth of a metre. (*Abbreviation:* mm.)

Millimicron. One-thousandth of a micron. Nanometre. (*Abbreviation:* mμ.)

Millimole. One-thousandth of a mole. (*Abbreviation:* mmol.)

Milliosmole. One-thousandth of an osmole. (*Abbreviation:* mosmol.)

Millirad. One-thousandth of a rad. (*Abbreviation:* mrad.)

Millivolt. One-thousandth of a volt. (*Abbreviation:* mV.)

Minepentate. The B.P. Commission approved name for 2-(2-dimethyl-aminoethoxy)ethyl 1-phenyl-cyclopentanecarboxylate. An anti-parkinsonian drug.

Mineralocorticoid. A corticoid that influences salt (sodium and potassium) metabolism.

Minim. One-sixtieth of one fluid drachm. The volume at 16·7°C of 0·91146 grain of water.

Mio- (Gk *meion:* less). Prefix signifying less or decreasing.

Miosis. Abnormal contraction of the pupil of the eye.

Miotic. An agent that contracts the

pupil of the eye. Causing the pupil to contract.

Miracidium. The free-swimming larva of a trematode. (*Plural:* miracidia.)

Miscarriage. Abortion. Premature expulsion of the fertilized ovum before the foetus is viable: i.e. before the 28th week of pregnancy.

Miscegenation. Interbreeding between races, particularly black and white.

Miscible. Capable of being mixed.

Miso- (Gk *misein:* to hate). Prefix meaning hatred.

Mithramycin. The B.P. Commission approved name for an antibiotic derived from *Streptomyces argillaceus*, *Streptomyces plicatus* and *Streptomyces tanashiensis*, which has a cytotoxic action and is used as an antineoplastic drug.

Mitis. Mild.

Mito- (Gk *mitos:* thread). Prefix signifying a thread or thread-like structure.

Mitobronitol. The B.P. Commission approved name for 1,6-dibromo-1, 6-dideoxy-D-mannitol. An antineoplastic agent.

Mitochondria. Thread-like bodies (0·5 to 5μ by 0·3 to 0·7μ) in the cytoplasm of the cell, which are the 'power plant of the cell'. (*Singular:* mitochondrion.)

Mitoclomine. The B.P. Commission approved name for *NN*-di-(2-chloroethyl)- 4 -methoxy- 3 -methyl-1-naphthylamine. An antineoplastic agent.

Mitogenic. Causing cell division, or mitosis.

Mitomycin C. A cytotoxic antibiotic derived from *Streptomyces caespitosus*, which is used in the treatment of certain neoplastic conditions.

Mitopodozide. The B.P. Commission approved name for *N'*-ethylpodophyllohydrazide. An antineoplastic agent.

Mitosis. The common method of cell division in higher animals, characterized by a series of complex changes in the nucleus, leading to its subdivision, and followed by cleavage of the cell cytoplasm. Karyokinesis.

Mitotenamine. The B.P. Commission approved name for 5-bromo-3-[*N*-(2-chloroethyl) ethylaminomethyl]-benzo[*b*]thiophen. An antineoplastic agent.

Mitral. Shaped like a mitre. **Mitral incompetence**, functional or organic widening of the mitral valve. **Mitral stenosis**, pathological narrowing of the mitral valve. **Mitral valve, the**

atrioventricular valve separating the left atrium and the left ventricle.

Mittelschmerz. Intermenstrual pain.

Modality. A form of sensation. (*Plural:* modalities.) Touch, warmth, cold and pain are the four 'modalities' of cutaneous sensation.

Modiolus. The conical-shaped central axis of the cochlea.

Mogi- (Gk *mogis:* with difficulty). Prefix signifying with difficulty, difficult.

Mogigraphia. Writer's cramp.

Molar. Pertaining to moles. Grinding. **Molar solution,** a solution containing 1 mole of solute per litre. **Molar teeth,** the terminal three permanent teeth on each side of each jaw.

Molarity. The number of moles of a solute per litre of solution.

Mole. A localized aggregation of naevus cells. A degenerative mass in the uterus. The amount of substance of a system which contains as many elementary units as there are carbon atoms in 12 grammes of ^{12}C. **Carneous mole,** an ovum which has been destroyed by multiple haemorrhages between the decidua and chorion during the first twelve weeks of pregnancy. **Hairy mole,** a mole incorporating coarse, dark hairs, present at birth. **Hydatidiform mole,** an ovum that has undergone changes in the chorionic villi resulting in the formation of a mass of vesicles. **Junction mole,** a mole developing at a dermo-epidermal junction, which appears in childhood. **Tubal mole,** a carneous mole occurring in the uterine tube. **Vesicular mole,** hydatiform mole.

Molecular. Pertaining to a molecule. **Molecular weight,** the sum of the weights of the atoms constituting a molecule.

Molecule. The smallest combination of two or more atoms that can exist independently and maintain its characteristics.

Mollities. Softness or softening. **Mollities ossium,** osteomalacia.

Mollusca. The phylum of Metazoa that includes snails.

Molluscum. A disease characterized by soft rounded tumours in the skin. **Molluscum contagiosum,** a virus infection of the skin, characterized by small, pearly white epithelial tumours. **Molluscum fibrosum,** a form of von Recklinghausen's disease or neurofibromatosis. **Molluscum sebaceum,** Keratoacanthoma.

Molybdenum. A metallic element.

Symbol Mo. Atomic weight 95·94. Atomic number 42.

Mon-, Mono- (Gk *monos:* single). Prefixes meaning single, one, alone.

Monaural. Pertaining to one ear.

Monaxial. Having one axon.

Mongolism. The congenital form of mental subnormality, due to chromosomal abnormality, and associated with characteristic physical defects: Mongolian-like eyes, a snub nose, high cheek bones, a large tongue, a small round skull, short thick hands and feet, and a characteristic palm print. Down's syndrome (or disease).

Monilethrix. A disorder of hair in which the hairs appear beaded and constricted at intervals, and are fragile.

Monilia. Candida.

Moniliasis. Candidiasis.

Monoamine. A substance derived from ammonia by the substitution of a hydrocarbon radical in each molecule for all or part of the hydrogen. **Monoamine oxidase,** an enzyme that catalyses the oxidative deamination of monoamines, such as adrenaline and noradrenaline, to the corresponding carboxylic acids.

Mono-arthritis. Arthritis involving only one joint.

Monoblast. The precursor of the monocyte.

Monocephalus. A foetal monster with two conjoined bodies but only one head.

Monochromat. A colour-blind subject who is unable to distinguish any colours at all.

Monocistronic. Pertaining to one gene. **Monocistronic messenger,** a mRNA (messenger ribonucleic acid) molecule that programmes the synthesis of one protein.

Monocular. Pertaining to one eye. Having only one eyepiece.

Monocyclic. Involving one cycle.

Monocyte. The largest of the leucocytes, with an eccentric nucleus and bluish staining cytoplasm. There are up to 800 per c. mm. of blood.

Monocytosis. An increase in the monocytes in the circulating blood above 800 per c. mm. Mononucleosis.

Monodactylism. A congenital condition in which there is only one finger or one toe on the hand or foot.

Monoiodotyrosine. One of the iodine-containing derivatives of tyrosine obtained on the hydrolysis of thyroglobulin, the characteristic protein of the colloid in the thyroid gland.

Monomania. A form of partial insanity,

in which the mental disturbance involves only one subject.

Mononeuritis. Inflammation of a single nerve.

Mononuclear. Having only one nucleus.

Mononucleosis. Monocytosis. Glandular fever.

Mononucleotide. A unit in the structure of nucleic acids. It consists of a purine or pyrimidine base linked to a pentose sugar which in turn is esterified with phosphoric acid.

Monophasic. Unidirectional.

Monophobia. Fear of being alone.

Monophyletic. Of common origin. Descended from a single cell type.

Monoplegia. Paralysis of one limb.

Monorchism. Absence of one testis from the scrotum.

Monosaccharide. A simple sugar that cannot be further hydrolysed. Glucose, galactose, fructose and mannose are monosaccharides.

Monostearin, self-emulsifying. B.P.C. 1968. A mixture of esters of stearic and palmitic acids, with small amounts of the corresponding esters of oleic and other fatty acids, which is used as an emulsifying agent.

Monosynaptic. Pertaining to one synapse, or involving only one synapse.

Monotropic. Affecting only one species or one variety of tissue.

Mons. (*Plural:* montes.) A mound. **Mons pubis,** the rounded eminence in front of the symphysis pubis in women.

Mood. A state of mind or emotion.

Moraxella. A genus of the family Brucellaceae, consisting of gram-negative, rod-shaped organisms. They occur most commonly in infections of the eye in the form of *Moraxella lacunata* and *Moraxella liquefaciens* (Morax-Axenfeld bacillus.)

Morazone. The B.P. Commission approved name for 2, 3-dimethyl-4-(3-methyl-2-phenylmorpholinomethyl)-1-phenyl-5-pyrazolone. An analgesic.

Morbid. Diseased. Pathological.

Morbidity. The state of disease in the community.

Morbific. Disease producing.

Morbilli. Measles.

Morbilliform. Resembling measles.

Morbus. A disease.

Mordant. A substance that makes fast a dye, as in staining tissues or bacteria.

Moribund. In the state of dying.

Moron. A feeble-minded person whose 'mental age' is between 8 and 12 years.

Moroxydine. The B.P. Commission

approved name for *N*-(guanidinoformimidoyl)morpholine. An antiviral agent.

Morpheme. A sequence of phonemes. Morphemes are put together to make words.

Morpheridine. The B.P. Commission approved name for ethyl 1-(2-morpholinoethyl)-4-phenylpiperidine-4-carboxylate. A narcotic analgesic.

Morphine hydrochloride. B.P. 1968. $C_{17}H_{20}ClNO_3,3H_2O$. The hydrochloride of morphine, the principal alkaloid of opium, which is a powerful analgesic and narcotic, characterized by the rapid development of dependence and habituation.

Morphine sulphate. B.P. 1968. $(C_{17}H_{19}NO_3)_2,H_2SO_4,5H_2O$. A powerful narcotic analgesic with the same action and undesirable effects as morphine hydrochloride.

Morpho- (Gk *morphē:* form). Prefix indicating relationship to form.

Morphoea. A localized or circumscribed form of scleroderma.

Morphology. That branch of science dealing with structure and form.

-morphous (Gk *morphē:* form). Suffix indicating relationship to form.

Mortality. The state of being mortal. The death rate or mortality rate. **Infant mortality rate,** deaths in infants under 1 year of age registered in a year and expressed as rate per 1000 live births. **Maternal mortality rate,** deaths per 1000 births (live and still) resulting from viable pregnancies (i.e. of not less than 28 weeks duration). **Mortality rate,** or **Death rate,** number of deaths registered in a year, expressed as rate per 1000 of population. This is usually referred to as the crude death (or mortality) rate. It is being partially replaced by the **Standardized Mortality Ratio (S.M.R.),** the number of deaths in a given year expressed as a percentage of those anticipated in that year if mortality (by age and sex) of the standard period (1950–1952) had operated on the population of sex and age structure of the year in question. **Neonatal mortality rate,** the ratio of deaths among new-born infants under 4 weeks of age per 1000 live births. **Perinatal mortality rate,** the number of stillbirths and of deaths in the first week of life per 1000 births (live and still).

Mortification. Gangrene.

Mortuary. A building in which the dead are placed awaiting burial or disposal.

Morula. The mass of cells formed by

repeated division and subdivision of the blastomeres following fertilization of the ovum.

Mosquito. A fly of the subfamily Culicinae.

Motion. Movement. The process of changing position. **Motion sickness,** the nausea and/or vomiting induced by travel, whether by land, sea, or air.

Motoneurone. A neurone with a motor function.

Mould. A filamentous or mycelial fungus that grows as long filaments (hyphae) which branch and interlace to form a meshwork (mycelium), and reproduces by the formation of various kinds of spores. A shaped receptacle for producing a given shape or size.

Mouth. An opening or aperture. The proximal opening of the alimentary canal, bounded externally by the lips and cheeks, and internally by the gums and teeth.

Mouth-wash. An aqueous solution of substances with antiseptic, local analgesic, or astringent properties. Collutorium. There are two in the *British Pharmaceutical Codex,* 1968: sodium chloride mouth-wash, compound; zinc sulphate and zinc chloride mouth-wash. **Mouth-wash solution tablets,** B.P.C. 1968, a tablet containing sodium bicarbonate, tartaric acid, sodium benzoate, amaranth, menthol, thymol, saccharin, eucalyptus oil and lemon oil.

Movement. The act of moving. **Accessory movements,** movements of joints which cannot be produced voluntarily, but can be produced (*a*) where resistance is encountered to active movements, or (*b*) only passively. **Active movement,** movement produced by one's own muscles. **Amoeboid movement,** the movement of an amoeba produced by protusion of pseudopodia. **Athetoid movements,** repeated deliberate movements of a purposeless character. **Brownian movement,** the dancing movement of particles in a liquid. **Choreiform movements,** irregular, jerky, purposeless movements of a muscle or group of muscles. **Circus movement,** the continuous movement in a circle that occurs, for example, in atrial fibrillation. **Foetal movements,** the movements of the foetus, usually first felt around the eighteenth week of pregnancy. **Passive movement,** movement perpetuated by an outside force. **Reflex movement,** an involuntary movement resulting from a sensory stimulus. **Saccadic movement,** the quick movement of the eyes over a given space while reading a line of print.

Muc-, Muco- (L *mucus:* mucus). Prefixes indicating relationship to mucus.

Mucid. Mucilaginous.

Mucilage. An aqueous viscid solution, or partial solution, of gum used for suspending insoluble substances.

Mucilaginous. Resembling mucilage. Viscid, slimy, sticky.

Mucin. The glycoprotein that forms the basis of mucus.

Mucinase. An enzyme that hydrolyses mucin.

Mucinogen. The precursor of mucus.

Mucocele. A cyst or dilated cavity containing an accumulation of mucus.

Mucoid. Resembling mucus.

Mucolytic. Possessing the property of destroying mucus.

Mucomembranous. Relating to mucous membrane. **Mucomembranous colic,** irritable colon. The condition evoked by anxiety in nervous individuals, and characterized by painful spasm of the colon.

Mucopolysaccharide. A complex macromolecular substance built up of units which include amino sugars and uronic acids.

Mucoprotein. A glycoprotein in which a protein is conjugated with a polysaccharide.

Mucopurulent. Containing mucoid material and pus.

Mucor. A genus of the class Phycomycetes, which forms delicate white tubular filaments.

Mucormycosis. A chronic fungous infection of the lungs, which may spread to other organs, caused by certain species of Mucor, and liable to occur in patients suffering from diabetes mellitus and other debilitating diseases.

Mucosa. Mucous membrane.

Mucosal. Pertaining to a mucus membrane.

Mucosanguineous. Containing mucus and blood.

Mucous. Pertaining to mucus.

Mucoviscidosis. Fibrocystic disease of the pancreas.

Mucus. The viscid secretion of mucous membrane.

Muliebrity. The state of being a woman.

Multi- (L *multus:* many, much). Prefix meaning many or much.

Multifocal. Pertaining to more than one focus.

Multigravida. A woman who is bearing her second or subsequent child.

Multipara. A woman who has borne two or more children.

Mummification. Dehydration of the body tissues.

Mumps. A virus infection involving primarily the parotid glands. Epidemic parotitis.

Mural. Referring to, or occurring in, the wall of a cavity.

Murine. Pertaining to rodents.

Murmur. A sound of varying intensity, pitch and character heard on auscultation over the heart. **Aortic murmur,** a murmur produced at the aortic valve. **Apical murmur,** a murmur heard maximally at the apex of the heart. **Austin Flint murmur,** the diastolic murmur occasionally heard at the apex of the heart in some cases of aortic incompetence. **Cardiorespiratory murmur,** a murmur produced by some physical interaction between the heart and the lungs. **Diastolic murmur,** a murmur heard during cardiac diastole. **Graham-Steell murmur,** a soft diastolic murmur heard in the pulmonary area, resulting from relative pulmonary incompetence. **Haemic murmur,** a systolic murmur heard in certain anaemic states in the absence of any heart disease. **Machinery murmur,** the continuous, rumbling murmur of patent ductus arteriosus. **Mitral murmur,** a murmur at the mitral valve. **Presystolic murmur,** a murmur heard immediately before the onset of cardiac systole. **Pulmonary murmur,** a murmur produced at the pulmonary area. **Systolic murmur,** a murmur heard during cardiac systole. **To-and-fro murmur,** a murmur heard during systole and diastole of the heart. **Tricuspid murmur,** a murmur produced at the tricuspid valve.

Muscae volitantes. Black specks floating before the eyes, and commonly seen by normal persons in favourable conditions. They are opacities of various kinds, such as minute specks in the vitreous.

Muscarine. The highly toxic alkaloid in *Amanita muscaria*, which has an acetylcholine-like action.

Muscle. Muscular tissue. Tissue which is involved with the property of contractility. A prescribed collection of muscle tissue. **Antagonist muscle,** one acting in opposition to, but in coordination with, another: e.g. the biceps and the triceps; the former contracts to flex the elbow and at the same time the triceps relaxes. Conversely, when the triceps contracts to extend the elbow, the biceps relaxes. **Bicipital muscle,** a muscle with two heads of origin. **Bipennate muscle,** a muscle whose fibres are inserted on two sides of a central tendon. **Cardiac muscle,** muscle of the heart. **Fixation muscle,** a muscle that fixes a joint in order to ensure that certain movements of it are carried out efficiently. **Fusiform muscle,** a spindle-shaped muscle. **Involuntary muscle,** unstriped muscle. **Multipennate muscle,** a muscle, such as the deltoid, in which a number of extensions pass upwards into the muscle from its tendon of insertion. **Plain muscle,** unstriped muscle. **Quadrilateral muscle,** a quadrilateral-shaped muscle, in which the fibres run parallel. **Red muscle,** muscle which appears red in the fresh state, due to the presence of the pigment myohaemoglobin in large amounts. **Smooth muscle,** unstriped muscle. **Striated muscle,** striped muscle. **Striped muscle,** muscle consisting of fibres which have a striated appearance in transmitted light, and which constitutes skeletal muscle under the control of the will. **Synergic muscle,** muscle which acts in conjunction with another muscle to allow it to act more efficiently. **Triangular muscle,** a muscle in which the fibres converge on an apical tendon. **Unstriped muscle,** muscle made of spindle-shaped cells which does not appear striated in transmitted light. It is not under the control of the will. **Vestigial muscle,** a muscle well developed in lower animals but only rudimentary in man. **Voluntary muscle,** striped muscle. **White muscle,** the pale-coloured muscle tissue found in skeletal muscle.

Muscul-, Musculo- [(L *musculus:* muscle). Prefixes signifying relationship with muscle.

Muscular. Relating to muscle. Possessing well-developed muscles. **Muscular dystrophy,** *see* Dystrophy.

Muscularis. The muscular layer of an organ. **Muscularis mucosae,** the layer of unstriped muscle in certain mucous membranes such as that of the alimentary tract.

Mushroom. The name given to certain fungi. Some, such as *Amanita phalloides*, are poisonous. Others, such as *Psalliota campestris*, are edible. Mushrooms have no nutritive value. They are a luxury food.

Musk. The dried preputial secretion of

the musk deer (*Moschus moschiferus*), which has a potent odour. Once widely used medicinally, now only used in the perfumery industry.

Mustard. The seeds of *Brassica nigra* (black mustard) and *Brassica alba* (white mustard). It is used externally as a counter-irritant plaster, and internally as an emetic. Its widest use is as a condiment. **Mustard gas,** dichlorodiethyl sulphide. **Nitrogen mustard,** mustine.

Mustine hydrocholoride. B.P. 1968, $C_5H_{12}Cl_3N$. Nitrogen mustard. A cytotoxic agent, which must be given intravenously **(Mustine injection,** B.P. 1968), and is of particular value in the treatment of Hodgkin's disease.

Mutant. An organism bearing a mutant and which is breeding true from it. A gene in which mutation has occurred.

Mutarotation. The property of certain optically active substances of changing their specific rotation.

Mutation. An alteration in the DNA base of a chromosome that is transmissible.

Mute. Unable to speak. A person who is unable to speak. **Deaf mute,** a person who is dumb because he is deaf.

Mutism. Dumbness.

Muton. The smallest unit of a chromosome that can effectively mutate.

Mutualism. Symbiosis.

Myalgia. Muscular pain. **Epidemic myalgia,** Bornholm disease.

Myasthenia. Muscular weakness. **Myasthenia gravis,** a chronic, progressive weakness of the muscles, particularly those innervated by the cranial nerves, occurring mainly in adults, and of unknown etiology.

Myc-, Mycet-, Myceto- (Gk *mykēs:* fungus). Prefixes signifying association with a fungus.

Mycelial. Referring to mycelium.

Mycelium. The meshwork formed by filamentous fungi, or moulds, one of the morphological group of Eumycetes, or true fungi. (*Plural:* mycelia.) **Aerial mycelium,** the portion of the mycelium that protrudes from the vegetative mycelium into the air. **Vegetative mycelium,** the major part of the mycelium that grows on, and penetrates into, the substrate.

Mycete. A fungus.

Mycetoma. A chronic granulomatous infection produced by a variety of fungi, including *Nocardia madurae*, *Streptomyces somaliensis*, and *Madurella mycetomi*, entering the foot through thorn pricks. Madura foot.

Myco- (Gk *mykēs:* fungus). Prefix signifying relationship with fungus.

Mycobacteriaceae. A family of the order Actinomycetales.

Mycobacterium. The only genus of the family Mycobacteriaceae. The members of the genus are slender rods, which are difficult to stain but, which once stained, resist decolorization with acid: i.e. are acid fast. (*Plural:* mycobacteria.) **Anonymous mycobacteria,** acid-fast bacilli which cannot be identified as either human or bovine tubercle bacilli and which may be associated with human disease. *Mycobacterium johnei,* the causative organism of a chronic enteritis in cattle and sheep. *Myco. leprae,* the causative organism of leprosy. *Myco. smegmatis,* a commensal organism found in smegma. *Myco. tuberculosis,* the causative organism of tuberculosis.

Mycology. The study of fungi.

Mycoplasma. A genus of the order Mycoplasmatales. Also known as pleuropneumonia-like organisms (PPLO). The cause of great epizootics of severe respiratory disease in cattle, sheep and goats. Commensals in the oral cavity and genital tract in man. *Mycoplasma pneumoniae,* the causative organism of primary atypical pneumonia. Eaton's agent.

Mycoplasmatales. The order of bacteria, also known as pleuropneumonia-like organisms, which are non-motile, gram-negative and reproduce by fission into coccoid elementary bodies that are filterable.

Mycosis. A disease caused by a fungus. (*Plural:* mycoses.) **Mycosis fungoides,** an invariably fatal type of reticulosis, characterized initially by a skin eruption followed later by multiple ulcerating skin tumours.

Mycotic. Relating to a mycosis.

Mydriasis. Abnormal enlargement of the pupil. **Paralytic mydriasis,** mydriasis due to paralysis of the oculomotor nerve. **Spastic mydriasis,** mydriasis due to sympathetic irritation. **Traumatic mydriasis,** mydriasis following a contusion.

Mydriatic. A drug that dilates the pupil.

Myel-, Myelo- (Gk *myelos:* marrow). Prefixes signifying association with the bone marrow or spinal cord.

Myelencephalon. The caudal slope of the embryonic hindbrain that develops into the medulla oblongata.

Myelin. The fatty substance present in

the sheath of medullated nerve fibres. It is composed of lipids and protein, and is doubly refractile.

Myelination. The process of acquiring a medullary sheath.

Myelitis. Inflammation of the spinal cord.

Myeloblast. A primitive granulocyte formed by division of a haemocytoblast.

Myelocyte. A young granulocyte occurring normally in the bone marrow, and not the circulating blood, and formed by division of a myeloblast.

Myelofibrosis. Myelosclerosis.

Myelography. Radiological visualization of the spinal cord by the injection of radio-opaque substances into the subarachnoid space.

Myeloid. Pertaining to: (a) bone marrow; (b) the spinal cord; (c) myelocytes. **Myeloid leukaemia,** the form of leukaemia characterized by excessive production of myelocytes.

Myelomalacia. Softening of the spinal cord.

Myeloma, multiple. A neoplastic proliferation of the plasma cells, known as myeloma cells, characterized by the development of multiple cells in the skeleton. Myelomatosis.

Myelomatosis. Multiple myeloma.

Myelomeningocele. Spina bifida with herniation of the spinal cord as well as meninges.

Myelorrhagia. Haemorrhage into the spinal cord.

Myelosclerosis. A condition characterized by sclerosis of the bone marrow, extramedullary haemopoiesis, leucoerythroblastic anaemia, and splenomegaly. Myelofibrosis.

Myenteric. Pertaining to the myenteron (i.e. the muscular coat of the intestine).

Myiasis. Infestation of a cutaneous wound or sore with fly larvae.

Myl-, Mylo- (Gk *myle:* mill). Prefixes signifying association with the molar teeth.

Mylohyoid. Pertaining to the lower molar teeth and the hyoid bone.

Myo-, My- (Gk *mys:* muscle). Prefixes signifying association with muscle.

Myoblast. The primitive muscle cell.

Myocardial. To do with the myocardium.

Myocarditis. Inflammation of the myocardium.

Myocardium. The heart muscle.

Myoclonus. The condition characterized by sudden shock-like contractions of the muscles.

Myocoele. The transient central cavity of the embryonic mesodermic somite.

Myocyte. A muscle cell.

Myodynia. Pain in the muscles.

Myo-epithelium. Specialized contractile epithelial cells concerned with the movements of secretion in certain organs, including the mammary, lacrimal, salivary and sweat glands.

Myofibril. The active contractile component in the muscle fibre. Sarcostyle.

Myofilament. The ultramicroscopic protein filament in a myofibril.

Myogenic. Of muscular origin.

Myoglobin. One of the respiratory pigments of muscle which function in the transport of oxygen from the blood to the oxidizing systems.

Myoglobinaemia. The presence of free myoglobin in the circulating blood.

Myoglobinuria. The presence of myoglobin in the urine, due to severe injury of muscle or acute renal failure. Occasionally occurs following very severe exercise.

Myogram. A record of muscular contraction.

Myograph. An instrument for recording muscular contraction.

Myoid. Resembling muscle.

Myoidema. A localized muscular contraction, manifested by a transitory lump, evoked by a light tap over the pectoral muscles, and occurring in poor nutritional conditions such as that produced by pulmonary tuberculosis.

Myology. The study of muscles.

Myoma. A benign tumour composed of muscle tissue.

Myomalacia. Softening of muscle as a result of necrosis. **Myomalacia cordis,** the necrotic liquefaction of myocardium following a coronary infarction.

Myomectomy. Extirpation of a myoma.

Myometrium. The muscular coat of the uterus.

Myopathy. Wasting of the muscles. Muscular dystrophy.

Myopia. Shortsightedness.

Myoplasm. The contractile portion of the muscle cell.

Myorrhexis. Tearing of a muscle.

Myosin. The main protein of muscle.

Myositis. Inflammation of a muscle. **Myositis ossificans progressiva,** a disease characterized by progressive ossification in aponeuroses, ligaments and tendons.

Myotatic. Referring to the stretching of a muscle. **Myotatic irritability,** the ability of a muscle to contract in response to stretching.

Myotome. The part of the embryonic mesodermic somite from which muscle arises. A knife for cutting muscle.

Myotomy. Surgical division of a muscle.

Myotonia. Slow relaxation of a muscle after contraction. **Dystrophia myotonia,** a rare familial disease characterized by muscular atrophy of certain muscles and difficulty in relaxing these and/or other muscles. **Myotonia congenita,** a rare heredofamilial disease of children characterized by marked slowness of relaxation of muscles after contraction.

Myotonic. Affected with myotonia. Referring to the element of tonus in muscle.

Myotonus. Muscle tone.

Myralact. The B.P. Commission approved name for N-(2-hydroxyethyl) tetradecylammonium lactate. An antiseptic.

Myringa, The tympanic membrane.

Myringitis. Inflammation of the tympanic membrane (or myringa). **Myringitis bullosa,** a virus infection of the tympanic membrane characterized by haemorrhagic bullae.

Myringoplasty. Plastic repair of a perforation in the tympanic membrane.

Myringotomy. Surgical incision of the tympanic membrane.

Myrophine. The B.P. Commission approved name for 3-benzyl-6-O-tetradecanoylmorphine. A narcotic analgesic.

Myrrh. B.P.C. 1968. An oleo-resin obtained from the stem of *Commiphora molmol*, which is an astringent to the mucous membrane, and also has a carminative action.

Myx-, Myxo- (Gk *myxa:* mucus). Prefixes signifying association with mucus.

Myxoedema. Adult hypothyroidism, characterized by mental and physical lethargy, dry skin, puffy appearance of the face, deepening of the voice and a low basal metabolic rate.

Myxofibroma. A benign tumour composed of mucoid and fibroid tissue.

Myxoma. A benign tumour composed of mucoid tissue.

Myxomatosis. A highly infectious disease of rabbits due to a virus morphologically identical with vaccinia virus.

Myxoviruses. A group of viruses that cause respiratory diseases in man, animals and poultry. They derive their name from their affinity for mucus. *Myxovirus influenzae* A, B, and C, the causal viruses of influenza. *Myxovirus multiforme.* the causative virus of Newcastle disease (a form of fowl pest). *Myxovirus para-influenzae* 1, 2 *and* 3, viruses associated with febrile respiratory disease in early life, including croup. *Myxovirus parotidis,* the causative virus of mumps. *Myxovirus pestis-galli,* the causative virus of fowl plague.

N

Nadide. The B.P. Commission approved name for nicotinamide adenine dinucleotide. An antagonist to alcohol and narcotic analgesics.

Naevoid. Like a naevus.

Naevoxantho-endothelioma. Juvenile xanthoma, a spontaneously recovering condition in infants, characterized by yellowish nodules on the limbs, neck and trunk.

Naevus. A developmental blemish of the skin. (*Plural:* naevi.) **Blue naevus,** a slaty-blue area of discoloration in the sacral region, that may be nodular. **Dermal naevus,** the type of naevus on the face, smooth, dome-like, and varying in colour from that of the skin to dark brown. **Junction naevus,** a brown or black well-defined macule, which appears in childhood. **Naevus flammeus,** port-wine stain. A haemangioma of dilated blood vessels present at birth.

Nafcillin. The B.P. Commission approved name for a semi-synthetic penicillin derived from penicillanic acid which is acid stable and active against penicillinase-producing strains of staphylococci.

Naftazone. The B.P. Commission approved name for 1, 2-naphthaquinone 2-semicarbazone. A haemostatic.

Nagana. Trypansomiasis in horses, other equidae, cattle and dogs in Africa.

Nail. A flattened, elastic structure of a horny nature placed on the distal part of the dorsal surface of the fingers and toes. **Nail bed,** the germinative zone and corium underlying the nail. **Nail fold,** the fold of skin overlapping the root of the nail. **Ingrowing nail,** a nail, one or other edge of which (or both) is overgrown by the nail wall. **Spoon nail,** koilonychia. **Nail wall,** the fold of skin overlapping the edges of the nail.

Nalidixic acid. B.P.C. 1968. $C_{12}H_{12}N_2O_3$. An antibacterial agent active orally against gram-negative organisms.

Nalorphine hydrochloride. B.P. 1968. $C_{19}H_{22}BrNO_3$. An antagonist to narcotic analgesics.

Nandrolone decanoate. B.P. 1968. $C_{28}H_{44}O_3$. An anabolic steroid given intramuscularly. **Nandrolone phenylpropionate,** B.P. 1968, $C_{27}H_{34}O_3$. An anabolic steroid with a shorter action than the decanoate.

Nanism. Dwarfism.

Nano- (Gk *nanos:* dwarf). Prefix indicating dwarf-like. Prefix used to signify one-billionth of a unit.

Nanocephalia. Abnormal smallness of the head.

Nanogram. A billionth of a gramme. Also known as a millimicrogram.

Nanoid. Dwarfish.

Nanomelia. Extreme smallness of the limbs.

Nanometre. A billionth of a metre. (*Abbreviation:* nm.)

Nape. Back of the neck.

Naphazoline hydrochloride. B.P.C. 1968. $C_{14}H_{15}ClN_2$. A potent vasoconstrictor used as nose-drops. **Naphazoline nitrate,** B.P.C. 1968, $C_{14}H_{14}N_2$, HNO_3. A potent vasoconstrictor used as eye-drops.

Naphtha. A volatile mixture of hydrocarbons distilled from petroleum.

Naphthalene. $C_{10}H_8$. A hydrocarbon derived from coal tar, once widely used as an antiseptic and as a vermifuge. Also used as a moth repellent.

Naphthol. $C_{10}H_7.OH$. A derivative of coal tar once widely used as a vermifuge and parasiticide.

Naprapathy. A system of treatment based on the principle that diseases are due to disordered ligaments.

Narcissism. Love of self. The abnormal mental or emotional state characterized by excessive love of oneself and self-interest.

Narco- (Gk *narkē:* numbness). Prefix signifying stupor or numbness.

Narco-analysis. Psychoanalysis with the influence of a narcotic.

Narcohypnosis. Hypnosis while the

patient is under the influence of a hypnotic drug.

Narcolepsy. The condition characterized by the sudden onset of irresistible sleep at irregular intervals and for no apparent reason.

Narcomania. A morbid craving for narcotics.

Narcosis. A state of profound stupor or insensibility.

Narcotic. A drug that induces insensibility or deep sleep.

Nares. The nasal apertures. (*Singular:* naris.)

Nasal. Pertaining to the nose.

Nasal bones. Two small, oblong bones placed side by side between the frontal processes of the maxillae, and forming the bridge of the nose.

Nasion. The point on the skull where the internasal and frontonasal sutures meet.

Naso- (L *nasus:* nose). Prefix indicating association with the nose.

Nasolabial. Relating to the nose and lip.

Nasolacrimal. Pertaining to the nose and the lacrimal duct.

Nasopharynx. The part of the pharynx lying behind the nose and above the level of the soft palate.

Natal. Pertaining to birth. Pertaining to the buttocks.

Natamycin. The B.P. Commission approved name for an antibiotic derived from *Streptomyces natalensis*, which is active against fungi and yeasts.

Nates. The buttocks.

Natraemia. The presence of sodium in the blood.

Natrium. Sodium.

Natriuresis. The excretion of sodium in the urine.

Natriuretic. A substance that induces diuresis by means of interfering with tubular reabsorption of sodium in the kidneys.

Naturopathy. A form of therapy that eschews medicinal and surgical agencies, and utilizes the so-called natural forces such as heat, light and massage.

Nausea. The sensation of sickness without actual vomiting.

Navel. The umbilicus.

Navicular. Shaped like a boat.

Navicular bone. The bone in the foot interposed between the head of the talus proximally and the cuneiform bones distally.

Nealbarbitone. B.P. 1968. $C_{12}H_{18}N_2O_3$. An intermediate-acting barbiturate.

Near point. The nearest point at which small objects can be clearly distinguished by the eyes.

Nearthrosis. Pseudoarthrosis.

Nebula. A slight opacity on the cornea. A preparation of a medicament in an aqueous, alcoholic or glycerin-containing medium intended for application to the nose or throat by means of an atomizer, or nebulizer. (*Plural:* nebulae.)

Nebulizer. Atomizer. Spray.

Necator. A genus of hookworms. *Necator americanus,* the American hookworm, which is widespread in the tropics in Africa, America and Asia.

Neck. That part of the body that extends from the upper limit of the chest to the base of the skull.

Necro- (Gk *nekros:* dead). Prefix signifying association with death, dying, the dead.

Necrobacillosis. Infection with *Sphaerophorus necrophorus*, which is responsible for necrotic and diphtheritic lesions in animals, and occurs occasionally in man.

Necrobiosis. Physiological death of cells or tissues. **Necrobiosis lipoidica**, a condition, often associated with diabetes mellitus, in which lipoid deposition occurs in areas of degenerate collagen.

Necrology. The science of mortality statistics.

Necromania. A morbid preoccupation with death or with dead bodies.

Necrophilism. A morbid pleasure in dead bodies. Sexual intercourse with a dead body.

Necrophobia. A morbid fear of death and dead bodies.

Necropsy. A post-mortem examination.

Necrosis. Circumscribed death of cells or tissues with structural evidence of death. **Chemical necrosis**, necrosis caused by a chemical agent. **Coagulative necrosis**, necrosis in which the tissue becomes opaque and, for a time, the cells retain their shape. **Colliquative necrosis**, necrosis with softening of the tissues. **Fat necrosis**, necrosis of adipose tissue, as in the breast or pancreas. **Fibrinoid necrosis**, necrosis characterized by the irregular deposition of fibrin in necrotic lesions associated with a florid cellular reaction. **Ischaemic necrosis**, necrosis arising as a result of the cutting off of the blood supply to the affected area. **Radiation necrosis**, necrosis following exposure to excessive irradiation. **Rena**

cortical necrosis, necrosis in the renal cortex which usually occurs as a complication of pregnancy, but may occur in any condition of shock such as extensive burns or fulminating intestinal infections.

Necrospermia. The condition in which all the spermatozoa in the semen are dead or motionless.

Necrotic. Referring to necrosis.

Necrotoxin. A bacterial toxin that causes necrosis of tissue.

Needle. A sharp-pointed instrument, usually made of metal, and used for stitching, puncturing, or aspirating. **Aneurysm needle,** a curved needle with the eye at the point, and handled, used in ligaturing blood vessels. **Aspirating needle,** a long hollow needle used for withdrawing fluids from cavities. **Atraumatic needle,** a needle to which the suture is prefixed. **Cataract needle,** the needle used in operating on a cataract. **Cutting needle,** a needle with a sharp edge. **Discission needle,** a special form of cataract needle. **Hypodermic needle,** the small hollow needle used in conjunction with a hypodermic syringe for the subcutaneous injection of drugs. **Intramuscular needle,** a large hollow needle for administering drugs intramuscularly. **Round needle,** a needle, circular in cross-section and with no cutting edge. **Spinal needle,** a long, hollow needle, with an obturator, used for lumbar (or cisternal) puncture or for the intraspinal administration of drugs. **Transfusion needle,** a needle for giving blood.

Needling. The process of breaking up a cataract in the process of removing it. Discission.

Negativism. The morbid state of tending to do the opposite of what one is requested to do, or what most people would do in the circumstances. It is one of the features of schizophrenia.

Neisseria. A genus of gram-negative cocci, usually arranged in pairs, which are strict parasites. *Neisseria gonorrhoea,* the gonococcus, the causative organism of gonorrhoea. *Neisseria meningitidis,* the meningococcus, the causative organism of meningococcal meningitis (cerebrospinal fever).

Neisseriaceae. A family of the order Eubacteriales.

Nematoda. The phyllum of roundworms. It includes the following genera: Acanthocheilonema; Ancylostoma; Ascaris; Dirofilaria; Dracuncuus; Enterobius; Loa; Mansonella; Onchocerca; Strongyloides; Toxacara; Trichinella; Tricocephalus.

Neo- (Gk *neos:* new). Prefix meaning new.

Neocerebellum. The middle lobe of the cerebellum with the exception of the pyramid and uvula.

Neocinchophen. The B.P. Commission approved name for ethyl 6-methyl-2-phenylquinolone-4-carboxylate. An analgesic and antipyretic.

Neodymium. One of the rare earth elements. Symbol Nd. Atomic weight 144·24. Atomic number 60.

Neomycin sulphate. B.P. 1968. An antibiotic obtained from a selected strain of *Streptomyces fradiae,* used topically and orally.

Neon. An inert gaseous element. Symbol Ne. Atomic weight 20·179. Atomic number 10.

Neonatal. Referring to the first month of life. **Neonatal mortality rate,** the number of deaths of infants under 4 weeks of age per 1000 live births.

Neonate. A new-born infant.

Neopallium. The cerebral cortex with the exception of the archipallium (part of the rhinencephalon).

Neoplasm. A new growth. A tumour.

Neostigmine bromide. B.P. 1968. $C_{12}H_{19}BrN_2O_2$. An inhibitor of cholinesterase, which is active orally. **Neostigmine methylsulphate,** B.P. 1968, $C_{13}H_{22}N_2O_6S$, an inhibitor of cholinesterase, which is given parenterally.

Neothalamus. The lateral nucleus of the thalamus.

Nephr-, Nephro- (Gk *nephros:* kidney). Prefixes signifying association with the kidney.

Nephralgia. Pain in the kidney.

Nephrectomy. Surgical excision of a kidney.

Nephritis. Inflammation of the kidney.

Nephroblastoma. A highly malignant renal tumour of childhood.

Nephrocalcinosis. The deposition of calcium salts in and around the renal tubules.

Nephrocele. A hernial protrusion of a kidney.

Nephrolithiasis. The presence of calculi in the kidney.

Nephrolithotomy. The surgical removal of renal calculi by means of incising the kidney.

Nephrology. The study of the kidneys.

Nephron. The functioning unit of the

kidney, consisting of the renal corpuscle and the renal tubule.

Nephropathy. Disease of the kidneys.

Nephropexy. The operation for fixation of a floating kidney.

Nephroptosis. A floating or ptosed kidney.

Nephrorrhagia. Renal haemorrhage.

Nephrorrhaphy. Fixation of a floating kidney.

Nephrosclerosis. Sclerosis of the kidneys resulting from arterial disease. **Malignant nephrosclerosis,** malignant hypertension.

Nephrosis. A degenerative condition of the kidney, characterized by gross albuminuria, oedema and anaemia. **Lipoid nephrosis,** a form of nephrosis in childhood characterized by marked lipoidal degeneration of the tubules.

Nephrostomy. The operation of making an opening into the renal pelvis for drainage purposes.

Nephrotic. Pertaining to nephrosis. **Nephrotic syndrome,** another name for nephrosis.

Nephrotomy. The operation of making an incision into the kidney.

Nephrotoxic. Having a toxic effect in the kidneys.

Nephro-ureterectomy. The operation of removing a kidney along with its ureter.

Nerve. A bundle of nerve fibres. **Adrenergic nerve,** a nerve that acts by the release of adrenaline or noradrenaline. **Afferent nerve,** a nerve that transmits impulses centripetally. **Autonomic nerve,** a nerve of the autonomic nervous system: i.e. an adrenergic or a cholinergic nerve. **Cholinergic nerve,** a nerve that acts by the release of acetylcholine. **Efferent nerve,** a nerve that transmits impulses centrifugally. **Motor nerve,** an efferent nerve that carries excitatory impulses. **Myelinated nerve,** a nerve with a myelin sheath. **Non-myelinated nerve,** a nerve that does not have a myelin sheath. **Parasympathetic nerve,** a nerve of the parasympathetic nervous system. **Peripheral nerves,** the cranial and spinal nerves, including elements of the autonomic nervous system. **Sensory nerve,** an afferent nerve that conveys sensory impulses to the central nervous system. **Somatic nerve,** a nerve, sensory or motor, supplying somatic structures, as opposed to an autonomic nerve. **Sympathetic nerve,** a nerve of the sympathetic nervous system. **Vasomotor nerve,** a nerve responsible for dilatation (*vasodilator nerve*) or

constriction (*vasoconstrictor nerve*) of a blood vessel.

Nerve gas. One of a series of volatile organic derivatives of phosphoric acid that inhibit the action of cholinesterase, thereby leading to a toxic accumulation of acetylcholine in the body.

Nervous. Relating to nerves. Apprehensible, timid.

Nettle-rash. Urticaria.

Neur-, Neuro- (Gk *neuron:* nerve). Prefixes indicating association with a nerve, or nerves, or the central nervous system.

Neural. Relating to the nerves.

Neuralgia. Pain in the course or distribution of a nerve.

Neuralgic. Relating to neuralgia.

Neurasthenia. Nervous exhaustion. A neurosis characterized by mental and physical irritability and a sense of fatigue.

Neurectomy. Surgical excision of part of a nerve.

Neurexeresis. The operation of evulsing a nerve.

Neurilemma. Neurolemma.

Neuritis. Inflammation of a nerve or nerves.

Neuroanatomy. Anatomy of the nervous system.

Neurobiotaxis. The phenomenon whereby a nerve cell will migrate in the direction from which most stimuli come.

Neuroblast. The embryonic precursor of the nerve cell or neurone.

Neuroblastoma. A tumour arising from the adrenal medulla and the sympathetic ganglia, which often develops in infancy.

Neurodermatitis. A disorder of the skin in which stress is the major, or at least an important, etiological factor.

Neurodermatosis. Neurodermatitis. (*Plural:* neurodermatoses.)

Neurofibril. One of the fine fibrils in the nerve cell and its processes.

Neurofibroma. A tumour of a nerve arising from Schwann cells.

Neurofibromatosis. A widespread hamartomatous overgrowth of nerve-sheath tissue characterized by neuro-fibromatous masses surrounding the peripheral nerves of the limbs and skin.

Neurogenesis. The development and growth of nerves and nervous tissue.

Neuroglia. The connective tissue of the central nervous system.

Neurohypophysis. The posterior lobe of the pituitary gland.

Neurolemma. The delicate sheath surrounding every peripheral cell, whether myelinated or non-myelinated.

Neurology. The study of the nervous system and its disorders.

Neuroma. A tumour composed of nervous tissue.

Neuromuscular. Pertaining to nerves and muscles. **Neuromuscular junction,** motor end-plate in which the nerve to a muscle ends.

Neuromyelitis. Inflammation of the spinal cord and of the nerves. **Neuromyelitis optica,** bilateral optic neuritis with myelitis.

Neurone. A nerve cell, including its various processes. **Alpha neurones,** the large anterior grey column neurones that innervate the extrafusal fibres of voluntary muscle. **Effector neurones,** motor neurones. The neurones of the motor nuclei of the cranial and spinal nerves. **Gamma neurones,** medium-sized anterior grey column neurones that innervate the intrafusal fibres of neuromuscular spindles. **Golgi neurones,** the multipolar neurones of the grey matter of the spinal cord. *Golgi type I* neurones have long axons that pass into the white matter. *Golgi type II* neurones have short axons that do not leave the grey matter. **Internuncial neurones,** neurones carrying impulses to the motor neurones of the anterior horn of grey matter of the same or adjacent segments of the spinal cord. **Intersegmental neurones,** neurones whose axons link adjacent parts of the spinal cord with each other. **Intrasegmental neurones,** neurones confined to one segment of the spinal cord. **Motor neurones,** effector neurones. **Postganglionic neurones,** neurones that arise in the ganglia of the autonomic nervous system. **Preganglionic neurones,** the neurones in the autonomic nervous system that arise in the central nervous system and terminate in ganglia. **Receptor neurones,** the neurones that constitute the afferent, or sensory, nerve fibres. **Sensory neurones,** receptor neurones.

Neuronophagia. Phagocytosis of neuronal debris by macrophages.

Neuroparalysis. Paralysis caused by disease of the nerve serving the affected part.

Neuropathy. Disease or disorder of the nervous system.

Neurophysin. An inert protein in the neurohypophysis to which the polypeptide hormones of the gland are attached.

Neuroretinitis. The form of papillitis in which the retina is seriously involved.

Neurosecretion. The process of elaboration and secretion of substances by nerve cells, as occurs in the hypothalamic nuclei, in which the neurohypophysial hormones are formed and then passed down the axons to the posterior lobe of the pituitary.

Neurosis. A mental or emotional disturbance, usually manifesting itself by some functional disturbance of the body without any structural lesion.

Neurosurgery. Surgery of the nervous system.

Neurosyphilis. Syphilis of the nervous system.

Neurotendinous. Pertaining to nerve and tendon. **Neurotendinal. Neurotendinous endings,** the proprioceptive nerve endings found near the junctions of tendons with muscles.

Neurotic. Referring to a neurosis or an individual suffering from a neurosis. An unduly highly strung person.

Neurotomy. Surgical division of a nerve.

Neurotoxic. Having a toxic effect on nervous tissue.

Neurotrophic. Pertaining to the influence of the nerves in maintaining the health and nutrition of the tissues.

Neurotropic. That which has an affinity for nervous tissue.

Neurovascular. Pertaining to the nervous and vascular systems.

Neutral. The state of being neither acid nor alkaline.

Neutron. One of the two particles of which nuclei consist.

Neutropenia. A reduction in the number of neutrophil leucocytes per cubic millimetre of circulating blood to a figure below that found in health.

Neutrophil. A mature granulocyte, or polymorphonuclear leucocyte, 10 to 12μ in diameter, which stains only faintly with the Romanowsky stains.

Newton. That force which, when applied to a body having a mass of 1 kilogram, gives it an acceleration of 1 metre per second per second. (*Abbreviation:* N.)

Nexus. A bond. Interlacing.

Nialamide. B.P. 1968. $C_{16}H_{18}N_4O_2$. A monoamine-oxidase inhibitor used for the treatment of depressive illness.

Nicametate. The B.P. Commission approved name for 2-diethylaminoethyl nicotinate. A peripheral vasodilator.

Niche. A depression or recession in a smooth surface.

Nickel. A metallic element. Symbol Ni.

Atomic weight 58·71. Atomic number 28.

Niclosamide. B.P. 1968. $C_{13}H_8Cl_2N_2O_4$. A taenicide.

Nicocodine. The B.P. Commission approved name for 6-O-nicotinoylcodeine. A narcotic analgesic.

Nicomorphine. The B.P. Commission approved name for 3, 6-di-O-nicotinoylmorphine. A narcotic analgesic.

Nicotinamide. B.P. 1968. $C_6H_6N_2O$. A component of the vitamin B complex, used as an alternative to nicotinic acid.

Nicotine. $C_{10}H_{14}N_2$. A liquid alkaloid obtained from the dried leaves of *Nicotiana tabacum*, the tobacco plant, which paralyses all autonomic ganglia, having first stimulated them.

Nicotinic acid. B.P. 1968. $C_6H_5NO_2$. A constituent of the vitamin B complex, essential for human nutrition in a daily requirement of 15 to 20mg. Lack of it causes pellagra. It is also a vasodilator.

Nicotinyl alcohol. The B.P. Commission approved name for 3-pyridylmethanol. A peripheral vasodilator.

Nicoumalone. B.P. 1968. $C_{19}H_{15}NO_6$. An oral anticoagulant.

Nictitation. Winking.

Nidation. Implantation. The embedding of the fertilized ovum in the uterus.

Nidus. A nest. A focus of infection.

Nifenazone. The B.P. Commission approved name for 2,3-dimethyl-4-nicotinamido-1-phenyl-5-pyrazolone. An anti-inflammatory drug and an analgesic.

Nifuratel. The B.P. Commission approved name for 5-methylthiomethyl-3-(5-nitrofurfurylideneamino) oxazolidin-2-one. A trichomonacide.

Nifurtimox. The B.P. Commission approved name for tetrahydro-3-methyl-4- (5-nitrofurfurylideneamino) -1, 4-thiazine 1, 1-dioxide. A trypanocide.

Night-terror. A type of nightmare, occurring in childhood.

Nightmare. A bad, or terrifying, dream.

Nikethamide. B.P. 1968. $C_{10}H_{14}N_2O$. A respiratory stimulant.

Niobium. A rare metallic element. Symbol Nb. Atomic weight 92·906 Atomic number 41.

Nipple. The cylindrical or conical eminence that projects from just below the centre of the anterior surface of the breast, into which the lactiferous ducts of the breast open.

Niridazole. The B.P. Commission approved name for 1-(5-nitrothiazol-2-yl) imidazolidin-2-one. A schistosomacide.

Nit. The larva of a louse.

Nitr-, Nitro- (Gk *nitron:* nitre). Prefixes indicating a compound containing the group $-NH_2$.

Nitrate. A salt of nitric acid.

Nitrazepam. B.P. Addendum 1971. $C_{15}H_{11}N_3O_3$. A tranquillizer and hypnotic.

Nitre. Potassium nitrate.

Nitric acid. B.P.C. 1968. HNO_3. A powerful corrosive.

Nitrilo-. A prefix indicating the presence of a cyanide group, $C\equiv N$.

Nitrite. A salt of nitrous acid.

Nitrobenzene. Nitrobenzol. A highly toxic substance, with a benzaldehyde (oil of almond) smell and a sweet taste, used in the manufacture of aniline, as a preservative in polishes, in cheap perfumery and scent, and as an insect repellent. Its most serious toxic manifestation is haemolytic anaemia.

Nitrofurantoin. B.P. 1968. $C_8H_6N_4O_5$. A bactericide used in the treatment of urinary-tract infections.

Nitrofurazone. B.P.C. 1968. $C_6H_6N_4O_4$. An antibacterial agent used as a local application.

Nitrogen. A gaseous element. Symbol N. Atomic weight 14·008. Atomic number 7. It exists free in the atmosphere, of which it constitutes approximately four-fifths by volume. **Nitrogen balance,** the difference between the nitrogen intake and excretion of an individual, **Nitrogen equilibrium,** the state of affairs when nitrogen intake = nitrogen output. **Nitrogen fixation,** the conversion of atmospheric nitrogen into nitrates by soil bacteria. **Nitrogen mustard,** mustine. **Nitrogen narcosis,** the narcosis induced by breathing nitrogen under increased pressure, as occurs in deep diving. **Non-protein nitrogen,** the nitrogen derived from urea, uric acid, creatine, creatinine, and amino-acids. The normal blood non-protein nitrogen (N.P.N.) is 25 to 40mg. per 100ml., and approximately 50 per cent of this is urea nitrogen. **Nitrogen trichloride,** agene.

Nitroglycerin. Glyceryl trinitrate.

Nitrosamines. Powerful chemical carcinogens.

Nitroso- (Gk *nitron:* nitre). Prefix indicating the presence of the univalent NO group, or nitrosyl.

Nitrous oxide. B.P. 1968. N_2O. Laughing gas. A short-acting general anaesthetic, used widely in dentistry and obstetrics.

Nitroxoline. The B.P. Commission

approved name for 8-hydroxy-5-nitroquinoline. An antibacterial agent.

Nocardia. A genus of actinomycetes, which are obligatory aerobes and often acid-fast. The majority are saprophytes. *Nocardia asteroides,* the causative organism of nocardiosis. *Nocardia farcina,* the causative organism of bovine farcy. *Nocardia madurae,* one of the causal organisms of mycetoma (madura foot).

Nocardiosis. A chronic suppurative disease of the lungs caused by *Nocardia asteroides,* which may metastasize to other organs of the body.

Noci- (L *nocere:* to hurt). Prefix indicating relationship to injury or a noxious influence.

Nociceptive. Capable of receiving or transmitting pain.

Noct- (L *nox (noctis):* night). Prefix indicating association with night or darkness.

Noctambulation. Sleep-walking. Somnambulism.

Noctiphobia. Abnormal fear of the night or darkness.

Nocturia. The passage of an abnormally large volume of urine during the night.

Node. A knob. A circumscribed mass. **Atrioventricular node,** the mass of specialized muscle fibres lying above the orifice of the coronary sinus, which gives rise to the atrioventricular bundle. **Heberden's nodes,** small, bony swellings which form on the dorsum of the terminal phalanges of the fingers in some cases of osteoarthrosis. **Lymph nodes,** lymph glands. **Primitive node,** a knob-like thickening at the headward end of the embryonic primitive streak, where the ectoderm is fused with the entoderm. **Ranvier's nodes,** regularly recurring constrictions in the myelin sheath of a nerve fibre. **Sinu-atrial node,** a small mass of specialized muscle fibres in the upper part of the sulcus terminalis of the right atrium, which acts as the pacemaker of the heart.

Nodose. Having knobs or nodes.

Nodule. A small node. **Cerebellar nodule,** the most anterior part of the inferior surface of the vermis. **Lentiform nodule,** a rounded projection at the end of the long process of the incus. **Lymph nodule,** lymphatic follicle. **Milkers' nodules,** red painless nodules that develop on the hands of milkers, and thought to be due to a virus. **Rheumatic nodules,** subcutaneous nodules that develop in rheumatoid arthritis. **Singers' nodules,** vocal nodules that develop in professional voice-users, particularly singers. **Subcutaneous nodules,** the nodules, up to 2 or 3cm. in diameter, that arise from tendons and aponeuroses in 20 per cent of children with rheumatic fever. **Vocal nodules,** nodules, formed by hyperplasia of the epithelium of the free edge of the vocal folds, that develop predominantly in professional voice-users as a result of abuse of the voice.

Noma. Cancrum oris. Gangrenous stomatitis.

Nomo- (Gk *nomos:* law). Prefix signifying association with law or usage.

Nomogram. A graph of graduated lines representing a series of variables, whereby the value of one variable can be obtained from a line connecting the other variables involved.

Non- (L *non:* not). Prefix meaning not.

Nonigravida. A woman pregnant for the ninth time.

Nonipara. A woman who has borne nine children.

Non-secretor. An individual who does not secrete in his saliva, or other body secretions, the blood group antigens.

Noracymethadol. The B.P. Commission approved name for 1-ethyl-4-methyl-amino-2, 2-diphenylpentyl acetate. A narcotic analgesic.

Noradrenaline. A precursor of adrenaline, which is present in the adrenal medulla, and is released, along with adrenaline, on stimulation of sympathetic adrenergic nerves. It is a powerful vasoconstrictor.

Noradrenaline acid tartrate. B.P. 1968. $C_{12}H_{17}NO_9H_2O$, A sympathomimetic drug given in the form of an intravenous infusion in the treatment of hypotension.

Norbutrine. The B.P. Commission approved name for 2-cyclobutylamino-1-(3,4-dihydroxyphenyl)ethanol. A bronchodilator.

Norcodeine. The B.P. Commission approved name for *N*-demethylcodeine. A narcotic analgesic.

Norethandrolone. B.P. 1968. $C_{20}H_{30}O_2$. An anabolic steroid.

Norethisterone. B.P. 1968. $C_{20}H_{26}O_2$. A progestational steroid which is active orally. **Norethisterone acetate,** B.P. 1968, $C_{22}H_{28}O_3$, a progestational steroid with the same action as norethisterone, but effective in half the dosage.

Norethynodrel. B.P. 1968. $C_{20}H_{26}O_2$. A

progestational steroid which is active orally.

Norgestrel. The B.P. Commission approved name for 13β-ethyl-17-hydroxy-18, 19-dinor-17α-pregn-4-en-20-yn-3-one. A progestational steroid.

Norlevorphanol. The B.P. Commission approved name for (—)-3-hydroxymorphinan. A narcotic analgesic.

Norma. The outline of a surface. **Norma basalis,** the lower surface of the base of the skull. **Norma frontalis,** the outline of the skull viewed from in front. **Norma lateralis,** the outline of the skull viewed from the side. **Norma occipitalis,** the outline of the skull as viewed from behind. **Norma verticalis,** the outline of the skull as seen from above.

Normethadone. The B.P. Commission approved name for 6-dimethylamino-4,4-diphenylhexan-3-one. A narcotic analgesic.

Normo- (L *norma:* rule). Prefix indicating conforming to the rule: i.e. normal.

Normoblast. The nucleated progenitor of the erythrocyte, normally only found in the bone marrow.

Normochromic. The term applied to an erythrocyte containing a normal amount of haemoglobin.

Normocyte. A normal shaped erythrocyte.

Normorphine. The B.P. Commission approved name for N-demethylmorphine. A narcotic analgesic.

Normotensive. Signifying a normal blood pressure.

Normothermia. A normal state of temperature.

Norpipanone. The B.P. Commission approved name for 4,4-diphenyl-6-piperidinohexan-3-one. An analgesic.

Nortriptyline hydrochloride. B.P. 1968. $C_{19}H_{22}ClN$. An antidepressant with anticholinergic properties, which does not inhibit monoamine oxidase.

Noscapine. B.P. 1968. $C_{22}H_{23}NO_7$. A cough suppressant.

Nose. The external organ of smell, and the first part of the respiratory tract, which forms the structurally variegated pyramidal prominence in the centre of the face.

Noso- (Gk *nosos:* disease). Prefix signifying association with disease.

Nosology. The scientific classification of disease.

Nosophobia. An inordinate fear of disease.

Nosopsyllus. A genus of fleas. *Nosopsyllus fasciatus,* the common rat flea.

Nostalgia. Homesickness.

Nostrils. The two elliptical apertures leading into the nasal cavities. The nares.

Nostrum. A quack medicine, or secret remedy.

Notch. A deep depression or indentation. **Acetabular notch,** the gap in the inferior projecting margin of the acetabulum. **Angular notch,** the notch on the lesser curvature of the stomach at its most dependent part. **Apical notch,** the notch just to the right of the apex of the heart where the two interventricular grooves meet. **Cardiac notch of lung,** the notch in the anterior border of the left lung, in which the heart lies. **Cardiac notch of stomach,** the acute angle at which the left margin of the oesophagus joins the greater curvature of the stomach. **Cerebellar notch, anterior,** the wide, shallow notch that lodges the pons and upper part of the medulla oblongata. **Cerebellar notch, posterior,** the deep, narrow notch that lodges the falx cerebelli of the dura mater. **Clavicular notch,** the depression on the upper part of the sternum articulating with the clavicle. **Costal notches,** four facets in the lateral border of the sternum that articulate with the cartilages of the 3rd–6th ribs. **Ethmoidal notch,** the gap between the orbital plates of the frontal bone. **Fibular notch,** the triangular notch on the lateral surface of the lower end of the tibia. **Frontal notch,** the small notch on the superior orbital margin medial to the supra-orbital notch. **Intercondylar notch,** the notch separating the two condyles at the lower end of the femur. **Intertragic notch,** the notch between the tragus and antitragus of the external ear. **Jugular notch of occipital bone,** the indentation in the front of the jugular process that forms the posterior part of the jugular foramen. **Jugular notch of the sternum,** the notch in the superior surface of the manubrium sterni. **Lacrimal notch,** a notch on the medial border of the orbital surface of the maxilla. **Mandibular notch,** the wide notch between the coronoid process and the condylar process. **Mastoid notch,** the deep groove on the medial side of the mastoid process from which the posterior belly of the digastric takes origin. **Nasal notch of the frontal bone,** the rough, serrated area on the nasal part of the frontal bone. **Nasal notch of the maxilla,** the well-marked notch on the maxilla which forms the lower border and adjoining part of the lateral border of the piriform aperture of the nose. **Pre-occipital notch,** an indentation on the inferolateral border of the cerebral hemisphere some 5cm. in front of the occipital pole. **Radial notch,** an oblong articular depression on the upper part of the lateral aspect of the coronoid process. **Sciatic notch, greater,** the deep notch on the posterior border of the ilium, bounded above by the ilium and below by the ilium and ischium. **Sciatic notch, lesser,** the notch in the posterior border of the ischium that lies between the ischial spine and the tuberosity. **Sphenoglenoid notch,** the notch lying between the free, lateral border of the spine of the scapula and the dorsal aspect of the neck of the bone. **Sphenopalatine notch,** the notch that separates the orbital and sphenoidal processes of the palatine bone. **Splenic notch(es),** one or two notches on the superior border of the spleen, indicating the lobulated character of the foetal spleen. **Supra-orbital notch,** the notch at the junction of the lateral two-thirds and medial one-third of the supra-orbital margin, which transmits the supra-orbital vessels and nerves. **Suprascapular notch,** the notch that separates the anterolateral end of the superior border of the scapula from the root of the coronoid process. **Suprasternal notch,** jugular notch. **Tentorial notch,** the large, oval opening between the anterior border of the tentorium cerebelli and the dorsum sellae of the sphenoid bone. **Thyroid notch,** the v-shaped notch that separates the laminae of the thyroid cartilage. **Trigeminal notch,** a shallow, smooth notch on the upper border of the petrous temporal in the middle cranial fossa. **Trochlear notch,** the notch between the anterior surface of the olecranon and the superior surface of the coronoid process of the ulna, which articulates with the trochlea of the humerus. **Ulnar notch,** a depression on the medial surface of the lower end of the radius. **Vertebral notch(es),** the concavities above and below the pedicles of the vertebral arches.

Noto- (Gk *noton:* back). Prefix signifying relationship to the back.

Notochord. The primitive axial skeleton of the embryo.

Novobiocin. An antibiotic derived from *Streptomyces niveus,* which is active against many gram-positive organ-isms, especially *Staphylococcus aureus,* and some strains of *Proteus vulgaris,* when given orally. It is available in two forms: **Novobiocin calcium, B.P. 1968,** and **Novobiocin sodium, B.P. 1968.**

Noxa. A harmful agent or influence.

Noxiptyline. The B.P. Commission approved name for 3-(2-dimethyl-aminoethyloxyimino)-1,2:4,5-dibenzo-cyclohepta-1,4-diene. An antidepressant.

Noxythiolin. The B.P. Commission approved name for *N*-hydroxymethyl-*N'*-methylthiourea. An antifungal agent.

Nubile. Of an age capable of childbearing.

Nucha. The back of the neck.

Nucle-, Nucleo- (L *nucleus:* kernel). Prefixes signifying association with a nucleus.

Nuclear. Relating to a nucleus. **Nuclear medicine,** the application of radioactive materials to diagnosis and treatment and the study of human disease.

Nuclease. An enzyme which splits nucleic acid by hydrolysis of inter-nucleotide bonds.

Nucleic acid. A substance of high molecular weight, containing phosphoric acid, sugars, and purine and pyrimidine bases, which constitutes the prosthetic groups of nucleoproteins. Two types of nucleic acid occur in nature: deoxyribonucleic acid (DNA), and ribonucleic acid (RNA).

Nucleolonema. The electron-dense network of the nucleolus.

Nucleolus. A dense spherical body, rich in ribonucleic acid (RNA), of which there is one or more in each nucleus. (*Plural:* nucleoli.)

Nucleons. A collective term for neutrons and protons.

Nucleoprotein. A conjugated protein, consisting of a simple protein combined with nucleic acid.

Nucleosidase. An enzyme that catalyses the hydrolysis of a nucleoside into sugar and phosphoric acid.

Nucleoside. A purine or pyrimidine base condensed with a sugar radicle.

Nucleotidase. An enzyme that catalyses the hydrolysis of a nucleotide into a nucleoside and phosphoric acid.

Nucleotide. The unit of the nucleic acid, consisting of a purine or pyrimidine base linked to a pentose sugar which in turn is esterified with phosphoric acid.

Nucleus. The densely staining meshwork, surrounded by a tough, double-layer membrane, and containing the chromosomes, which is the controller of the cell. The central positively charged core of the atom. A central core. A collection of living cells, usually nerve cells. (*Plural:* nuclei.) **Nucleus of the abducent nerve,** a small nucleus in the floor of the 4th ventricle that gives rise to the abducent nerve. **Nuclei of the accessory nerve,** two nuclei, one continuous with the nucleus ambiguus, from which the cranial root arises, and one on the lateral part of the anterior grey column of the spinal cord extending down to the level of the 5th cervical segment. **Nucleus ambiguus,** a group of large motor nerve cells sited deep in the reticular formation, from which fibres emerge to join the glosso-pharyngeal nerve, the vagus nerve and the accessory nerve. **Amygdaloid nucleus,** amygdaloid body. **Arcuate nuclei,** curved, interrupted bands of grey matter closely applied to the anterior and medial aspects of the pyramids, which give origin to the anterior external arcuate fibres. **Basal nuclei,** subcortical masses of grey matter within the cerebral hemisphere: the corpus striatum, the amygdaloid body and the claustrum. **Caudate nucleus,** part of the corpus striatum, which projects into the floor of the anterior horn and central part of the lateral ventricle and the roof of the inferior horn, an important component of the extrapyramidal system. **Central magnocellular nucleus,** an ill-defined column of large multipolar cells in the posterior grey column of the spinal cord. **Cervical nucleus,** a group of cells in the mid-cervical region of the spinal cord, occupying the postero-medial part of the base of the posterior column. **Cochlear nucleus, dorsal,** a nucleus on the dorsal aspect of the inferior cerebellar peduncle. **Cochlear nucleus, ventral,** a nucleus on the ventrilateral aspect of the inferior cerebellar peduncle. **Nucleus cuneatus,** the upper portion of the fasciculus cuneatus in the medulla oblongata. **Cuneate nucleus, accessory,** a group of cells lying dorsilateral to the cuneate nucleus which give origin to the posterior external arcuate fibres. **Nucleus dentatus,** the largest of the cerebellar nuclei. **Dorsal nucleus of the vagus,** a nucleus in the medulla oblongata, which gives origin to motor fibres to the involuntary muscle

of the bronchi, heart, oesophagus, stomach, small intestine and part of large intestine. Afferent fibres from the oesophagus and abdominal alimentary tract terminate in it. **Nucleus emboliformis,** one of the cerebellar nuclei, lying to the medial side of the dentate nucleus. **Nucleus of the facial nerve,** the nucleus in the reticular formation of the lower part of the pons, from which most of the motor fibres of the facial nerve are derived. **Nucleus fastigii,** phylogenetically the oldest of the cerebellar nuclei situated in the anterior part of the superior vermis. **Nucleus globosus,** one of the cerebellar nuclei, lying medial to the nucleus emboliformis. **Nucleus gracilis,** a nucleus on the dorsal aspect of the medulla oblongata, in which the fasciculus gracilis terminates. **Habenular nucleus,** a nucleus in the trigonum habenulae from which the fibres of the fasciculus retroflexus arise, and which is concerned with the sense of smell. **Nucleus of the hypoglossal nerve,** an elongated nucleus in the medulla oblongata. **Nucleus intercalatus,** a nucleus in the medulla oblongata, lying lateral to the hypoglossal nucleus. **Interpeduncular nucleus,** a nucleus in the floor of the 3rd ventricle, in which the fasciculus retroflexus from the habenular nucleus ends. **Interstitial nucleus,** a small collection of cells in the lateral wall of the 3rd ventricle. **Intralaminar nuclei,** a group of small nuclei in the internal medullary lamina of the thalamus. **Nucleus of lateral lemniscus,** a cell station in the rostral part of the lateral lemniscus. **Nucleus of the lens,** the firm central part of the lens of the eye. **Lentiform nucleus,** one of the basal nuclei, sited just lateral to the internal capsule, which is made up of the putamen and the globus pallidus. **Nuclei of mamillary body,** two nuclei in each of the mamillary bodies. **Marginal nucleus,** a collection of polygonal cells capping the posterior grey column of the spinal cord. **Mesencephalic nucleus,** a column of nerve cells in the midbrain, which gives origin to the mesencephalic root of the trigeminal nerve. **Nucleus of the oculomotor nerve,** a group of cells in the floor of the aqueduct of the midbrain. **Olivary nucleus,** the constituent of the olive, an oval elevation in the medulla oblongata. **Paraventricular nucleus,** a very vascular collection of large nerve cells in the hypophysis. **Nuclei pontis,** masses of grey matter scattered throughout the basilar part of the pons. **Pretectal nucleus,** a collection of grey matter in the superior colliculus, which forms part of the pathway for the light reflex. **Nucleus pulposus,** the soft, jelly-like content of the disc between adjacent vertebral bodies. **Red nucleus,** a large ovoid mass dorsal to the substantia nigra, which forms an important part of the extrapyramidal system. **Reticular nuclei,** a series of 5 masses of cells in the reticular formation of the brain stem. **Reticular nucleus of the thalamus,** a thin sheet of cells adjacent to the internal capsule. **Sacral nuclei,** groups of cells in the mid-sacral region of the spinal cord. **Salivary nucleus,** a collection of nerve cells lying close to the rostral end of the dorsal nucleus of the vagus. It is subdivided into *superior and inferior salivary nuclei* which send secretomotor fibres to the salivary and, perhaps, the lacrimal glands through the facial and glossopharyngeal nerves, respectively. **Nucleus of the spinal tract of the trigeminal nerve,** a nucleus that stretches from the apex of the posterior grey column of the spinal cord to the pons, where it becomes continuous with the superior sensory nucleus of the nerve. **Superior sensory nucleus of the trigeminal nerve,** lying on the lateral side of the motor nucleus, the main sensory nucleus of the nerve. **Subthalamic nucleus,** a small nucleus lying below the lateral part of the thalamus. **Supra-optic nucleus,** a nucleus in the hypophysis that covers the optic chiasma, which gives origin to the supraoptichypophysial tract to the posterior lobe of the hypophysis. **Supraspinal nucleus,** the nucleus, continuous above with the nucleus of the hypoglossal nerve, that gives origin to the efferent fibres of the 1st cervical nerve. **Thalamic nuclei,** the anterior nucleus and the medial nucleus as well as lateral nuclei, and ventral nuclei, and the intralaminar nuclei, the reticular nucleus, and the midline nuclei. **Thoracic nucleus,** a well-defined column of nerve cells stretching from the 8th cervical to the 3rd lumbar segments. **Nucleus of the tractus solitarius,** a nucleus practically coextensive with the dorsal nucleus of the vagus nerve. **Nuclei of the trigeminal nerve:** *motor nucleus,* which lies in the upper part of the pons; *superior sensory nucleus; nucleus of the spinal tract of the trigeminal nerve;*

mesencephalic nucleus. **Trochlear nucleus,** a nucleus situated in the floor of the cerebral aqueduct opposite the upper part of the inferior colliculus. **Nuclei of vagus nerve,** *ambiguus; dorsal; nucleus of the tractus solitarius.*

Nuclide. A particular variety of atom characterized by its atomic number and mass number.

Nulli- (L *nullus:* none). Prefix meaning none.

Nullipara. A woman who has not borne children.

Number. A numeral. A specified quantity. **Atomic number,** the number of protons in the nucleus of the atom. **Diploid number,** the number of chromosomes present in the cell of a diploid individual (46 in man). **Haploid number,** half the number of cells present in the normal somatic cell. **Iodine number,** the number of grammes of iodine absorbed by each 100 grammes of fat: an indication of the amount of unsaturated fat in the given specimen. **Mass number,** the total number of neutrons and protons in the nucleus of an isotope.

Numbness. Loss or impairment of sensation, often restricted to touch.

Nummular. Coin shaped.

Nurse. One who looks after the sick or an infant. To take care of the sick. To suckle.

Nut. The seed or fruit of various trees.

Nutation. Nodding.

Nutmeg. B.P.C. 1968. The dried kernels of the seeds of *Myristica fragrans,* a carminative now largely used as a culinary flavouring agent. It acts as a stimulant when ingested in excess as by certain addicts. It is also available as **Nutmeg oil,** B.P.C. 1968.

Nutrition. The sum of the processes involved in the ingestion and absorption of food. Nutriment or food. The study of the processes involved in nutrition.

Nux vomica. B.P. 1968. The dried ripe seeds of *Strychnos nux-vomica,* the active constituents of which are strychnine and brucine. It is available as **Nux vomica liquid extract, B.P.** 1968, which contains 3mg. of strychnine in 0·2ml., and **Nux vomica tincture,** B.P. 1968, which contains 2·5mg. of strychnine in 2ml.

Nychthemeral. Circadian.

Nyctalopia. Night blindness.

Nycto- (Gk *nyx* (*nypt-*): night). Prefix signifying relationship to darkness or night.

Nyctophilia. Preference for the night.

Nyctophobia. An abnormal fear of the night or darkness.

Nyctophonia. Loss of voice during the day, but not at night.

Nycturia. Nocturia.

Nympha. One of the labia minora. (*Plural:* nymphae.)

Nympho- (Gk *nymphē:* a bride or maiden). Prefix signifying relationship to the nymphae or labia minora.

Nymphomania. Excessive sexual desire in a woman.

Nystagmoid. Resembling nystagmus.

Nystagmus. Rapid oscillatory movements of the eyes, independent of the normal movements of the eye which are not affected. **Labyrinthine nystagmus,** nystagmus occurring in disease of the middle ear, in which the semicircular canals are involved. **Miners' nystagmus,** nystagmus occurring in those who have worked long at the coal face.

Nystatin. B.P. 1968. The antibiotic derived from *Streptomyces noursei,* which is an antifungal agent.

O

Ob- (L *ob:* against). Prefix signifying against, in front of.

Obese. Fat. Overweight.

Obesity. Fatness. An excessive accumulation of weight. Corpulence.

Obex. A small curved fold that covers the inferior angle of the 4th ventricle.

Obfuscation. Confusion. Obscureness.

Objective. The lens of a microscope nearest the object under observation. Aim. Perceptible, external, to the individual.

Obligate. Essential.

Obnubilation. Clouded consciousness.

Obsession. A fixed idea or delusion.

Obstetrician. One who practises obstetrics.

Obstetrics. The art of midwifery.

Obstipation. Intractable constipation.

Obtund. Blunt. To blunt or dull.

Obturator. A structure to occlude an opening or aperture.

Obtuse. Dull. Stupid. Blunt.

Occipital. Pertaining to the occiput or the back of the head.

Occipital bone. The trapezoid bone that forms the back of the head, and is pierced by the foramen magnum.

Occiput. The back of the head.

Occlusion. The act of closing or being closed.

Occult. Hidden. Concealed.

Ocellus. The simple eye of an insect. (*Plural:* ocelli.)

Ochronosis. A rare condition, in which the ligaments and cartilages, and sometimes the conjunctiva, become stained by black or dark brown pigment.

Octa-, Oct- (L *octo:* eight). Prefixes meaning eight.

Octacosactrin. The B.P. Commission approved name for a synthetic corticotrophin.

Octaphonium chloride. The B.P. Commission approved name for benzyl-diethyl-2-[4-(1,1,3,3-tetramethylbutyl) phenoxy]-ethylammonium chloride. An antiseptic.

Octatropine methylbromide. The B.P. Commission approved name for 8-methyl-O-(2-propylvaleryl)tropinium bromide. An anticholinergic agent.

Octavalent. Denoting an element with a valency of eight.

Octaverine. The B.P. Commission approved name for 6, 7-dimethoxy-1-(3,4,5-triethoxyphenyl) isoquinoline. An antispasmodic.

Octigravida. A woman pregnant for the eighth time.

Octipara. A woman who has borne eight children.

Octyl gallate. B.P. 1968. $C_{15}H_{22}O_5$. An antioxidant for preserving oils and fats.

Octyl nitrite. B.P. 1968. $C_8H_{17}NO_2$. A vasodilator, given by inhalation for the relief of the pain of angina pectoris.

Ocular. Relating to the eye.

Oculentum. An eye ointment.

Oculist. An ophthalmologist.

Oculogyric. Referring to movements of the eye. **Oculogyric crises,** spasmodic, conjugate deviations of the eyes, such as may occur as a sequel to encephalitis lethargica.

Oculomotor. Causing, or relating to, movements of the eye: **Oculomotor nerve,** the 3rd cranial nerve.

Odditis. Inflammation of the sphincter of Oddi.

-ode, -odes (Gk *eidos:* like). Suffixes meaning having the form.

Odont-, Odonto- (Gk *odous (odont-):* tooth). Prefixes meaning a tooth.

Odontalgia. Toothache.

Odontic. Relating to teeth.

Odontitis. Inflammation of a tooth.

Odontoblast. One of the cells from which dentine is formed.

Odontogenesis. The development of teeth.

Odontoid. Toothlike.

Odontology. The study of the teeth and their diseases.

Odontome. A tumour or cyst of dental origin which arises from the whole tooth germ, or from either the enamel organ or the connective tissue part alone.

Odyn-, Odyno- (Gk *odynē:* pain). Prefixes meaning pain.

-odynia (Gk *odynē:* pain). Suffix meaning pain.

Oeciacus. A genus of bugs parasitic on swallows, which occasionally attack man.

Oedema. Dropsical swelling due to an excess of fluid in the intercellular tissues. **Angioneurotic oedema,** the form of urticaria characterized by large weals or swellings. Giant urticaria. **Cardiac oedema,** oedema due to congestive heart failure. **Epidemic oedema,** a condition characterized by oedema and heart failure, due to ingestion of the seeds of *Argemone mexicana,* and seen predominantly in India. Epidemic dropsy. **Famine oedema,** oedema due to hypoproteinaemia due to an inadequate intake of protein. Nutritional oedema. **Renal oedema,** oedema due to nephrosis or glomerulonephritis.

Oedipus complex. Abnormal attachment of a child to the parent of the opposite sex, with an accompanying hostility to the parent of the same sex.

Oesophag-, Oesophago- (Gk *oisophagos:* gullet). Prefixes indicating association with the oesophagus.

Oesophagectomy. Surgical excision of the oesophagus.

Oesophagitis. Inflammation of the oesophagus.

Oesophagocele. Herniation of the oesophagus.

Oesophagodynia. Pain in the oesophagus. Oesophagalgia.

Oesophagoscope. An endoscopic instrument for examining the oesophagus.

Oesophagostomum. A genus of nematodes. *Oesophagostomum apiostomum,* a species sometimes found in man in Nigeria and Central Africa, and causing dysentery.

Oesophagostomy. The making of an artificial opening into the oesophagus.

Oesophagotomy. The making of an incision into the oesophagus.

Oesophagus. The muscular canal, 25 cm. long, stretching from the pharynx to the stomach. The gullet. (*Plural:* oesophagi.)

Oestradiol. The most active of the naturally occurring oestrogenic hormones formed in the ovarian follicles. Oestradiol, B.P.C. 1968, $C_{18}H_{24}O_2$. Oestradiol benzoate, B.P. 1968, $C_{25}H_{28}O_3$, given in oily solution by intramuscular injection.

Oestrane. The parent hydrocarbon of the oestrogens.

Oestridae. The family of Diptera that includes warble flies and bat flies.

Oestriol. An oestrogen which has been obtained from human ovaries and placenta and pregnancy urine. It is more soluble in water than other oestrogens. One of the three naturally occurring oestrogens, the others being oestradiol and oestrone.

Oestriol sodium succinate. The B.P. Commission approved name for oestra-1,3,5(10)-triene-3, 16α, 17β-triol 16,17-di(sodium succinate). A drug for the treatment of thrombocytopenic haemorrhage. **Oestriol succinate,** the B.P. Commission approved name for oestra-1,3,5-(10)-triene-3,16α,17β-triol 16,17-di(hydrogen succinate). A drug for the treatment of thrombocytopenic haemorrhage.

Oestrogen. A substance with the physiological property of producing oestrus.

Oestrone. The first oestrogen to be crystallized. It has been isolated from blood, urine and placental tissue. It differs from oestradiol in having an oxygen atom instead of a hydroxyl group at carbon-17. Oestrone and oestradiol are freely interconvertible in the body.

Oestrus. The phase of the female sexual cycle in which the female is prepared to accept the male for copulation. Heat.

Oestrus ovis. The 'sheep nostril fly', which may cause myiasis in the eye, nose and mouth in man.

-ogenous, -ogeny (Gk *genein:* to produce). Suffixes meaning produced in or by.

Ohm. The unit of electrical resistance, being the resistance between two points of a conductor when a constant difference of potential of 1 volt, applied between these points, produces in the conductor a current of 1 ampere, the conductor not being the source of any electromoctive force.

-oid (Gk *eidos:* form). Suffix signifying like or resembling.

Oil. A liquid immiscible in water but soluble in ether, and usually combustible. **Fixed oil,** an oil that cannot be distilled without decomposition. **Volatile oil,** a hydrocarbon, which is highly aromatic, and mostly prepared by distillation. **Essential oil,** a mixture of esters, aldehydes, alcohols, ketones and terpenes. Ethereal oil.

Ointment. A semisolid preparation, consisting of a fatty substance mixed with an active drug, for external use.

-ol. A suffix denoting that the substance is an alcohol or a phenol.

Oleandomycin. The B.P. Commission approved name for an antibiotic derived from *Streptomyces antibioticus*, which is active against a wide range of micro-organisms.

Oleate. A salt or ester of oleic acid.

Olecranon. The uppermost part of the ulna, which is bent forwards at its summit to articulate with the olecranon fossa of the humerus.

Oleic acid. $C_{18}H_{34}O_2$. The commonest of the naturally occurring fatty acids, being present in most fats and oils. **Oleic acid, B.P.** 1968, obtained by the hydrolysis of fats or fixed oils.

Oleo- (L *oleum:* oil). Prefix indicating relationship to oil.

Oleopalmitate. A compound of a base with oleic and palmitic acids.

Oleoresin. A natural solution of a resin in a volatile oil.

Oleostearate. A compound of a base with oleic and stearic acids.

Oleothorax. Compression of the lung by means of the injection of oil into the pleural cavity.

Oleum. Oil. (*Plural:* olea.)

Olfaction. The sense of smell.

Olfactory. Associated, or to do, with the sense of smell. **Olfactory nerve,** the 1st cranial nerve.

Olig-, Oligo- (Gk *oligos:* little). Prefixes meaning little or few.

Oligaemia. Deficiency in the volume of the blood.

Oligodactylia. A congenital deficiency of fingers or toes.

Oligodendrocyte. One of the three main types of neuroglia cells. It is ectodermal in origin and occurs in both the grey and white matter of the central nervous system, where it is the counterpart of the Schwann cell. Oligodendroglia.

Oligodendroglia. Oligodendrocytes.

Oligodendroglioma. A form of glioma, characterized by uniform sheets of rectangular, box-like cells, with a clear cytoplasm and darkly staining nuclei.

Oligodipsia. Absence of, or grossly diminished, thirst.

Oligodontia. The condition characterized by lack of the complete set of teeth.

Oligohydramnios. Deficiency of liquor amnii.

Oligomenorrhoea. Scanty or infrequent menstruation.

Oligophrenia. General lack of mental ability, the result of imperfect, or incomplete, development of the brain.

Oligospermia. Abnormally low number of spermatozoa in the semen.

Oliguria. Abnormally low excretion of urine.

Olivary. Relating to the olive. Shaped like an olive.

Olive. A smooth, oval elevation on the anterolateral surface of the medulla oblongata, caused by the olivary nucleus.

Olive oil. B.P. 1968. The fixed oil expressed from the ripe fruits of *Olea europaea*. It consists of glycerides, the chief fatty acid of which is oleic acid. It also contains linoleic, myristic, palmitic, and stearic acids. It is a staple article of diet in all the olive-growing countries, and is used for culinary purposes throughout the western world. Medicinally it is used internally as a demulcent and laxative, externally as a soothing application to the skin.

-ology (Gk *logos:* word). Suffix signifying a science, or study.

-oma (Gk *ōma:* swelling). Suffix signifying a swelling or tumour.

Omentectomy. Surgical excision of part of the omentum.

Omentopexy. The operation of scarifying, and then suturing the omentum to the abdominal wall, to establish an anastomosis between the portal circulation and that of the vena cava.

Omentoplasty. The use of the omentum as grafts.

Omentum. A fold of peritoneum, extending between abdominal organs. (*Plural:* omenta.) **Greater omentum,** the double sheet of peritoneum folded on itself to make four layers, hanging down from the greater curvature of the stomach over the front of the small intestine, and then turning back on itself to the anterosuperior surface of the transverse colon. **Lesser omentum,** the fold of peritoneum that extends to the liver from the lesser curvature of the stomach.

Omo- (Gk *ōmos:* shoulder). Prefix indicating association with the shoulder.

Omphal-, Omphalo- (Gk *omphalos:* the navel). Prefixes signifying association with the umbilicus.

Omphalitis. Inflammation of the umbilicus.

Omphalus. The umbilicus.

Onanism. Coitus interruptus.

Onchocerca. A genus of filarial worms. *Onchocerca volvulus,* the species responsible for onchocerciasis in Equatorial Africa, West and East Africa, Guatemala and Mexico.

Onchocerciasis. The disease caused by *Onchocerca volvulus*, and characterized by subcutaneous nodules and blindness. It is transmitted by species of Simulium, or black flies.

Onco- (Gk *onkos:* mass). Prefix signifying tumour.

Oncogenesis. The production of tumours.

Oncogenic. Giving rise to tumours.

Oncology. The study of new growths or tumours.

Oncolysis. The destruction of a tumour.

Oncomelania. A genus of snails which transmits *Schistosoma japonicum.*

Oncotic. Pertaining or relating to swelling or oedema. **Oncotic pressure,** the effective osmotic pressure of plasma, representing the difference between the osmotic pressure of blood and that of lymph or tissue fluid.

Oneirism. A dreamlike, waking state.

Oneiro- (Gk *oneiros:* dream). Prefix signifying relationship to dreams or dreaming.

Oneirophrenia. A form of schizophrenia, or of toxic-exhaustive psychosis with schizoid features, on recovering from which the patient describes it as a dream.

Onoma- (Gk *onoma:* name). Prefix signifying relationship with names or words.

Onomatology. Terminology. The science of names and nomenclature.

Onomatophobia. Morbid fear of a certain word or name.

Onomatopoiesis. The formation of meaningless words.

Ontogeny. Ontogenesis. The changes through which an organism passes from the fertilization of the ovum until the fully adult form is attained.

Onych-, Onycho- (Gk *onyx:* nail). Prefixes signifying association with a nail.

Onychauxis. Thickening of the nails.

Onychia. Inflammation of the nails.

Onychogryphosis. The thickened, disturbed state of a nail (usually a toenail), resulting from chronic irritation and inflammation. Claw-nail.

Onychoheterotopia. Abnormally placed, or ectopic, nails.

Onycholysis. Separation of the nail from its bed.

Onychomadesis. Shedding of all the nails.

Onychophagia. Nail biting.

Onychoptosis. Detachment of the nail from the nail-bed.

Onychoschizia. Splitting of the nails into lamellae.

Onychotillomania. Neurotic picking of the nails.

Oo- (Gk *ōon:* egg). Prefix signifying relationship to an egg.

Oocephalus. An individual with an egg-shaped head.

Oocyesis. Ovarian pregnancy.

Oocyst. The encysted ookinete in the wall of a mosquito's stomach.

Oocyte. The immature ovum.

Oogonium. The primordial cell from which the oocyte arises.

Ookinete. The zygote of the malarial parasite as it develops movement to become embedded in the wall of the stomach of the mosquito, where it forms the oocyst.

Oophor-, Oophoro- (Gk *ōophoros:* egg-bearing). Prefixes signifying relationship to ovary.

Oophorectomy. Surgical excision of an ovary.

Oophoritis. Inflammation of an ovary.

Oophoron. The ovary.

Oophoropexy. Surgical fixation of the ovary to the abdominal wall.

Oophorrhagia. Ovarian haemorrhage.

Ooplasm. The yolk of the ovum.

Operation. A surgical procedure. The mode of action of a drug.

Operculum. A cover or lid. (*Plural:* opercula.) **Opercula of the insula,** three areas of the cerebral cortex (*frontal, frontoparietal,* and *temporal*) that overlap the insula. **Trophoblastic operculum,** the trophoblast that covers over the embedded ovum.

Ophidiophobia. Morbid dread of snakes.

Ophthalm-, Ophthalmo- (Gk *ophthalmos:* eye). Prefixes signifying relationship to the eye.

Ophthalmectomy. Surgical enucleation of an eye (or eyes).

Ophthalmia. Inflammation of the eye. **Ophthalmia neonatorum,** inflammation of the eye in the newborn due to maternal infection, and acquired at birth. **Ophthalmia nodosa,** a nodular conjunctivitis due to the irritation of the hairs of certain caterpillars.

Ophthalmic. Relating to the eye.

Ophthalmitis. Ophthalmia. **Sympathetic ophthalmitis,** the condition in which serious inflammation attacks the second eye after injury of the other.

Ophthalmodynamometry. The measurement of blood pressure in the retinal artery.

Ophthalmodynia. Pain in the eye.

Ophthalmologist. A medically qualified specialist in diseases of the eye.

Ophthalmology. The study of the eye and its disorders and diseases.

Ophthalmometer. Keratometer.

Ophthalmoplegia. Paralysis of one or more of the eye muscles. **Chronic ophthalmoplegia,** paralysis due to myopathy of the eye muscles. **Congenital ophthalmoplegia,** primary aplasia of the eye muscles which occurs congenitally. **Exophthalmic ophthalmoplegia,** the condition characterized by protrusion of the eyes with paresis of the eye muscles. Thyrotropic exophthalmos. **External ophthalmoplegia,** ophthalmoplegia involving only the external eye muscles. **Internal ophthalmoplegia,** ophthalmoplegia involving only the internal muscles of the eye (sphincter pupillae and ciliary muscle). **Total ophthalmoplegia,** ophthalmoplegia involving all the extrinsic and intrinsic muscles of one or both eyes. **Toxic ophthalmoplegia,** ophthalmoplegia induced by toxic agents such as diphtheria, influenza, and lead.

Ophthalmorrhexis. Rupture of the eyeball.

Ophthalmoscope. An instrument for examining the interior of the eye.

-opia, -opy (Gk *ōps:* eye). Suffixes meaning vision or defect of the eye.

Opiate. A preparation of opium.

Opipramol. The B.P. Commission approved name for 5-⟨ 3-[4-(2-hydroxyethyl)piperazin-1-yl]propyl ⟩-dibenz [b, f] azepine. An antidepressant.

Opisth-, Opistho- (Gk *opisthess:* behind). Prefixes signifying backwards, or referring to the back.

Opisthognatism. Recession of the lower jaw.

Opisthorchiasis. Infection with the liver flukes, *Opisthorcis felineus* or *Opisthorcis viverrini.*

Opisthorchidae. A family of flukes which includes the genus Clonorchis.

Opisthotonos. A tetanic spasm characterized by intense hyperextension of the head and back.

Opium. B.P. 1968. The latex obtained by incision from the unripe capsules of *Papaver somniferum.* It contains not less than 9·5 per cent of morphine. Basically it has the same action as morphine. **Camphorated opium tincture,** B.P. 1968, a preparation containing 0·05 per cent w/v of morphine, and used to relieve cough. **Paregoric.** Opium tincture, B.P. 1968, a preparation containing 1·0 per cent w/v of morphine. Laudanum. **Powdered opium**

B.P. 1968, a preparation containing 10·0 per cent of morphine.

Opo- (Gk *ōps:* face, eye). Prefix signifying relationship to the face or eyes. (Gk *opos:* juice). Prefix meaning juice.

Opodidymus. A conjoined twin with one body, but two heads partially fused at the back, and two faces.

Opponens. Opposing.

-opsia, -opsy (Gk *opsis:* vision). Suffixes denoting a condition of vision.

Opsonin. A thermolabile substance in normal serum which facilitates phagocytosis.

Optic. Pertaining to the eye or vision. **Optic nerve,** the 2nd cranial nerve.

Optician. A maker of optical instruments, including spectacles.

Optics. The science of the properties of light in all its aspects.

Opto- (Gk *optos:* seen). Prefix meaning visible or related to vision.

Optometer. An instrument for measuring the refraction of the eye.

Ora. Margin. **Ora serrata,** the jagged margin of the retina just behind the ciliary body.

Oral. Pertaining to the mouth.

Orange. A citrus fruit with a high vitamin C content: 100 millilitres contain 50mg. of vitamin C. **Dried bitter-orange peel,** B.P. 1968, the dried, outer part of the pericarp of the ripe, or nearly ripe, fruit of *Citrus aurantium,* which is used as a flavouring agent and as a bitter and carminative. **Fresh bitter-orange peel,** B.P.C. 1968, the outer part of the pericarp of the ripe, or nearly ripe, *Citrus aurantium,* which has the same uses as the dried peel. A colour of the visible spectrum, wave-length 5850 to 6470 Ångström units. **Orange II, III and IV,** dyes used as indicators of pH.

Orbicular. Circular.

Orbit. The pyramidal hollow in the skull, situated on each side of the nose, that contains the eyeball.

Orbitotomy. Surgical incision of the orbit.

Orchi-, Orchido-, Orchio- (Gk *orchis:* testis). Prefixes signifying relationship to the testis.

Orchichorea. Involuntary twitching movements of the testis.

Orchidalgia. Pain in the testis.

Orchidectomy. Surgical removal of a testis.

Orchidodoptosis. Ptoris, or sagging, of the testis.

Orchido-epididymectomy. Surgical excision of the testis and epididymis.

Orchidotomy. Surgical incision of the testis.

Orchiopexy. Surgical fixation of a testis.

Orchitis. Inflammation of the testis.

Orchodynia. Pain in the testis.

Orciprenaline sulphate. B.P. 1968. $C_{22}H_{36}N_2O_{10}S$. A sympathomimetic amine used in the treatment of asthma.

Order. In biological classification the group below a class and above a family.

Ordinate. The vertical line in a graph.

Ordure. Excrement.

Orf. A widespread virus infection of sheep, sometimes transmitted to man in the form of a pustular eruption of the fingers, hands, forearms and face.

Organ. A differentiated part of the body that performs a specific function. **Spiral organ of Corti,** a series of epithelial structures on the zona arcuata of the basilar membrane of the cochlea that act as the sensory receptors for hearing.

Organelle. A specialized part of an animal cell, such as the centrosome.

Organic. Pertaining to organs or to living substances.

Organism. A living entity.

Organizer. A group of cells having a controlling influence in embryonic development.

Organo- (Gk *organon:* organ). Prefix signifying relationship to an organ. In chemistry a prefix signifying organic.

Organochloride insecticides. Chlorinated insecticides. These include aldrin, benzene hexachloride, DDT, and dieldrin.

Organophosphorus insecticides. Powerful cholinesterase inhibitors. They include malathion and parathion.

Orgasm. The climax of sexual intercourse.

Orifice. Opening or aperture.

Ornithodoros. A genus of argarid ticks, which include the vectors of the spirochaetes of tick-borne relapsing fever.

Ornithonyssus. A species of laelaptid mites, several of which attack man.

Ornithosis. A virus infection of man acquired from birds.

Oro- (L *os, oris:* mouth). Prefix signifying association with the mouth.

Oropsylla. A genus of fleas.

Oroya fever. Bartonellosis.

Orphenadrine citrate. B.P. 1968. $C_{24}H_{31}NO_8$. A drug used in the treatment of parkinsonism. **Or**

phenadrine hydrochloride, B.P. 1968, $C_{18}H_{23}NO$, HCl, a drug with the same action as the citrate.

Orrho- (Gk *orrhos:* serum). Prefix signifying relationship to serum.

Ortho- (Gk *orthos:* straight). Prefix signifying straight, normal. In chemistry it signifies attachment to a benzene ring in adjacent (1:2) positions.

Orthochromic. Normally stained or coloured. Orthochromatic. **Orthochromic anaemia,** anaemia with a normal colour index.

Orthodiagram. The record obtained with an orthodiagraph.

Orthodiagraph. An X-ray apparatus for the accurate recording of the contour of structures in the body by the elimination of all oblique rays.

Orthodontics. The branch of dentistry concerned with the prevention and treatment of dental irregularities and malocclusion.

Orthograde. Walking or standing erect.

Orthopaedics. The branch of surgery concerned with diseases of the locomotor system.

Orthophoria. The state in which at rest the visual axes of the two eyes are in alignment.

Orthopnoea. The form of difficulty in breathing which is so severe that the patient cannot lie down but must sit, or stand, up.

Orthoptera. The order of Insecta that includes cockroaches, crickets, grasshoppers and locusts.

Orthoptics. The treatment of strabismus by means of specially designed exercises for the muscles of the eye.

Orthoptoscope. An instrument for the examination of binocular vision, the capacity of fusion and the balance of the ocular muscles. Synoptophore.

Orthostatic. Pertaining, or due, to the erect posture. **Orthostatic albuminuria,** albuminuria that only occurs when the individual is up and about, not when he is recumbent.

Os. Bone. (*Plural:* ossa.)

Os. Mouth. (*Plural:* ora.) **External os of the uterus,** the aperture through which the cavity of the cervix communicates with that of the vagina. **Internal os of the uterus,** the aperture between the cervix and the body of the uterus.

Osche-, Oscheo-(Gk *oscheon:* scrotum). Prefixes signifying relationship to the scrotum.

Oscillation. To-and-fro movement, like a pendulum.

Oscillator. An apparatus used in physical medicine to give massage.

Oscillo- (L *oscillare:* to swing). Prefix meaning swinging.

Oscillograph. An instrument that records electric oscillations.

Oscillometer. An instrument for recording any form of oscillation.

Osculation. Kissing.

Osculum. A small opening or aperture. (*Plural:* oscula.)

-osis (Gk *ōsis:* general suffix forming verb nouns of action or condition). Suffix signifying a state, condition, or increase.

Osmic acid. OsO_4. An acid used as a fat stain, and as a tissue fixative in electron microscopy. Osmium tetroxide.

Osmiophilic. Readily stained with osmic acid.

Osmium. A metallic element of the platinum group. Symbol Os. Atomic weight 190·2. Atomic number 76.

Osmo- (Gk *osmē:* smell). Prefix indicating relationship to smell. (Gk *ōsmos:* impulse). Prefix indicating relationship to impulse or osmosis.

Osmolality. The osmotic concentration of a solution expressed as osmoles per kilogram of water.

Osmolar. Osmotic.

Osmolarity. The osmotic concentration of a solution expressed as osmoles per litre of solution.

Osmole. The unit of osmotic pressure, being the number obtained by dividing the molar concentrations of a solute by the number of ions formed in the dissociation of the solute.

Osmoreceptor. A receptor of smell stimuli. A receptor in the hypothalamus sensitive to changes in osmotic pressure and one of the controlling factors of thirst. A similar receptor in the duodenum which helps to control the emptying time of the stomach.

Osmosis. The passage of a solvent through a membrane from a dilute solution to a more concentrated one.

Osmotic. Relating to osmosis. **Osmotic pressure,** the pressure that must be applied to a solution to prevent the passage into it of solvent when the two are separated by a semipermeable membrane. **Colloid osmotic pressure,** the osmotic pressure exerted by colloids, such as plasma protein.

Osphresio- (Gk *osphrēsis:* smell). Prefix indicating relationship to odours.

Osseomucin. The ground substance of bone, consisting of a mucoprotein matrix.

Osseous. Bony.

Ossicle. A small bone. **Auditory ossicles,** three movable ossicles in the tympanic cavity: *malleus, incus,* and *stapes.* **Mental ossicles,** small ossicles which form in the mandible about the 7th month of foetal life. **Pterion ossicle,** a sutural bone between the sphenoidal angle of the parietal bone and the greater wing of the sphenoid bone. **Suprasternal ossicles,** ossicles fused to the manubrium in around 7 per cent of skeletons.

Ossification. The process of bone formation. **Intracartilaginous ossification,** the process whereby most bones are formed, the bone being preformed in cartilage. **Intramembranous ossification,** the process of ossification which occurs in a meshwork of collagenous fibres, as in the skull. **Ossification centres,** the areas in which the process of ossification begins.

Ossify. To change into bone.

Oste-, Osteo- (Gk *osteon:* bone). Prefixes signifying relationship to bone.

Ostectomy. Surgical excision of a bone, or part of a bone.

Osteitis. Inflammation of bone. **Osteitis deformans,** a chronic disease, in which the bones become thickened, softened and bent, thereby producing considerable deformity in advanced cases. **Osteitis fibrosa cystica generalisata,** a disease characterized by the presence of cysts in the bone, due to excessive production of parathormone. If the rarefaction of bone is not accompanied by cyst formation, the condition is known as *osteitis fibrosa generalisata.*

Osteoarthropathy. Disease of the joints. **Hypertrophic osteoarthropathy,** a disorder characterized by clubbing of the fingers and toes and painful swelling of the ends of long bones, accompanied by characteristic X-ray changes in the lungs.

Osteoarthrosis. A chronic degenerative condition of the joints, usually most marked in the weight-bearing joints.

Osteoarthrotomy. Surgical excision of the articular end of a bone.

Osteoblast. The cell from which bone is made.

Osteochondritis. Inflammation of both bone and cartilage. **Osteochondritis dissecans,** a condition in adolescents characterized by the detachment of fragments of articular cartilage or bone into the cavity of a joint—usually the knee.

Osteochondromatosis. The condition

characterized by the occurrence of multiple nodules of cartilage. **Synovial osteochondromatosis,** the condition characterized by the presence of nodules of cartilage in the synovial membrane, usually of the knee.

Osteochondrosis. The term used to designate disturbances of epiphyseal ossification of unknown cause that occur in childhood.

Osteoclasis. Surgical fracturing of a bone to correct a deformity. Absorption of bone substance.

Osteoclast. The cell responsible for the absorption and removal of bone. A surgical instrument for breaking bone.

Osteoclastoma. A tumour usually at the metaphysis of a long bone which occurs in children and young adults. Now usually known as *giant-cell tumour of bone.*

Osteocyte. A bone cell.

Osteodystrophy. Defective bone formation.

Osteogenesis. The formation of bone. **Osteogenesis imperfecta,** a congenital, hereditary condition, characterized by fragility of the bones, resulting in multiple fractures and subsequent gross skeletal deformity.

Osteoid. The organic matrix of bone. Bone-like.

Osteology. The study of bones.

Osteolysis. The absorption of bone.

Osteolytic. Pertaining to, or causing, osteolysis.

Osteoma. A benign tumour of bone. When it protrudes from the bone it constitutes an exostosis. (*Plural:* osteomas.)

Osteomalacia. A condition characterized by softening of the bones, with resultant skeletal deformity. It is more common in women than in men, and is often associated with lack of vitamin D in adult life.

Osteomyelitis. Inflammation of the bone marrow.

Osteone. The Haversian cell and its surrounding lamellae.

Osteopaedion. A dead foetus which has undergone calcification.

Osteopathy. Disease of bone. A code of the practice of medicine, in which manipulation plays a leading part.

Osteopetrosis. A rare hereditary and congenital condition, characterized by replacement of the normal structure of bone by dense structureless bone.

Osteophyte. A bony excrescence. An exostosis.

Osteoporosis. Increased porousness of bone due to lack of calcium salts. It

may be generalized or localized and due to various causes. Not the least of these is the ageing process.

Osteosarcoma. A common, and notoriously malignant, form of sarcoma, which usually starts at the metaphysis, and tends to occur in later childhood.

Osteosclerosis. Abnormal hardening of bone. **Osteosclerosis fragilis,** osteopetrosis.

Osteotome. A surgical instrument for cutting bone.

Osteotomy. The operation of cutting a bone.

Osteotribe. A surgical instrument for removing carious bone.

Ostiofolliculitis. A superficial form of staphylococcal folliculitis.

Ostium. Orifice or opening. (*Plural:* ostia.) **Ostium primum,** the original opening in the foetal interatrial septum. **Ostium secundum,** the precursor of the foramen ovale in the foetal heart, which normally closes at, or soon after, birth.

-ostomy (Gk *stoma:* mouth). Suffix indicating an artificial opening into the organ that constitutes the first part of the word.

Ostreogrycin. The B.P. Commission approved name for antibiotics produced by *Streptomyces ostreogriseus.*

Ot-, Oto- (Gk *ous, ōtos:* ear). Prefixes signifying relationship to the ear.

Otalgia. Earache.

Otectomy. Surgical excision of the contents of the ear.

Otic. Aural.

Otitic. Pertaining to otitis.

Otitis. Inflammation of the ear. **Mucous otitis,** the condition characterized by a mucinous exudate in the middle ear. *'Glue ear'.* **Otitis externa,** inflammation of the outer ear. **Otitis media,** inflammation of the middle ear.

Otoconium. Otolith. (*Plural:* otoconia.)

Otocyst. The embryonic auditory vesicle.

Otolarngology. The branch of medicine dealing with diseases of the ear and larynx.

Otolith. One of several minute crystalline bodies, consisting of a mixture of calcium carbonate and protein, in the maculae of the utricle and saccule, which play a part in the orientation of the body. Octoconium.

-otomy (Gk *tomē:* incision). Suffix indicating an incision into the organ that constitutes the first part of the word.

Otomycosis. Mycotic infection of the outer ear.

Otoplasty. Plastic surgery of the external ear.

Otorhinolaryngology. The branch of medicine dealing with diseases of the ear, nose and throat.

Otorrhagia. Bleeding from the external ear.

Otorrhoea. Discharge from the ear.

Otosclerosis. The form of deafness due to new formation of spongy bone in the middle and internal ear.

Otoscope. Auriscope.

Ototoxic. Having a toxic effect in the ear or on hearing.

Ouabain. A cardiac glycoside obtained from the seeds of *Strophanthus gratus*, or from the wood of *Acokanthera schimperi* or *A. ouabaio*. It has an action similar to that of digitalis.

Ovari-, Ovario- (L *ovarium:* ovary). Prefixes signifying relationship to the ovary.

Ovarian. Relating to the ovaries or an ovary.

Ovariectomy. Surgical excision of an ovary.

Ovariocele. Hernia of an ovary.

Ovariocyesis. Ovarian pregnancy.

Ovariorrhexis. Rupture of an ovary.

Ovariotomy. The surgical excision of an ovary or of an ovarian tumour.

Ovaritis. Inflammation of an ovary.

Ovary. The female gonad or sexual gland. (*Plural:* ovaries.)

Overbite. The extent to which the upper teeth overlap the lower teeth with the mouth at rest.

Overt. Open.

Ovi-, Ovo- (L *ovum:* egg). Prefixes signifying relationship to an egg or ovum.

Oviduct. The tube through which the ovum passes to the uterus or the exterior.

Oviparous. Egg-laying. Producing offspring in the form of eggs.

Ovoviviparous. Producing eggs which hatch within the body.

Ovulation. The process whereby the mature ovum is released from the fully ripened vesicular follicle into the uterine tube.

Ovum. The female sexual cell, or egg. (*Plural:* ova.)

Oxacillin. The B.P. Commission approved name for a semi-synthetic penicillin: which is active orally against penicillin-resistant strains of staphylococci.

Oxalate. A salt or ester of oxalic acid.

Oxalic acid. $C_2H_2O_4$, H_2O. An acid used for removing ink stains and iron mould, and the colour from calico.

Oxalosis. Congenital oxaluria. An inborn error of metabolism.

Oxaluria. The exceretion of abnormally large amounts of oxalates in the urine.

Oxandrolone. The B.P. Commission approved name for 17β-hydroxy-17α-methyl-2-oxa-5α-androstan-3-one. An anabolic steroid.

Oxazepam. The B.P. Commission approved name for 7-chloro-1,3-dihydro-3-hydroxy-5-phenyl-1, 4-benzodiazepin-2-one. A tranquillizer.

Oxeladin. The B.P. Commission approved name for 2-(2-diethylamino-ethoxy) ethyl 2-ethyl-2-phenylbutyrate. A cough suppressant.

Oxethazine. The B.P. Commission approved name for 2-di-[α-N-trimethylphenethyl carbamoyl)methyl]-aminoethanol. A local anaesthetic.

Oxidase. An enzyme that brings about biological oxidation.

Oxidation. The process whereby a compound (*a*) loses one or more electron, (*b*) loses some atom or atoms, such as hydrogen or a metal, which have a relatively weak attraction for electrons, or (*c*) combines with one or more atoms such as chlorine or oxygen which have a relatively strong attraction for electrons.

Oxide. A compound of an element or radical with oxygen.

Oxidized cellulose. B.P.C. 1968. A sterilized polyanhydroglucuronic acid. It is an absorbable haemostatic available in the form of white or creamy-white gauze.

Oxidoreductase. An enzyme that catalyses the transfer of electrons from one molecule to another.

Oximeter. A photoelectric instrument for determining the oxygen content of the blood.

Oxogenic steroids. Urinary 17-oxogenic steroids, derivatives of cortisol and its metabolites, which provide an index of glucocorticoid function.

Oxolinic acid. The B.P. Commission approved name for 5-ethyl-5,8-dihydro-8-oxo-1,3-dioxolo[4,5-g]quinoline-7-carboxylic acid. An antiproteus agent.

Oxosteroids. Urinary neutral 17-oxo-steroids which are compounds derived from androgenic and glucocorticoid hormones.

Oxprenolol. The B.P. Commission approved name for 1-(o-allyloxy-phenoxy)-3-isopropylaminopropan-2-ol. A beta-adrenergic receptor blocking agent.

Oxy- (Gk *oxys:* sharp). Prefix meaning sharp, keen, or acute, or the presence in a compound of oxygen or of a hydroxyl group.

Oxybuprocaine. The B.P. Commission approved name for 2-diethylaminoethyl 4-amino-3-butoxybenzoate. A local anaesthetic.

Oxycephaly. A cranial deformity characterized by a high forehead sloping to a peak.

Oxycinchophen. The B.P. Commission approved name for 3-hydroxy-2-phenylquinoline-4-carboxylic acid. A uricosuric agent.

Oxycodone. The B.P. Commission approved name for 7, 8-dihydro-14-hydroxycodeinone. A narcotic analgesic.

Oxyfedrine. The B.P. Commission approved name for L-3-[(β-hydroxy-*a*-methylphenethyl)amino] -3′- methoxypropiophenone. A coronary vasodilator.

Oxygen. A colourless, odourless, tasteless gaseous element. Symbol O. Atomic weight 15·994. Atomic number 8. It is essential for animal and plant life, and constitutes approximately one-fifth of the atmosphere. It combines with most elements to form oxides. **Oxygen,** B.P. 1968, prepared by fractional distillation of liquid air or by electrolysis of water. It contains not less than 99·0 per cent v/v of oxygen.

Oxygenator. A machine for the extracorporeal oxygenation of venous blood.

Oxyhaemoglobin. The easily dissociated compound of haemoglobin and oxygen, which is responsible for the transport of oxygen from the lungs to the body tissues.

Oxymel. An old-fashioned remedy for coughs and sore throats, consisting of vinegar and honey.

Oxymesterone. The B.P. Commission approved name for 4, 17β-dihydroxy-17*a*-methylandrost-4-en-3-one 4-hydroxy-17*a*-methyltestosterone. An anabolic steroid.

Oxymetazoline. The B.P. Commission approved name for 2-(4-t-butyl-3-hydroxy-2, 6-dimethylbenzyl)-2-imidazoline. A vasoconstrictor.

Oxymetholone. The B.P. Commission approved name for 17β-hydroxy-2-hydroxymethylene-17*a*-methyl-5*a*-androstan-3-one. An anabolic steroid.

Oxymorphone. The B.P. Commission approved name for 7,8-dihydro-14-hydroxymorphinone. A narcotic analgesic.

Oxyntic. Acid-secreting.

Oxypertine. The B.P. Commission approved name for 1-[2-(5,6-dimethoxy-2-methylindol-3-yl)ethyl]-4-phenylpiperazine. A psychotropic agent.

Oxyphenbutazone. B.P. 1968. $C_{19}H_{20}N_2O_3,H_2O$. A metabolite of phenylbutazone. An analgesic and antipyretic used particularly in the treatment of gout and rheumatoid arthritis.

Oxyphencyclimine hydrochloride. B.P. 1968. $C_{20}H_{29}ClN_2O_3$. An anticholinergic drug used as an antispasmodic.

Oxyphenisatin acetate. B.P.C. 1968. $C_{24}H_{19}NO_5$. A laxative.

Oxyphenonium bromide. The B.P. Commission approved name for 2-(*a*-cyclohexylmandeloyloxy) ethyldiethylmethyl-ammonium bromide. An antispasmodic.

Oxyphil. Acidophil.

Oxypurinol. The B.P. Commission approved name for 1*H*-pyrazolo [3, 4-*d*]pyrimidin-4,6-diol. A xanthine oxidase inhibitor.

Oxytetracycline dihydrate. B.P. 1968. The dihydrate of an antibiotic derived from *Streptomyces rimosus*. A broad-spectrum antibiotic with a range of action comparable to that of tetracycline. **Oxytetracycline tablets,** B.P. 1968, tablets containing 250mg. of oxytetracycline dihydrate. **Oxytetracycline hydrochloride,** B.P. 1968, an antibiotic derived from *Streptomyces rimosus*. It is the constituent of **Oxytetracycline capsules,** B.P. 1968, and **Oxytetracycline injection,** B.P. 1968.

Oxytocia. Rapid childbirth.

Oxytocic. Hastening childbirth. An agent that achieves this.

Oxytocin. A hormone of the neurohypophysis that reinforces the contractions of the uterus during parturition, increases the motility of the uterus during coitus, and gives rise to the rapid ejection of milk from a secreting mammary gland by stimulation of the myoepithelial cells in the ducts of the gland. **Oxytocin injection,** B.P. 1968, a sterile aqueous solution containing the oxytocic principle of the neurohypophysis, which may be obtained from the pituitary glands of oxen or other mammals, or by synthesis. **Oxytocin tablets,** B.P. 1968, tablets containing synthetic oxytocin.

Oxytocinase. An enzyme in the plasma of pregnant women that destroys oxytocin.

Oxyuroidea. A superfamily of the Nematoda which includes the genus Enterobius.

Ozaena. A form of chronic atrophic rhinitis associated with the formation of extremely foul-smelling crusts in the nares.

Ozone. An allotropic form of oxygen, with the chemical symbol O_3. It is a potent oxidizer.

P

Pabulum. Food. Nutriment.

Pacemaker. The term applied in medicine to the sinu-atrial node in the right atrium which normally controls the rate of the heart. **Artificial pacemaker,** a battery which is used to control the rate of the heart when the normal pacemaker is unable to function. **Ectopic pacemaker,** an initiating source outside the sinu-atrial node. **Idioventricular pacemaker,** an initiating source in the ventricles. **Wandering pacemaker,** the condition in which the initiating site moves about from the siunatrial node to some other site in the atrium or the atrioventricular node.

Pachy- (Gk *pachys:* thick). Prefix meaning thick.

Pachydactyly. Abnormal thickness of the tips of the fingers and toes.

Pachydermia. Abnormally thick skin.

Pachyglossia. Abnormal thickness of the lips.

Pachymeningitis. Inflammation of the dura mater.

Pachyonychia. Gross thickening of the nail.

Pachyotia. Thickening of the ear. Boxer's ear.

Pachytene. The third stage of meiosis, in which the homologous chromosomes become coiled round each other and shortened.

Pack. A dressing.

Pad. A cushion, or cushion-like thickening. **Infrapatellar pad,** the pad of fat that separates the synovial membrane of the knee joint from the ligamentum patellae. **Retropubic pad,** the pad of fat that separates the antero-lateral surface of the bladder from the pubis.

Paed-, Paedo- (Gk *pais, paidos:* child). Prefixes signifying association with a child.

Paederasty. Sodomy practised by adults with boys.

Paediatrics. The branch of medicine dealing with the diseases and disorders of childhood.

Pain. A sensation of discomfort, suffering or distress, of varying degree up to the level of being agonizing and unbearable. **Afterpains,** the cramp-like painful contractions of the uterus following childbirth. **Hunger pains,** the epigastric pain occurring several hours after a meal and relieved by the ingestion of food. **Labour pains,** the contraction of the uterus during labour. **Lightning pains,** the radiating pains that occur in tabes dorsalis. **Referred pain,** pain arising in a viscus that is felt in an area of skin, the sensory nerves from which enter the same segments of the spinal cord as those which receive pain fibres from the viscus in question. **Root pain,** pain caused by disease of the sensory nerve roots. **Visceral pain,** pain felt vaguely in the region of the viscus which is responsible for it.

Paint. In pharmacy, a liquid preparation intended for application to the skin or mucous surfaces. It is usually medicated with a substance, or substances, having analgesic, antiseptic, astringent, or caustic properties. There are seven in the *British Pharmaceutical Codex* 1968: Brilliant green and crystal violet paint; Coal tar paint; Crystal violet paint; Compound iodine paint; Magenta paint; Compound mastic paint; Compound podophyllin paint.

Palaeo- (Gk *palaios:* old). Prefix signifying ancient, primitive, or early.

Palaeocerebellum. The predominantly spinocerebellar part of the cerebellum, consisting of the anterior lobe, excluding the lingula, the pyramid and the uvula.

Palaeontology. The study of external forms of life in the form of their fossil remains.

Palaeopathology. The study of disease as exemplified in fossils, bones and mummies.

Palaeostriatum. The globus pallidus.

Palaeothalamus. Phylogenetically, the oldest part of the thalamus, consisting of the anterior and medial parts.

Palate. The roof of the mouth. **Hard (bony) palate,** the front part of the palate consisting of the palatine processes of the maxillae and the horizontal plates of the palatine bones. **Soft palate,** the rear portion of the palate consisting of a fold of mucous membrane enclosing an aponeurosis, muscular fibres, blood vessels, nerves, lymphoid tissue and mucous glands, suspended from the posterior border of the hard palate, and extending downwards and backwards between the oral and nasal parts of the pharynx. **Cleft palate,** a congenital deformity caused by incomplete closure of the lateral halves of the palate.

Palatine. Relating to the palate.

Palatine bones. Two bones situated at the posterior part of the nasal cavity, between the maxillae and the pterygoid processes of the sphenoid bone.

Palato- (L *palatum:* palate). Prefix signifying relationship with the palate.

Palatoplasty. Plastic surgery of the palate.

Palatorraphy. Suturing of the palate, as in the operation for a cleft palate.

Pali-, Palin- (Gk *palin:* backwards). Prefixes meaning again.

Palindromic. Recurrent or relapsing. **Palindromic rheumatism,** a form of rheumatism characterized by recurring attacks of acute peri-articular pain without, as a rule, any permanent involvement of the joint.

Palingraphia. Involuntary repetition of words or phrases in writing.

Paliphrasia. Involuntary repetition of words or phrases.

Palladium. A metallic element. Symbol Pd. Atomic weight 106·4. Atomic number 46.

Pallaesthesia. Sensibility to vibration.

Pallanaesthesia. The loss of the ability to recognize the sensation of vibrations.

Palliative. Mitigating, but not curing. A medication that relieves.

Pallidum. Globus pallidus.

Pallium. The cerebral cortex.

Palm. The front, or anterior surface, of the hand.

Palmitic acid. $C_{15}H_{31}COOH$. A saturated fatty acid derived from palm oil.

Palpation. The method of clinical examination by means of the laying on of hands to establish the size and shape of underlying organs or tumours, the state of the skin and so forth.

Palpebral. Pertaining to the eyelid.

Palpitation. Fluttering. Consciousness of the beating of the heart, usually evoked by unduly rapid, or irregular, action of the heart.

Palsy. Paralysis.

Paludism. Malaria.

Pampiniform. Shaped like a tendril.

Pan- (Gk *pan:* all). Prefix meaning all, entire.

Panacea. Cure-all.

Pancarditis. Inflammation of the pericardium, myocardium and endocardium.

Pancreas. A soft, lobulated, gland, 12 to 15cm. long, extending transversely across the posterior abdominal wall behind the stomach, from the duodenum to the spleen. It secretes into the duodenum 1200 to 1500ml. of juice every day, which contains trypsinogen, chymotrypsinogen, carboxypeptidases, amylase, lipase and nucleases. It contains the cells (islets of Langerhans) that produce insulin.

Pancreatectomy. Surgical excision of the pancreas.

Pancreatin. B.P. 1958. A preparation of pancreas containing trypsin, lipase, and amylase, which is used in the treatment of pancreatic insufficiency.

Pancreatitis. Inflammation of the pancreas.

Pancreatotomy. Surgical incision of the pancreas.

Pancreozymin. A factor, or hormone, isolated from duodenal mucosa that produces a flow of pancreatic juice rich in enzymes.

Pancuronium bromide. The B.P. Commission approved name for $3\alpha,17\beta,$ diacetoxy-$2\beta,16\beta$-dipiperidino-5α-androstane dimethobromide. A neuromuscular blocking agent.

Pancytopenia. Diminution in number of all the cellular elements in the circulating blood.

Pandemic. The term applied to a disease affecting a wide area such as a whole country or continent.

Pangoninae. A subfamily of the family Tabanidae, popularly known as 'horse flies' or 'clegs'.

Panhypopituitarism. Defective function of the whole of the adenohypophysis.

Panhysterectomy. Complete surgical removal of the uterus, including the cervix.

Panidazole. The B.P. Commission approved name for 2-methyl-5-nitro-1-[2-(4-pyridyl)ethyl]imidazole. An amoebicide.

Panniculitis. Inflammation of the subcutaneous fat.

Panniculus. A sheet or membrane. **Panniculus adiposus,** the layer of subcutaneous fat.

Pannus. Superficial vascularization of

the cornea. **Phlyctenular pannus,** the development of superficial blood-vessels at the periphery of the cornea. **Trachomatous pannus,** the vascularization of the cornea that occurs in trachoma.

Panophthalmitis. Inflammation involving the whole of the eye.

Panstrongylus. A genus of Triatomine bugs. *Panstrongylus megistus* transmits *Trypanosoma cruzi,* the cause of human trypansomasis in Brazil.

Pant-, Panto- (Gk *pas, pantos:* all). Prefixes signifying the whole, all.

Panthenol. The B.P. Commission approved name for ($\pm$)-2,4-dihydroxy-N-(3-hydroxypropyl)-3,3-dimethyl-butyramide. A drug used in the treatment of paralytic ileus and postoperative distension.

Pantotheine. Derived from pantothenic acid, this is a precursor of coenzyme A which plays an essential role in the metabolism of fat and carbohydrate.

Pantothenic acid. Part of the vitamin B complex, sometimes known as vitamin B_3. Little is known about its significance to man, except that it is an essential constituent of the diet.

Papain. A proteolytic enzyme derived from the unripe fruit of *Carica papaya,* which is used as a meat tenderizer.

Papaveretum. B.P.C. 1968. The hydrochlorides of alkaloids of opium. It has the sedative and soporific properties of morphine.

Papaverine hydrochloride. B.P. 1968. $C_{20}H_{22}ClNO_4$. The hydrochloride of papaverine, one of the alkaloids of opium, which has little, if any, hypnotic or analgesic action, but a spasmolytic action.

Papilla. A small, nipple-shaped projection. (*Plural:* papillae.) **Dermal papillae,** the numerous sensitive and vascular eminences in the papillary layer of the corium. **Duodenal papilla,** the projection on the descending part of the duodenum at the junction of its medial and posterior walls, on the summit of which opens the hepato-pancreatic ampulla. **Filiform papillae,** the conical papillae that cover the anterior two-thirds of the dorsum of the tongue. **Foliate papillae,** four or five vertical folds on the border of the tongue just in front of the palatoglossal arch. **Fungiform papillae,** relatively large, round, deep red papillae found chiefly at the sides and apex of the tongue. **Hair papilla,** a small, conical, vascular papilla at the bottom of each hair follicle. **Lacrimal papilla,** the

small conical elevation in the medial angle of the eye, the apex of which is pierced by the punctum lacrimale. **Renal papillae,** numerous nipple-like elevations that indent the wall of the renal sinus. **Simplex papillae,** papillae similar to dermal papillae, that cover the whole of the mucous membrane of the tongue. **Vallate papillae,** 8 to 12 papillae which form a V-shaped row on the dorsum of the tongue immediately in front of, and parallel with, the sulcus terminalis.

Papilliform. Like a papilla.

Papillitis. Inflammation affecting the part of the optic nerve opthalmo-scopically visible at the optic disc.

Papilloedema. Oedema of the optic disc.

Papilloma. A benign tumour of surface epithelium, appearing as a warty or papillary overgrowth. (*Plural:* papillomas.)

Papillomatosis. The widespread growth of papillomas.

Papillomatous. Having the characteristics of a papilloma.

Papovavirus. The group of viruses that contains the papilloma (the cause of warts in man) and polyoma viruses and a vacuolating agent of monkeys. (Hence the name: PA-PO-VA.)

Papule. A pimple, or small, circumscribed elevation on the skin.

Papulo-erythematous. The presence of papules on a reddened, or erythematous, skin.

Papulopustular. Characterized by the presence of both papules and pustules.

Papulosquamous. Characterized by being both papular and scaly.

Papulovesicular. Characterized by the presence of both papules and vesicles (or blisters).

Para- (Gk *para:* beyond). Prefix signifying, beside, near, or beyond.

Parabiosis. Union of two organisms, as in conjoined twins.

Paracentesis. Tapping or puncture of a body cavity with a trocar and cannula for the purpose of withdrawing fluid.

Paracentral. Lying close to the centre.

Paracetamol. B.P. 1968. $C_8H_9NO_2$ (*p*-acetamidophenol). An analgesic and antipyretic with an action comparable to, though weaker than, that of aspirin.

Paracholia. Disordered bile secretion.

Parachordodes. A genus of Gordiacea, or hairworms, which may accidentally infect man.

Paracoccidioides brasiliensis. The dimorphic fungus that causes South American blastomycosis.

Paracortical. Around or near the cortex. **Paracortical zone,** a zone in lymphatic glands lying between the cortex and medulla, and packed with lymphocytes.

Paracusis. Perversion of the sense of hearing.

Paradidymis. A small collection of convoluted tubules situated in front of the lower part of the spermatic cord above the head of the epididymis.

Paraesthesia. A sensation of numbness and tingling.

Paraffin. A saturated hydrocarbon of the methane series. A mixture of solid hydrocarbons obtained from petroleum. **Hard paraffin,** B.P. 1968, a mixture of solid hydrocarbons obtained from petroleum or shale oil. It is used to stiffen ointment bases, and in the preparation of wax baths. **Liquid paraffin,** B.P. 1968, a mixture of liquid hydrocarbons obtained from petroleum. It is used internally as a laxative, and externally as an emollient. **White soft paraffin,** B.P. 1968, a semi-solid mixture of hydrocarbons obtained from petroleum and bleached, which is used as a basis for medicaments which are not intended to be absorbed. **Yellow soft paraffin,** B.P. 1968, a semi-solid mixture of hydrocarbons obtained from petroleum. Its uses are as for white soft petroleum. **Paraffin ointment,** B.P. 1968, an ointment containing hard paraffin and white or yellow soft paraffin.

Paraffinoma. A nodular subcutaneous thickening, due to the injection of paraffin or camphorated oil.

Paraformaldehyde. B.P.C. 1968. A solid polymer of formaldehyde which is used as a source of the latter.

Paraganglion. A microscopic spherical mass of chromaffin cells found in close proximity to a ganglion of the sympathetic trunk. (*Plural:* paraganglia.)

Parageusia. Perverted or abnormal sense of taste.

Paragonimus. A genus of lung flukes. *Paragonimus westermani* the oriental lung fluke which infects man in the Far East, South America, and parts of West Africa.

Paragordius. A genus of Gordiacea, or hairworms, which may occasionally infect man.

Paragranuloma. A variant of lymphadenoma which remains localized to one group of lymph nodes for many years and does not affect the general health. Reticular lymphoma.

Paragraphia. Misplacement of words or of letters in words, or use of wrong words. The inability to write from dictation.

Para-influenza viruses. Four viruses, so named because they are similar in size to the influenza virus. They form a subgroup of the myxoviruses, and are responsible for infections of the upper respiratory tract.

Parakeratosis. Retention of nuclei of the desquamating keratinized cells, such as occurs in many scaly dermatoses.

Paraldehyde. B.P. 1968. $(CH_3.CHO)_3$. A powerful and quick-acting hypnotic and anticonvulsant, with a potent unpleasant odour.

Paralysis. Loss of muscular power due to interference with its nerve supply. Palsy. (*Plural:* paralyses.) **Paralysis agitans,** Parkinsonism. **Bulbar paralysis,** paralysis resulting from a lesion in the medulla oblongata. **Crutch paralysis,** paralysis of the upper limb due to compression of the brachial plexus in the axilla by a crutch. **Facial paralysis,** paralysis resulting from involvement of the facial nerve. **Familial periodic paralysis,** a rare form of temporary recurring flaccid paralysis affecting the muscles of the trunk and limbs, with loss of reflexes. **Flaccid paralysis,** paralysis accompanied by loss of tone of the affected muscles and absent reflexes, due to a lower motor neurone lesion. **Spastic paralysis,** paralysis accompanied by spasticity of the affected muscles and exaggerated reflexes due to an upper motor neurone lesion.

Paramedian. Located near the midline.

Paramedical. Related to the science or practice of medicine.

Paramesial. Paramedian.

Paramethadone. B.P. 1968. $C_7H_{11}NO_3$. An anticonvulsant.

Paramethasone. The B.P. Commission approved name for a corticosteroid which is about ten times as active as hydrocortisone.

Parametritis. Inflammation of the parametrium.

Parametrium. The cellular tissue separating the supravaginal portion of the cervix uteri from the bladder, and extending on to the sides of the cervix and laterally between the layers of the broad ligament.

Paramnesia. Perversion of memory, characterized by faulty recollection of events, places or people.

Paramyclonus. A condition characterized by paroxysmal, jerking contractions of the muscles of the limbs.

Paramyoclonus multiplex, myoclonus.

Paramyotonia. Failure to relax a muscle after contraction. **Paramyotonia congenita,** a rare condition in which myotonia, induced by exposure to cold, is accompanied by episodes of muscular weakness.

Paranasal. Around or near the nose.

Paranoia. The mental affliction characterized by the appearance and persistence in a clear sensorial setting, without obvious affective disturbance such as elation or depression, of closely knit intelligibly related delusions.

Paranoid. The term applied to illnesses or syndromes characterized by unwarranted suspiciousness, often accompanied by persecutory ideas.

Paraphasia. Incomplete aphasia characterized by the misuse of words.

Paraphenylenediamine. A hair dye that is liable to cause contact dermatitis.

Paraphilia. Sexual perversion.

Paraphimosis. Retraction of the foreskin with constriction of the glans penis.

Paraphrenia. A paranoid disorder, in which the content of thought abounds in loosely knit delusions and hallucinations.

Paraplegia. Paralysis of the lower part of the body and of the lower limbs.

Paraponera clavata. A species of ants, whose bite is agonizingly painful and may cause tissue necrosis.

Paraproteins. Atypical proteins which do not normally occur in the blood.

Parapsoriasis. An erythemato-squamous condition of the skin characterized by well-defined linear plaques on the trunk and upper parts of the limbs.

Parapsychology. The study of extrasensory phenomena.

Pararenal. Near the kidney.

Parasite. An organism that lives on another at the expense of the latter (or host).

Parasiticide. An agent or substance that is lethal to parasites.

Parasitology. The scientific study of parasites.

Parasitophobia. Abnormal fear of parasites.

Parasternal. Near or alongside the sternum.

Parasympathetic. Pertaining to the cranio-sacral division of the autonomic nervous system.

Parasympatholytic. Having an action antagonistic to the parasympathetic nervous system.

Parasympathomimetic. Simulating the action of the parasympathetic nervous system.

Paratenon. The fatty and aveolar tissue surrounding a tendon in its sheath.

Parathion. An organophosphorus insecticide, which acts by virtue of being a potent cholinesterase inhibitor.

Parathormone. The hormone secreted by the parathyroid glands, which controls calcium and phosphorus metabolism.

Parathyroid glands. Four small ductless glands lying on the back of the thyroid gland that secrete the hormone controlling the metabolism of calcium and phosphorus.

Parathyroidectomy. Surgical removal of a parathyroid gland.

Paratope. The antigen-combining site on an antibody molecule, complementary to an epitope.

Paratyphoid. Paratyphoid fever, a disease caused by infection with *Salmonella paratyphi* A, B, or C.

Paravertebral. Situated near or alongside the vertebral column.

Paregoric. Camphorated opium tincture, B.P.

Parenchyma. The functional elements of an organ, as opposed to its structural elements.

Parenteral. Introduced other than by the mouth.

Paresis. Partial or temporary paralysis.

Paretic. Relating to, or affected by, paresis.

Parfossularus. A genus of fresh-water snails, which are hosts of *Clinoritis sinensis*, the Chinese liver fluke.

Pargyline. The B.P. Commission approved name for *N*-benzyl-*N*-methylprop-2-ynylamine. A hypotensive agent.

Paries. Wall. (*Plural:* parietes.)

Parietal. Relating to the wall of an organ. **Parietal lobe,** part of the cerebral hemisphere.

Parietal bone. An irregularly quadrilateral bone, lying between the frontal bone in front, the occipital bone behind, and the temporal bone below, and forming a large part of the cranial vault.

Parity. The condition of having borne children.

Parkinsonism. A progressive disease characterized by muscular stiffness, rhythmic tremor, characteristic gait, and loss of facial expression. Usually a disease of later life. Parkinson's disease. Paralysis agitans.

Paromomycin sulphate. B.P. 1968. An

antibiotic derived from *Streptomyces rimosus*, which is used for the treatment of localized intestinal infections.

Paronychia. Inflammation around the nail.

Paroöphoron. A few scattered remnants of the tubules of the mesonephros, situated in the broad ligament between the epoöphoron and the uterus.

Parosmia. Perverted sense of smell.

Parotid gland. The largest of the salivary glands, lying below the external acoustic meatus, between the mandible and the sternocleidomastoid.

Parotitis. Inflammation of the parotid gland. **Epidemic parotitis,** mumps.

Paroxysm. A sudden onset or recurrence. A spasm or convulsion.

Paroxysmal. Occurring in, or having the attributes of, a paroxysm. **Paroxysmal cold haemoglobinuria,** a disease, usually a complication of tertiary syphilis, characterized by episodes of severe haemolysis, and haemoglobinuria, due to cold haemolysins. **Paroxysmal nocturnal haemoglobinuria,** an episodic haemolytic anemia in adults, manifested by attacks of haemoglobinuria, usually occurring at night, and due to a defect in the red cells. **Paroxysmal tachycardia,** a paroxysm of tachycardia with sudden onset and sudden termination. It may be atrial, ventricular, or nodal in origin.

Pars. A part. (*Plural:* partes.) **Pars amorpha,** a space of low electron opacity in the nucleolonema of the nucleolus. **Pars ciliaris retinae,** the double layer of pigmented and non-pigmented cells continued from the nervous part of the retina over the posterior surfaces of the ciliary processes. **Pars distalis,** the greater part of the adenohypophysis. **Pars dorsalis diencephali,** the thalamus and epithalamus. **Pars intermedia,** the part of the hypophysis between the adenohypophysis and the neurohypophysis. **Pars iridica retinae,** the thin pigmented continuation of the retina over the iris. **Pars membranacea septi,** the thin, fibrous, upper part of the ventricular septum. **Pars opercularis,** the portion of the middle frontal gyrus lying behind the ascending ramus. **Pars orbitalis,** the portion of the middle frontal gyrus lying below the anterior ramus. **Pars plana,** the smooth, posterior part of the inner surface of the ciliary body. **Pars plicata,** the anterior, corrugated part of the inner surface of the ciliary body. **Pars triangularis,** the portion of the middle frontal gyrus

lying between the ascending and anterior rami. **Pars tuberalis,** the upward prolongation of the adenohypophysis that surrounds the infundibulum and covers the tuber cinereum. **Pars ventralis diencephali,** the hypothalamus.

Parthenogenesis. Asexual reproduction.

Partogram. A record of cervical dilatation, in which the dilatation of the cervix (in cm.) is plotted against the duration of labour, and compared with an average curve.

Parturition. The process of childbirth.

Parulis. Gumboil.

Parvi- (*L parvus:* small). Prefix signifying small.

Paste. A semisolid preparation intended for external application, and consisting of finely powdered medicaments mixed with soft or liquid paraffin, or with a non-greasy base made with glycerin, mucilage or soap. There are eight in the *British Pharmaceutical Codex,* 1968: Compound aluminium paste; Coal tar paste; Dithranol paste; Magnesium sulphate paste; Resorcinol and sulphur paste; Titanium dioxide paste; Triamcinolone dental paste; Zinc and coal tar paste.

Pasteurella. A genus of bacteria belonging to the family Brucellaceae, which are gram-negative rods showing bipolar staining. *Pasteurella pestis,* the causative organism of plague. *Pasteurella tularensis,* the causative organism of tularaemia.

Pasteurization. The method of sterilizing milk by raising it to a temperature of either $72°C$ for at least 15 seconds, or $63°$ to $65°C$ for half-an-hour, and then cooling immediately.

Pastille. A medicament incorporated in a base containing gelatin and glycerin, or acacia and sugar, and intended to dissolve slowly in the mouth. There is one in the *British Pharmaceutical Codex,* 1968: Opiate squill pastille (Gee's linctus pastille).

Past-pointing. Failure to touch a given point, with the eyes shut. A sign of vestibular disturbance.

Patch. A small circumscribed area. **Mucous patch,** a slightly raised, sodden, greyish patch, with an irregular edge, that occurs on mucous membranes in secondary syphilis. **Patch test,** a skin test for the detection of an allergen. **Peyer's patches,** the aggregated lymphatic follicles in the small intestine.

Patella. The flat, triangular sesamoid bone situated in front of the knee joint. The knee cap.

Path-, Patho- (Gk *pathos:* disease). Prefixes signifying disease.

Pathogen. A micro-organism or substance causing disease.

Pathogenic. Disease producing. Pathogenetic.

Pathognomonic. Characteristic, or indicative of, a given disease.

Pathology. The science of the study of the causes of disease and the morbid changes they produce in the body.

Pathophobia. Morbid dread of disease.

-pathy (Gk *pathos:* disease). Suffix signifying a morbid condition or disease.

Patulous. Open. Distended.

Pavementation. The phenomenon in the inflammatory process, characterized by the white blood cells becoming adherent to the endothelium of the blood vessels.

Peau d'orange. The dimpled appearance of the skin over the breast in certain cases of cancer of the breast.

Pecazine. The B.P. Commission approved name for 10-(1-methyl-3-piperidylmethyl)phenothiazine. A tranquillizer.

Pecilocin. The B.P. Commission approved name for an antifungial antibiotic derived from *Paecilomyces varioti banier* var. *antibioticus.*

Pecten. The middle third of the anal canal. **Pecten pubis,** the sharp upper boundary of the pectineal surface of the superior ramus of the pubis.

Pectin. A purified carbohydrate product obtained from the acid extract of the inner portion of the rind of citrus fruits or from apple pomace. It is largely responsible for the jellying of fruit.

Pectineal. Pertaining to the pubis.

Pectoral. Pertaining to the chest.

Pectoriloquy. The clear transmission of the spoken word heard on auscultation over consolidated lung or a lung cavity. **Whispering pectoriloquy,** the clear transmission of the whispered word in such circumstances.

Pedicel. A small process springing from the long processes of a podocyte, which surrounds the capillary in the renal corpuscle.

Pedicle. A stalk, or narrow stem.

Pediculicide. An agent or substance that destroys lice.

Pediculoides. A genus of mites. *Pediculoides ventricosus,* a species of mite responsible for grain itch, or straw itch. Also known as *Pyemotes ventricosus.*

Pediculosis. Infestation with lice. **Pediculosis capitis,** infestation of the hair

by *Pediculus humanus* var. *capitis* (usually known as *Pedicus capitulsi*). **Pediculosis corporis,** infestation of the body with *Pediculus humanus* var. *corporis* (usually known as *Pediculus corporis*). Vagabond's disease. **Phthiriasis pubis,** infestation of the pubic hair (in severe cases, also of the eyelashes and axillary hair) by *Phthirus pubis,* the crab louse.

Pediculus. A genus of lice. *Pediculus humanus* var. *capitis* (*Pediculus capitis*), head louse. *Pediculus humanus* var. *corporis* (*Pediculus corporis*), the body louse.

Pedometer. An instrument for recording the number of steps taken in walking.

Peduncle. A stalk or pedicle. **Cerebellar peduncles,** three bundles of nerve fibres on each side, issuing from the anterior cerebellar notch. The *superior* peduncles connect the cerebellum to the midbrain; the *middle* peduncles connect it to the pons; the *inferior* peduncles connect it to the medulla oblongata. **Cerebral peduncles,** the two lateral halves of the midbrain. Each consists of a dorsal part (*tegmentum*) and a ventral part (*crus cerebri*) separated by the *substantia nigra.* **Peduncle of the flocculus,** a narrow band of white fibres (afferent and efferent) that emerges from the medial end of the flocculus. **Peduncle of the mamillary body,** a band of afferent fibres that connect each mamillary body with the tegmentum.

Pellagra. A disease caused by lack of nicotinic acid in association with protein deficiency, and characterized by dermatitis, diarrhoea, and dementia. (The three D's.)

Pellicle. A thin skin or film.

Pelmatogram. A footprint.

Pelo- (Gk *pelos:* mud). Prefix meaning mud.

Pelotherapy. The therapeutic use of mud: e.g. mud baths.

Pelvic. Concerned with, or related to, the pelvis.

Pelvimeter. A pair of calipers specially designed for measuring the diameters of the pelvis.

Pelvimetry. Measurement of the pelvis.

Pelvis. A basin-like cavity. (*Plural:* pelves.) **Android pelvis,** a female pelvis with male features. **Anthropoid pelvis,** a female pelvis with a long conjugate and a relatively short transverse diameter. **Assimilation pelvis,** a pelvis in which either the last lumbar vertebra has become fused into the sacrum, or the 1st sacral vertebra partakes of the characters of a lumbar vertebra. **Axis of the pelvis,** an imaginary straight line drawn perpendicular to the plane of the brim at its centre, which would show the position of the centre of the foetal head in its passage through the pelvis. **Bony pelvis,** the massive bony ring interposed between the movable segments of the vertebral column, which it supports, and the lower limbs, upon which it rests. It is composed of the two hip bones laterally and in front, and the sacrum and coccyx behind. **Brim of the pelvis,** the plane of division between the false and the true pelvis, bounded in front by the top of the symphysis pubis, behind by the promontory of the sacrum, and laterally by the ala of the sacrum, the sacro-iliac joints, the ilio-pectineal line and the pubic crest. **Cavity of the pelvis,** the space between the plane of the brim above and the plane of the outlet below. **Contracted pelvis,** a pelvis in which any diameter of the inlet or outlet is shortened by more than 0·5cm. **Coxalgic pelvis,** deformity of the pelvis resulting from disease of the hip joint. **Diameters of the pelvis,** three in number. *Anteroposterior* (*conjugate*) *diameter,* from the lumbosacral angle to the symphysis pubis (average of 110mm. in female). *Oblique diameter,* from the iliopectineal eminence to the opposite sacro-iliac joint (average of 125mm. in female). *Transverse diameter,* from the middle of the brim on one side to the same point on the opposite side (average of 135mm. in female). **Dolicocephalic pelvis,** an oval pelvis with a short transverse and a relatively long conjugate diameter. **False pelvis,** greater pelvis. **Flat pelvis,** a pelvis in which there is shortening of the transverse diameter. **Floor of the pevis,** the soft parts that fill in the pelvic outlet. **Funnel-shaped pelvis,** the male pelvis which is heavier, deeper and narrower than the female pelvis. **Greater pelvis,** the expanded portion of the cavity above and in front of the superior pelvic aperture. **Gynaecoid pelvis,** the normal female pelvis. **Inclination of the pelvis,** the relation of the plane of the pelvic brim to the horizontal. **Inlet of the pelvis,** the brim of the pelvis. **Kyphotic pelvis,** the transverse contraction of the pelvic outlet induced by kyphosis in the lumbar region. **Lesser pelvis,** that part of the pelvic cavity that lies below and behind the superior pelvic aperture. **Metasipellic pelvis,** a round pelvis with

conjugate and transverse diameters approximately equal. **Oblique (or asymmetrical) pelvis,** distortion of the pelvis produced by shortening of one leg before puberty, or from defective development of the lateral mass of one side of the sacrum (*Naegele's pelvis*). **Osteomalacic pelvis,** distortion of the pelvis resulting from osteomalacia. Triradiate pelvis. **Outlet of the pelvis,** the lower pelvic strait bounded anteriorly by the lower margin of the symphysis pubis and the sub-pubic arch, posteriorly by the coccyx, and laterally by the ischial tuberosities and the sacro-sciatic ligaments. **Planes of the pelvis,** four in number: of the brim, the cavity, the outlet, and the plane of least pelvic dimensions. **Platypellic pelvis,** an oval pelvis with a relatively long transverse diameter. **Platypelloid pelvis,** or *simple flat pelvis,* a pelvis with a short antero-posterior and a wide transverse diameter of the inlet. **Rachitic pelvis,** the abnormal pelvis produced by rickets, characterized by gross flattening. **Renal pelvis,** the pelvis of the ureter. **Scoliotic pelvis,** the asymmetrical pelvis produced by scoliosis. **Spondyloslisthetic pelvis,** the distorted pelvis produced by forward displacement of the 5th lumbar vertebra. **Triradiate pelvis,** osteomalacic pelvis. **True pelvis,** the lesser pelvis. **Pelvis of the ureter,** the funnel-shaped dilatation within the renal sinus.

Pemoline. The B.P. Commission approved name for 2-imino-5-phenyloxazolidin-4-one. A central nervous system stimulant.

Pemphigoid. Resembling, or of the nature of, pemphigus. A bulbous disease of the aged.

Pemphigus. A skin eruption characterized by blebs or bullae. **Benign pemphigus,** a bulbous eruption affecting mainly the eyes and mouth. Ocular pemphigus. **Pemphigus erythematodes,** a form of pemphigus in which localized exfoliation is the most prominent feature. **Familial benign pemphigus,** a chronic, benign form of pemphigus occurring at friction sites (e.g. collar line) in members of the same family. **Pemphigus foliaceus,** a form of pemphigus in which diffuse exfoliation is the most prominent feature. **Ocular pemphigus,** benign pemphigus. **Pemphigus vegetans,** a chronic form of pemphigus in which vegetations develop at the base of the bullae. **Pemphigus vulgaris,**

a chronic and potentially fatal disease.

Pempidine tartrate. B.P. 1968. $C_{14}H_{27}NO_6$. A ganglion-blocking hypotensive agent.

Penamecillin. The B.P. Commission approved name for acetoxymethyl 6-phenylacetamidopenicillianate. A semisynthetic penicillin.

Pendecamaine. The B.P. Commission approved name for NN-dimethyl-(3-palmitamidopropyl)aminoacetic acid betaine. A surface-active agent.

Penethamate hydriodide. The B.P. Commission approved name for benzylpenicillin 2-diethylaminoethyl ester hydriodide. A penicillin derivative for the treatment of respiratory-tract infections.

-penia (Gk *penia:* poverty). Suffix meaning lack of, shortage of.

Penicillamine. B.P. 1968. $C_5H_{11}NO_2S$. A chelating agent, used mainly in the treatment of hepato-lenticular degeneration.

Penicillin. The name given by Sir Alexander Fleming in 1929 to an antibacterial substance, or antibiotic, produced by the mould *Penicillium notatum*, and which is active against a wide range of micro-organisms. It is now available in many forms— natural and semisynthetic.

Penicillinase. An enzyme produced by certain micro-organisms which inactivates penicillin. The B.P. Commission approved name for an enzyme from cultures of *Bacillus cereus* or *B. subtilis* which hydrolyses benzylpenicillin to penicilloic acid, and is used in the treatment of allergic reactions to penicillin.

Penicillium. A genus of fungi of the class Ascomycetes. Penicillin is obtained from *Penicillium chrysogenum* and *Penicillium notatum*.

Penicillus. A terminal arteriole in the spleen. (*Plural:* penicilli.)

Penis. The male organ of copulation.

Pent-, Penta- (Gk *pente:* five). Prefixes meaning five.

Pentacosactride. The B.P. Commission approved name for a synthetic corticotrophin.

Pentacynium methylsulphate. The B.P. Commission approved name for a hypotensive agent.

Pentaerythritol tetranitrate. $C_5H_8N_4O_{12}$. A coronary vasodilator.

Pentagastrin. B.P. Addendum 1971. $C_{37}H_{49}N_7O_9S$. A synthetic polypeptide used for the stimulation of gastric secretion.

Pentalamide. The B.P. Commission approved name for 2-pentyloxybenzamide. A fungicide.

Pentamethonium bromide. The B.P. Commission approved name for pentamethylenedi(trimethylammonium bromide). A hypotensive agent.

Pentamethonium iodide. The B.P. Commission approved name for pentamethylenedi(trimethylammonium iodide). A hypotensive agent.

Pentamidine isethionate. B.P. 1968. $C_{23}H_{36}N_4O_{10}S_2$. A trypanocide.

Pentapiperide. The B.P. Commission approved name for an anticholinergic drug.

Pentaquine. The B.P. Commission approved name for 8-(5-isopropyl-aminopentylamino)-6-methoxyquinoline. An antimalarial drug.

Pentastomide. A class of worm-like arthropods, two genera of which, *Linguatula* and *Porocephalus*, are of medical importance.

Pentavalent. Having a valency of five.

Pentazocine. The B.P. Commission approved name for 1,2,3,4,5,6-hexahydro-8-hydroxy-6,11-dimethyl-3-(3-methylbut-2-enyl)-2,6-methano-3-benzazocine. An analgesic.

Penthienate. The B.P. Commission approved name for 2-diethylaminoethyl α-cyclopentyl-α-hydroxy-α-(2-thienyl) acetate. An antispasmodic.

Penthrichloral. The B.P. Commission approved name for 5,5-di(hydroxy-methyl)-2-trichloromethyl-1,3-dioxan. A hypnotic.

Pentobarbitone sodium. B.P. 1968. $C_{11}H_{17}N_2NaO_3$. An intermediate-acting barbiturate.

Pentolinium tartrate. B.P. 1968. $C_{23}H_{42}N_2O_{12}$. A ganglion-blocking hypotensive agent.

Pentose. A monosaccharide with only five carbon atoms in the molecule. The most important pentose is ribose.

Pentosuria. The presence of a pentose in the urine. An inborn error of metabolism characterized by the excretion of the pentose, xylulose, in the urine.

Pepper. The fruit of various species of *Piper*. Black pepper, the unripe fruit of *Piper nigrum*. Cayenne pepper, capsicum. White pepper, the ripe fruit of *Piper nigrum*. All are used as condiments.

Peppermint oil. B.P. 1968. The oil distilled from the fresh flowering tops of *Mentha piperita* (L). It is a carminative. Concentrated peppermint water, B.P. 1968, 20ml. of peppermint oil, 600ml.

of 90 per cent alcohol, with purified water to 1000ml.

Pepsin. The proteolytic enzyme of the gastric juice that converts proteins into peptones and proteoses.

Pepsinogen. The precursor of pepsin.

Peptic. Pertaining to digestion or to pepsin.

Peptide. The compound formed by the combination of two or more amino-acids, the carboxyl group of one being united with the amino group of the other, with the elimination of a molecule of water. **Peptide bond,** the —CO—NH group joining the amino-acid residues in a peptide.

Peptone. The product of the partial hydrolysis of protein during the process of digestion with, mainly, the proteolytic enzymes.

Peptonize. To convert protein into peptone by enzyme action.

Peptonuria. The presence of peptones in urine.

Peptostreptococcus. A genus of anaerobic streptococci.

Per- (L *per:* through). Prefix signifying through, throughout, thoroughly. In chemistry denoting the highest valency of a series.

Perborate. A salt of perboric acid. Perborates are strong oxidizing agents with bleaching and disinfectant actions.

Perboric acid. HBO_3. An unstable acid, from which perborates are derived.

Percentile. One of 100 equal parts of a series divided in order of their measurable magnitude.

Percept. The object perceived. The mental image of an object in space.

Perception. The mental interpretation of a sensory stimulus. **Extrasensory perception,** perception other than by the sense organs.

Perchlorate. A salt of perchloric acid.

Perchloric acid. $HClO_4$. A powerful oxidizing agent.

Perchloride. A chloride containing the highest possible amount of chlorine.

Percolation. The extraction of the soluble portion of a substance by allowing a solvent to pass slowly through it.

Percussion. The diagnostic procedure of tapping the surface of the body with a finger or small hammer known as a plessor, to determine the resonance of the underlying parts. This may be immediate or direct by tapping directly on the body surface, or mediate or indirect by the intervention of a finger.

Percutaneous. Administration through the skin.

Perencephaly. The condition characterized by the presence of multiple cysts in the brain.

Perfusion. The introduction of fluids into the body by passage through the blood vessels.

Peri- (Gk *peri:* around). Prefix meaning around.

Periadenitis. Inflammation affecting the tissues around a gland.

Perianal. Surrounding the anus.

Periapical. Around the apex of a tooth.

Periarteritis. Inflammation of the outer coat of an artery.

Periarthritis. Inflammation of the tissues surrounding a joint.

Peribronchial. Situated around a bronchus.

Pericardectomy. Surgical removal of the pericardium.

Pericardiocentesis. Puncture of the pericardium for aspiration of the contents of the pericardial sac.

Pericardiolysis. Division of pericardial adhesions.

Pericardiorrhaphy. Suture of a pericardial wound.

Pericardiostomy. The operation of making an opening into the pericardial sac in order to drain the sac.

Pericarditis. Inflammation of the pericardium. **Chronic constrictive pericarditis,** chronic inflammation of the pericardium resulting in great thickening of the pericardium with resultant constriction of the heart.

Pericardium. The conical, fibroserous sac that contains the heart and the roots of the great vessels. **Fibrous pericardium,** the outer sac of the pericardium, consisting of fibrous tissues. **Serous pericardium,** the inner sac of the pericardium which consists of a delicate membrane.

Pericardotomy. Making an incision in the pericardium.

Pericellular. Situated around a cell.

Perichondritis. Inflammation of the perichondrium.

Perichondrium. The fibrous membrane which covers hyaline cartilage except where the latter coats the articular ends of bones.

Pericoronitis. Inflammation of the gingiva surrounding the crown of a partially erupted tooth.

Pericranium. The periosteum on the outer surface of the skull.

Pericyazine. The B.P. Commission approved name for 2-cyano-10-[3-(4-

hydroxypiperidino)propyl]phenothiazine. A tranquillizer.

Pericyte. A cell, resembling a fibroblast, found around blood vessels.

Perifolliculitis. Inflammation around a pilosebaceous follicle.

Perihepatitis. Inflammation of the peritoneal covering of the liver.

Perikaryon. The cell body of a neurone.

Perilymph. The fluid, identical in composition, and confluent with the cerebrospinal fluid, that fills the bony labyrinth.

Perimeter. Diameter. An instrument for measuring the fields of vision.

Perimetritis. Inflammation of the perimetrium.

Perimetrium. The outer, serous coat of the uterus.

Perimetry. Measuring the field of vision.

Perimysium. The connective-tissue sheath surrounding each fasciculus, or bundle, of muscular fibres in skeletal muscle.

Perinatal. Pertaining to the period shortly before, during, and after birth. **Perinatal mortality,** deaths of the foetus after the 28th week of pregnancy and deaths of the new-born child during the first week of life.

Perineorrphapy. Suture of a laceration of the perineum.

Perinephric. Situated around a kidney.

Perineum. The area between the scrotum (or vagina) in front, the buttocks behind and the medial sides of the thighs laterally.

Perineurium. The connective-tissue sheath surrounding a funiculus, or bundle of nerve fibres.

Period. An interval of time. **Childbearing period,** the time of life between the menarche and the menopause when a woman is capable of bearing children. **Gestation period,** the duration of pregnancy. **Incubation period,** the time elapsing between the time of infection and its first clinical manifestation. **Lag period** (or phase), the period between the inoculation of a medium with micro-organisms before multiplication begins. **Menstrual period,** the menses. The time during which menstruation persists. **Quarantine period,** the period of time equal to the longest incubation period of a disease, during which restrictions are placed on the movements of those who have been in contact with those infected with the disease. **Refractory period,** the period following activity in a muscle or nerve when there is no response to a further stimulus. It may

be *absolute* or *relative*. **Safe period,** the period of time (pre-ovulatory and post-ovulatory) during menstruation when intercourse is least likely to lead to conception. **Silent period,** the phase during the auscultatory recording of blood pressure when the sounds disappear—to re-appear again. The auscultatory gap. **Wenckebach period,** the periodical lengthening of the P-R interval that occurs prior to a dropped beat.

Periodic. Recurring at intervals. **Periodic fever,** periods of pyrexia separated by afebrile intervals. **Periodic table,** an arrangement of the chemical elements in order of their atomic numbers.

Periodontal. Lying around a tooth. Periodontic. **Periodontal membrane,** the membrane that attaches the root of a tooth to the alveolar bone.

Periodontitis. Inflammation of the periodontal membrane.

Perioral. Around the mouth.

Periorbital. Around the eye.

Periosteum. The fibrous membrane which covers all but the articular cartilage of bone.

Periostitis. Inflammation of the periosteum.

Peripheral. Relating to, or situated at, the periphery.

Periphlebitis. Inflammation of the outer coat of the veins.

Peripolesis. Free movement of one cell around the perimeter of another.

Perisplenitis. Inflammation of the peritoneal coat of the spleen.

Peristalsis. The worm-like movement of the intestine and other tubular organs, characterized by alternate waves of relaxation and contraction. **Mass peristalsis,** short forcible movements of the colon that occur three or four times a day. **Reversed peristalsis,** a wave of contraction in a direction the reverse of normal.

Peritendineum. The thin, fibro-elastic sheath that surrounds a tendon.

Peritendinitis. Inflammation of a tendon sheath.

Peritomy. The operation for pannus by excising a collar of conjunctiva round the corneal margin.

Peritoneal. Pertaining to the peritoneum. **Peritoneal cavity,** the potential space between the parietal and visceral layers of the peritoneum.

Peritoneoscope. An endoscopic instrument for examining the peritoneal cavity and its contents.

Peritoneum. The sac of serous membrane that lines the abdominal wall and is reflected over the contained viscera. **Parietal peritoneum,** the part that lines the abdominal wall. **Visceral peritoneum,** the part that is reflected over the contained viscera.

Peritonsillar. Around a tonsil. **Peritonsillar abscess,** an abscess around a tonsil. Quinsy.

Peritrichous. Relating to cilia, or to bacteria which have flagella projecting over the entire surface.

Perivenous. Around a vein.

Periungual. Around a nail.

Periureteric. Situated around the ureter.

Perlapine. The B.P. Commission approved name for 6-(4-methylpiperazin-1-yl)-11H-dibenz[b,e]azepine. A hypnotic.

Perle. A capsule for the administration of medicine.

Perlèche. Maceration and fissuring of the epithelium at the corner of the mouth in children.

Perlingual. Through the tongue.

Permanganate. A salt of permanganic acid. Permanganates are strong oxidizing agents.

Permanganic acid. $HMnO_4$. An unstable acid which rapidly decomposes to MnO_2 and oxygen.

Pernasal. Through the nose.

Pernicious. Vicious. Destructive. **Pernicious anaemia,** a megaloblastic anaemia due to deficiency of vitamin B_{12}.

Pernio. Chilblain.

Perniosis. The group of skin affections caused by the effect of persistent moderate degrees of cold on a skin with susceptible blood vessels.

Pero- (Gk *pēros:* maimed). Prefix signifying maimed or deformed.

Peromelia. Malformation of the extremities.

Peroneal. Pertaining to the fibula.

Peroneo- (Gk *peronē:* brooch, fibula). Prefix signifying association with the fibula.

Peroneus. One of several muscles on the fibular side of the leg.

Peroral. Through the mouth.

Peroxidase. An enzyme that catalyses the transfer of oxygen from an organic peroxide to a suitable substrate, thus causing oxidation.

Peroxide. A compound with the linkage —O—O—. **Hydrogen peroxide,** H—O—O—H, is the classical example.

Peroxisome. A particle somewhat smaller than a mitochondrium, and corresponding to the micro-bodies seen in electron micrographs of the liver, which contains the enzymes, urate

oxidase, D-amino acid oxidase, and catalase.

Perphenazine. B.P. 1968. $C_{21}H_{26}ClN_3OS$. A tranquillizer and anti-emetic.

Perseveration. The condition characterized by the senseless repetition of words or deeds.

Perspiration. Sweat. **Insensible perspiration,** the water that passes through the skin by diffusion and osmosis, and not as the result of activity of the sweat glands.

Persulphate. A salt of persulphuric acid.

Persulphide. A sulphide which contains more sulphur than any other sulphide.

Persulphuric acid. $H_2S_2O_8$. A strong oxidizing agent.

Pertussis. Whooping-cough.

Peru balsam. B.P.C. 1968. The balsam exuded from the trunk of the South American tree *Myroxylon pereirae.*

Perversion. A turning away from the normal course.

Pes. The foot. **Pes cavus,** clawfoot, the deformity characterized by an abnormally high longitudinal arch. **Pes equino-varus,** club foot, in which the heel is drawn up, with inversion of the foot. **Pes hippocampi,** the anterior extremity of the hippocampus. **Pes planus,** flat foot.

Pessary. An instrument or appliance for insertion into the vagina to support a prolapsed uterus. A solid body suitably shaped for vaginal administration and containing medicaments intended to act locally. (*Plural:* pessaries.) There are seven pessaries in the *British Pharmaceutical Codex* 1968: Acetarsol pessaries; Crystal violet pessaries; Di-iodohydroxyquinoline pessaries; Ichthammol pessaries; Lactic acid pessaries; Nystatin pessaries; Stilboestrol pessaries.

Pest. Plague.

Pesticide. A substance or agent that is lethal to fungi, insects and the like.

Pestle. An implement for crushing powders and the like in a mortar.

Petechia. A minute haemorrhagic spot on the skin. (*Plural:* petechiae.)

Pethidine hydrochloride. B.P. 1968. $C_{15}H_{22}ClNO_2$. A narcotic analgesic.

Petit mal. Minor epilepsy.

Petrolatum. Soft paraffin.

Petrosal. Pertaining to the petrous portion of the temporal bone.

Petrous. Resembling a rock. Petrosal.

-pexy (Gk *pēxis:* a fixing). Suffix signifying fixation.

Peyote. Mescaline.

Phaco- (Gk *phakos:* a lentil or lentil-shaped object). Prefix signifying relationship to a lens.

Phaeo- (Gk *phaios:* grey, dusky). Prefix meaning grey.

Phaeochromocyte. The cell in the chromaffin system, which secretes adrenaline and noradrenaline. Chromaffin cell.

Phaeochromocytoma. A tumour of the adrenal medulla, composed of chromaffin cells, which secretes adrenaline.

Phage. Bacteriophage.

-phage (Gk *phagein:* to eat). Suffix meaning an eater.

Phagedaena. A rapidly spreading form of ulceration.

Phago- (Gk *phagein:* to eat). Prefix signifying eating or consuming.

Phagocyte. A cell that has the property of ingesting microbes, foreign particles and other cells.

Phagocytin. The bactericidal factor in phagocytes.

Phagocytosis. The process of ingestion and digestion by cells. The response of phagocytes to invasion by microbes and the like.

Phako- (Gk *phakos:* a lentil or lentil-shaped object). Prefix signifying relationship to a lens.

Phakomatosis. A group of diseases with a familial incidence and a congenital basis with a tendency for the development of lens-like neoplasms in the central nervous system and elsewhere.

Phalangeal. Pertaining to a phalanx.

Phalangectomy. Surgical extirpation of a phalanx.

Phalangitis. Inflammation of a phalanx.

Phalanx. One of the bones of the fingers or toes. (*Plural:* phalanges.)

Phallic. Pertaining to the penis.

Phallo- (Gk *phallos:* penis). Prefix signifying relationship with the penis.

Phalloplasty. Plastic surgery of the penis.

Phallus. The embryonic progenitor of the penis in the male and the clitoris in the female. Commonly used now as a synonym for the penis.

Phanero- (Gk *phaneros:* visible). Prefix meaning visible.

Phaneromania. Constant preoccupation with touching some external part as manifested by plucking a beard or moustache, or picking at a pimple.

Phanerosis. The act of becoming visible.

Phanquone. The B.P. Commission approved name for 4,7-phenanthroline-5, 6-quinone. An amoebicide.

Phantasy. Visionary imagination.

Phantom. An apparition. **Phantom**

limb, the sensation as if a limb were still present after amputation. **Phantom pregnancy,** false pregnancy.

Pharmaceutical. Pertaining to pharmacy.

Pharmacist. A dispensing chemist, a chemist and druggist.

Pharmaco- (Gk *pharmakon:* drug). Prefix signifying relationship to drugs.

Pharmacogenetics. The study of genetically determined variations in the response to drugs.

Pharmacognosy. The branch of pharmacology that deals with the study of crude drugs.

Pharmacologist. One who studies the action of drugs.

Pharmacology. The science and study of the action of drugs on the body.

Pharmacomania. An abnormal craving for drugs.

Pharmacophobia. Morbid fear of drugs.

Pharmacopoeia. A book published by some authorized body, generally constituted by law, which describes most of the drugs in common use, with directions for their preparation, identification, standardization and dosage.

Pharmacy. The science and art of the preparation, combination and dispensing of drugs. The premises where such dispensing is performed.

Pharyng-, Pharyngo- (Gk *pharynx, pharyng-:* throat). Prefixes indicating relationship with the pharynx.

Pharyngismus. Spasm of the muscles of the pharynx.

Pharyngitis. Inflammation of the pharynx.

Pharyngocoele. A pharyngeal diverticulum.

Pharyngoconjunctivitis. Infection of the pharynx and conjunctiva by an adenovirus, most commonly found in children. Pharyngoconjunctival fever.

Pharyngoglossal. Pertaining to the pharynx and tongue.

Pharyngolaryngectomy. Surgical excision of the pharynx and larynx.

Pharyngopalatine. Relating to the pharynx and the palate.

Pharyngoplasty. Plastic surgery of the pharynx.

Pharyngoplegia. Paralysis of the muscles of the pharynx.

Pharyngoscope. An instrument for examining the pharynx.

Pharyngotomy. Surgical incision of the pharynx.

Pharynx. The part of the digestive tube that is placed behind the nasal cavities, the mouth and the larynx. A musculomembranous tube, 12 to 14 cm. long, which extends from the under-surface of the skull to the level of the 6th cervical vertebra opposite the lower border of the cricoid cartilage.

Phen-, Pheno- (Gk *phainein:* to show). Prefixes signifying derivation from benzene, or to show or appear.

Phenacemide. The B.P. Commission approved name for (phenylacetyl) urea. An anticonvulsant.

Phenacetin. B.P. 1968. $C_{10}H_{13}NO_2$. An analgesic and antipyretic with a tendency to damage the kidneys.

Phenactropinium chloride. The B.P. Commission approved name for N-phenacylhomatropinium chloride. A hypotensive agent.

Phenadoxone. The B.P. Commission approved name for 6-morpholino-4,4-diphenylheptan-3-one. An analgesic and hypnotic.

Phenaglycodol. The B.P. Commission approved name for 2-(4-chlorophenyl)-3-methylbutane-2,3-diol. A central nervous system depressant.

Phenampromide. The B.P. Commission approved name for N-(l-methyl-2-piperidinoethyl)propionanilide. A narcotic analgesic.

Phenate. A compound of phenol and a base.

Phenazocine hydrobromide. B.P. Addendum, 1969. $C_{22}H_{28}BrNO$, $\frac{1}{2}H_2O$. A morphine-like analgesic.

Phenazone. B.P.C. 1968. $C_{11}H_{12}N_2O$. An antipyretic and analgesic, whose indiscriminate use is not without danger.

Phenazopyridine. The B.P. Commission approved name for 2,6-diamino-3-phenylazopyridine. An analgesic.

Phenbenicillin. The B.P. Commission approved name for an acid-resistant, orally active, semi-synthetic penicillin, similar to phenethicillin.

Phenbutrazate. The B.P. Commission approved name for 2-(3-methyl-2-phenylmorpholino) ethyl 2-phenylbutyrate. An appetite suppressant.

Phencyclidine. The B.P. Commission approved name for 1-(1-phenylcyclohexyl) piperidine. An analgesic and anaesthetic.

Phendimetrazine. The B.P. Commission approved name for (+)-3,4-dimethyl-2-phenylmorpholine. An appetite suppressant.

Phenelzine sulphate. B.P. 1968. $C_8H_{14}N_2O_4S$. A monoamine-oxidase inhibitor antidepressant.

Phenethicillin potassium. B.P. 1968. A semisynthetic penicillin which is not inactivated by acid and can therefore be given orally.

Phenethyl alcohol. The B.P. Commission approved name for 2-phenylethanol. An antiseptic.

Pheneturide. The B.P. Commission approved name for 2-phenylbutyryl urea. An anticonvulsant.

Phenformin hydrochloride. B.P. Addendum 1971. $C_{10}H_{16}ClN_5$. An oral hypoglycaemic agent.

Phenglutarimide. The B.P. Commission approved name for 2-(2-diethylamino-ethyl)-2-phenylglutarimide. An antiparkinsonian drug.

Phenindamine tartrate. B.P. 1968. $C_{23}H_{25}NO_6$. An antihistaminic.

Phenindione. B.P. 1968. $C_{15}H_{10}O_2$. An oral anticoagulant.

Pheniprazine. The B.P. Commission approved name for α-methylphenethylhydrazine. A monoamine oxidase inhibitor.

Pheniramine. The B.P. Commission approved name for 3-dimethylamino-1-phenyl-1-(2-pyridyl)propane. An antihistamine.

Phenmetrazine hydrochloride. B.P. 1968. $C_{11}H_{16}ClNO$. An appetite suppressant.

Phenobarbitone. B.P. 1968. $C_{12}H_{12}N_2O_3$. Probably the most widely used barbiturate as a sedative and anticonvulsant. **Phenobarbitone sodium,** B.P. 1968, $C_{12}H_{11}N_2NaO_3$, a preparation that can be given by injection.

Phenobutiodil. The B.P. Commission approved name for a radio-opaque substance.

Phenol. B.P. 1968. $C_6H_5.OH$. Carbolic acid. A bactericide and an antipruritic. Liquefied phenol, B.P. 1968, 80 per cent w/w of phenol in purified water, B.P.

Phenology. The study of the effects of climate on living things.

Phenolphthalein. B.P. 1968. $C_{20}H_{14}O_4$. An irritant purgative.

Phenolsulphonphthalein. B.P. 1968. $C_{19}H_{14}O_5S$. Phenol red. A dye used as the basis of a renal function test.

Phenomorphan. The B.P. Commission approved name for 3-hydroxy-N-phenethylmorphinan. A narcotic analgesic.

Phenoperidine. The B.P. Commission approved name for ethyl 1-(3-hydroxy-3-phenylpropyl) - 4 - phenylpiperidine - 4-carboxylate. A narcotic analgesic.

Phenotype. The visible traits that characterize the members of a group. The same phenotype may appear when the genotype is different, just as different phenotypes may appear when the genotype is the same.

Phenoxy-. The prefix indicating the presence of the group OC_6H_5: i.e. phenyl and an atom of oxygen.

Phenoxybenzamine hydrochloride. B.P. 1968. $C_{18}H_{23}Cl_2NO$. An adrenaline antagonist used to control the hypertension induced by a phaeochromocytoma.

Phenoxyethanol. B.P.C. 1968. $C_8H_{10}O_2$. A preparation which has an antibacterial action against *Pseudomonas aeruginosa*, and to a lesser extent against *Proteus vulgaris*.

Phenoxymethylpenicillin. B.P. 1968. 6-phenoxyacetamidopenicillanic acid, produced by certain strains of *Penicillium notatum* or related organisms and active when given by mouth. **Phenoxymethylpenicillin calcium,** B.P. 1968, a derivative of phenoxymethylpenicillin that is absorbed more readily. **Phenoxymethylpenicillin potassium,** B.P. 1968, a preparation with an action comparable to the calcium derivative.

Phenoxypropazine. The B.P. Commission approved name for (1-methyl-2-phenoxyethyl)hydrazine. A monoamine oxidase inhibitor.

Phenprobamate. The B.P. Commission approved name for 3-phenylpropyl carbamate. A skeletal muscle relaxant.

Phenprocoumon. The B.P. Commission approved name for an anticoagulant.

Phensuximide. B.P.C. 1968. $C_{11}H_{11}NO_2$. An anticonvulsant used in the treatment of petit mal.

Phentermine. The B.P. Commission approved name for $\alpha\alpha$-dimethylphenethylamine. An anorexiant.

Phentolamine mesylate. B.P. 1968. $C_{18}H_{23}N_3O_4S$. An adrenaline antagonist used in the diagnosis of phaeochromocytoma.

Phenyl. The monovalent organic radical C_6H_5.

Phenylalanine. α-amino-β-phenyl-propionic acid. One of the essential amino-acids.

Phenyl aminosalicylate. The B.P. Commission approved name for an antituberculosis drug.

Phenylbutazone. B.P. 1968. $C_{19}H_{20}N_2O_2$. An analgesic and antipyretic.

Phenylene. The divalent radical C_6H_9.

Phenylephrine hydrochloride. B.P. 1968. $C_9H_{14}ClNO_2$. A sympathomimetic used topically as a vasoconstrictor, and systemically, mainly in anaesthesia, to prevent hypotension.

Phenylketonuria. A form of mental deficiency due to the inability of the individual to metabolize phenylalanine as a result of the congenital absence of the enzyme phenylalanine hydroxylase.

Phenylmercuric acetate. B.P.C. 1968. $C_8H_8HgO_2$. A preparation with bacteriostatic and antifungal properties. **Phenylmercuric nitrate,** B.P. 1968, $C_{12}H_{11}Hg_2NO_4$. A preparation with the same properties as the acetate. Both are used as bactericides in parenteral preparations.

Phenylpropanolamine hydrochloride. B.P.C. 1968. $C_9H_{14}ClNO$. A sympathomimetic amine with an action similar to that of ephedrine.

Phenylpyruvic acid. A metabolic product of phenyalanine, found in the urine in cases of phenylketonuria.

Phenylthiocarbamide. A substance that has an intensely bitter taste to 70 per cent of the population, and is tasteless to the remainder. The differentiation is genetically determined. Phenylthiorurea.

Phenyltoloxamine. The B.P. Commission approved name for N-2-(2-benzylphenoxy)ethyldimethylamine. An antihistaminic.

Phenyramidol. The B.P. Commission approved name for 1-phenyl-2-(2-pyridylamino)ethanol. An analgesic.

Phenytoin. B.P.C. 1968. $C_{15}H_{12}N_2O_2$. An anticonvulsant. **Phenytoin sodium,** B.P. 1968, $C_{15}H_{11}N_2NaO_2$. An anticonvulsant with relatively little hypnotic action.

Pherohormone. A substance secreted by an individual or animal which releases a specific reaction in another member of the same species. Ectohormone.

Phial. A small glass container for liquid medicine. Vial.

-philia (Gk *philein:* to love). Suffix signifying attraction, or craving, for.

Philtrum. The shallow vertical groove in the middle of the outer surface of the upper lip.

Phimosis. Narrowing of the preputial orifice.

Phleb-, Phlebo- (Gk *phleps, phlebos:* vein). Prefixes signifying relationship with veins.

Phlebectomy. Surgical excision of a vein or of a section of it.

Phlebitis. Inflammation of a vein.

Phlebography. Radiological visualization of the veins by means of the injection of radio-opaque substances. The recording of the venous pulsation.

Phlebolith. A concretion in a vein, usually a calcified thrombus.

Phleborrhagia. Haemorrhage from a vein.

Phleborrhexis. Rupture of a vein.

Phlebosclerosis. Thickening of the wall of a vein.

Phlebothrombosis. Clotting, or thrombosis, in a vein without preliminary phlebitis.

Phlebotomus. A genus of small, very hairy flies of the family Psychodidae. Sandflies. They are the vectors of several forms of leishmaniasis, sandfly fever, and Oroya fever.

Phlebotomy. Venesection.

Phleg- (Gk *phlegma:* inflammation). Prefix meaning inflammation.

Phlegm. Mucus, particularly that expectorated from the respiratory tract.

Phlegmasia. Inflammation. **Phlegmasia alba dolens,** white leg. Tense, painful swelling of the leg following childbirth, due to iliofemoral thrombosis. **Phlegmasia caerula dolens,** a rare form of iliofemoral thrombosis, marked by sudden intense venous engorgement of the limb, followed by gangrene.

Phlegmatic. Dull, morose, apathetic.

Phlegmon. Inflammation of the connective tissue.

Phlogo- (Gk *phlogōsis:* inflammation). Prefix signifying relationship to inflammation.

Phlorizin. A glycoside obtained from the root bark of apple, cherry, pear and plum trees, which is used experimentally to induce glycosuria in animals.

Phlycten. A small blister or vesicle. A small bleb on the conjunctiva or cornea, which goes on to ulceration.

Phlyctenular. Characterized by the presence of phlyctens.

-phobe (Gk *phobos:* fear). Suffix denoting one having a phobia.

Phobia. Unreasonable fear or dread.

-phobia (Gk *phobos:* fear). Suffix signifying fear or dread.

Phoco- (Gk *phŏkē:* seal). Prefix indicating absence of, or imperfect development of.

Phocomelia. Defective development of the limbs so that the hands and feet are attached close to the body.

Pholcodine. B.P. 1968. $C_{23}H_{30}N_2O_4$, H_2O. An antitussive.

Pholedrine. The B.P. Commission approved name for 4-(2-methylaminopropyl)phenol. A sympathomimetic agent.

Phon. A unit of the subjective loudness of a sound.

Phon-, Phono- (Gk *phōnē:* voice). Prefixes indicating relationship to sound.

Phonasthenia. Weakness of the voice, usually due to fatigue or overuse or abuse of the voice.

Phonation. The production of sounds by the vocal cords.

Phoneme. The basic unit of sound in spoken language. There are just over 40 phonemes in the English language.

Phonetic. Pertaining to the voice or speech.

Phonetics. The science of speech and sound production.

Phonoautograph. An instrument that records the vibrations of the voice or any other sound.

Phonocardiogram. An instrument for the graphic recording of heart sounds and murmurs.

Phonometer. An instrument for measuring the pitch and intensity of sounds.

Phoresis. The transmission of chemical ions into the tissues by means of an electric current.

-phoria (Gk *phorein:* to bear). Suffix signifying, in ophthalmology, any deviation of the eyes from normal, or any turning of the visual axis.

Phormia. A genus of flies of the temperate and sub-arctic zones. *Phormia regina,* a species that may infect suppurating wounds.

Phos- (Gk *phōs:* light). Prefix meaning light.

Phosgene. Carbonyl chloride. A poisonous asphyxiating gas.

Phosphagen. Creatine phosphate.

Phosphataemia. An excess of phosphates in the blood.

Phosphatase. An enzyme that liberates inorganic phosphate from phosphoric esters. **Acid phosphatase,** one of the constituents of prostatic secretion, which is grossly increased in carcinoma of the prostate with a resultant increase in its serum level. **Alkaline phosphatase,** an enzyme whose level in the serum is increased in liver and bone disease, and certain cases of carcinoma of the breast. **Phosphatase test,** a test for the efficiency of the pasteurization of milk.

Phosphate. A salt of phosphoric acid.

Phosphatidylcholine. Lecithin.

Phosphatidylethanolamine. Cephalin.

Phosphatidylinositol. A phospholipid found mainly in plants and nervous tissue.

Phosphaturia. An excess of phosphates in the urine.

Phosphide. A compound of phosphorus with another element.

Phosphocreatin. Creatine phosphate.

Phosphofructokinase. One of the enzymes concerned in the process of glycolysis.

Phosphogalactose uridyl transferase. The enzyme concerned in the metabolism of galactose, the congenital absence of which is responsible for the hereditary disease galactosaemia.

Phosphoglucomutase. An enzyme concerned in the breakdown of glycogen to glucose.

Phosphoglycerate kinase. An enzyme concerned in the process of glycolysis.

Phosphoglyceromutase. An enzyme concerned in the process of glycolysis.

Phospholipid. A class of lipids which contain phosphoric acid and a nitrogenous organic base such as choline or ethanolamine. They include the lecithins and cephalin.

Phosphonecrosis. Necrosis of the jaw that may occur in those who work with phosphorus. Phossy jaw.

Phosphopyruvate hydratase. An enzyme concerned in the process of glycolysis. Enolase.

Phosphorated. Forming a compound with phosphorus.

Phosphoric acid. B.P. 1968. H_3PO_4. A constituent of some mixtures prescribed to stimulate appetite.

Phosphorus. A non-metallic, poisonous, highly inflammable element. Symbol P. Atomic weight 30·9738. Atomic number 15.

Phosphoryl. The trivalent radical $\equiv$PO.

Phosphorylase. The enzyme that catalyses the breakdown of glycogen to glucose and phosphate.

Phosphorylation. The addition of phosphate to an organic molecule by means of phosphorylase.

Phosphuretted. Phosphorated.

Phot-, Photo- (Gk |*phōs, phōtos:* light). Prefixes meaning light.

Photic. Pertaining to light.

Photochrogenic. Possessing the ability, or faculty, of forming pigment on exposure to light.

Photodermatitis. An eruption on areas of the skin exposed to light induced by sensitization of the skin by certain drugs and occurring on exposure to sunlight.

Photoelectric. Pertaining to the electric effects of light or other radiations.

Photometer. An instrument for measuring the intensity of light.

Photometric. Pertaining to the measurement of light.

Photomicrograph. The photograph of an object as seen through a microscope.

Photon. A quantum of electromagnetic radiation.

Photophobia. Abnormal fear of light. The blepharospasm induced by corneal irritation.

Photophthalmia. Ophthalmia induced by intense light, such as ultraviolet rays.

Photopia. Day vision.

Photopic. Pertaining to vision in bright light. **Photopic vision,** vision in bright light when the cones come into play.

Photopsiae. Subjective flashes of light due to retinal irritability.

Photo-retinitis. Retinitis induced by bright light, as after looking at an eclipse of the sun with unprotected eyes.

Photosensitive. Sensitive to light.

Photosynthesis. The process whereby, under the influence of light, compounds are built up, particularly in green plants in which, using chlorophyll, carbohydrates are formed from carbon dioxide and water.

Phototaxis. The reaction of microorganisms and cells to light, which may be *negative* (repulsion) or *positive* (attraction).

Photuria. The passage of luminous, or phosphorescent, urine.

Phren- (Gk *phrēn:* diaphragm, heart, mind). Prefix indicating association with the diaphragm or the mind.

Phrenetic. Frenzied.

-phrenia (Gk *phrēn:* diaphragm, heart, mind). Suffix indicating association with the mind or the diaphragm.

Phrenic. Pertaining to the diaphragm. Pertaining to the mind.

Phrenicectomy. The operation for removal of part of the phrenic nerve.

Phrenico-exeris. Avulsion of the phrenic nerve.

Phrenology. The study of the mind from the shape of the head.

Phryno- (Gk *phrynos:* a toad). Prefix signifying toad-like.

Phrynoderma. The state of the skin, characterized by dryness, roughness, hyperkeratosis, and follicular papules, induced by lack of vitamin A. Toad skin.

Phthalate. A salt of phthalic acid.

Phthalein. One of a group of dyes prepared from phthalic anhydride and a phenol.

Phthalic acid. $C_6H_4(COOH)_2$. An acid used in the manufacture of dyes and in organic synthesis.

Phthalylsulphathiazole. B.P. 1968. $C_{17}H_{13}N_3O_5S_2$. An insoluble sulphonamide used in the treatment of intestinal infections such as bacillary dysentery.

Phthiriasis. Infestation with the crab louse, *Phthirus pubis.*

Phthirus. A genus of lice. *Phthirus pubis,* the crab louse, a common parasite of man, infesting predominantly the pubic hairs.

Phthisis. Any wasting disease, but usually restricted to the progressive wasting associated with chronic active pulmonary tuberculosis.

Phyco- (Gk *phykos:* seaweed). Prefix signifying relationship to seaweed.

Phycomycetes. The class of fungi which form non-septate hyphae, asexual sporangiospores, and sexual spores of the zygospore or oospore varieties.

Phycomycosis. The subcutaneous infection caused by the phycomycete *Basidiolus ranarum,* which occurs in tropical and subtropical countries.

Phylo- (Gk *phylon:* tribe). Prefix signifying relationship to a group.

Phylogenesis. The developmental history of a species or order of animals or plants. The ancestral history of an individual.

Phylum. A primary division of the animal kingdom. (*Plural:* phyla.)

Physaloptera. A genus of roundworms.

Physical. Pertaining to the body, material matter, or physics.

Physics. The branch of science that deals with the properties of matter and of the forces governing it.

Physio- (Gk *physis:* nature). Prefix indicating relationship to physiology or nature.

Physiognomy. The countenance.

Physiology. That branch of science that deals with the function of the living body.

Physiotherapy. The employment of physical measures, such as exercise, heat and massage, in the treatment of disease. Physical medicine.

Physo- (Gk *physa:* air). Prefix signifying relationship to air or gas.

Physopsis. A sub-genus of snails of the genus Bulinus.

Physostigmine. B.P.C. 1968. $C_{15}H_{21}N_3O_2$. An anticholinesterase agent used as a miotic in eye-drops. **Physostigmine salicylate,** B.P. 1968, $C_{15}H_{21}N_3O_2,C_7H_6O_3$. An anticholinesterase used as a miotic. **Physostigmine sulphate,** B.P.C. 1968, $(C_{15}H_{21}N_3O_2)_2,H_2SO_4$, an anticholinesterase used as a miotic.

Phyt-, Phyto- (Gk *phyton:* plant). Prefixes signifying relationship to plants.

Phytase. The enzyme that catalyses the hydrolysis of phytic acid, as in the process of bread making.

Phytate. A salt of phytic acid.

Phytic acid. Inositol hexaphosphate, a constituent of cereals which forms insoluble salts with calcium and iron, and thereby interferes with their absorption.

Phytohaemagglutinin. Material from plants which agglutinate erythrocytes.

Phytomenadione. B.P. 1968. $C_{31}H_{46}O_2$. Vitamin K_1. A naturally occurring vitamin K which maintains a normal level of prothrombin in the blood. It is used in the treatment of haemorrhage due to hypoprothrombinaemia.

Phytopathology. The study of plant diseases.

Phytophotodermatitis. A form of dermatitis produced on exposure to the sun after having been in contact with the juice of certain plants.

Phytotoxin. A toxin derived from a plant.

Pia mater. The vascular membrane that closely invests the brain and the spinal cord.

Pian. Yaws.

Pica. Abnormal craving for unusual food or substances not fit for food.

Picloxydine. The B.P. Commission approved name for a bactericide and fungicide.

Pico- (Ital *piccolo:* small). Prefix meaning small. In the international system of units (SI) it means one-trillionth.

Picornavirus. The group of viruses which includes the enteroviruses and rhinoviruses. The name is derived from pico (small) and RNA (because they contain ribonucleic acid).

Picrate. A salt of picric acid.

Picric acid. $C_6H_3N_3O_7$. Trinitrophenol. A strong antiseptic

Picro- (Gk *pikros:* bitter). Prefix meaning bitter.

Piedra. A fungus disease of the hair.

Piedraia. A genus of fungus. *Piedraia hortai,* the causative fungus of black piedra.

Pifenate. The B.P. Commission approved name for an analgesic.

Pigeon breeder's lung. A form of pneumonia resulting from sensitization to pigeons.

Pigment. A colouring matter. A medicinal preparation for application to the skin or mucous surfaces.

Pigmentation. Coloration or discoloration by the deposition of pigment.

Pile. Haemorrhoid.

Piliform. Hair-like.

Pill. A spherical or ovoid mass containing one or more medicaments.

Pillar. An elongated, supporting structure.

Pilo- (L *pilus:* hair). Prefix indicating association with hair.

Pilocarpine hydrochloride. B.P.C. 1968. $C_{11}H_{17}ClN_2O_2$. The hydrochloride of pilocarpine, an alkaloid obtained from the leaves of *Pilocarpus microphyllus* and other species of Pilocarpus. **Pilocarpine nitrate, B.P.** 1968, the nitrate of pilocarpine. Both hydrochloride and nitrate are miotics, having the muscarine actions of acetylcholine.

Pilomotor. Causing movement of the hair.

Pilonidal. Denoting a growth of hair in a cyst.

Pilosebaceous. Pertaining to the hair follicles and sebaceous glands.

Pilosis. Excessive or abnormal growth of hair.

Pilula. A small pill. (*Plural:* pilulae.)

Pilus. A hair. (*Plural:* pili). **Pili torti,** a rare congenital condition characterized by twisting of the hair shaft which is friable and gives an over-all impression of stubble.

Pimelo- (Gk *pimelē:* fat). Prefix signifying relationship to fat.

Pimimodine. The B.P. Commission approved name for ethyl 4-phenyl-1-(3-phenylaminopropyl)piperidine-4-carboxylate. A narcotic analgesic.

Pimozide. The B.P. Commission approved name for 1-⟨1-[4,4-bis(4-fluorophenyl)butyl] - 4 - piperidyl⟩ - benzimidazolin-2-one. A tranquillizer.

Pimple. A papule or pustule.

Pincement. Pinching or nipping of the tissues in massage.

Pineal body. A small structure, about 8×4mm., lying on the dorsal aspect of the superior quadrigeminal bodies.

Pinguecula. A yellow triangular patch on the conjunctiva, usually found in elderly people, especially those exposed to strong sunlight, dust, and wind.

Pink disease. Erythroedema. Acrodynia.

Pink eye. Acute catarrhal or mucopurulent conjunctivitis.

Pinocytosis. The active incorporation of fluid into a cell by the formation of minute intracytoplasmic vesicles.

Pint. A measure of capacity: 20 fluid ounces; one-eighth of a gallon; 568ml.

Pinta. A spirochaetal infection caused by *Treponema carateum*, occurring in Central and South America.

Pintid. The dermal lesion of pinta.

Pinworm. Threadworm. *Enterobius vermicularis.*

Pipamazine. The B.P. Commission approved name for 10-[3-(4-carbamoyl-piperidino)propyl]-2-chlorophenothiazine. A tranquillizer and antiemetic.

Pipamperone. The B.P. Commission approved name for 1-[3-(4-fluorobenzoyl)propyl]-4-piperidinopiperidine-4-carboxamide. A tranquillizer.

Pipazethate. The B.P. Commission approved name for 2-(2-piperidinoethoxy) ethyl 10-thia-1,9-diaza-anthracene-9-carboxylate. A cough suppressant.

Pipenzolate bromide. The B.P. Commission approved name for 3-benziloyloxy-1-ethyl-1-methylpiperidinium bromide. An antispasmodic.

Piperazine adipate. B.P. 1968. $C_4H_{10}N_2$, $C_6H_{10}O_4$. **Piperazine calcium edetate,** the B.P. Commission approved name for a chelate produced by treating ethylenediamine-*NNN'N'*-tetra-acetic acid with calcium carbonate and piperazine. **Piperazine citrate, B.P.** 1968, $(C_4H_{10}N_2)_3,2C_6H_8O_7$. **Piperazine hydrate, B.P.C.** 1968, $C_4H_{10}N_2$, $6H_2O$. **Piperazine phosphate, B.P.** 1968, $C_4H_{10}N_2,H_3PO_4,H_2O$. All five preparations are anthelmintics used in the treatment of roundworm and threadworm infestation.

Piperidolate. The B.P. Commission approved name for 1-ethyl-3-piperidyl diphenyl acetate. A parasympatholytic agent.

Piperocaine. The B.P. Commission approved name for 3-(2-methylpiperidino) propyl benzoate. A local anaesthetic.

Piperoxan. The B.P. Commission approved name for 2-piperidinomethyl-1,4-benzodioxan. An adrenergic blocking agent.

Pipette. A glass tube used to measure and transfer liquids or gases in the laboratory.

Pipoxolan. The B.P. Commission approved name for 5,5-diphenyl-2-(2-piperidinoethyl)-1,3-dioxolan-4-one. An antispasmodic.

Pipradrol. The B.P. Commission approved name for α-2-piperidylbenzhydrol. A central nervous system stimulant.

Piprinhydrinate. The B.P. Commission approved name for an antihistaminic.

Piqûre. Puncture.

Piriform. Pear-shaped.

Piritramide. The B.P. Commission approved name for 4-(4-carbamoyl-4-piperidinopiperidino)-2,2-diphenyl-butyronitrile. An analgesic.

Pisiform. The most medial of the four bones in the proximal row of the carpus.

Pit. An indentation. **Auditory pit,** the depression in the embryo which marks the beginning of the internal ear. **Granular pits,** the irregular depressions on the interior of the skull caused by the arachnoid granulations. **Olfactory pit,** the embryonic beginning of the nasal cavity.

Pitch. The quality of a sound, depending on the rapidity of the vibrations of the body producing the sound.

Pith. To pierce the spinal cord or brain, with a view to destroying it, as in the experimental animal, preliminary to certain experiments.

Pithiatism. The treatment of disease by suggestion, or the state of mind induced by suggestion.

Pitting. The induction of pits by pressure over an area of subcutaneous oedema.

Pituicyte. The characteristic cell of the neurohypophysis.

Pituitary. The hypophysis cerebri.

Pituitary, powdered (posterior lobe). B.P.C. 1968. A powder prepared from the posterior lobe of mammalian pituitary bodies. It has oxytocic, pressor, antidiuretic and hyperglycaemic actions.

Pityriasis. A bran-like skin eruption. **Pityriaris alba,** pityriasis simplex. **Pityriasis capitis,** dandruff. Seborrhoea capitis. **Pityriasis lichenoides,** a papular eruption with certain features resembling psoriasis. **Pityriasis rosea,** a common disease characterized by oval pink macules on the trunk and proximal parts of the limbs. **Pityriasis rubra pilaris,** a rare chronic disorder of the skin characterized by extensive areas of red scaly skin. **Pityriasis simplex,** a common condition in children, characterized by patches of fine scaling. **Pityriasis steatoides,** seborrhoea corporis. **Pityriasis versicolor,** a café au-lait eruption, usually on the upper part of the trunk due to *Malassezia furfur*.

Pityrosporum ovale. A small gram-negative yeast, which is a common commensal of normal skin.

Pivampicillin. The B.P. Commission approved name for a semi-synthetic penicillin.

Pivhydrazine. The B.P. Commission approved name for *N*-benzyl-*N*′-pivaloylhydrazine. A monoamine oxidase inhibitor.

Placebo. A pharmacologically inert substance given to a patient either to gratify him or as a control to some active drug undergoing clinical trial.

Placenta. The organ which connects the foetus to the uterine wall, by means of which the respiratory, nutritive and excretory functions of the foetus are performed. **Abruptio placentae,** premature separation of a normally sited placenta. **Placenta accreta,** the condition resulting from absence of the decidua basalis, as a result of which the uterine muscle is exposed to invasion by the trophoblast and to penetration by the chorionic villi, thereby constituting one form of adherent placenta. **Adherent placenta,** a placenta which does not come away spontaneously in the third stage of labour. **Battledore placenta,** a placenta to which the umbilical cord is attached eccentrically. **Placenta bilobata,** a placenta divided into lobes. **Placenta bipartita,** a placenta in two parts. **Placenta diffusa,** a placenta formed over the whole area of the chorion. **Placenta multipartita,** a placenta in several parts. **Placenta praevia,** a placenta implanted in the lower uterine segment. **Placenta succenturia,** a placenta with small outlying portions. **Placenta tripartita,** a placenta in three parts.

Placentography. Radiological demonstration of the placenta *in utero*.

Placode. An embryonic ectodermal thickening. **Auditory placodes,** the first rudiments of the internal ear. **Epibranchial placodes,** thickened ectodermal patches at the dorsal ends of the 1st, 2nd, and 4th clefts, which are intimately related to the underlying ganglia of the 7th, 9th and 10th cranial nerves. **Olfactory placodes,** the ectodermal thickenings which represent the rudiments of the nasal cavity.

Plagio- (Gk *plagios:* oblique). Prefix meaning oblique or asymmetrical.

Plagiocephaly. A lopsided skull due to asynchronous fusion of the bones.

Plague. A bacterial infection caused by *Pasteurella pestis*. **Bubonic plague,** the common form, characterized by enlargement of the lymphatic nodes (buboes). **Pneumonic plague,** the form in which the lungs are the primary site of infection.

Plane. A flat surface. **Coronal plane,** a vertical plane at right angles to the median plane, which passes through or parallel to the coronal suture of the skull, dividing the body into anterior and posterior parts. **Horizontal plane,** a plane drawn at right angles to both coronal and sagittal planes. **Lateral planes, left and right,** lines drawn vertically through points halfway between the anterior superior iliac spines and the symphysis pubis. **Median plane,** a vertical plane which passes through the centre of the trunk and divides the body into superficially symmetrical right and left halves. **Sagittal plane,** any plane parallel to the median plane. **Subcostal plane,** a line drawn through the body on a level with the most dependent parts of the 10th costal cartilages. **Supracristal plane,** on the posterior surface of the body a transverse line joining the highest parts of the two iliac crests, cutting through the spinous process of the 4th lumbar vertebra in the midline. **Transpyloric plane,** a line encircling the body at a level midway between the suprasternal notch and the symphysis pubis. **Transtubercular plane,** a line carried round the trunk at the level of the tubercle on the iliac crest.

Planigraphy. Body section radiography.

Plano- (L *planus:* flat). Prefix meaning flat or level.

Planoconcave. Flat on one side, concave on the other.

Planoconvex. Flat on one side, convex on the other.

Planorbis. A species of snails or molluscs.

Planta. The sole of the foot. (*Plural:* plantae.)

Plantar. Pertaining to the sole of the foot.

Plantigrade. Walking on the whole of the sole of the foot, as man does.

Plaque. A patch.

-plasia (Gk *plassō:* to form). Suffix signifying formation.

Plasm-, Plasmo- (Gk *plasma:* anything formed). Prefixes indicating a relationship to a cell or plasma.

Plasma. The fluid portion of the blood. **Plasma cell,** a connective-tissue cell which is particularly abundant in the lamina propria of the gastro-intestinal tract. **Dried human plasma, B.P. 1968,** prepared by drying a pool of the supernatant fluids which are separated by centrifuging or by standing from quantities of whole human blood. **Dried human plasma protein fraction,** B.P. 1968, prepared by freeze-drying human plasma protein fraction. **Human plasma protein fraction, B.P.** 1968, a solution of the proteins of liquid human plasma, containing albumin and certain globulins which retain their solubility on heating. **Plasma membrane,** the thin wall that surrounds most cells. Cell membrane. **Plasma proteins,** the proteins in plasma: albumin, globulin, and fibrinogen.

Plasmalogens. A group of phospholipids abundant in brain and muscle.

Plasmapheresis. The process in which blood is withdrawn, centrifuged and the resulting separated red blood corpuscles are returned to the animal by intravenous injection, thus depriving the animal of plasma proteins, but not haemoglobin.

Plasmin. The proteolytic enzyme in plasma responsible for dissolving fibrin clots and other clotting factors.

Plasminogen. The inactive precursor of plasmin.

Plasmodium. The genus of the class Sporozoa, of the phyllum Protozoa, which includes the causative organisms of malaria. (*Plural:* plasmodia.) *Plasmodium falciparum,* the cause of malignant tertian malaria. *Plasmodium knowlesii,* the natural cause of chimpanzee malaria which may be capable of transmission to man. *Plasmodium malariae,* the cause of quartan malaria. *Plasmodium ovale,* the cause of some cases of malaria in Africa. *Plasmodium vivax,* the cause of benign tertian malaria.

Plasmolysis. Shrinking of a cell as a result of dehydration by osmotic action.

Plasmoptysis. Rupture of a cell with escape of protoplasm.

-plast (Gk *plastos:* formed). Suffix signifying a primitive cell.

Plaster. A substance intended for external application, as a support, as a means of applying medicaments, or for the purpose of taking an impression of a part. **Plaster of Paris,** calcium sulphate dihydrate, which solidifies on the addition of water, and is used widely in the treatment of fractures. **Self-adhesive plasters,** plasters prepared by spreading a self-adhesive mass on a supporting material which consists of plain or elastic cloths or plastic films. There are eight self-adhesive plasters in the *British Pharmaceutical Codex* 1968: Belladonna self-adhesive plaster; Extension plaster; Perforated plastic self-adhesive plaster; Salicylic acid self-adhesive plaster; Waterproof microporous plastic self-adhesive plaster;

Waterproof plastic self-adhesive plaster; Zinc oxide elastic self-adhesive plaster; Zinc oxide self-adhesive plaster.

Plastics. Synthetic and semi-synthetic polymeric materials, comprising a basic polymeric macromolecule, the polymer resin, and additives such as fillers, plasticizers, stabilizers and antistatics.

Plastron. The sternum and the costal cartilages.

-plasty (Gk *plassein:* to shape or mould). Suffix signifying moulding or shaping.

Plat-, Platy- (Gk *platys:* broad). Prefixes meaning broad or flat.

Plate. A flat structure or layer. A narrow flattened bar used in the treatment of certain fractures of bone. A shallow dish as used in bacteriology. **Basal plate of placenta,** the outer wall of the intervillous space. **Chordal plate,** notochordal plate. **Cribriform plate,** the part of the ethmoid bone in the floor of the anterior cranial fossa which helps to form the roof of the nasal cavity. **Ectodermal plate,** the plate formed by the cells of the germ disc within the trophoblastic shell. **Dental plate,** artificial denture. **Epiphysial plate,** the plate of cartilage between the epiphysis and the metaphysis of a growing bone. **Horizontal plate of the palatine bone,** the quadrilateral part of the palatine bone that forms the posterior part of the floor of the nasal cavity and posterior part of the bony palate. **Limiting plate,** the sheet formed by the liver cells where they adjoin the portal canals or hepatic vein tributaries; a similar limiting plate lies beneath the capsule of the liver. **Medullary plate,** the middle ectodermal thickening of the embryonic disc that later becomes the neural tube. **Motor end plate,** the specialized ending in skeletal muscle of the axons of effector neurones of the somatic system. **Muscle plate,** myotome. **Notochordal plate,** the predecessor of the notochord. **Occipital plate,** the membrane predecessor of the basilar part of the occipital bone. **Orbital plate of ethmoid bone,** the part of the bone that covers the middle and posterior ethmoidal sinuses and forms much of the medial wall of the orbit. **Orbital plates of the frontal bone,** two thin triangular lamellae that form the greater part of the roofs of the orbits. **Perpendicular plate of the ethmoid bone,** the thin quadrilateral plate that forms the upper part of the nasal septum. **Perpendicular plate of the palatine bone,** a thin, oblong plate that forms part of the inferior nasal meatus, and the medial wall of the maxillary sinus. **Prochordal plate,** a thickening of the yolk sac in front of the notochord which becomes the bucco-pharyngeal membrane. **Pterygoid plate, lateral,** the part of the bone that forms the medial wall of the infratemporal fossa. **Pterygoid plate, medial,** the part of the bone that forms the lateral boundary of the posterior nasal aperture and part of the lateral wall of the nasal part of the pharynx. **Skin plate,** dermatome. **Sternal plates,** the embryonic rudiments of the sternum. **Tarsal plate,** tarsus. **Tympanic plate,** the bony sides and floor of the external auditory meatus.

Platelet. An oval colourless blood cell, originating from megakaryocytes, which is concerned in the process of coagulation. The normal range is 250,000 to 500,000 per c.mm. Thrombocyte.

Platinum. A metallic element. Symbol Pt. Atomic weight 195·09. Atomic number 78.

Platy-. (Gk *platys:* broad). Prefix signifying broad or flat.

Platybasia. A developmental anomaly of the occipital bone and upper cervical spine.

Paltycephaly. Broadness of the skull.

Platyhelminth. A flatworm.

Platyhelminthes. A phylum which includes four classes: Turbelliria; Trematoda; Cestoda; Nemertea.

Platypelloid. Having a pelvis with a short antero-posterior and a wide transverse diameter of the inlet.

Platyrhine. Having a broad, flat nose.

Platysma. A thin sheet of muscle in the neck.

Pledget. A small piece of cotton-wool or gauze used as a swab.

-plegia (Gk *plēgē:* a blow, stroke). Suffix signifying a stroke or paralysis.

Pleio-, Pleo- (Gk *pleōn:* more). Prefixes meaning more.

Pleocytosis. An excess of cells. Often used to denote a lymphocytosis in the cerebrospinal fluid.

Pleomastia. The presence of supernumerary breasts or nipples.

Pleomorphism. The occurrence of several distinct types in the same species. Polymorphism.

Pleoptics. A method of treating amblyopia with particular reference to securing optimal binocular coordination.

Plessor. A small rubber-tipped hammer used to elicit tendon reflexes. Plexor.

Plethora. General congestion.

Plethysm- (Gk *plethysmos:* enlargement). Prefix meaning enlargement or fulness.

Plethysmograph. An instrument for recording changes in size of the part placed in it.

Pleur-, Pleuro- (Gk. *pleura:* rib, side). Prefixes indicating relationship to the pleura, a rib or a side.

Pleura. The serous membrane that invests each lung in the form of a closed, invaginated sac. (*Plural:* pleurae.) **Parietal pleura,** the part of the pleura that lines the inner surface of the corresponding half of the chest wall, covers a large part of the diaphragm, and is reflected over the structures occupying the middle part of the thorax. **Pulmonary pleura,** visceral pleura. **Visceral pleura,** the part of the pleura that covers the surface of the lung and lines the fissures between its lobes.

Pleuracotomy. Surgical incision into the pleural cavity. Pleurotomy.

Pleural. Relating to the pleura. Pleuritic.

Pleurectomy. Surgical excision of a portion of the pleura.

Pleurisy. Inflammation of the pleura. **Dry pleurisy,** pleurisy without an effusion. **Pleurisy with effusion,** pleurisy accompanied by the outpouring of a serous effusion.

Pleuritic. Relating to the pleura. Pleural.

Pleurocentesis. Puncture of the pleural cavity for diagnostic or therapeutic purpose.

Pleurodynia. A painful condition of the chest wall.

Pleurolysis. Pneumolysis.

Pleuropericardial. Relating to the pleura and the pericardium.

Pleuroperitoneal. Relating to the pleura and the peritoneum.

Pleuropneumonia. A combination of pleurisy and pneumonia with a predominance of pleuritic pain.

Pleurotomy. Pleuracotomy.

Pleurotyphoid. Typhoid fever which is preceded or accompanied by acute pleurisy.

Plexiform. Resembling a plexus.

Pleximeter. A mediate, usually made of bone or ivory, but may be a finger, placed on the chest wall in the process of percussion.

Plexor. Plessor.

Plexus. A network of blood vessels, lymphatics or nerves. (*Plural:* plexuses.) **Anular plexus,** the plexus of nerves around the periphery of the cornea. **Aortic plexus, abdominal,** a plexus of sympathetic nerve fibres around the abdominal aorta. **Aorticus thoracalis plexus,** a delicate plexus of sympathetic nerve fibres on the thoracic aorta. **Basilar venous plexus,** several interconnecting venous channels situated between the layers of the dura mater. **Brachial plexus,** a plexus in the posterior triangle of the neck and the axilla, formed by the union of the ventral rami of the lower four cervical nerves and the greater part of the ventral ramus of the 1st thoracic nerve. **Cardiac plexus,** a plexus situated at the base of the heart and divided into a *superficial* part formed by the cardiac branch of the superior cervical ganglion of the left sympathetic trunk, and the lower of the two cervical branches of the left vagus nerve; and the *deep* part formed by the cardiac nerves derived from the cervical and upper thoracic ganglia of the sympathetic trunk and the cardiac branches of the vagus and recurrent laryngeal nerves. **Carotid plexus, internal,** a plexus of sympathetic nerve fibres surrounding the internal carotid artery and formed by the two branches of the internal carotid nerve. **Carotid venous plexus, internal,** a plexus of veins that unites the cavernous sinus with the internal jugular vein. **Cavernous plexus,** a venous plexus beneath the mucous membrane of the nose. **Cervical plexus,** a plexus situated opposite the upper four cervical vertebrae, and formed by the ventral rami of the upper four cervical nerves. **Choroid plexus,** a highly vascular fringe of pia mater which projects into the lateral ventricle. There is a similar choroid plexus in the 3rd and the 4th ventricles. **Coccygeal plexus,** a small plexus formed by the ventral rami of the 5th sacral and the coccygeal nerves and a branch from the 4th sacral nerve. **Coeliac plexus,** a plexus situated at the level of the 12th thoracic, and 1st lumbar, vertebra, surrounding the coeliac artery, and formed by the greater and lesser splanchnic nerves and some filaments from the vagus and phrenic nerves. **Coronary plexus, left,** a plexus that accompanies the left coronary artery, or is formed by filaments from the cardiac plexus. **Coronary plexus,**

right, a plexus that accompanies the right coronary artery, and is formed by filaments from the cardiac plexus. **Dental plexus, inferior,** a plexus formed by the branches of the inferior alveolar nerve to the molar and premolar teeth of the mandible. **Dental plexus, superior,** a plexus formed by branches of the anterior, middle, and posterior, alveolar nerves. **Gastric plexus, left,** a secondary plexus connected with the coeliac plexus, which accompanies the left gastric artery. **Hepatic plexus,** the largest offset of the coeliac plexus, which accompanies the hepatic artery and the portal vein. **Hypogastric plexuses, inferior,** formed by the hypogastric nerve. In the male each plexus is situated on the side of the rectum, seminal vesicle, prostate, and posterior part of the bladder. In the female it is on the side of the rectum, cervix uteri, vaginal fornix, and posterior part of the bladder. **Hypogastric plexus, superior,** situated in front of the bifurcation of the abdominal aorta, and formed by branches of the aortic plexus and the 3rd and 4th lumbar splanchnic nerves. **Infraorbital plexus,** a plexus formed by the buccal branches of the facial nerve and superior labial branches of the infraorbital nerve. **Lumbar plexus,** a plexus lying within the psoas major in front of the transverse processes of the lumbar vertebrae, and formed by the ventral rami of the first three lumbar nerves and the greater part of the 4th. **Lymphatic plexuses of diaphragm,** one on the abdominal surface and one on the thoracic surface. **Lymphatic plexuses of intestines,** a *periglandular,* and a *submucous,* plexus. **Lymphatic plexus of mammary gland,** a plexus in the interlobular spaces and in the walls of the lactiferous ducts. **Mesenteric plexus, inferior,** a plexus surrounding the inferior mesenteric artery and derived from the aortic plexus. **Mesenteric plexus, superior,** a plexus surrounding the superior mesenteric artery, which is a continuation of the coeliac plexus. **Myenteric plexus,** a plexus of nerves and ganglia situated between the circular and longitudinal layers of the small intestine. **Oesophageal plexus,** a plexus between the muscular and submucous coats of the oesophagus, derived from the branches of the vagus and sympathetic nerves. **Ovarian plexus,** a plexus accompanying the ovarian artery and formed by branches from the renal and aortic plexuses.

Ovarian plexus of veins, a plexus formed by the ovarian vein between the layers of the broad ligament. **Pampiniform plexus,** in the male a convoluted plexus of veins which constitutes the chief mass of the spermatic cord. **Parotid plexus,** a plexus in the parotid gland formed by branches of the facial nerve. **Patellar plexus,** a plexus on the lateral side of the knee, formed by branches of the saphenous nerve and the lateral cutaneous nerve of the thigh. **Pharyngeal plexus,** a plexus at the upper border of the middle constrictor of the pharynx, formed by the pharyngeal branch of the vagus nerve, and branches of the sympathetic trunk, the glossopharyngeal and the external laryngeal nerves. **Pharyngeal venous plexus,** the venous plexus on the outer surface of the pharynx, from which the pharyngeal veins rise. **Phrenic plexus,** a plexus that accompanies the inferior phrenic artery, and arises from the coeliac ganglion. **Prostatic plexus,** a plexus that arises from the inferior hypogastric plexus. **Prostatic venous plexus,** a plexus lying behind the arcuate pubic ligament and the symphysis pubis and in front of the bladder and prostate. Its chief tributary is the deep dorsal vein of the penis, and it drains into the vesical and internal iliac veins. **Pterygoid venous plexus,** a plexus situated between the temporal and lateral pterygoid muscles and between the two pterygoid muscles, which receives a large number of veins and anastomoses with the facial vein and cavernous sinus. **Pulmonary plexuses, anterior** and **posterior,** plexuses lying on the anterior and posterior aspects of the roots of the lungs, and formed by branches from the vagus nerve and the sympathetic trunk. **Rectal plexus, middle,** a plexus that arises from the inferior hypogastric plexus. **Rectal venous plexus,** a plexus that surrounds the rectum and communicates in front with the vesical plexus in the male and the uterovaginal plexus in the female. **Renal plexus,** a plexus lying around the renal artery and its branches, and formed by filaments from the coeliac ganglion, coeliac plexus, lowest thoracic splanchnic nerve, 1st lumbar splanchnic nerve, and aortic plexus. **Sacral plexus,** a plexus formed by the lumbosacral trunk, the ventral rami of the 1st, 2nd and 3rd sacral nerves, and part of the ventral ramus of the 4th sacral nerve, and situated on the posterior wall of the pelvic cavity. **Solar plexus,** coeliac plexus. **Splenic plexus,** a plexus formed by branches from the coeliac plexus, left coeliac ganglion and right vagus nerve, which accompanies the splenic artery. **Submucous plexus,** a secondary plexus of the myenteric plexus. **Subsartorial plexus,** a plexus formed by the anterior branch of the obturator nerve and branches of the femoral nerve, and situated at the lower border of the adductor longus.

-plexy (Gk *plexus:* a stroke). Suffix signifying a stroke or seizure.

Plica. A fold or plait. (*Plural:* plicae.) **Plica fimbriata,** a fringed fold of mucous membrane on each side of the inferior surface of the tongue. **Plica lacrimalis,** a fold of mucous membrane just above the opening of the naso-lacrimal duct into the nose. **Plica semilunaris,** a semilunar fold of conjunctiva lateral to the caruncle. **Plica triangularis,** in the foetus a free fold of mucous membrane covering the anterior inferior part of the tonsil.

Plication. The operation of reducing the size of an organ or muscle by taking in folds in it.

-ploid (L *-ploideus:* multiple). Suffix signifying multiple in form.

Plombage. The surgical procedure of filling the pleural cavity with inert material as a form of collapse therapy.

Plumbism. Lead poisoning.

Pluri- (L *plus:* more). Prefix meaning more or several.

Pluriglandular. Pertaining to, or derived from, several glands.

Plutonium. A radioactive element. Symbol Pu. Atomic weight 242. Atomic number 94.

Pneu- (Gk *pnein:* to breathe). Prefix signifying relationship to breathing or respiration.

Pneu-, Pneuma-, Pneumat- (Gk *pneuma:* air, breath). Prefixes signifying relationship with air, gas, respiration.

Pneumarthrosis. Air or gas in a joint.

Pneumatic. Pertaining to air or gas.

Pneumatization. The development of air-filled cavities in bone or other tissues.

Pneumatocardia. The presence of gas or air in the heart.

Pneumatocele. Hernial protrusion of the lung. A gas-filled cavity.

Pneumatophore. An oxygen-breathing apparatus used in rescue work, as in coal mines.

Pneumaturia. The passing of air or gas in the urine.

Pneu-, pneumo-, pneumono- (Gk *pneumōn:* lung). Prefixes signifying relationship to the lungs.

Pneumocephalus. The presence of air or gas in the cranial cavity.

Pneumococcaemia. The presence of pneumococci in the blood.

Pneumococcal. Pertaining to the pneumococcus.

Pneumococcus. The causative organism of lobar pneumonia. An oral or lanceolate gram-positive coccus occurring in pairs. *Diplococcus pneumoniae.*

Pneumoconiosis. Fibrous induration of the lungs due to chronic inhalation of irritant dusts. (*Plural:* pneumoconioses.)

Pneumoencephalography. Radiological examination of the brain by injection of air into the ventricles.

Pneumoencephalomyelography. Radiological examination of the brain and spinal cord by means of injecting air into the subarachnoid space.

Pneumogastric. Pertaining to the lungs and the stomach.

Pneumograph. An instrument for recording the movements of the chest during respiration.

Pneumohaemopericardium. The presence of air and blood in the pericardial cavity.

Pneumohaemothorax. The presence of air and blood in the pleural cavity.

Pneumohydropericardium. The presence of air and fluid in the pericardial cavity.

Pneumohydrothorax. The presence of air and fluid in the pleural cavity.

Pneumolysis. The surgical procedure of separating the lung and parietal pleura from the endothoracic fascia, as in collapsing the lung.

Pneumomalacia. Softening of the lung.

Pneumonectomy. Surgical excision of a lung.

Pneumonia. Inflammation of the lung. **Aspiration pneumonia,** pneumonia caused by aspiration of infected material. **Bacterial pneumonia,** pneumonia due to bacterial invasion of the affected part. **Bronchopneumonia,** pneumonia characterized by involvement of scattered areas in the lungs. **Hypostatic pneumonia,** pneumonia due to infection of congested bases of the lungs. **Lipoid pneumonia,** pneumonia caused by inhalation of oily material. **Lobar pneumonia,** pneumonia involving a whole lobe (or lobes); 90 per cent of cases are due to infection by the pneumococcus. **Mycoplasma pneumonia,** pneumonia caused by *Myco-*

POLE

plasma pneumoniae. Primary atypical pneumonia. **Postoperative pneumonia,** pneumonia, usually hypostatic, occurring during the postoperative period. **Primary atypical pneumonia,** mycoplasma pneumonia. **Viral pneumonia,** pneumonia caused by a virus.

Pneumonitis. Inflammation of the lung that does not proceed to the stage of consolidation.

Pneumonopexy. Fixation of the lung to the chest wall.

Pneumopericardium. The presence of air or gas in the pericardial cavity.

Pneumoperitoneum. The presence of air or gas in the peritoneal cavity. **Artificial pneumoperitoneum,** the deliberate introduction of air into the peritoneal cavity for the purpose of reducing pulmonary excursion.

Pneumothorax. The presence of air or gas in the pleural cavity. **Artificial pneumothorax,** a pneumothorax deliberately induced for the purpose of collapsing the underlying lung. **Spontaneous pneumothorax,** a pneumothorax induced by rupture of a bulla in the lung. **Tension pneumothorax,** a pneumothorax in which a flap of torn pleura acts as a check valve allowing more air to enter during inspiration than can escape during expiration.

Pnigophobia. Fear of choking.

Pock. The characteristic pustule of smallpox.

Pod-, Poda- (Gk *pous, pod-:* foot). Prefixes signifying relationship to the foot.

Podagra. Gout affecting the big toe.

Podalic. Pertaining to the feet.

Podiatrist. Chiropodist.

Podocyte. The epithelial cell of the glomerular capsule.

Podogram. A tracing of the foot.

Podophyllum. B.P.C. 1968. The dried rhizome and roots of *Podophyllum peltatum* L., used for the preparation of the resin. **Indian podophyllum,** B.P.C. 1968, the dried rhizome and roots of *Podophyllum hexandrum,* which grows in India. **Podophyllum resin,** B.P. 1968, the resin, obtained from Indian podophyllum or, more rarely, podophyllum. A caustic with a cytotoxic action.

Podopompholyx. Pompholyx of the toes and feet.

Poikilo- (Gk *poikilos:* varied). Prefix meaning varied or irregular.

Poikilocyte. An erythrocyte showing irregularity of shape.

Poikilocytosis. The presence of poikilocytes in the circulating blood.

Poikilodentosis. Mottled dental enamel.

Poikiloderma. An atrophic state of the skin accompanied by pigmentation

Poikilothermy. The state in which the body temperature varies with the environmental temperature.

Point. A spot or small area. **Boiling point,** the temperature at which a liquid has a vapour pressure equal to barometric pressure. **Corresponding points,** retinal areas coordinated visually in the occipital cortex so that an object is seen with both eyes as a single object. **Dew point,** the temperature at which atmospheric moisture is deposited as dew. **Disparate points,** retinal areas which are not corresponding points. **Far point,** the farthest point of distinct vision. Remote point. **Freezing point,** the temperature at which a liquid solidifies. **McBurney's point,** the junction of the lateral and middle thirds of the line joining the anterior superior iliac spine to the umbilicus. It marks the base of the vermiform appendix, and the site of maximal tenderness in cases of acute appendicitis involving a normally sited appendix. **Near point,** the nearest point of distinct vision. **Nodal points,** two points on the common optical axis corresponding to the optical centre of a single lens. **Remote point,** far point.

Pointillage. Massage with the tips of the fingers.

Poison. A noxious substance. **Poison ivy,** a climbing vine, *Rhus toxicodendron,* which is acutely toxic on contact with the skin.

Polarimeter. An instrument for measuring the rotation of polarized light. Polerimeter.

Polariscope. Polarimeter.

Polarity. Having two opposite poles.

Polarization. The change produced in a ray of light on passing through certain media. The accumulation of bubbles of hydrogen gas on the negative plate of a galvanic battery.

Polaroid. The trade name for a synthetic plastic film, used for reducing glare through lenses and windshields.

Poldine methylsulphate. B.P. 1968. $C_{22}H_{29}NO_7S$. An anticholinergic drug used in the treatment of hyperchlorhydria and associated pyloric spasm. It is longer lasting than atropine.

Pole. Either extremity of an axis. **Abembryonic pole,** the most recently embedded pole of the blastocyst. **Anterior pole of the eyeball,** the central point of the anterior curvature of the eyeball. **Anterior pole of the lens,** the central point of the anterior surface of the lens. **Embryonic pole,** the area of deepest penetration of the blastocyst. **Frontal pole,** the anterior end of the cerebral hemisphere. **Negative pole,** the cathode. **Occipital pole,** the posterior end of the cerebral hemisphere. **Positive pole,** the anode. **Posterior pole of the eyeball,** the central point of the posterior curvature of the eyeball. **Posterior pole of the lens,** the central point of the posterior surface of the lens. **Temporal pole,** the anterior end of the temporal lobe.

Poli-, Polio- (Gk *polios:* grey). Prefixes denoting relationship to the grey matter of the nervous system.

Polioencephalitis. Inflammation of the grey matter of the brain.

Polioencephalomeningomyelitis. Inflammation of the grey matter and meninges of the brain and the spinal cord.

Polioencephalomyelitis. Inflammation of the grey matter of the brain and the spinal cord.

Poliomyelitis. Inflammation of the grey matter of the spinal cord. **Acute anterior poliomyelitis,** an infection by the polioviruses involving the anterior horn cells of the spinal cord.

Poliosis. Premature greying of the hair.

Poliovirus. The virus responsible for poliomyelitis. There are three polioviruses (types 1, 2, and 3) which constitute a subgroup of enteroviruses.

Politerization. Inflation of the middle ear by the Politzer bag.

Pollen. The microspores of seed plants.

Pollex. The thumb.

Pollicization. Surgical reconstruction of a thumb.

Pollinosis. Hay fever.

Polonium. The radioactive element originally separated from pitchblende by the Curies. Symbol Po. Atomic number 84. Atomic weight 210.

Poloxalkol. The B.P. Commission approved name for a polymer of ethylene oxide, propylene oxide and propylene glycol. A surface active agent.

Poloxyl lanolin. The B.P. Commission approved name for a polyoxyethylene condensation product of anhydrous lanolin. An emollient.

Poly- (Gk *polys:* many). Prefix meaning many or much.

Polyarteritis. Simultaneous inflammation of a number of arteries. **Polyarteritis nodosa,** a disease of unknown origin, characterized by local inflammatory lesions in small and medium-sized arteries.

Polyarthritis. Arthritis involving several joints simultaneously.

Polycheiria. The condition of having a supernumerary hand (or hands).

Polychromasia. The bluish, or bluish-red, staining which characterizes immature erythrocytes, as in pernicious anaemia. Polychromatophilia.

Polychromatic. Multicoloured.

Polychromatophilia. Polychromasia.

Polycistronic. Pertaining to several cistrons, or genes. **Polycistronic messenger,** an RNA molecule that programmes the synthesis of two or more proteins.

Polycoria. The condition in which there are holes in the iris besides the pupil.

Polycystic. Composed of many cysts.

Polycythaemia. The condition characterized by an excess of erythrocytes in the circulating blood.

Polydactylism. The presence of supernumerary digits on the hands or feet.

Polydipsia. Excessive thirst.

Polydontia. The presence of more than the normal number of teeth.

Polyethylene. A long-chain synthetic resin, used widely as a plastic material in surgery.

Polygeline. The B.P. Commission approved name for a polymer of urea and polypeptides derived from denatured gelatin. A restorer of blood volume.

Polygenic. Pertaining to, or influenced by, several genes.

Polyglandular. Pertaining to several glands.

Polygnathus. A foetal monster in which a parasitic twin is attached to the chin of the autosite.

Polygraph. An instrument for the simultaneous recording of arterial and venous pulsations.

Polyhedral. Having many sides.

Polymastia. The presence of supernumerary breasts.

Polymelia. The presence of more than the normal number of limbs.

Polymer. A compound formed by the combination of simpler molecules, the molecular weight being a whole multiple of the molecular weight of the original compound.

Polymer fume fever. An influenza-like illness that occurs in people who work with polytetrafluoroethylene (PTFE).

Polymorph. A polymorphonuclear granulocyte or leucocyte.

Polymorphonuclear. Having a lobated

nucleus. A polymorphonuclear leuco-cyte.

Polymorphous. Occurring in different forms. Polymorphic.

Polymyalgia. Pain in several muscles. **Polymyalgia rheumatica,** a condition characterized by the acute onset of pain in the shoulder and pelvic girdles, usually in elderly women.

Polymyositis. A condition of unknown etiology, characterized by weakness of the proximal muscles of the limbs.

Polymyxin B sulphate. B.P. 1968. A mixture of the sulphates of antimicrobial peptides produced by various strains of *Bacillus polymyxa* or by any other means. An antibiotic active against a wide range of gram-negative organisms.

Polyneuritis. Inflammation of many nerves. Multiple peripheral neuritis.

Polynuclear. Having, or pertaining to, several nuclei.

Polyopia. Perception of more than one image of the object looked at.

Polyorchidism. The presence of super-numerary testes.

Polyostotic. Affecting many bones. **Polyostotic fibrous dysplasia,** the condition characterized by focal loss of intramedullary bone structure, with fibrous proliferation, occurring in many bones.

Polyoxyl 8 stearate. Polyoxyl 40 stearate. The B.P. Commission approved names for two surface-active agents.

Polypeptide. A peptide formed by the condensation of a large number of amino-acids.

Polyphagia. Gluttony. Overeating.

Polypharmacy. The inclusion of many drugs in one prescription.

Polyphyletism. The theory that blood cells are formed from more than one stem cell.

Polyploid. Having three or more sets of the haploid number of chromosomes in somatic cell nuclei.

Polypoid. Like a polypus.

Polyposis. A rare, familial, pre-cancerous condition, in which the colon is studded with polypi. **Polyposis coli.**

Polypus. A pedunculated growth. (*Plural:* polypi.) Polyp.

Polyradiculitis. Inflammation of the roots of the spinal nerves.

Polyribosome. Polysome.

Polysaccharide. A sugar formed by the condensation of a large number of monosaccharide units.

Polyserositis. Inflammation of several serous membranes, usually the peri-toneum and pericardium.

Polysome. In nucleic acid biosynthesis the complex of several ribosomes bound to a molecule of mRNA. Each component ribosome of the poly-some is engaged in protein synthesis but is at a different stage of translation of the molecule of mRNA.

Polysomus. A monster with one head and several bodies.

Polysorbate 20, 60, 80. B.P.C. 1968. Three non-ionic surface-active agents used in the preparation of emulsions, creams, ointments and suppository bases. Other members of the series to which the B.P. Commission has given approved names are: **Polysorbate 40, Polysorbate 65, Polysorbate 85.**

Polyspermia. An abnormally profuse seminal secretion. Polyspermy.

Polyspermy. The entry of more than one spermatozoon into the ovum.

Polythelia. The presence of super-numerary nipples.

Polythiazide. The B.P. Commission approved name for 6-chloro-3,4-di-hydro-2-methyl-3-(2,2,2-trifluoroethyl-thiomethyl)-1,2,4-benzothiadiazine-7-sulphonamide 1,1-dioxide. A diuretic.

Polyuria. The passage of excessive amounts of urine.

Polyuronide. A substance composed of uronic acid units.

Polyvalent. Having several valencies.

Polyvinox. The B.P. Commission approved name for poly(butyl vinyl-ether). A skin application.

Pompholyx. A vesicular eruption on the sides and fronts of the fingers and the palm of the hand and the sides and fronts of the toes and the soles of the feet.

Ponderal. Pertaining to weight.

Pono- (Gk *ponos:* toil). Prefix signi-fying relationship to hard work or pain.

Pons. A bridge. The part of the brain lying between the medulla oblongata and the midbrain.

Ponticulus. A little bridge. The ridge on the cranial surface of the eminentia conchae, to which the auricularis posterior muscle is attached.

Popliteal. Pertaining to the space behind the knee.

Pore. A minute opening. **Gustatory pore,** the opening of a taste bud on to the tongue.

Porencephaly. The presence of cysts on the surface of the brain resulting from birth injury or a failure of develop-ment. It is commonly associated with severe mental subnormality and cerebral palsy.

Porfiromycin. The B.P. Commission approved name for an antineoplastic antibiotic derived from *Streptomyces ardus*.

Porocephaliasis. Infection with Porocephalus.

Porocephalus. A genus of Pentastorrida which may invade man by the swallowing of the eggs, which mature in the liver. The resulting, often symptomless, condition is known as porocephaliasis.

Poroplastic. Porous and plastic.

Porphin. The parent substance, or nucleus, of the porphyrins.

Porphobilinogen. A porphyrin precursor that is excreted in large amounts in the urine in acute porphyria.

Porphyria. An inborn error of metabolism associated with the excretion of porphyrins in the urine. There are two main forms of the disease: congenital porphyria and acute intermittent porphyria. Both are due to an inherited defect.

Porphyrin. One of a group of biological pigments composed of four pyrrole nuclei joined together by $=CH-$ bridges. The many porphyrins are characterized by different substituent groups in positions 1 to 8 in the porphin ring system.

Porphyrinuria. The excretion of porphyrin in the urine.

Porta. A gateway, or hilus. **Porta hepatis,** the deep fissure on the inferior surface of the liver, between the quadrate lobe in front and the caudate lobe behind, through which pass the portal vein, the hepatic artery, and the right and left hepatic ducts.

Portacaval. Pertaining to the portal vein and the inferior vena cava.

Portal. Porta. Pertaining to a porta. **Anterior intestinal portal,** the communication between the embryonic foregut and midgut.

Portio. A part.

-posia (Gk *posis:* drinking). Suffix signifying relationship to drinking or the intake of fluids.

Positron. A particle of the same mass as an electron.

Poskine. The B.P. Commission approved name for *O*-propionylhyoscine. A central nervous system depressant.

Posology. The science of dosage.

Post- (L *post:* after). Prefix meaning after or behind.

Postcentral. Behind a centre.

Postcibal. After the ingestion of food.

Posterior. Behind or after.

Postero- (L *posterus:* behind). Prefix meaning posterior.

Postero-anterior. From the back to the front.

Posterolateral. Behind and to the lateral side.

Posteromedial. Behind and to the medial side.

Posterosuperior. Situated behind and above.

Postganglionic. Distal to a ganglion.

Postgraduate. One who has graduated in a university. Following graduation.

Postholith. A preputial concretion.

Postmaturity. Beyond the normal date of maturity.

Postmenopausal. After the menopause.

Post mortem. After death. **Post-mortem examination,** examination of a body after death. Necropsy.

Postoperative. Following an operation.

Postpartum. After parturition or birth.

Postprandial. After a meal. Postcibal.

Postpuberal. After puberty.

Postsystolic. Occurring at the end of cardiac systole.

Post-traumatic. Following, or the result of, trauma.

Potash. Impure potassium carbonate.

Potassium. An alkaline metallic element. Symbol K. Atomic weight 39·102. Atomic number 19.

Potassium acid tartrate. B.P.C. 1968. $C_4H_5KO_6$. Cream of tartar. A saline purgative.

Potassium bicarbonate. B.P.C. 1968. $KHCO_3$. An antacid, used to treat or prevent acidosis, and to reduce the acidity of the urine.

Potassium bromide. B.P. 1968. KBr. A sedative.

Potassium chlorate. B.P.C. 1968. $KClO_3$. A mild astringent and sialagogue, commonly used in gargles.

Potassium chloride. B.P. 1968. KCl. Used in the treatment of potassium deficiency.

Potassium citrate. B.P. 1968. $C_6H_5K_3O_7,H_2O$. A systemic alkalinizing agent.

Potassium gluconate. B.P.C. 1968. $C_6H_{11}KO_7$. Used in the treatment of potassium deficiency.

Potassium hydroxide. B.P. 1968. KOH. Caustic potash. A powerful caustic. **Potassium hydroxide solution,** B.P. 1968, potash solution. It contains 5 per cent w/v of total alkali, calculated as KOH.

Potassium hydroxyquinoline sulphate.

B.P.C. 1968. An equimolecular mixture of $(C_9H_7NO)_2,H_2SO_4$, and K_2SO_4. It has antibacterial and deodorant properties.

Potassium iodide. B.P. 1968. KI. Used in the preoperative management of thyrotoxicosis, in the treatment and prevention of simple goitre, and as an expectorant. It is a constituent of aqueous iodine solution B.P. (Lugol's solution).

Potassium menaphthosulphate. The B.P. Commission approved name for a vitamin K analogue.

Potassium perchlorate. B.P.C. 1968. $KClO_4$. Used in the treatment of thyrotoxicosis.

Potassium permanganate. B.P. 1968. $KMnO_4$. An oxidizing antiseptic.

Potassium sorbate. B.P.C. 1968. $C_6H_7KO_2$. A bactericide and fungicide used as a preservative.

Potato. *Solanum tuberosum*, the tuber of which contains around 20 grammes of carbohydrate per 100 grammes, and from 10 to 30 mg. of ascorbic acid per 100 grammes, and which is a major item of diet in many parts of the western world.

Potential. A state of tension. **Action potential,** the electrical activity set up in excitable tissue during its activity. **Injury potential,** the difference in potential recorded when one electrode is in contact with an uninjured part of a nerve and the other is in contact with a cut or crushed point. **Membrane potential,** the difference in potential across the walls of a cell. **Resting potential,** the steady potential difference between the inside and the outside of a resting nerve cell.

Potentiometer. An instrument for measuring voltage.

Pouch. A sac or pocket. **Hepatorenal pouch,** the portion of the peritoneal cavity behind the right lobe of the liver and in front of the right kidney and right transverse mesocolon. **Pharyngeal pouch,** one of the five paired sacculations of the embryonic pharynx. **Rathke's pouch,** the rudiment of the anterior lobe of the hypophysis. **Recto-uterine pouch,** the peritoneal pouch between the rectum and the posterior surface of the uterus. **Rectovesical pouch,** the peritoneal pouch between the rectum and the bladder in the male. **Vesico-uterine pouch,** the peritoneal pouch between the uterus and the bladder.

Poultice. A soft, moist, pultaceous hot or warm mass for application to the surface of the body as a means of applying heat. Cataplasm.

Pound. A unit of weight. **Avoirdupois pound,** 16 ounces, equivalent to 453·6 grammes. **Apothecaries pound,** 12 ounces, equivalent to 373·2 grammes.

Povidone. B.P.C. 1968. Polyvinyl pyrrolidone. A suspending and dispersing agent in aqueous oral medicaments, a tablet binder, and also used in the film coating of tablets.

Povidone-iodine. The B.P. Commission approved name for a complex produced by reacting iodine with polyvinylpyrrolidone. A topical antiseptic.

Powder. A mixture of two or more powdered medicaments. There are two powders in the *British Pharmocopoeia* 1968: Absorbable dusting powder; Compound tragacanth powder. There are 12 powders in the *British Pharmaceutical Index* 1968: Compound bismuth powder; compound calcium carbonate powder; Aromatic chalk powder; Aromatic chalk powder with opium; Compound effervescent powder; Compound effervescent powder, double-strength; Ipecacuana and opium powder (Dover's powder); Compound liquorice powder; Compound magnesium carbonate powder; Compound magnesium trisilicate powder; Compound rhubarb powder; Mitigated silver nitrate.

Poxviruses. A group of viruses within the size range, 200×300 mμ to 265×350 mμ, which have a predilection for infecting epithelial cells. They include the viruses of smallpox, chickenpox and vaccinia.

Practolol. The B.P. Commission approved name for 4-(2-hydroxy-3-isopropylaminopropoxy)acetanilide. A β-adrenergic receptor blocking agent.

Prae- (L *prae*: before). Prefix signifying before, in front.

Praeputium clitoridis. The fold which overhangs the glans clitoridis.

Praevia. Going before.

Pramiverine. The B.P. Commission approved name for a spasmolytic.

Pramoxine. The B.P. Commission approved name for 4-[3-(4-butoxyphenoxy)propyl]morpholine. A local anaesthetic.

Prampine. The B.P. Commission approved name for *O*-propionylatropine. A drug with an atropine-like action used in the treatment of peptic ulcer.

Praseodymium. An element of the rare earth group. Symbol Pr. Atomic weight 140·907. Atomic number 59.

Prazepam. The B.P. Commission

approved name for 7-chloro-1-(cyclo-propylmethyl)-1, 3-dihydro-5-phenyl-1,4-benzodiazepin-2-one. A muscle relaxant.

Prazitone. The B.P. Commission approved name for 5-phenyl-5-(2-piperidyl)methylbarbituric acid. An antidepressant.

Pre- (L *prae:* before). Prefix signifying before, in front.

Pre-agonal. Immediately preceding death.

Pre-axial. In front of an axis of the body or a limb.

Precancerous. Preceding the onset of cancer. With a tendency to develop cancer.

Precipitin. An antibody to a soluble antigen, which it causes to precipitate.

Preciptinogen. An antigen which stimulates the formation of a precipitin.

Precordial. Related to the precordium.

Precordium. The area of the chest wall overlying the heart.

Precuneus. The quadrilateral area on the medial surface of the cerebral hemisphere, bounded in front by the upturned end of the sulcus cinguli, behind by the parieto-occipital sulcus, above by the supero-medial margin and below by the supraspherical sulcus.

Predentine. The clear layer lying between the odontoblasts and the fully formed dentine in young teeth where dentine is being formed.

Predigestion. The partial digestion of food by artificial means before it is eaten.

Prednisolamate. The B.P. Commission approved name for prednisolone 21-dimethylaminoacetate. A corticosteroid.

Prednisolone. B.P. 1968. $C_{21}H_{28}O_5$. A synthetic glucocorticoid which has the same chemical relationship to prednisone as hydrocortisone has to cortisone, and is used for the same purposes as prednisone. **Prednisolone pivalate,** B.P. 1968, $C_{26}H_{36}O_6$, a prednisolone derivative used as an anti-inflammatory ointment, and as an intra-articular microcrystalline suspension. **Prednisolone sodium phosphate,** B.P. 1968, $C_{21}H_{27}Na_2O_8P$, a prednisolone derivative used in eye-drops, other preparations for topical use, and intravenously.

Prednisone. B.P. 1968. $C_{21}H_{26}O_5$. A synthetic glucocorticoid which has the same action and uses as cortisone acetate but is effective in a dosage one-quarter to one-fifth of that of cortisone. It is used mainly for its anti-inflammatory action. **Prednisone acetate,** B.P. 1968, $C_{23}H_{28}O_6$, a preparation with the same properties as prednisone.

Prednylidene. The B.P. Commission approved name for a synthetic corticosteroid.

Pre-eclampsia. A disease of late pregnancy characterized by hypertension, proteinuria and often oedema, which, if untreated, progresses to eclampsia.

Pre-erythrocytic. The term applied to the phase in malaria when the sporozoite develops into the schizont and then the merozoite in the tissue cells, especially those of the liver.

Preganglionic. Preceding a ganglion.

Pregnancy. The state of being with child. Gestation. The period from conception to birth. **Abdominal pregnancy,** the development of the fertilized ovum within the abdominal cavity. **Ectopic pregnancy,** the development of the fertilized ovum outwith the uterine cavity. Ectopic gestation. Extra-uterine pregnancy. **Extra-uterine pregnancy,** ectopic pregnancy. **Intra-ligamentary pregnancy,** pregnancy within the broad ligament. **Intra-peritoneal pregnancy,** abdominal pregnancy. **Multiple pregnancy,** the condition in which more than one foetus is present in the uterus. **Ovarian pregnancy,** implantation of the fertilized ovum in the ovary. **Tubal pregnancy,** the development of the fertilized ovum in the uterine tube.

Pregnanediol. The excretion product of progesterone, which is excreted in the urine during menstruation and pregnancy.

Pregnant. With child. Gravid.

Pregnenolone. The B.P. Commission approved name for a drug used in the treatment of rheumatoid arthritis.

Prehensile. Capable of grasping.

Pre-ictal. Before a stroke, or an attack.

Pre-icteral. Before the development of jaundice.

Premalignant. Precancerous.

Premenstrual. Preceding menstruation.

Premenstruum. The period of the menstrual cycle immediately preceding menstruation.

Premolar. In front of the molar teeth. **Premolar teeth,** the two teeth on either side of both jaws (8 in all) between the molar teeth and the canine teeth. Biscuspid.

Premyelocyte. Promyelocyte.

Prenatal. Preceding birth. Antenatal.

Prenylamine. The B.P. Commission

approved name for N-(3,3-diphenyl-propyl)-α-methylphenethylamine. A coronary vasodilator.

Preoperative. Occurring before a surgical operation.

Prepatellar. In front of the patella.

Prepuce. The fold of skin at the neck of the penis that is folded on itself and overlaps the glans penis for a variable distance. The foreskin. **Prepuce of the clitoris,** praeputium clitoridis.

Preputial. Pertaining to the prepuce.

Prepyloric. Proximal to the pylorus.

Prepyramidal. In front of the pyramid of the medulla oblongata.

Presby- (Gk *presbys:* old). Prefix meaning old or indicating relationship to old age.

Presbyacusis. The deterioration of hearing which occurs with increasing age.

Presbyopia. The impairment of vision which occurs with advancing years.

Prescription. An order for drugs, preparations or appliances, given in relation to a named person by a duly qualified medical practitioner, or registered dentist.

Presenility. Premature old age.

Presentation. The presenting part of the foetus at the cervix uteri. **Breech presentation,** when the buttocks present. **Brow presentation,** when the brow presents. **Face presentation,** when the face presents. **Shoulder presentation,** when a shoulder presents.

Presphenoid. The anterior part of the body of the sphenoid bone.

Pressor. A substance that raises the blood pressure.

Pressure. The force or stress exerted by a body, gas or liquid. **Arterial pressure,** blood pressure. **Atmospheric pressure,** the pressure exerted by the atmosphere at sea level. **Colloid osmotic pressure,** the proportion of the osmotic pressure of the blood due to the plasma proteins. **Blood pressure,** the pressure of the blood on the walls of the arteries. **Diastolic pressure,** the lowest arterial pressure during diastole. **Hydrostatic pressure,** pressure within a closed fluid system. **Intra-ocular pressure,** the pressure within the eyeball. **Intra-ventricular pressure,** the pressure within the ventricles of the heart. **Oncotic pressure,** the difference between the osmotic pressure of [the blood and that of lymph or tissue fluid. **Osmotic pressure,** the pressure developed when a solution and its solvent are separated by a semipermeable membrane. **Partial pressure,** the

pressure exerted by any one of the components of a mixture of gases. **Pulse pressure,** the difference between the systolic and the diastolic pressure. **Systolic pressure,** the maximal arterial pressure during systole. **Venous pressure,** the blood pressure in the veins.

Presymptomatic. Existing before the appearance of symptoms.

Presystole. The interval in the cardiac cycle immediately preceding systole.

Pretibial. In front of the tibia.

Priapism. Persistent erection of the penis.

Prickly heat. Miliaria.

Prilocaine. The B.P. Commission approved name for N-(2-propylamino-propionyl)-o-toluidine. A local anaesthetic.

Primaquine phosphate. B.P. 1968. $C_{15}H_{27}N_3O_9P_2$. An antimalarial drug.

Primidone. B.P. 1968. $C_{12}H_{14}N_2O_2$. An anticonvulsant widely used in the treatment of grand mal epilepsy.

Primigravida. A woman who is pregnant for the first time.

Primipara. A woman who has given birth to one child.

Prism. A solid, triangular or polygonal in section, and bounded by parallelograms. **Prism dioptre,** the unit indicating the strength of a prism which will produce a linear apparent displacement of 1 cm. of an object situated 1 metre away.

Pristinamycin. The B.P. Commission approved name for an antibiotic produced by *Streptomyces pristina spiralis.*

Pro- (Gk *pro:* before). Prefix signifying before, in front of, in place of.

Proband. The index case or individual who is responsible for the initiation of a genetic study. Propositus.

Probang. A flexible rod with a globular tip used for making local applications to, or removing foreign bodies from, the oesophagus and larynx.

Probe. An exploratory instrument.

Probenecid. B.P. 1968. $C_{13}H_{19}NO_4S$. A uricosuric agent used in the treatment of gout. As it reduces the tubular excretion of penicillin, it is therefore sometimes used as an adjunct to penicillin therapy, to ensure high levels of penicillin.

Procainamide hydrochloride. B.P. 1968. $C_{13}H_{22}ClN_3O_2$. A myocardial depressant which is used in the treatment of certain cardiac arrhythmias.

Procaine hydrochloride. B.P. 1968. $C_{13}H_{21}ClN_2O_2$. A short-acting local anaesthetic.

Procaine penicillin. B.P. 1968. A sparingly soluble salt of benzylpenicillin, which is administered intramuscularly to provide a depot from which benzylpenicillin is released slowly into the bloodstream.

Procarbazine. The B.P. Commission approved name for *N*-4-isopropylcarbamoylbenzyl-*N'*-methylhydrazine. A drug used in the treatment of lymphadenoma.

Procephalic. Pertaining to the front of the head.

Process. A prominence or outgrowth. A course of action or events. **Articular processes of the vertebrae,** two superior and two inferior processes which spring from the junctions of the pedicles and laminae and control and restrict the vertebra's range of movement. **Caudate process of liver,** a narrow tongue of liver substance lying behind the porta hepatis and in front of the inferior vena cava. **Ciliary processes,** inward foldings of the choroid which form a frill behind the iris around the margin of the lens. **Clinoid process, anterior,** the medial extremity of the posterior border of the lesser wing of the sphenoid bone. **Clinoid process, middle,** a small eminence which completes the anterior border of the sella turcica laterally. **Clinoid process, posterior,** a tubercle on each side of the sella turcica. **Cochleariform process,** the pulley in the tympanic cavity over which the tendon of the tensor tympani bends. **Condylar process,** the stout articular process of the mandible. **Coracoid process,** a curved process arising from the upper surface of the neck of the scapula. **Coronoid process of mandible,** the projection from the upper anterior part of the ramus of the mandible. **Coronoid process of ulna,** a bracketlike projection from the front of the ulna immediately below the olecranon. **Ethmoidal process,** a thin plate in the inferior nasal concha that joins the uncinate process of the ethmoid. **Falciform process,** the portion of the sacrotuberous ligament that is continued along the ramus of the ischium. **Frontal process of the maxilla,** the part of the maxilla that projects upwards and backwards between the nasal and lacrimal bones. **Frontal process of the zygomatic bone,** the part of the zygomatic bone that articulates with the zygomatic process of the frontal bone above and the greater wing of the sphenoid behind. **Process**

of the incus, long, the process of the incus that articulates with the head of the stapes. **Process of the incus, short,** the backward projecting, conical process of the incus. **Intrajugular process,** the bony spicule that divides the jugular notch of the occipital bone in two. **Jugular process,** the quadrilateral part of the occipital bone that forms the posterior part of the jugular foramen. **Lacrimal process of the inferior nasal concha,** a small pointed process that forms part of the canal for the naso-lacrimal duct. **Process of the malleus, anterior,** a forward-directed delicate spicule. **Process of the malleus, lateral,** a conical projection attached to the tympanic membrane. **Mamillary process,** a rough elevation on the posterior border of the superior articular processes of the lumbar vertebrae. **Mastoid process,** the conical projection of the mastoid portion of the temporal bone. **Maxillary process of the inferior nasal concha,** a thin lamella that forms part of the medial wall of the maxillary sinus. **Muscular process of the arytenoid cartilage,** the rounded lateral angle of the cartilage. **Palatine process of maxilla,** the thick medial projection from the lowest nasal surface of the bone that forms a considerable part of the floor of the nasal cavity and the roof of the mouth. **Papillary process of the liver,** a small rounded projection below and to the left of the caudate lobe. **Petrosal process,** a small projection on each side of the body of the sphenoid bone below the dorsum sellae. **Phalangeal processes of the spiral organ,** thin flattened plates which are continuations of the outer rods and unite with the phalangeal processes of Deiters' cells to form the reticular lamina. **Pterygoid process,** a process jutting downwards from the junction of the body and greater wing of the sphenoid bone. **Pyramidal process,** a projection of the palatine bone that fits into the interval between the lower end of the pterygoid plates of the pterygoid process. **Septal process,** the medial part of the lower nasal cartilage. **Sphenoidal process of the nasal septum,** a narrow process that extends backwards between the vomer and the perpendicular plate of the ethmoid bone. **Sphenoidal process of the palatine bone,** a thin plate that is directed upwards and medially. **Spinous process,** the spine of a vertebra, which projects backwards and downwards from the junction of the laminae. **Styloid process of the fibula,** a blunt elevation on the head of the fibula. **Styloid process of the 3rd metacarpal bone,** a short projection on the radial side of the dorsal surface of the base. **Styloid process of the radius,** a downward projection on the lateral side of the lower end of the radius. **Styloid process of the temporal bone,** a slender, tapering process projecting downwards and backwards from the under-surface of the bone. **Styloid process of the ulna,** a short, rounded projection at the lower end of the ulna. **Temporal process of the zygomatic bone,** a backward projection that forms part of the zygomatic arch. **Transverse processes,** the lateral projections from the junctions of the pedicles and laminae of the vertebrae. **Uncinate process of the ethmoid bone,** a thin, curved bar of bone that curves downwards and backwards in the lateral wall of the middle nasal meatus. **Uncinate process of the pancreas,** a prolongation of the head of the pancreas. **Vaginal process of the sphenoid,** a thin projection on the under-surface of the body of the sphenoid bone that articulates with the ala of the vomer. **Vocal process of the arytenoid cartilage,** the anterior angle that gives attachment to the vocal ligament. **Xiphoid process,** the lowest of the three pieces of the sternum. **Zygomatic process of the frontal bone,** the lateral boundary of the supra-orbital margin that articulates with the zygomatic bone. **Zygomatic process of the maxilla,** a rough pyramidal projection that articulates with the zygomatic bone. **Zygomatic process of the temporal bone,** the zygoma.

Processus. Process. **Processus cochleariformis,** the pulley in the tympanic cavity, over which the tendon of the tensor tympani bends. **Processus vaginalis of the peritoneum,** a peritoneal process in the foetus, the distal portion of which becomes the tunica vaginalis.

Prochlorperazine maleate. B.P. 1968. $C_{28}H_{32}ClN_3O_8S$. A phenothiazine tranquillizer and anti-emetic administered orally. **Prochlorperazine mesylate,** B.P. 1968, $C_{22}H_{32}ClN_3O_6S_3$, an intramuscular preparation.

Procidentia. Prolapse.

Proclonol. The B.P. Commission approved name for 4,4'-dichloro-α-cyclopropylbenzhydrol. An acaricide and fungicide.

Proct-, Procto- (Gk *prōktos:* anus).

Prefixes signifying association with the anus and/or rectum.

Proctalgia. Pain in the rectum or anus. **Proctalgia fugax,** a condition characterized by the sudden onset of short bouts of severe pain in the rectum without demonstrable cause. Paroxysmal proctalgia.

Proctectasia. Dilatation of the anus or rectum.

Proctectomy. Surgical excision of the rectum.

Proctitis. Inflammation of the rectum.

Proctocele. Prolapse of the rectum.

Proctocolitis. Inflammation of the rectum and colon.

Proctodaeum. The primitive anus.

Proctodynia. Pain in or around the anus.

Proctology. That branch of medicine concerned with diseases of the rectum and anus.

Proctorrhagia. Bleeding from the rectum.

Proctorrhaphy. Suturing of a lacerated rectum.

Proctoscope. A speculum for examining the rectum.

Proctotomy. Incision into the rectum or anus for repair of a stricture or an imperforate anus.

Procyclidine hydrochloride. B.P. 1968. $C_{19}H_{30}ClNO$. A parasympatholytic agent used in the treatment of parkinsonism.

Prodromal. Premonitory.

Prodrome. A premonitory symptom.

Proenzyme. The precursor of an enzyme.

Proerythroblast. The earliest identifiable specific cell in the erythrocyte series.

Profadol. The B.P. Commission approved name for 1-methyl-3-propyl-3-(3-hydroxyphenyl)pyrrolidine. An analgesic and antitussive.

Proflavine hemisulphate. B.P. 1968. $C_{26}H_{24}N_6O_4S,2H_2O$. An acridine antiseptic active against many gram-positive and gram-negative bacteria. **Proflavine cream,** B.P.C. 1968, a cream containing 0·1 per cent proflavine hemisulphate.

Profunda. Deepseated.

Progeria. Premature old age.

Progesterone. $C_{21}H_{30}O_2$. The hormone secreted by the corpus luteum which converts the proliferative endometrium to the secretory phase. If pregnancy ensues, it helps to maintain the decidua. **Progesterone injection,** B.P. 1968, a sterile solution (10 mg. in 1 ml.) of progesterone in ethyl oleate or some other suitable ester or fixed oil, for intramuscular injection.

Proglottis. The segment of a tapeworm.

Prognathism. Excessive projection of one or both jaws.

Prognosis. A forecast as to the probable cause and outcome of a disease.

Proguanil hydrochloride. B.P. 1968. $C_{11}H_{17}Cl_2N_5$. An antimalarial drug.

Proheptazine. The B.P. Commission approved name for hexahydro-1,3-dimethyl-4-phenylazepin-4-yl propionate. A narcotic analgesic.

Prolactin. The lactogenic hormone of the anterior pituitary that stimulates the secretion of milk. Luteotrophin.

Prolapse. The sinking down, or falling, of an organ.

Proligerous. Germinating. Producing offspring.

Prolintane. The B.P. Commission approved name for 1-(α-propylphenethyl)pyrrolidine. A 'tonic'.

Promazine hydrochloride. B.P. 1968. $C_{17}H_{21}ClN_2S$. A phenothiazine tranquillizer.

Promegakaryocyte. A primitive megakaryocyte.

Prometaphase. The stage of mitosis between prophase and metaphase, when the nuclear membrane disappears and the spindle sinks inwards so that its axis lies on a line joining the two centrosomes.

Promethazine hydrochloride. B.P. 1968. $C_{17}H_{21}ClN_2S$. An antihistaminic. **Promezathine theoclate,** B.P. 1968, $C_{24}H_{27}ClN_6O_2S$, a promezathine salt with the same action as the hydrochloride.

Promethoestrol. The B.P. Commission approved name for 3,4-di-(4-hydroxy-3-methylphenyl)hexane. An oestrogen.

Prominence. An elevation. **Prominence of the facial nerve canal,** an elevation in the tympanic cavity, marking the position of the upper part of the bony canal in which the facial nerve is contained. **Laryngeal prominence,** the subcutaneous prominence produced by the angle of junction of the two laminae of the thyroid cartilage. Adam's apple.

Promontory. A projection. **Sacral promontory,** the anterior projecting edge of the 1st sacral vertebra. **Tympanic promontory,** the prominence on the medial wall of the tympanic cavity formed by the outward projection of the cochlea.

Promoxolan. The B.P. Commission

approved name for 4-hydroxymethyl-2,2-di-isopropyl-1,3-dioxolan. A sedative.

Promyelocyte. A primitive granular leucocyte, intermediate between a myeloblast and a myelocyte.

Pronation. The movement whereby the radius is carried obliquely across the front of the ulna, and the hand faces palm downwards.

Prone. Lying face downwards.

Pronephros. The collection of rudimentary and transient nephric tubules that represent the commencing development of the kidney in the embryo.

Pronethalol. The B.P. Commission approved name for 2-isopropylamino-1-(2-naphthyl)ethanol. An adrenaline antagonist.

Pronormoblast. Proerythroblast.

Pronucleus. The nuclear material of the ovum and the spermatozoon after fertilization. **Female pronucleus,** the reticulum formed by the chromosomes of the ovum after fertilization. **Male pronucleus,** the head of the spermatozoon after penetration of the ovum.

Propamidine. The B.P. Commission approved name for 1, 3-di-(4-amidinophenoxy)propane. A bactericide and fungicide.

Propanidid. The B.P. Commission approved name for propyl 4-diethylcarbamoylmethoxy-3-methoxyphenylacetate. An anaesthetic.

Propantheline bromide. B.P. 1968. $C_{23}H_{30}BrNO_3$. A parasympatholytic drug used for the control of gastric secretion and intestinal mobility.

Propatylnitrate. The B.P. Commission approved name for 1,1,1-trisnitratomethylpropane. A coronary vasodilator.

Properdin. A β-globulin in plasma which is the protein component of the properdin system which is responsible for the non-specific killing of gram-negative bacteria and the neutralization of viruses.

Prophase. The first stage of mitosis.

Prophylaxis. Prevention. Preventive treatment.

Propicillin. The B.P. Commission approved name for an acid-resistant, orally active, semi-synthetic penicillin, with only slight activity against penicillinase-producing staphylococci.

Propiolactone. The B.P. Commission approved name for an antiseptic.

Propiomazine. The B.P. Commission approved name for 10-(2-dimethylaminopropyl)-2-propionylphenothiazine. A sedative.

Propionate. A salt or ester of propionic acid.

Propionic acid. $C_3H_6O_2$. A saturated fatty acid with a fungicidal action.

Propiram fumarate. The B.P. Commission approved name for N-(1-methyl-2-piperidinoethyl)-N-(2-pyridyl)-propionamide fumarate. An analgesic.

Propositus. Proband. Premise. (*Plural: propositi.*)

Propranolol hydrochloride. B.P. 1968. $C_{16}H_{22}ClNO_2$. An adrenergic beta-receptor blocking agent, which is used in the treatment of cardiac arrhythmias and angina pectoris.

Proprioceptor. A receptor end organ on the somatic afferent components of the nervous system. Proprioceptors are found in muscles, tendons, joints and the labyrinth, and give information concerning the movements and position of the body in space.

Proptometer. An instrument for measuring the degree of proptosis.

Proptosis. Undue prominence of the eyeball. Exophthalmos.

Propyl docetrizoate. The B.P. Commission approved name for propyl 3-diacetylamino-2,4,6-tri-iodobenzoate. A radio-opaque substance.

Propylene glycol. B.P. 1968. $C_3H_8O_2$. A useful solvent of low toxicity.

Propyl gallate. B.P. 1968. $C_{10}H_{12}O_5$. An antioxidant for preserving fats and oils.

Propylhexedrine. B.P.C. 1968. $C_{10}H_{21}N$. A volatile sympathomimetic amine, with a local vasoconstrictor action, used in inhalers for the relief of nasal congestion.

Propyl hydroxybenzoate. B.P. 1968. $C_{10}H_{12}O_3$. A preservative for aqueous preparations, creams and emulsions.

Propyliodone. B.P. 1968. $C_{10}H_{11}I_2NO_3$. A contrast medium used in bronchography.

Propylthiouracil. B.P. 1968. $C_7H_{10}N_2OS$. An antithyroid drug used in the treatment of thyrotoxicosis.

Propyphenazone. The B.P. Commission approved name for 4-isopropyl-2,3-dimethyl-1-phenyl-5-pyrazolone. An analgesic.

Proquamezine. The B.P. Commission approved name for 10-(2,3-bisdimethylaminopropyl)phenothiazine. A bronchial spasmolytic.

Proscillaridin. The B.P. Commission approved name for a cardiac glycoside.

Prosencephalon. The forebrain.

Proso- (Gk *prosō:* forward). Prefix meaning forward or anterior.

Prosop-, Prosopo- (Gk *prosōpon:* face). Prefixes signifying relationship to the face.

Prosopagus. Conjoined twins with the parasitic twin attached to the face of the other elsewhere than in the jaw.

Prosopothoracopagus. Conjoined twins united by the upper abdomen, chest and face.

Prostaglandins. Unsaturated hydroxy acids, originally isolated from the prostate and seminal vesicles, but now known to occur in a wide variety of tissues. They stimulate smooth muscle including that of the female genital tract, and also have a vasodepressor action.

Prostate. A firm, partly glandular, partly muscular, body, surrounding the commencement of the urethra in the male. It is about the size of a chestnut.

Prostatectomy. Surgical excision of the prostate.

Prostatitis. Inflammation of the prostate.

Prostatolith. A calculus in the prostate.

Prosthesis. An artificial replacement: e.g., an artificial limb. (*Plural: prostheses.*)

Prot-, Proto- (Gk *prōtos:* first). Prefixes meaning first.

Protamine sulphate injection. B.P. 1968. A sterile solution of protamine sulphate prepared from the sperm or mature testes of fish belonging to the families Clupeidae or Salmonidae. It is used as an antidote to heparin.

Protanopia. The partial form of colour blindness, in which the red end of the spectrum is much less bright than for normal people, and is often shortened.

Protease. A proteolytic enzyme that breaks down protein by splitting the peptide linkage.

Protein. A very large and elaborate polypeptide made up of almost infinite combinations of amino-acids. Proteins are widely distributed in the animal and vegetable kingdom, and form the principal constituents of the cell protoplasm.

Proteinuria. The presence of protein in the urine.

Proteolysis. The splitting up of protein.

Proteolytic. That which induces proteolysis.

Proteose. An intermediate product of proteolysis between protein and peptone.

Proteus. A genus of gram-negative bacilli, belonging to the family

Enterobacteriaceae. The most important members of the genus are *Proteus morganii* and *Proteus vulgaris*.

Prothionamide. B.P.C. 1968, Supplement 1971. $C_9H_{12}N_2S$. A tuberculostatic agent.

Prothrombin. The precursor of thrombin. It is present in the circulating blood and is changed to thrombin in the presence of calcium ions and thromboplastin.

Protodiastole. The earliest phase of cardiac diastole, immediately following the reduced ejection phase of ventricular systole.

Protokylol. The B.P. Commission approved name for 1-(3,4-dihydroxyphenyl)-2-(α-methyl-3,4-methylenedioxyphenethylamino)ethanol. A sympathomimetic agent.

Proton. One of the two particles of which nuclei consist.

Protopathic. Primary. **Protopathic pain,** pain of a particularly unpleasant nature and not well localized. **Protopathic sensitivity,** sensitivity to pain and temperature which is rather ill defined.

Protoplasm. The highly complex colloidal material of which animal and vegetable tissues are formed.

Protoplast. The whole body of living material of a bacterial cell, as bounded peripherally by the plasma or cytoplasmic, membrane.

Protoporphyrin. The porphyrin constituent of haemoglobin, myoglobin and various respiratory pigments.

Protozoa. The phylum of the animal kingdom, consisting of unicellular parasites and made up of four classes: Sporozoa, Zoomastigophora, Ciliata, and Rhizopoda.

Protriptyline hydrochloride. B.P. Addendum 1971. $C_{19}H_{22}ClN$. An antidepressant.

Protuberance. Projection or prominence. **Mental protuberance,** the prominence of the chin. **Occipital protuberance, external,** the bony protuberance at the upper end of the median furrow at the back of the neck. **Occipital protuberance, internal,** a blunt protuberance in the middle of the internal surface of the squamous part of the occipital bone.

Providencia. A group of gram-negative motile bacilli closely allied to the genus Proteus.

Provitamin. Precursor of a vitamin. **Provitamin A,** carotene.

Proximal. Nearer the centre of the body or the median line.

Proxymetacaine hydrochloride. B.P.C. 1968. $C_{16}H_{27}ClN_2O_3$. An ophthalmic local anaesthetic.

Proxyphylline. The B.P. Commission approved name for 7-(2-hydroxypropyl)theophylline. A bronchodilator.

Prune. The dried ripe fruit of the plum, *Prunus domesticus*, which has a mildly laxative action.

Prurigo. A chronic disease of the skin characterized by the appearance of papules or pimples that itch intensely. **Besnier's prurigo,** a form of prurigo associated with hay fever and/or asthma.

Pruritus. Itching. **Pruritus ani,** itching at the anus. **Pruritus vulvae,** itching of the vulva.

Prussic acid. Hydrocyanic acid.

Psammo- (Gk *psammos:* sand). Prefix indicating relation to sand, sand-like.

Psammoma. A calcified spherule found in certain meningiomas.

Psellism. Stuttering.

Pseud-, Pseudo- (Gk *pseudēs:* false). Prefixes signifying deceptive or false.

Pseudarthrosis. A false joint, as between the fragments of an ununited fracture.

Pseudo-agglutination. The rouleaux formation of erythrocytes.

Pseudocholinesterase. An enzyme that differs from cholinesterase in that it hydrolyses non-choline esters.

Pseudocryptorchidism. The condition in which a normally sited testis is retractile and can be drawn upwards by the cremasteric muscle into the inguinal canal.

Pseudocyesis. Spurious pregnancy. A condition in which all or some of the manifestations of pregnancy appear without conception having occurred.

Pseudoephedrine hydrochloride. B.P.C. 1968. $C_{10}H_{16}ClNO$. A sympathomimetic amine with an action like that of ephedrine.

Pseudoglobulin. A globulin which is water-soluble.

Pseudogout. Chondrocalcinosis.

Pseudohermaphroditism. The condition in which the gonads are of one sex but the external manifestations of sex are contradictory.

Pseudohypertrophic muscular dystrophy. The form of muscular dystrophy, in which the muscles, though weak, appear hypertrophied as a result of fatty infiltration.

Pseudohypertrophy. Enlargement without genuine hypertrophy.

Pseudohypoparathyroidism. The congenital condition in which the renal tubules are unresponsive to parathormone.

Pseudologia fantastica. Pathological lying.

Pseudolymphoma. The development of lymphoid nodules in the skin, orbit and rectum, which resemble follicular lymphomas, but are not malignant.

Pseudomembranous. Characterized by the presence of a false membrane. **Pseudomembranous entercolitis,** acute necrosis of the mucosa of the ileum and colon.

Pseudomonadaceae. The family of the order Pseudomonadales.

Pseudomonadales. An order of bacteria which includes two families: Pseudomonadaceae and Spirillaceae.

Pseudomonas. A genus of the family Pseudomonadaceae. *Pseudamonas pyocyanea,* the only species pathogenic to man. A gram-negative, non-sporing bacillus often present in the normal intestinal flora.

Pseudomyxoma peritonei. A mucus-secreting lesion, usually of the appendix or ovary, that ruptures and discharges its contents into the peritoneal cavity.

Pseudoneuritis. The blurring of the optic disc that occurs in some hypermetropic eyes.

Pseudophyllidea. The order of tapeworms which includes the genus Diphyllobothrium, the most important member of which is the fish tapeworm *Diphyllobothrium latum.*

Pseudopodium. A protoplasmic process extruded as a means of propulsion, or as a means of ingesting food, by an amoeba. *(Plural:* pseudopodia.**)**

Pseudopolyposis. The presence of multiple pseudopolypi, as in certain cases of ulcerative colitis.

Pseudopolypus. A tab of mucous membrane produced by inflammatory change, and resembling a polypus.

Pseudosarcoma. A proliferative condition of fibrous tissue in which histological assessment of malignancy is difficult.

Pseudoxanthoma elasticum. A condition characterized by the appearance of elevated yellow plaques in the skin, angioid streaks in the retina, and degenerative changes in the arteries.

Psilocybin. The B.P. Commission approved name for 3-(2-dimethylaminoethyl)indol-4-yl dihydrogen phosphate. A psychotomimetic.

Psilosis. Sprue. Falling out of the hair.

Psittacosis. An epizootic disease of birds which may affect man. The causative organism is a virus belonging to the psittacocis-lymphogranuloma-trachoma group of viruses.

Psoriasis. A chronic skin disease of unknown origin, characterized by sharply defined patches of erythema covered by silvery scales, usually on extensor surfaces. **Arthopathic psoriasis,** the form of the disease associated with chronic arthritis. **Flexural psoriasis,** the form in which the disease appears mostly in the body folds. **Guttate psoriasis,** the form, usually in children, in which the lesions are small and globular. **Pustular psoriasis,** the form in which the disease appears as sterile pustules, usually on the thenar and hypothenar eminencies and the soles.

Psych-, Psycho- (Gk *psychē:* soul, mind). Prefixes signifying association with the mind.

Psychasthenia. A psychoneurosis characterized by fears and anxieties.

Psyche. The mind.

Psychiatry. The study of diseases and disorders of the mind.

Psychic. Pertaining to the mind.

Psycho-analysis. The theories and practice of the Freudian school of psychology.

Psychodelic. Characterized by freedom from anxiety and by the enjoyment of highly creative, coloured thought patterns.

Psychogenic. Of emotional or mental origin.

Psychology. The branch of science concerned with the working of the mind and mental processes.

Psychomotor. Pertaining to the motor effects of mental activity.

Psychoneurosis. An emotional disturbance in which the individual suffers from persisting unwarranted fears and anxieties, lack of self-confidence and general interest in life. *(Plural:* psychoneuroses.**)**

Psychopath. An individual who is suffering from a persistent disorder or disability of mind which results in abnormally aggressive or seriously irresponsible conduct.

Psychopathology. The pathology of mental disease.

Psychopharmacology. The study of the effects of drugs on the mind.

Psychosensory. Pertaining to mental perception of sensory stimuli.

Psychosexual. Pertaining to the emotional or psychic aspects of sex.

Psychosis. Severe mental illness. Insanity. *(Plural:* psychoses.**)**

Psychosomatic. Pertaining to the mind and the body.

Psychotherapy. Any form of therapy that operates through the mind.

Psychotic. Relating to a psychosis.

Psychotropic. Exerting an action on the mind.

Psychro- (Gk *psychros:* cold). Prefix meaning cold or relationship to cold.

Psychrophilic. Preferring the cold. **Psychrophilic bacteria,** bacteria that grow best at low temperatures.

Psyllium. B.P.C. 1968. The dried ripe seed of *Plantago psyllium* L. or *P. indica* L. In virtue of its property of absorbing and retaining water, it is used in the treatment of chronic constipation.

Pterion. The point on the skull where the frontal, the sphenoid, the parietal, and the squamous part of the temporal bone meet.

Pteroylglutamic acid. Folic acid.

Pterygium. A degenerative condition of the subconjunctival tissues which proliferate as vascularized tissue to invade the cornea.

Pterygo- (Gk *pteryx:* wing). Prefix signifying wing-like, or relationship to the pterygoid process.

Pterygoid. Wing-shaped.

Ptomaine. A term originally applied to toxic amines produced in the course of protein decomposition.

Ptosis. Drooping of the upper eyelid. Prolapse of any organ.

-ptosis (Gk *ptōsis:* fall). Suffix signifying a lowered position or drooping.

Ptyal-, Ptyalo- (Gk *ptyalon:* spittle, saliva). Prefixes signifying association with saliva.

Ptyalin. Salivary amylase that converts starch into maltose.

Ptyalism. Excessive secretion of saliva.

Ptyalith. A salivary calculus.

Ptyalography. Sialography.

Puberal. Relating to puberty.

Pubertal. Relating to puberty.

Puberty. The span of years during which the sex glands become capable of exercising their reproductive functions.

Pubescence. Puberty.

Pubic. Relating to the pubis or the pubic region.

Pubiotomy. Surgical division of the pubic bone to one side of the midline.

Pubis. The anterior part of the hip bone which meets the pubis of the opposite side in the median plane to form the symphysis pubis. (*Plural:* pubes.)

Pudendum. The external genitalia.

Puerperal. Pertaining to the puerperium. **Puerperal pyrexia,** any febrile condition occurring in a woman in whom a temperature of 100·4°F (38°C) has occurred within fourteen days of childbirth or miscarriage.

Puerperium. The period succeeding labour, during which the genital organs return to their pre-pregnancy state. The duration is usually six to eight weeks.

Pulex. A genus of fleas. *Pulex irritans,* the common or human flea. (*Plural:* pulices.)

Pulheems. A medical system of classification used in the British Armed Services: P = physical capacity; U = upper limbs; L = lower limbs; H = hearing; EE = eyesight; M = mental capacity; S = stability (emotional).

Pulicide. An agent that kills fleas.

Pullulation. Sprouting or germinating.

Puer- (L *puer:* child). Prefix signifying association with a child.

Pulmo-, Pulmono- (L *pulmo:* lung). Prefixes indicating relationship with the lungs.

Pulmolith. A calculus in the lung.

Pulmonary. Pertaining to the lungs.

Pulpectomy. Removal of pulp from a tooth.

Pulpitis. Inflammation of the pulp of a tooth.

Pulse. The rhythmic dilatation of an artery produced by ventricular systole. **Alternating pulse,** pulsus alternans. **Anacrotic pulse,** a pulse with a perceptible notch in the ascending limb, as in aortic stenosis. **Arterial pulse,** the pulse. **Capillary pulse,** the pulse visible in the capillaries in the nail-bed in aortic incompetence. **Bigeminal pulse,** pulsus bigeminus. **Collapsing pulse,** a pulse with a sharp rise and fall, as occurs in aortic incompetence due to the large pulse pressure. Waterhammer pulse. **Pulse deficit,** the difference between the ventricular rate and the arterial pulse rate in atrial fibrillation. **Dicrotic pulse,** a pulse with an exaggerated dicrotic wave, as in hypotension. **Jugular pulse,** the pulse as seen or palpated in the jugular vein. **Paradoxical pulse,** pulsus paradoxicus. **Pulse pressure,** the difference between the systolic and the diastolic pressure. **Thready pulse,** a scarcely perceptible pulse. **Venous pulse,** the pulsation in a vein. **Waterhammer pulse,** collapsing pulse.

Pulsus. Pulse. **Pulsus alternans,** a regular pulse in which alternating pulsations are strong and weak. A sign of advanced heart failure. **Pulsus bigeminus,** a pulse in which the beats occur in pairs. **Pulsus paradoxicus,** a pulse that decreases in size during inspiration.

Pulvinar. The expanded posterior end of the thalamus.

Pumilio pine oil. B.P.C. 1968. The distillate from the fresh leaves of *Pinus mugo,* which is used as an inhalant to relieve cough and nasal congestion.

Punctate. Marked with points or dots.

Punctum. Point. (*Plural:* puncta.) **Punctum lacrimale,** the minute orifice near the medial angle of the eye, through which tears enter the lacrimal canaliculus.

Puncture. A hole made by a fine pointed instrument. **Cisternal puncture,** puncture of the cisterna magna with a trocar and cannula for diagnostic or therapeutic purposes. **Lumbar puncture,** puncture of the subarachnoid space with a trocar and cannula passed between the 4th and 5th lumbar vertebrae for diagnostic or therapeutic purposes. **Splenic puncture,** puncture of the spleen with a trocar and cannula for diagnostic purposes. **Sternal puncture,** puncture of the sternum with a special needle to obtain a sample of bone marrow for diagnostic purposes. **Ventricular puncture,** puncture of a cerebral ventricle with a trocar and cannula for diagnostic or therapeutic purposes.

Pupil. The circular aperture just to the nasal side of the iris through which light rays enter the eye. **Argyll Robertson pupil,** the pupil which responds to accommodation but not light. A syphilitic stigma.

Pupillary. Pertaining to the pupil.

Purgation. Evacuation of the bowels by means of purgatives.

Purgative. A drug for causing evacuation of the bowels. Cathartic.

Purine. The heterocyclic compound containing a pyrimidine ring and ʃan imidazole ring fused together, which constitutes the base of the purine bases adenine and guanine. Other naturally occurring purine derivatives are xanthine and uric acid.

Puromycin. The B.P. Commission approved name for an antibiotic derived from *Streptomyces albo-niger,* which has an amoebicidal and trypanocidal action.

Purple. A colour formed by a mixture of red and blue. **Visual purple,** rhodopsin.

Purpura. A condition characterized by the occurrence of purple spots in the skin, due to extravasation of blood in the skin. **Anaphylactoid purpura,** Henoch's purpura. **Purpura artefacta,** self induced purpura. **Haemorrhagic purpura,** idiopathic thrombocytopenic purpura. **Henoch's purpura,** non-thrombocytopenic purpura, occurring usually in children, and accompanied by articular or digestive manifestations. Anaphylactoid purpura. Purpura simplex. **Idiopathic thrombocytopenic purpura,** a severe form of purpura characterized by a reduced platelet count, a prolonged bleeding time and a normal coagulation time. Essential thrombocytopenia. Purpura haemorrhagica. **Senile purpura,** purpura occurring in old people.

Purulent. Concerned with, or containing, pus.

Pus. The liquid product of inflammation, containing leucocytes, dead or dying micro-organisms and cellular debris.

Pustule. A small elevation of the skin containing pus. **Malignant pustule,** cutaneous anthrax.

Putamen. The larger, lateral, dark coloured portion of the lentiform nucleus.

Putrefaction. The decomposition of living matter, particularly protein, usually by bacteria assisted by enzymatic action.

Putrescine. An amine found in decaying meat.

Pyaemia. A form of septicaemia in which abscesses develop throughout the body.

Pyel-, Pyelo- (Gk *pyelos:* pelvis). Prefixes signifying relationship to the pelvis of the kidney.

Pyelitis. Inflammation of the pelvis of the kidney.

Pyelocystitis. Inflammation of the pelvis of the kidney and the bladder.

Pyelogram. An X-ray picture of a kidney visualized with a radio-opaque medium.

Pyelography. Radiological visualization of the kidneys with a radio-opaque medium. **Intravenous pyelography,** pyelography after intravenous administration of the radio-opaque medium. **Retrograde pyelography,** pyelography after introduction of the radio-opaque medium through ureteric catheters.

Pyelonephritis. Inflammation of the kidney, including the pelvis.

Pyemotidae. A family of mites. *Pyemotes ventricosus* (*Pediculoides ventricosus*), the mite responsible for the dermatitis known as grain itch or straw itch.

Pygmalionism. Falling in love with an object made by oneself: e.g. a statue.

Pygo- (Gk *pygē:* rump). Prefix signifying association with the buttocks.

Pygopagus. Conjoined twins joined at the buttocks back to back.

Pyknic. Having a short, stocky, thick build with a tendency to obesity.

Pykno- (Gk *pyknos:* thick, frequent). Prefix meaning thick or frequent.

Pyknolepsy. A form of epilepsy characterized by frequent attacks of petit mal.

Pyknosis. The process whereby the degenerating nucleus becomes smaller and thicker.

Pyknotic. Pertaining to pyknosis.

Pyle- (Gk *pylē:* gate). Prefix signifying association with the portal vein.

Pylephlebitis. Inflammation of the portal vein.

Pylethrombophlebitis. Thrombosis and inflammation of the portal vein.

Pylorectomy. Surgical excision of the pylorus.

Pyloric. Pertaining to the pylorus.

Pyloro- (Gk *pylōros:* gate-keeper). Prefix signifying relationship to the pylorus.

Pyloroplasty. A plastic operation on the pylorus with a view to widening it when stenosed.

Pylorospasm. Spasm of the pylorus.

Pylorus. The opening through which the stomach communicates with the duodenum.

Py-, Pyo- (Gk *pyon:* pus). Prefixes meaning pus.

Pyocele. Distension of a cavity or tube as a result of the accumulation of pus.

Pyocolpos. A collection of pus in the vagina.

Pyocyanin. The bluish-green pigment produced by *Pseudomonas pyocyanea*.

Pyoderma. A pustular skin eruption.

Pyogenic. Producing pus.

Pyometra. A collection of pus in the uterus.

Pyometritis. Purulent inflammation of the uterus.

Pyomyositis. Inflammation of the muscles with abscess formation.

Pyopneumothorax. The presence of pus and air in a pleural cavity.

Pyorrhoea. A discharge of pus. **Pyorrhoea alveolaris,** periodontal disease with a purulent discharge.

Pyosalpingitis. Purulent inflammation of the uterine tube.

Pyosalpinx. An accumulation of pus in the uterine tube.

Pyosis. Suppuration.

Pyothorax. The presence of pus in the pleural cavity. Empyema.

Pyo-ureter. A collection of pus in the ureter.

Pyramid. A conical eminence. **Pyramid of the cerebellum,** the part of the inferior surface of the vermis between the tuber vermis and the uvula. **Decussation of the pyramids,** the decussation of the great motor tracts in the medulla oblongata. **Pyramid of the medulla oblongata,** one of the two elevations formed by the pyramidal tracts on the ventral surface of the medulla oblongata. **Renal pyramids,** the pale, striated, conical masses in the medulla of the kidney. **Pyramid of the vestibule,** the anterior end of a vestibular crest of the bony labyrinth.

Pyrantel. The B.P. Commission approved name for an anthelmintic.

Pyrazinamide. B.P. 1968. $C_5H_5N_3O$. A tuberculostatic drug used in the treatment of tuberculosis.

Pyreto- (Gk *pyretos:* fever). Prefix signifying relationship to fever.

Pyrexia. Fever.

Pyridostigmine bromide. B.P. 1968. $C_9H_{13}BrN_2O_2$. An anticholinesterase with the same action as neostigmine, but only one-fourth as active. It is used in the treatment of myasthenia gravis.

Pyridoxine hydrochloride. B.P. 1968. $C_8H_{12}ClNO_3$. Vitamin B_6. A vitamin present in yeast, liver, cereals and wheat, which plays a part in protein metabolism, haemopoiesis, and the nutrition of the skin.

Pyrimethamine. B.P. 1968. $C_{12}H_{13}Cl N_4$. An antimalarial drug largely used as a prophylactic.

Pyrithione zinc. The B.P. Commission approved name for a drug for the treatment of seborrhoea.

Pyritinol. The B.P. Commission approved name for a sedative.

Pyro- (Gk *pyr:* fire). Prefix signifying association with fire.

Pyrogen. A fever-producing substance.

Pyrogenic. Fever inducing.

Pyromania. A morbid preoccupation with, and desire to produce, fires.

Pyrophobia. Morbid fear of fire.

Pyrosis. Heartburn.

Pyroxylin. B.P. 1968. A nitrated cellulose used in the preparation of collodions.

Pyrrobutamine. The B.P. Commission

approved name for 1-[4-(4-chloro-phenyl)-3-phenylbut-2-enyl]pyrrolidine. An antihistaminic.

Pyrrocaine. The B.P. Commission approved name for N-(pyrrolidin-1-ylacetyl)-2,6-xylidine. A local anaesthetic.

Pyruvate. A salt or ester of pyruvic acid.

Pyruvate kinase. The enzyme which catalyses the transfer of phosphate from phosphoenolpyruvate to adenosine diphosphate, and lack of which is one of the causes of hereditary non-spherocytic haemolytic anaemia.

Pyruvic acid. An intermediate compound in the metabolism of carbohydrate. $CH_3—CO—COOH$.

Pyuria. The presence of pus in the urine.

P wave. The wave in the electrocardiogram, representing atrial activity.

Q

Q fever. An acute febrile illness caused by *Rickettsia burnetii*, and characterized by pyrexia, headache and pneumonitis.

Quadrantanopia. Loss of vision in one quadrant of the field of vision.

Quadratus. Four-sided.

Quadri- (L *quattor:* four). Prefix meaning four or fourfold.

Quadriceps. Four-headed.

Quadrigeminal. Fourfold. Composed of four points.

Quadripara. A woman who has given birth to four children.

Quadriplegia. Paralysis of all four limbs.

Quadrivalent. Having a valency of four.

Quadruplet. One of four children born at one birth.

Quarantine. Enforced retention (originally for 40 days) by international law of individuals entering a country from another country where they may have been in contact with certain infectious diseases. Isolation of individuals who have been in contact with highly infectious diseases.

Quart. A unit of capacity equivalent to 2 pints or 1·136 litres.

Quartan. Recurring every 72 hours.

Quassia. B.P.C. 1968. The dried stem-wood of *Picrasma excelsa*, which is used as a bitter.

Quellung. The capsular swelling that occurs in bacteria when mixed with specific antibody.

Quickening. The first foetal movements felt by the mother, usually in the 4th or 5th month of pregnancy.

Quicklime. Calcium oxide. CaO.

Quicksilver. Mercury.

Quillaia. B.P. 1968. The dried inner bark of *Quillaja saponaria* and other species of Quillaja, which is used as an emulsifying agent.

Quinacillin. The B.P. Commission approved name for a semi-synthetic penicillin.

Quinalbarbitone sodium. B.P. 1968. $C_{12}H_{17}N_2NaO_3$. An intermediate-acting barbiturate.

Quinestradol. The B.P. Commission approved name for 3-cyclopentyloxy-oestra-1,3,5(10)-triene-16α,17β-diol. An oestrogen.

Quinestrol. The B.P. Commission approved name for 3-cyclopentyloxy-19-nor-17α-pregna-1,3,5(10)-trien-20-yn-17-ol. An oestrogen.

Quinethazone. The B.P. Commission approved name for 7-chloro-2-ethyl-1,2-dihydro-6-sulphamoylquinazolin-4-one. A diuretic and hypotensive agent.

Quingestanol. The B.P. Commission approved name for 3-cyclopentyloxy-19-nor-17α-pregna-3,5-diene-20-yn-17-ol. A progestational steroid.

Quinidine. An alkaloid obtained from the bark of various species of Cinchona. **Quinidine sulphate,** B.P. 1968, $C_{40}H_{50}N_4O_8S,2H_2O$, a myocardial depressant used in the treatment of paroxysmal ventricular tachycardia and atrial fibrillation.

Quinine. An alkaloid derived from the bark of various species of Cinchona, which was widely used in the prevention and treatment of malaria, but has now been replaced to a large extent, though not completely, by less toxic and more effective modern anti-malarial drugs. Quinine sulphate is also used as a bitter. The following salts are included in the *British Pharmacopoeia* 1968: quinine bisulphate; quinine dihydrochloride; quinine hydrochloride; quinine sulphate.

Quinque- (L *quinque:* five). Prefix meaning five.

Quinquivalent. Having a valency of five.

Quinsy. Peritonsillar abscess.

Quintuplet. One of five children born at the same birth.

Quotidian. Recurring daily.

Quotient. The number obtained by dividing one number by another. **Intelligence quotient,** a rating of intellectual attainment obtained by dividing an individual's mental age as ascertained by given tests, by his chronological age, and then multiplying by 100. (*Abbreviation:* I.Q.) **Respiratory quotient,** the volume of carbon dioxide produced in respiration divided by the volume of oxygen used in the same time. (*Abbreviation:* R.Q.)

Q wave. The initial wave of the QRS complex, representing ventricular activity, in the electrocardiogram.

R

Rabid. Afflicted by, or related to, rabies.

Rabies. A viral infection of the brain of certain animals, particularly dogs and wolves, which is transmitted to man by the bite of an infected animal, and causes an illness characterized by mental changes and spasm of the muscles of swallowing and respiration. Hydrophobia. **Rabies Antiserum, B.P. 1968,** a preparation from native serum containing the antiviral globulins or their derivatives which have the specific power of neutralizing the virus of rabies. It contains not less than 80 units per ml. **Rabies vaccine, B.P. 1968,** a suspension, in a saline or other appropriate solution isotonic with blood, of a suitable killed rabies virus in uncontaminated brain tissue, derived from animals previously infected intracerebrally with rabies virus.

Racemethorphan. The B.P. Commission approved name for a narcotic analgesic.

Racemic. Optically inactive, being composed of equal parts of dextrorotatory and laevorotatory forms.

Racemoramide. The B.P. Commission approved name for a narcotic analgesic.

Racemorphan. The B.P. Commission approved name for a narcotic analgesic.

Racemose. Resembling a bunch of grapes.

Rachi-, Rachio- (Gk *rachis:* spine). Prefixes signifying relationship to the spine.

Rachianaesthesia. Spinal anaesthesia.

Rachiotome. A surgical instrument for dividing vertebral laminae.

Rachiotomy. Surgical incision of vertebral laminae.

Rachipagus. Conjoined twins joined together by a fused vertebral column.

Rachitic. Related to rickets.

Rachitis. Rickets.

Rachitogenic. Inducing rickets.

Rad. *R*adiation *A*bsorbed *D*ose. The unit of measurement of the absorbed dose of ionizing radiation, equal to 100ergs per gramme.

Radiation. Electromagnetic waves or energy. The emission of such energy. Divergence from a central point. **Acoustic radiation,** a tract of fibres that run from the medial geniculate nucleus to the temporal lobe. **Optic radiation,** a tract of fibres that run from the lateral geniculate body to the occipital lobe.

Radical. Root. A group of atoms that act as a unit.

Radicle. A rootlet.

Radicular. Pertaining to a root or radicle.

Radiculectomy. Surgical excision of the posterior root of a spinal nerve.

Radiculitis. Inflammation of the root of a spinal nerve.

Radio- (L *radius:* ray). Prefix signifying relationship to radiation.

Radioactivity. The property of emitting radiation by the spontaneous disintegration of certain nuclides or their nuclei.

Radio-autography. The detection of radio-isotopes by the ability of the emitted radiation to blacken a photographic emulsion.

Radiography. The making of a photographic record by means of x-rays. Roentgenography.

Radio-isotope. An isotope that is radioactive.

Radiology. The science of x-rays and their use for diagnostic purposes in medicine.

Radiometer. An instrument for measuring the intensity of radiation.

Radionuclide, A radioactive nuclide.

Radio-opaque. Not permitting the passage of x-rays.

Radioscopy. Examination of the image thrown by x-rays on a fluorescent screen.

Radiotherapy. The use of ionizing radiations in the treatment of disease.

Radium. A radioactive element. Symbol Ra. Atomic weight 226. Atomic number 88. It emits α-, β-, and γ-rays, and was at one time, and to a certain extent still is, used in the treatment of various forms of cancer.

Radius. The lateral bone of the forearm.

Radix. A root. (*Plural:* radices.)

Radon. A colourless, radioactive gaseous emanation of radium. Chemical symbol Rn. Atomic weight ;222. Atomic number 86.

Raisin. A partially dried grape.

Rale. A pulmonary adventitious sound.

Ramus. A branch. (*Plural:* rami.) **Ramus communicans, grey,** the branch which the ventral ramus of each spinal nerve receives from the corresponding ganglion of the sympathetic trunk. It conveys postganglionic fibres from the ramus to the nerve for distribution to the blood vessels, sweat glands and arrectores pilorum muscles in its area. **Ramus communicans, white,** the branch which the ventral ramus of the thoracic and the 1st and 2nd lumbar nerves each contributes to the corresponding sympathetic ganglion. It conveys efferent preganglionic fibres from the nerve to the sympathetic trunk, and transmits afferent visceral fibres from the trunk to the nerve. **Dorsal ramus of the spinal nerves,** the smaller of the two branches of each spinal nerve. It supplies the muscles and skin of the appropriate area of the posterior part of the neck and trunk. **Ventral ramus of the spinal nerves,** the larger of the two branches of each spinal nerve. It supplies the limbs and the anterior and lateral aspects of the trunk in the appropriate area.

Ranula. A cyst on the floor of the mouth which usually arises as a result of distension of a mucous or salivary gland.

Rape. Unlawful sexual intercourse with a woman without her consent, by force, fear or fraud.

Raphe. A seam. **Palpebral raphe, lateral,** the interlacing of the lateral ends of the palpebral fibres of the orbicularis oculi. **Pharyngeal raphe,** the strong fibrous band in the middle of the posterior wall of the pharynx. **Pterygomandibular raphe,** a tendinous band which stretches from the hamulus of the medial pterygoid plate to the posterior end of the mylohyoid line of the mandible. **Raphe of the scrotum,** the ridge in the midline of the scrotum.

Rash. A skin eruption.

Rate. Measurement of speed or frequency. **Basal metabolic rate,** the amount of energy produced per unit of surface area per hour at complete mental and physical rest. **Birth rate,** the live births per annum per 1000 of estimated population at the middle of the year. **Circulation rate,** the volume of blood discharged by the heart per minute. **Death rate, crude,** the total deaths per annum per 1000 of estimated population at the middle of the year. **Death rate, standardized,** the death rate at all ages calculated for comparative purposes in such a way that allowance is made for the sex and age composition of the population involved. **Erythrocyte sedimentation rate,** the rate of settling or sedimentation of erythrocytes carried out under prescribed conditions. **Fertility rate,** the live births occurring, divided by the female population at childbearing age (usually taken as 15 to 44 years). **Glomerular filtration rate,** the rate at which a given substance (e.g. inulin) is cleared from the blood as it passes through the glomeruli. **Infant mortality rate,** the deaths under 1 year of age occurring in the calendar year, divided by the total live births occurring in the calendar year (usually expressed per 1000.) **Maternal mortality rate,** the deaths ascribed to puerperal causes divided by the total live births and stillbirths (usually expressed per 1000). **Morbidity incidence rate,** the number of illnesses (number of spells of illness or number of persons sick, as applicable) beginning within a specified period of time related to the average number of persons exposed to risk during that period (or at its midpoint). **Mortality rate,** death rate. **Neonatal mortality rate,** the number of deaths of infants under 4 weeks of age per 1000 live births. **Peak flow rate,** the maximum volume of air expired during a forced expiration. Maximum expiratory flow rate. **Perinatal mortality rate,** stillbirths plus deaths in the first week of life per 1000 total births. **Period prevalence morbidity rate,** the number of illnesses (number of spells of illness or number of persons sick, as applicable) existing at any time within a specified period of time related to the average number of persons exposed to risk during that period of time (or at its midpoint). **Point prevalence morbidity rate,** the number of illnesses (number of spells of illness or number of persons sick as applicable) existing at a specified point of time related to the number of persons exposed to risk at that point of time. **Proportional**

mortality rate, the ratio of deaths from a given cause to the total deaths (usually expressed as a percentage). Pulse rate, the number of beats palpable (usually in the radial artery at the wrist) per minute. Respiration rate, the number of respiratory (inspiration plus expiration) movements of the chest per minute. Stillbirth rate, the number of stillbirths per 1000 total births.

Ratio. Relation of one thing to another. Albumin-globulin ratio, the relation of the serum albumin to the serum globulin. (Normal = 1·5.) Bodyweight ratio, body weight (in grammes) divided by body height (in centimetres). Cardiothoracic ratio, the ratio of the transverse diameter of the heart to the transverse diameter of the chest at its widest point above the dome of the diaphragm. Standardized mortality ratio, the number of deaths registered in the year of experience as a percentage of those which would have been expected in that year had the sex/age mortality of a standard period (1950–1952) operated on the sex/age population of the year of experience.

Rauwolfia serpentina. B.P.C. 1968. The dried roots of Rauwolfia serpentina, which contains several hypotensive alkaloids. Rauwolfia vomitoria, B.P.C. 1968, the dried roots of Rauwolfia vomitoria, or African rauwolfia, which is used for the preparation of reserpine.

Ray. A straight line or beam of radiation. Actinic rays, light rays that produce chemical changes. Alpha rays, high-speed, low-penetrating helium nuclei ejected by radioactive substances. Beta rays, high-velocity, penetrating electrons emitted from radioactive substances. Cathode rays, the stream of electrons emitted from the cathode (negative electrode) of a vacuum tube which, impinging on a target, give rise to x-rays. Gamma rays, electromagnetic radiation of short wave-length but high penetrating power, emitted from radioactive substances. Grenz rays, very soft, poor-penetrating x-rays. Hertzian rays, electromagnetic waves of long wavelength; radio waves. Incident ray, the ray of light that impinges on a surface before reflection. Infra-red rays, radiations just beyond the red end of the spectrum (wave-lengths 7700 to 500,000 Å). Reflected ray, the ray of light after it has been reflected from the surface of a denser medium. Roentgen rays, x-rays. Ultraviolet rays, invisible rays beyond the violet end of the spectrum (wave-lengths 4000 to 2000). X-rays, the short-wave, penetrating electromagnetic vibrations emitted from a vacuum tube by the bombardment of the anode with cathode rays.

Raynaud's disease. Intermittent pallor or cyanosis of the extremities induced by exposure to cold, caused by spasm of the digital blood vessels, and occurring usually in women. Raynaud's phenomenon, constriction of the digital blood vessels as in Raynaud's disease, but occurring with associated and contributing conditions and diseases.

Re- (L re: again). Prefix meaning back, again.

Reaction. A response to a stimulus. Interaction between chemical compounds. Allergic reaction, the response of the tissues to an antigen to which they have been sensitized. Anaphylactic reactions, the antigen-antibody reaction in a hypersensitive individual. Cold agglutination reaction, the agglutination, by the serum of patients with primary atypical pneumonia, at low temperatures of human erythrocytes of blood group O. Reaction of degeneration, the reaction of muscle to electrical stimuli after its nerves have degenerated. Diazo reaction, the pink discoloration of the froth of urine on adding a given reagent, which occurs in the 2nd week of typhoid fever. It is merely a confirmatory test and by no means occurs in every case. Graft reaction, the response of the tissues to an incompatible graft. Herxheimer reaction, the exacerbation of syphilitic symptoms and signs that occurs in some patients when given antisyphilitic treatment. Immunity reaction, the response of an immune host to an antigen. Lepra reaction, an inflammatory phase, usually acute, in leprosy which occurs as a manifestation of hypersensitivity to Myco. leprae. Leukaemoid reaction, an unusual form of leucocytosis, in which myelocytes and immature polymorphs are present, thus resembling the blood picture of leukaemia. Pfeiffer's reaction, the lysis induced in cholera vibrios when they are injected intraperitoneally along with an anticholera serum devoid of complement. Prausnitz-Küstner reaction, an allergic test based on passive transfer of allergic sensitivity. Stormy clot reaction, the breaking up of clot in litmus milk medium produced by *Cl. welchii*, but not specific for this organism. **Strauss reaction,** a diagnostic test for glanders. **Transfusion reaction,** the body's response to the transfusion of incompatible blood. **Vaccinoid reaction,** the minor response to smallpox vaccination in an individual who has a partial immunity to the disease. **Wassermann reaction,** a diagnostic test for syphilis. **Weil-Felix reaction,** a diagnostic test for typhus fever. **Widal reaction,** a diagnostic test for typhoid fever which usually becomes positive about the 7th to 10th day.

Reagin. A type of antibody which has a particular ability to become fixed in the skin or mucous membranes.

Receptor. A specialized sensory nerve ending.

Recess. A small hollow or cavity. **Caecal recesses,** the three peritoneal recesses in the neighbourhood of the caecum. **Cochlear recess,** a small recess on the inner wall of the vestibule. **Costo-diaphragmatic recess,** a recess between the costal and diaphragmatic pleurae. **Costomediastinal recess,** the slit-like cavity between the costal and mediastinal pleurae. **Dorsal recess, lateral, of 4th ventricle,** a backward extension, on both sides, lying above the inferior medullary velum and below the cerebellar nuclei. **Dorsal recess, median, of 4th ventricle,** an extension dorsally into the white core of the cerebellum above the nodule. **Duodenal recess, superior,** a small peritoneal pocket on the left side of the upper portion of the ascending part of the duodenum, present in about 50 per cent of people. **Duodenojejunal recess,** a peritoneal pouch between the duodenojejunal junction and the root of the transverse mesocolon, which occurs in about 20 per cent of people. **Elliptical recess,** the recess in the vestibule that lodges the utricle. **Epitympanic, recess,** the portion of the tympanic cavity above the level of the tympanic membrane. **Ileocaecal recess, inferior,** the recess, produced by the ileocaecal fold of peritoneum which extends from the anterior and inferior surfaces of the terminal part of the ileum to the mesoappendix. It is well marked in the young but tends to disappear with age. **Ileocaecal recess, superior,** a narrow chink bounded in front by the vascular fold of the caecum, behind by the mesentery of the ileum, below by the terminal ileum, on the right by the ileocaecal junction. It is best developed in children. **Infundibular recess,** the funnel-shaped recess of the 3rd ventricle as it is prolonged downwards into the infundibulum, with the hypophysis attached to the apex. **Intersigmoid recess,** a peritoneal recess behind and below the sigmoid colon which tends to disappear with age. **Lateral recess of 4th ventricle,** a narrow curved pouch on each side between the inferior cerebellar peduncle and the peduncle of the flocculus. **Mesentericoparietal recess,** a peritoneal pouch just below the horizontal part of the duodenum usually only present in young children. **Mesocolic recess,** duodenojejunal recess. **Optic recess,** an angular recess of the 3rd ventricle immediately above the optic chiasma. **Paraduodenal recess,** a peritoneal pouch behind the paraduodenal fold and to the left of the ascending duodenum, usually only present up to early childhood. **Pharyngeal recess,** a slit-like depression behind the auditory tube. **Pineal recess,** a small recess of the 3rd ventricle that projects into the stalk of the pineal body. **Retrocaecal recess,** the peritoneal pouch behind the caecum, in which the appendix often lies. **Retroduodenal recess,** a peritoneal pouch lying behind the fourth part of the duodenum; it is only occasionally present. **Sacciformis recess,** an upward protrusion of the capsule of the distal radio-ulnar joint. **Sphenoethmoidal recess,** the triangular fossa above the superior concha of the nasal cavity, which receives the opening of the sphenoidal sinus. **Spherical recess,** the recess in the vestibule that lodges the saccule. **Splenic recess,** the part of the omental bursa projecting, between the lienorenal and gastrosplenic ligaments, towards the spleen. **Subpopliteal recess,** a cul-de-sac of the synovial membrane of the knee joint extending between the lateral meniscus and the tendon of the popliteus. **Suprapineal recess,** a diverticulum of the 3rd ventricle running back above the pineal body.

Recessive. Not dominant. Tending to recede.

Recidivist. A person who tends to relapse, particularly a criminal who returns to his criminal career after punishment.

Rectal. Pertaining to the rectum.

Recto- (L *rectus:* straight). Prefix indicating relationship to the rectum.

Rectocele. Prolapse of the rectum.

Rectosigmoid. Pertaining to the rectum and the sigmoid colon.

Rectovesical. Pertaining to the rectum and the urinary bladder.

Rectum. The terminal portion of the alimentary tract, about 12cm. long, stretching from the sigmoid colon to the anal canal.

Rectus. Straight.

Recumbent. Lying down.

Recuperation. Recovery.

Recurrent. Returning. Turning back in its course.

Red. One of the primary colours, at the opposite end of the visible spectrum to violet, and with a wavelength of around 6500 ångstrom units.

Redox. A reduction-oxidation reaction. **Redox-potential,** the affinity of an oxidation-reduction system for electrons. Oxidation-reduction potential.

Reduction. The removal of oxygen from, or the addition of hydrogen to, a compound. Replacing the two parts of a fractured limb in alignment.

Reduplication. Doubling. Applied particularly to the doubling of heart sounds.

Reflex. Involuntary response to a stimulus. **Abdominal reflex,** contraction of the abdominal muscles in response to scratching of the skin. **Accommodation reflex,** reflex contraction of the pupils on accommodation. **Ankle reflex,** ankle jerk. **Arc, reflex,** the pathway of receptor, neurones and effector involved in producing a reflex. **Axon reflex,** a reflex which occurs without the impulse entering a nerve cell body. **Biceps reflex,** biceps jerk. **Blinking reflex,** closure of the eyes on the sudden approach of an object. **Carotid sinus reflex,** the influence exerted on blood pressure and heart rate by alterations in the pressure in the carotid sinus. **Conditioned reflex,** a reflex acquired or induced by repetitive training or conditioning. **Conjunctival reflex,** the blinking induced by lightly touching the conjunctiva. **Consensual light reflex,** contraction of one pupil on applying a light stimulus to the other. **Corneal reflex,** reflex blinking on touching the cornea. **Cremasteric reflex,** reflex contraction of the cremasteric muscle on stroking the medial side of the thigh. **Deep reflex,** any one of the tendon reflexes. **Gastro-colic reflex,** the mass contraction of the colon that follows the entry of food into the stomach. **Grasp reflex,** reflex closure of the hand on stimulating the palm. **Jaw reflex,** jaw jerk. **Knee reflex,** knee jerk. **Labyrinthine reflex,** one of the reflexes induced by stimulation of the vestibular apparatus. **Light reflex,** contraction of the pupil on exposure to light. **Mass reflex,** the complex response that occurs in patients with complete transection of the spinal cord on a stimulus being applied below the site of the lesion. **Monosynaptic reflex,** the simplest form of reflex, involving only two neurones: a sensory and a motor neurone. **Multisynaptic reflex,** a reflex involving internuncial neurones, as well as a sensory and a motor neurone. **Plantar reflex,** flexion of the great toe on stimulation of the lateral aspect of the sole of the foot. **Righting reflex,** one of the labyrinthine reflexes whereby the upright posture is maintained. **Scratch reflex,** the scratching induced in animals by stimulating the skin on the back or side. **Spinal reflex,** a reflex involving the spinal cord but not the brain. **Startle reflex,** the reaction of an infant to sudden noise or movement. **Statiokinetic reflex,** one of the labyrinthine reflexes, induced through the ampullary crests of the semicircular canal by movements of the head, for the maintenance of kinetic balance. **Statiotonic reflex,** one of the labyrinthine reflexes for the maintenance of muscle tone, and induced by stimulation of the maculae of the saccule and utricle by the position of the head. **Stretch reflex,** reflex contraction of a muscle when it is stretched, as in the various tendon reflexes or jerks. **Superficial reflex,** a reflex induced by stimulation of the skin. **Tendon reflex,** a reflex contraction of muscle induced by tapping a tendon. Deep reflex. **Triceps reflex,** triceps jerk. **Visceral reflex,** a reflex induced by stimulus of a viscus. **Withdrawal reflex,** the reflex withdrawal of a limb on receiving a harmful stimulus.

Reflux. Regurgitation. Backward flow.

Refraction. The deflexion of a ray of light on passing from one medium to another of different optical density. Determining the refractive error in the eye with a view to correcting it.

Refractometer. An instrument for measuring the refractive power of the eye and other translucent substances.

Refractory. Obstinate. Resistant to treatment or stimuli.

Refrangible. Capable of being refracted.

Refrigeration. The act of inducing a low temperature.

Refringent. Refractive.

Regimen. A prescribed course of treatment.

Regurgitation. A backward flow.

Rehabilitation. Restoration to health and working capacity.

Reiter's disease. A syndrome of arthritis, conjunctivitis, and non-gonococcal urethritis, of unknown etiology.

Relapse. Return of a disease after apparent recovery.

Relapsing fevers. Fevers caused by Borrelia, and characterized by attacks of remittent fever. **Louse-borne relapsing fever,** an infection by *Borrelia recurrentis*, which is transmitted by the human body louse, *Pediculus humanus* var. *corporis*, and occurs in temperate climes. **Tick-borne relapsing fever,** an infection by *Borrelia duttoni*, which is transmitted by ticks, and occurs in tropical and subtropical regions mainly, but also in Eastern Europe and the Mediterranean littoral.

Relaxant. Causing relaxation. An agent or drug causing relaxation.

Relaxation. Easing or lowering of tension.

Relaxin. A water-soluble polypeptide isolated from the corpus luteum of the ovaries of pregnant sows, which induces relaxation of the symphysis pubis and softening of the cervix uteri.

Reluxation. Redislocation.

Rem. *R*oentgen *E*quivalent *M*an (or *M*ammal). That dose of any ionizing radiation absorbed per gramme of living matter such that the biological effectiveness is the same as 1 rad of 200–250 kV$_p$ x-rays.

Remission. A temporary abatement of symptoms and signs during an illness.

Renal. Pertaining to the kidney.

Renin. A peptide secreted by cells of the juxtaglomerular apparatus in the kidney, which has enzymic properties and catalyses the transformation of a plasma protein, angiotensinogen, into the vasoconstrictor substances angiotensin I and II.

Rennet, A preparation obtained from the stomach of the calf, containing rennin, and used for curdling milk in cheese-making and in the making of junket.

Rennin. The milk-curdling ferment in the gastric juice of the calf, that converts caseinogen into casein.

Renography. Radiography of the kidney.

Reovirus. One of a group of viruses, first given the name *R*espiratory *E*nteric *O*rphan viruses; hence the name. They were originally classified as ECHO viruses, but are now recognized as a separate group with three serological types.

Replication. A turning back or folding back.

Repolarization. Restoration of the polarized state in muscle or nerve during recovery from conduction of an excitatory process.

Repositor. An instrument for replacing displaced organs.

Rescinnamine. The B.P. Commission approved name for methyl *O*-(3,4,5-trimethoxycinnamoyl)reserpate. A tranquillizer and hypotensive agent.

Resection. Surgical removal of part of the body.

Resectoscope. A modified cystoscope for the transurethral resection of the prostate.

Reserpine. B.P. 1968, $C_{33}H_{40}N_2O_9$. An alkaloid obtained from the roots of species of Rauwolfia, and used as a hypotensive agent and as a tranquillizer.

Reserve. Remainder. In store for future use. **Alkali reserve,** carbon dioxide combining power of the plasma.

Resin. A product of oxidation of volatile oils, soluble in alkalis (forming resin soaps) and alcohol; insoluble in water. **Gum resins,** extracts from plants consisting of gums and resins. **Ion-exchange resin,** a synthetic organic polymer, to which ionizable groups are attached and which has the property of being able to exchange its labile ions for ions present in the solution with which it is in contact. There are two types of ion-exchange resins: *anion-exchange resins*, in which the ionizable group is basic; and *cation exchange resins*, in which the ionizable group is acidic. **Oleo-resin,** a solution of resin in volatile oil.

Resolution. The subsidence of inflammation. The degree to which detail can be distinguished visually.

Resonance. The sound produced on percussion over a part that can vibrate freely: e.g. the lungs. **Amphoric resonance,** the sound like blowing over the top of an empty bottle, that is produced on percussion over a pulmonary cavity. **Cracked-pot resonance,** the sound produced on percussion over a pulmonary cavity that communicates with a small bronchus. **Skodaic resonance,** the high-pitched sound produced on percussion over the relaxed lung immediately above a pleural effision. **Vocal resonance,** the sound heard on auscultation over the lungs as the individual speaks.

Resorcinol. B.P. 1968. $C_6H_6O_2$. A keratolytic.

Respiration. The act of breathing, whereby oxygen is taken into the lungs, and carbon dioxide is expelled. **Abdominal respiration,** breathing carried out predominantly by the abdominal muscles. **Artificial respiration,** respiration which is maintained by artificial means in the absence of natural breathing. **Cheyne-Stokes respiration,** respiration which waxes and wanes, with alternating periods of apnoea and deep breathing. **Cogwheel respiration,** jerky or interrupted respiration. **Paradoxical respiration,** deflation of the lung during inspiration, and inflation of the lung during expiration.

Respirator. An apparatus for maintaining respiration, as in patients with paralysed muscles of respiration.

Restiform. Rope-like. Corded.

Retching. Ineffective movements of vomiting.

Rete. A mesh or network. (*Plural: retia.*) **Rete testis,** the network of anastomosing tubes that connect the straight seminiferous tubules with the efferent ductules.

Reticular. Resembling a net.

Reticulin. Bundles of collagen fibrils which form a network in many organs.

Reticulocyte. The earliest non-nucleated red blood cell.

Reticulocytosis. The presence of an excessive number of reticulocytes in the circulating blood.

Reticulo-endothelial. Pertaining to tissues which have both reticular and endothelial attributes.

Reticulo-endotheliosis. A condition in which the reticulo-endothelial cells become filled with metabolites of a lipid nature.

Reticulum. A network. (*Plural: reticula.*) **Endoplasmic reticulum,** a reticulum of membranous structure scattered throughout the cytoplasm. **Lymphatic reticulum,** the meshwork of reticular tissue in the lymph nodes. **Sarcoplasmic reticulum,** the reticular tissue in muscle tissue closely associated with the sarcolemma.

Retiform. Resembling a network.

Retina. The inner nervous coat of the eye, which is specially adapted for the reception of light stimuli.

Retinaculum. A retaining band. An instrument for holding back tissues during an operation. (*Plural:* retinacula.) **Retinacula of the ankle:** *Inferior extensor retinaculum,* a y-shaped band placed in front of the talocrural joint. *Superior extensor retinaculum,* a band stretching from the anterior border of the fibula to the anterior border of the tibia. *Flexor retinaculum,* a band stretching from the tibial malleolus to the calcaneus. **Retinacula of the hip joint,** longitudinal bands in the fibrous capsule of the joint. **Patellar retinacula, lateral and medial,** expansions from the vastus medialis and vastus lateralis, which are attached to the margins of the patella and the ligamentum patellae and extend to the corresponding collateral ligament and the tibial condyles. **Peroneal retinacula,** two fibrous bands (*inferior* and *superior*) that retain the tendons of the peroneus longus and brevis in position as they cross the lateral side of the ankle. **Retinacula of the wrist:** *Extensor retinaculum* a strong fibrous band that extends across the back of the wrist. *Flexor retinaculum,* a strong fibrous band that crosses the front of the carpus.

Retinal. Vitamin A aldehyde. A prosthetic in the retinal pigment rhodopsin or visual purple. Pertaining to the retina.

Retinitis. Inflammation of the retina. **Photo-retinitis,** retinitis induced by exposure to bright sunlight: e.g. looking at an eclipse of the sun with inadequately protected eyes. **Retinitis pigmentosa,** a degenerative disease of the retina, which is bilateral, begins in childhood, and often results in blindness.

Retino- (L *rete:* net). Prefix signifying relationship to the retina.

Retinoblastoma. A developmental tumour of the retina which appears in infancy, and which metastasizes unless enucleated promptly.

Retinol. One of the two forms of vitamin A. Vitamin A alcohol.

Retinopathy. Degenerative disease of the retina.

Retinoscope. The instrument used in retinoscopy.

Retinoscopy. The method of determining the refraction of the eye by observation of the movements of the shadow produced when a light is projected into the retina. Skiascopy. The shadow test.

Retractor. An instrument for holding back the edges of an operating wound.

Retro- (L *retro:* backward). Prefix meaning backward or behind.

Retrobulbar. Behind the eyeball. Behind the medulla oblongata. **Retrobulbar neuritis,** inflammation of the optic nerve proximal to the retina.

Retrocaecal. Situated behind the caecum.

Retrocedent. Moving backwards. Plunging inwards.

Retroflexion. Backward bending.

Retrograde. Moving backwards.

Retrolental. Behind the lens of the eye. **Retrolental fibroplasia,** a condition characterized by proliferation of the retinal blood vessels into the vitreous with excess formation of fibrous tissue and blindness, induced in new-born infants by oxygen poisoning.

Retroperitoneal. Behind the peritoneum.

Retropulsion. Involuntary act of running which occurs in patients with parkinsonism. Pushing back.

Retrosternal. Behind the sternum.

Retroversion. Bending backwards of an organ.

Rhabditoidea. The superfamily of the class Phasmidia that includes the genus Strongyloides.

Rhabdo- (Gk *rhabdos:* rod). Prefix indicating relationship to a rod, or rod-shaped.

Rhabdomyolysis. Dissolution or disintegration of muscle accompanied by myoglobinuria.

Rhabdomyoma. A tumour of striated muscle.

Rhabdomyosarcoma. A highly malignant tumour in children due to neoplastic proliferation of mesenchymal connective tissue.

Rhabdophobia. Morbid fear of the rod and of being punished.

Rhagades. Fissures or cracks at mucocutaneous junctions.

-rhaphy (Gk *rhaphē:* seam). Suffix meaning joining in a seam or junction.

-rhea (Gk *rhein:* to flow). Suffix signifying a flux or flow.

Rhenium. A metallic element of the platinum group. Symbol Re. Atomic weight 186·22. Atomic number 75.

Rheo- (Gk *rheos:* current). Prefix signifying relationship to an electric current, or flow.

Rheobase. The minimal amount of electric current that will produce a response.

Rheology. The study of the flow of liquids.

Rhesus. A species of Catarrhine monkey of the genus Macaca. **Rhesus factor,** *see* Factor.

Rheumatic. Pertaining to rheumatism. **Rheumatic fever,** acute rheumatism.

Rheumatism. A generic term used to describe pain of unknown origin affecting the connective and muscular tissues and joints. **Acute rheumatism,** an acute illness of unknown etiology. characterized by pyrexia and flitting joint pains, and liable to lead to involvement of the heart. Predominantly a disease of childhood and adolescence.

Rheumatoid. Resembling rheumatism. **Rheumatoid arthritis,** *see* Arthritis.

Rheumatology. The study of rheumatic diseases.

Rhexis. Rupture of an organ or vessel.

Rhin-, Rhino- (Gk *rhis:* nose). Prefixes signifying relationship to the nose.

Rhinencephalon. Those portions of the cerebrum concerned with the reception and conduction of olfactory impressions: the olfactory bulb, the olfactory tract, the anterior perforated substance, the amygdaloid body, the piriform area, the hippocampal formation, the paraterminal gyrus, the fornix, and the habenular gyrus.

Rhinitis. Inflammation of the nasal mucous membrane.

Rhinolith. A nasal calculus.

Rhinologist. A specialist in diseases of the nose.

Rhinomycosis. A fungal infection of the nasal mucous membrane.

Rhinophyma. A form of rosacea characterized by gross hypertrophy of the sebaceous glands of the nose. Cauliflower nose.

Rhinoplasty. Plastic repair of the nose.

Rhinorrhoea. A profuse watery nasal discharge.

Rhinoscleroma. A disease characterized by a hard infiltration of the mucous membrane of the upper air passages, with secondary invasion of the lips and nose and accompanying great disfigurement. Respiratory scleroma.

Rhinoscopy. Examination of the nasal cavities.

Rhinosporidiosis. A chronic polypforming infection, with *Rhinosporidium seeberi,* of the nose, eyes, ears and larynx, and occasionally the genitalia and skin.

Rhinosporidium. A genus of fungi that has never been cultured. *Rhinosporidium seeberi,* the causative organism of rhinosporidiosis.

Rhinovirus. One of a group of viruses

responsible for many cases of the common cold.

Rhipicephalus sanguineus. The common dog tick which transmits the rickettsia of typhus in various parts of the world.

Rhiz-, Rhizo- (Gk *rhiza:* root). Prefixes signifying relationship to a root.

Rhizopoda. The class of protozoa that includes the genus Entamoeba.

Rhizopus. A species of filamentous fungi.

Rhizotomy. Surgical division of a nerve root.

Rhodium. A metallic element. Symbol Rh. Atomic weight 102·91. Atomic number 45.

Rhodo- (Gk *rhodon:* rose). Prefix meaning red.

Rhodopsin. The photo-sensitive purple pigment in the retinal rods, which is bleached by light. It is a conjugated protein. Visual purple.

Rhombencephalon. The medulla oblongata, pons and cerebellum. The hindbrain.

Rhomboid. Shaped like a rhomb: i.e. an oblique parallelogram.

Rhonchus. The coarse rattling sound heard on auscultation over a lung in which there is partial obstruction in the bronchi and bronchioles, as in bronchitis.

Rhubarb. B.P. 1968. The rhizome of *Rheum palmatum* L., deprived of most of its bark and dried. On account of the anthraquinone derivatives it contains it has a purgative action.

-rhysis (Gk *rhysis:* a flow). Suffix signifying flowing out.

Rhythm. Regular recurring movement or action. **Alpha rhythm,** the dominant rhythmic waves in the normal electroencephalogram, with an average frequency of 10 per second. **Beta rhythm,** low potential waves, with a frequency of 25 per second, in the electroencephalogram. **Gallop rhythm,** the triple cardiac rhythm heard on auscultation, and usually indicating advanced heart failure when accompanying a tachycardia. **Nodal rhythm,** heart rhythm initiated at the atrioventricular node. **Sinus rhythm,** the normal heart rhythm, initiated at the sinu-atrial node.

Rib. One of 12 pairs of elastic arches of bone, which are connected behind with the vertebral column. *True ribs* the first seven ribs, that are connected in front, via costal cartilages, with the sternum. *False ribs,* the remaining five ribs; the costal cartilages of the first three of these are connected with the cartilage of the rib immediately above.

Floating ribs, the last two ribs which are free at their anterior end.

Riboflavine. B.P. 1968. $C_{17}H_{20}N_4O_6$. A member of the vitamin B complex which may be obtained synthetically or by fermentation. It occurs as a water-soluble pigment in many foodstuffs such as milk, eggs, liver, malted barley and yeast. Lack of it results in angular stomatitis, glossitis and anogenital dermatitis. The recommended daily intake is 1·5 to 3mg. for adults and 0·6 to 1·8mg. for children. **Riboflavine phosphate (sodium salt),** B.P.C. 1968, Supplement 1971, $C_{17}H_{20}N_4O_9NaP,2H_2O$. A soluble compound of riboflavine used for the preparation of injections.

Ribonuclease. An enzyme that catalyses the hydrolysis of ribonucleic acid.

Ribonucleic acid. RNA. A nucleic acid present in all cells, mainly in the cytoplasm. **Messenger (mRNA),** the category of RNA which conveys genetic information from the cell nucleus to the protein-synthesizing centres in the cell. It accounts for about 1 per cent of the total RNA in the cell. **Ribosomal RNA,** the RNA found in ribosomes. It accounts for about 80 per cent of the total cell RNA. **Transfer (tRNA),** the category of RNA that functions as a carrier of activated amino-acids during protein synthesis.

Ribose. One of the pentose sugars found in nucleotides.

Ribosome. One of the small, round electron-dense particles, consisting of equal amounts of protein and RNA, in the cytoplasm of cell.

Ribovirus. One of the group of animal viruses which contain RNA as opposed to DNA.

Rice. The seed of *Oryza sativa*, one of the main sources of food in many parts of the world. **Rice diet,** a low-sodium diet used in patients with heart failure and/or hypertension. **Rice-water,** a diluent drink for invalids containing rice and sweetening or flavouring.

Ricin. A highly toxic protein present in castor-oil seeds.

Rickets. A disease principally of childhood, characterized by various deformities of bone resulting from softening of the bone due to lack of vitamin D. **Renal rickets,** rickets induced by renal dysfunction.

Rickettsia. A genus of the order Rickettsiales, which biologically is intermediate between the smaller bacteria and the larger viruses. The members of the genus are visible by the light microscope, divide by binary fission and are obligate intracellular parasites.

Rickettsia. An organism belonging to the genus Rickettsia. (*Plural:* rickettsiae.)

Rickettsiales. An order of the class Microtatobiotes. Individual organisms in the order are over 0·2*u* in diameter.

Rickettsialpox. A mild disease with a chickenpox-like eruption, caused by *Rickettsia akari*, which is conveyed to man from the mouse by the mouse mite. It occurs in U.S.A., U.S.S.R., and West and South Africa.

Ridge. A crest. A linear elevation. **Alveolar ridge,** the ridge left on the alveolar border of the mandible which has been rendered edentulous. **Germ ridge,** the projection into the coelomic cavity, from which the gonads arise. **Interureteric ridge,** the ridge in the bladder that connects the two ureteric orifices. **Supracondylar ridge, lateral,** the lower end of the lateral border of the humerus. **Supracondylar ridge, medial,** the lower end of the medial border of the humerus.

Rifamide. The B.P. Commission approved name for rifamycin B diethylamide, one of the antibiotics derived from *Streptomyces mediterranei*. It is active mainly against gram-positive micro-organisms.

Rifampicin. The B.P. Commission approved name for an orally active derivative of rifamycin used in the treatment of tuberculosis.

Rifamycin. The B.P. Commission approved name for antibiotics derived from *Streptomyces mediterranei*, which are active against a wide range of micro-organisms.

Rift Valley fever. A virus infection of sheep in Africa, which may be acquired by farmers and veterinarians.

Rigidity. Stiffness. Inflexibility. **Cadaveric rigidity,** rigor mortis. **Cerebellar rigidity,** rigidity of the spinal muscles resulting from a lesion of the middle lobe of the cerebellum. **Clasp-knife rigidity,** the stiffness of the muscles in spastic paralysis, which suddenly gives way. **Cog-wheel rigidity,** the jerky movement of the muscles in parkinsonism. **Decerebrate rigidity,** the rigidity of the muscles induced by transection of the brain stem between the red nucleus and the lateral vestibular nucleus.

Rigor. A shivering fit. Rigidity. **Rigor**

mortis, the gradual stiffening of the muscle tissue that occurs after death.

Rima. A slit or cleft. (*Plural:* rimae.) **Rima glottidis,** the fissure between the vocal folds. **Rima vestibuli,** the fissure between the vestibular folds of the larynx.

Rimose. Marked by many cracks and fissures.

Rinderpest. An acute, highly infectious viral disease of ruminants and swine, endemic in Africa and Asia.

Ring. A circular structure. **Anorectal ring,** the ring of muscle at the anorectal junction. **Atrioventricular rings,** the fibrous ring surrounding the atrioventricular orifices. **Ciliary ring,** the part of the ciliary body continuous with the choroid. **Femoral ring,** the base of the femoral canal. **Fibrocartilaginous ring,** the thickened circumference of the tympanic membrane. **Fibrous rings,** the rings surrounding the atrioventricular and arterial orifices of the heart. **Inguinal ring, deep,** the opening in the transversalis fascia, midway between the anterior superior iliac spine and the symphysis pubis that transmits the spermatic cord in the male and the round ligament of the uterus in the female. **Inguinal ring, superficial,** an interval in the aponeurosis of the external oblique muscle just above and lateral to the crest of the pubis, that transmits the spermatic cord in the male and the round ligament of the uterus in the female. **Retraction ring,** the palpable furrow that forms in the lower segment of the uterus in obstructed labour. **Scleral ring,** the narrow white ring round the optic disc seen in many old people. **Tendinous ring, common,** a fibrous ring surrounding the upper, medial and lower margins of the optic canal, from which the four recti muscles arise **Terminal ring,** the junction of the body and the tail in the spermatozoon. **Tracheal ring,** tracheal cartilage.

Ringworm. Infection with three related dermatophytic fungi: Microsporum, Tricophyton, and Epidermophyton. Tinea.

Ristocetin. The B.P. Commission approved name for antibiotics derived from *Nocardia lurida*, which are active against gram-positive micro-organisms.

Risus. A laugh. **Risus sardonicus,** the grinning distortion of the facial muscles that occurs in tetanus.

Riziform. Resembling grains of rice.

Rocky Mountain spotted fever. A disease caused by *Rickettsia rickettsii*, which is transmitted by the tick *Dermacentor andersoni*, and occurs in the Rocky Mountains and in South America. The characteristic rash is morbilliform in type.

Rod. A thin slender structure. **Rods of Corti,** two rows of rod-like bodies (the *inner* and *outer* rods of Corti) in the spiral organ of the cochlea. **Retinal rods,** rhodopsin-containing cells in the retina, constituting with the cones the light-sensitive elements in the retina.

Roentgen. The unit of exposure dose of x- or gamma-radiation, being that quantity of x- or gamma-radiation such that the associated corpuscular emission per 0·001293 gramme of air produces, in air, ions carrying 1 electrostatic unit of electricity of either sign. Symbol R.

Roentgenology. The branch of radiology concerned with the use of x-rays in diagnosis and treatment.

Rolitetracycline. The B.P. Commission approved name for an antibiotic.

Rombergism. The inability to stand steadily with the eyes closed, the result of loss of sensory inflow as in tabes dorsalis.

Rongeur. A bone-gouging forceps.

Rosacea. A condition characterized by congestive erythema over the forehead, nose, cheeks and shin, dependent upon changes in the bloodvessels of the skin.

Rose. A plant or flower of the species *Rosa*. **Attar of rose,** the volatile oil obtained by distilling the fresh flowers of *Rosa damascena*. **Rose water,** a preparation obtained by soaking rose petals in water and distilling over part of the fluid.

Rosemary oil. B.P.C. 1968. The oil obtained by distillation from the flowering tops or leafy twigs of *Rosmarinus officinalis*. It is used: (*a*) as a carminative; (*b*) as a rubefacient; (*c*) as a food seasoner and perfumery agent.

Roseola. A rose-coloured eruption.

Rosin. Colophony.

Rostellum. The anterior, hook-bearing portion of the head of a tapeworm. (*Plural:* rostella.)

Rostral. Cephalic or cephalad: e.g. the mid-brain is rostral to the medulla oblongata. Pertaining to a rostrum.

Rostrum. A beak, projection or ridge. (*Plural:* rostra.) **Rostrum of the corpus callosum,** the anterior end of the corpus callosum. **Rostrum of the sphenoid bone,** the prominent ridge on the inferior surface of the sphenoid bone.

Rotenone. $C_{23}H_{22}O_6$. An insecticide derived from derris root. It has also been used in the treatment of scabies.

Roughage. The insoluble indigestible material in food, which promotes peristaltic action.

Rouleaux. A heap, or roll, of erythrocytes, as seen in shed blood. (*Plural:* rouleaux.)

Roundworm. Ascaris.

-rrhage-, -rrhagia (Gk *rhegnynai:* to burst forth). Suffixes signifying excessive flow or discharge.

-rrhaphy (Gk *rhaphē:* suture). Suffix meaning suturing.

-rrhoea (Gk *rhoia:* flow). Suffix signifying flow or discharge.

Rubedo. Flushing of the skin. Blushing.

Rubefacient. Causing redness of the skin. An agent that reddens the skin.

Rubella. German measles. A mild infectious disease, due to a virus, with a characteristic rash. Its main hazard is that the virus can spread to the foetus, if a pregnant mother becomes infected, and cause foetal deformity. **Rubella vaccine (live attenuated).** B.P. Addendum 1971, an aqueous suspension of a suitable live attenuated strain of rubella virus grown in suitable cell cultures.

Rubidium. An alkaline element. Symbol Rb. Atomic weight 85·48. Atomic number 37.

Rubor. Redness.

Rubrospinal. Pertaining to the red nucleus and the spinal cord.

Rufocromomycin. The B.P. Commission approved name for an antibiotic produced by *Streptomyces rufochromogenus*.

Ruga. A ridge. (*Plural*: rugae.) Rugae are found in the bladder, stomach and vagina, and on the scrotum.

Rugose. Marked by rugae. Wrinkled.

Rum. A spirit distilled from the fermented juice of molasses.

Rumen. The first stomach of a ruminant.

Rumination. Chewing the cud physically or metaphorically.

Rump. The buttocks.

Rupia. An encrusted eruption occurring sometimes in syphilis.

Rupture. A break in continuity. Hernia.

Ruthenium. A rare metal of the platinium group. Symbol Ru. Atomic weight 101·1. Atomic number 44.

Rye. The grain of *Secale cereale*. One of the major bread foodstuffs of mankind.

S

Sac. A pouch. **Aortic sac,** the mammalian homologue of the ventral aorta, from which the aortic arches arise. **Hernial sac,** the peritoneal covering of a hernia. **Lacrimal sac,** the upper blind end of the naso-lacrimal duct. **Peritoneal sac, greater,** the main portion of the peritoneal cavity. **Peritoneal sac, lesser,** the omental bursa. **Preputial sac,** the potential sac that separates the prepuce from the glans penis. **Yolk sac,** the vascular sac attached to the mid-gut of the embryo, constituting one of the foetal membranes.

Sacchar-, Saccharo- (L *saccharum:* sugar). Prefixes signifying relationship to sugar.

Saccharated. Containing sugar.

Saccharin. B.P. 1968. $C_7H_5NO_3S$. A sweetening agent and substitute for sugar. **Saccharin sodium,** B.P. 1968, $C_7H_4NNaO_3S,2H_2O$. A sweetening agent, which is used in preference to saccharin as it is more palatable. It is also used intravenously as a test for the determination of circulation time.

Saccharolytic. Capable of breaking down or splitting sugars.

Saccharomyces. A genus of budding fungi, or yeasts.

Saccharomycetaceae. A family of Astomycetales, the members of which are unicellular fungi.

Sacculation. The formation of a sac or pouch.

Saccule. The smaller of the two vestibular sacs in the membranous labyrinth of the inner ear.

Saccus. A sac. (*Plural:* sacci.) **Saccus endolymphaticus,** the blind pouch in which the ductus endolymphaticus of the inner ear ends.

Sacral. Pertaining to the sacrum.

Sacralization. Fusion of the sacrum to the 5th lumbar vertebra.

Sacro- (L *sacrum:* sacred). Prefix signifying relationship to the sacrum.

Sacrococcygeal. Pertaining to the sacrum and the coccyx.

Sacro-iliac. Pertaining to the sacrum and the ilieum.

Sacrum. A large triangular bone formed by fusion of the 5 sacral vertebrae, inserted like a wedge between the two hip bones, and situated at the upper and posterior part of the pelvic cavity.

Sadism. The form of sexual perversion in which pleasure is derived from inflicting cruelty on another.

Sadomasochism. The coexistence of sadism and masochism.

Saffron. The yellow powder derived from the dried stigmas and styles of *Crocus sativus,* which is used as a colouring agent in foodstuffs.

Sagittal. In an anteroposterior plane, parallel to the sagittal suture of the skull.

Sago. A starch derived mainly from the pith of the sago palms, and used as a foodstuff.

Sal. A salt or a substance resembling a salt. **Sal ammoniac,** ammonium chloride. **Sal volatile solution,** aromatic ammonia solution, B.P.C. 1968. **Sal volatile spirit,** aromatic ammonium spirit, B.P.C. 1968.

Salazosulphadimidine. The B.P. Commission approved name for 4'-(4,6-dimethylpyrimidin -2 -ylsulphamoyl) - 4 - hydroxyazobenzene - 3 - carboxylic acid. A sulphonamide.

Salbutamol. B.P. Addendum 1971. $C_{13}H_{21}NO_3$. A bronchodilator administered as an aerosol.

Salicin. A glucoside obtained from the bark of young shoots of various species of poplars and willows, which has analgesic and antipyretic properties.

Salicylamide. $C_7H_7NO_2$. An antipyretic and analgesic, with an action comparable to that of acetylsalicylic acid.

Salicylate. A salt of salicylic acid.

Salicylic acid. B.P. 1968. $C_7H_6O_3$. A keratolytic agent with bacteriostatic and fungicidal properties. **Salicylic acid ointment,** B.P. 1968, a preparation containing 2 per cent salicylic acid.

Salicylism. Poisoning by salicylic acid or a salicylate.

Salinazid. The B.P. Commission approved name for *N*-isonicotinoyl-*N'*-salicylidenehydrazine. An anti-tuberculous drug.

Saline. Salty. Containing sodium chloride. **Hypertonic saline,** a solution of sodium chloride exceeding 0·9 per cent in strength. **Normal saline,** a solution containing 0·9 gramme of sodium per 100ml. of water. Sodium chloride solution, B.P.C. 1968. **Saline mixture,** B.P.C. 1968, a mixture containing sodium citrate, sodium nitrite and strong ammonium acetate solution. **Saline purgatives,** purgatives such as magnesium sulphate (Epsom salts), which act by producing bulky fluid contents that distend the bowel. **Saline solution for injection, normal,** sodium chloride injection, B.P. 1968.

Saliva. The mixed secretion of the salivary glands.

Salivation. An excessive secretion of saliva.

Salmefamol. The B.P. Commission approved name for 1-(4-hydroxy-3-hydroxymethylphenyl)-2-(4-methoxy-α-methylphenethylamino) ethanol. A bronchodilator.

Salmine. A protamine present in the sperm of salmon.

Salmonella. A genus of the family Enterobacteriaceae, which contains more than 400 types. They are gram-negative, non-sporing bacilli. The most important members of the genus are *S. typhi,* the causative organism of typhoid fever, and *S. paratyphi* A, B, and C, the causative organisms of paratyphoid fever. Many of the other members of the genus are responsible for outbreaks of food poisoning.

Salpingectomy. Surgical excision of a uterine tube.

Salpingitis. Inflammation of a uterine tube.

Salpingo- (Gk *salpinx:* tube). Prefix signifying relationship to a tube, particularly the uterine tube and the auditory tube.

Salpingo-oöphorectomy. Surgical excision of a uterine tube and an ovary.

Salt. Sodium chloride. A compound formed by the interaction of an acid and a base. **Carlsbad salt,** a mixture of sodium sulphate, potassium sulphate, sodium chloride and sodium bicarbonate. **Common salt,** sodium chloride. **Epsom salts,** magnesium sulphate. **Glauber's salt,** sodium sulphate. **Rochelle salt,** sodium potassium tartrate.

Smelling salts, aromatized ammonium carbonate.

Saltpetre. Potassium nitrate.

Salve. Ointment.

Samarium. A metallic element. Symbol Sm. Atomic weight 150·35. Atomic number 62.

Sample. Specimen. **Random sample,** a selection so made that every individual in the population concerned has an equal and independent chance of appearing in the sample.

Sanatorium. An establishment for the treatment of sick individuals, more particularly those requiring prolonged treatment.

Sandfly. A term applied to several types of flies, but more particularly the genus Phlebotomus. **Sandfly fever,** a virus infection transmitted by the sandfly.

Sane. Of sound mind.

Sangui- (L. *sanguis:* blood). Prefix signifying relationship to blood.

Sanguine. Plethoric. Optimistic.

Sanguineous. Pertaining to blood. Plethoric.

Sanies. A thin, evil-smelling discharge from an ulcer or wound.

Sanitation. The science of maintaining a healthy environment.

Sanity. Soundness of mind.

Sap. The fluid part of a cell or a plant. **Nuclear sap,** the clear medium in a nucleus.

Saponification. Conversion into soap.

Sapr-, Sapro- (Gk *sapros:* rotten). Prefixes meaning rotting or decaying.

Sapraemia. Toxaemia resulting from the absorption into the circulation of the toxins of putrefaction, but not the actual micro-organisms.

Saprophyte. An organism that lives upon dead or dying organic matter.

Sarc-, Sarco- (Gk *sarx, sarkos:* flesh). Prefixes meaning flesh-like.

Sarcina. A genus of the family Micrococcaceae, which grows in packets of eight and occur widely as saprophytes in nature. (*Plural*: sarcinae.)

Sarcocystis. A genus of the family Sarcosporidia, which invades muscle tissue. *S. lindemanni,* the only member of the genus known to invade man— and then only rarely.

Sarcoid. Flesh-like. Pertaining to sarcoma. Pertaining to sarcoidosis.

Sarcoidosis. A systemic disease of unknown etiology, in which characteristic epithelioid-cell follicles are scattered throughout many organs.

Sarcolemma. The cell or plasma membrane of a muscle fibre.

Sarcoma. A malignant tumour of connective tissue. (*Plural:* sarcomata.)

Sarcomere. The fundamental contractile unit of a striped muscle fibril, being the section between two successive Z discs.

Sarcophaga. A genus of the sub-family Sarcophaginae, which occasionally causes myiasis.

Sarcophaginae. A subfamily of the family Calliphoridae, commonly known as 'flesh flies'.

Sarcoplasm. The semifluid matrix of a muscle fibre in which the other constituents are embedded.

Sarcoptes. A genus of Acarina. *Sarcoptes scabiei,* the causative mite of scabies.

Sarcosome. Mitochondrium.

Sarcosporidia. An order of Protozoa, which is parasitic in muscles.

Sarcostyle. Myofibril.

Saturnism. Chronic lead poisoning. Plumbism.

Satyriasis. Excessive sexual impulse in men.

Saucerization. The laying open of a wound so as to produce a shallow depression.

Scab. The crust that forms on superficial injured areas.

Scabicide. An agent or drug that is lethal to *Sarcoptes scabiei.*

Scabies. A highly contagious, itching infestation of the skin with *Sarcoptes scabiei.*

Scala. A staircase or spiral. (*Plural:* scalae.) **Scala tympani,** the perilymphatic passage in the cochlea below the osseous spiral lamina. **Scala vestibuli,** the perilymphatic passage in the cochlea above the osseous spiral lamina.

Scald. The burn caused by hot liquid or vapour.

Scale. An instrument for measuring. An agreed upon scheme of measuring. An aggregation of superficial epidermal cells. To remove superficial material from a surface, as in removing tartar from teeth.

Scalene. Having unequal sides. Pertaining to one of the scalenus muscles.

Scalenectomy. Surgical excision of a scalenus muscle.

Scalenotomy. Surgical division of the fibres of a scalenus muscle.

Scaler. An instrument for counting the impulses produced by detectors of radioactivity such as Geiger counters.

Scalp. The integument of the skull.

Scalpel. A pointed knife with a convex edge.

Scandium. A metallic element. Symbol Sc. Atomic weight 44·96. Atomic number 21.

Scanning. The determination of the activity of a given radioactive element by recording the emitted ray.

Scapho- (Gk *skaphē:* skiff). Prefix meaning boat-like.

Scaphocephaly. A cranial deformity characterized by a long narrow skull, with a ridge along the line of the saggital suture.

Scaphoid. The largest and most lateral bone in the proximal row of the carpus. Boat-shaped.

Scapula. The large, flattened, triangular bone on the posterolateral aspect of the chest wall, stretching from the 2nd to the 7th rib.

Scapulo- (L *scapulae:* the shoulder blades). Prefix indicating relationship to the scapula or shoulder.

Scapus. The shaft of hair extending beyond the surface of skin.

Scar. The mark left by a healed wound, ulcer or breach of tissue.

Scarification. The making of a number of superficial incisions in the skin.

Scarlatina. Scarlet fever. An acute infectious disease caused by strains of haemolytic streptococci and characterized by a typical rash.

Scarlet fever. Scarlatina.

Scato- (Gk *skūr skatos:* dung). Prefix indicating relationship to faeces.

Scatology. The study of faeces.

Schick test toxin. B.P. 1968. A sterile filtrate from a culture in nutrient broth of *Corynebacterium diphtheriae,* which is used as a reagent for the diagnosis of susceptibility to diphtheria. **Schick control,** B.P. 1968, Schick test toxin which has been heated at a temperature between 70° and 85°C for not less than five minutes.

Schindylesis. A joint where a ridge fits into a grooved surface. A wedge-and-groove suture.

-schisis (Gk *schisis:* cleavage). Suffix signifying a cleft, fissure, or split.

Schisto- (Gk *schistos:* cleft). Prefix signifying a cleft, fissure, or split.

Schistocephalus. A monster with a fissured skull.

Schistoglossia. A congenitally cleft tongue.

Schistomelia. 'A congenitally cleft limb.

Schistosoma. A genus of Trematodes, or blood flukes. *S. haematobium,* the species responsible for urinary schistosomiasis. *S. mansoni* and *S. japonicum,* the species responsible for intestinal schistosomiasis.

Schistosomiasis. A widespread disease in Africa, the Eastern Mediterranean, the Far East and part of the Americas, caused by infestation with those species of schistosomes that are transmitted by fresh-water snails. It may involve the urinary or the intestinal tract.

Schistosomicide. A drug that kills schistosomes.

Schiz-, Schizo- (Gk *schizein:* to divide). Prefixes meaning split or a division.

Schizogony. The process whereby the trophozoite of the malaria parasite becomes a schizont.

Schizoid. Resembling schizophrenia.

Schizomycetes. A class of unicellular organisms that multiply by fission, including the bacteria. It includes five orders: Pseudomonadales, Eubacteriales, Actinomycetales, Spirochaetales, Mycoplasmatales.

Schizont. The stage of development of the malaria parasite following the trophozoite.

Schizontocide. A drug that kills the malaria parasite at the schizont stage.

Schizophrenia. A psychosis characterized by disturbance in reality relationships and disintegration in the personality.

Sciage. A to-and-fro, sawing movement in massage.

Sciatica. Pain in the distribution of the sciatic nerve.

Scinti- (L *scintilla:* spark). Prefix meaning a spark.

Scintigram. A record of the distribution of radioactivity in the tissues.

Scintillascope. An instrument for observing the scintillations produced by radioactive emanations. A scintillation counter.

Scintillation. Emission of sparks.

Scintiscan. A record of the gamma rays emitted by a radio-isotope.

Scirrho- (Gk *skirrhos:* hard). Prefix meaning hard.

Scirrhous. Relating to a scirrhus. Hard or indurated.

Scirrhus. A hard cancer due to infiltration with fibrous tissue.

Scissura. A cleft or fissure. (*Plural:* scissurae).

Scler-, Sclero- (Gk *skeleros:* hard). Prefixes meaning hard, or relationship to the sclera.

Sclera. The firm fibrous posterior coat of the eyeball.

Sclerectomy. Surgical excision of the sclera or part of it.

Scleredema. Oedematous thickening of the skin.

Sclerema. Thickening of the skin. **Sclerema neonatorum,** a generalized thickening of the skin, which is cold and livid, in the newborn.

Scleritis. Inflammation of the sclera.

Sclerodactyly. Scleroderma of the fingers.

Scleroderma. Thickening of the skin. It takes three forms: **Lichen sclerosus et atrophicus,** in which the changes take place immediately below the epidermis. **Morphoea,** in which the whole dermis is affected. Localized scleroderma. **Systemic sclerosis,** in which there is widespread involvement of the skin as well as of various organs. Generalized scleroderma.

Scleroma. A hardened patch or induration.

Scleromalacia. Degeneration or softening of the sclera.

Scleronychia. Thickness and dryness of the nails.

Sclerosis. Induration or hardening. **Amyotrophic lateral sclerosis,** a form of motor neurone disease characterized by wasting in the upper limbs and spasticity in the lower limbs. **Diffuse sclerosis,** a group of progressive diseases characterized by widespread demyelination of the white matter of the cerebral hemispheres, accompanied by blindness, mental deterioration and spastic paralysis. **Disseminated sclerosis,** multiple sclerosis. **Multiple sclerosis,** a disease of unknown etiology, characterized by spastic paralysis, intention tremor, nystagmus, difficulty in micturition and emotional instability, due to a demyelinating process in the central nervous system. **Primary lateral sclerosis,** sclerosis of the lateral columns of the spinal cord. **Systemic sclerosis,** generalized scleroderma. **Tuberose sclerosis,** a hereditary condition characterized by multiple cutaneous tumours of face, mental defectiveness and epilepsy.

Sclerotic. Hard. Pertaining to the sclera. The sclera. **Blue sclerotics,** a hereditary condition characterized by a pronounced blue coloration of the sclera, associated often with fragilitas ossium and deafness.

Sclerotome. A knife for incising the sclera. The part of a somite that enters into the formation of a vertebra.

Sclerotomy. Surgical incision of the sclera.

Scolex. The head of a tapeworm.

Scolio- (Gk *skolios:* twisted). Prefix meaning twisted or crooked.

Scoliosis. Lateral curvature of the spine.

-scope (Gk *skopein:* to examine). Suffix denoting an instrument for seeing or examining.

Scopolamine. Hyoscine.

Scorbutic. Relating to scurvy.

Scoto- (Gk *skotos:* darkness). Prefix indicating relationship to darkness.

Scotoma. A blind or partially blind spot in the visual field. (*Plural:* scotomata.)

Scotometer. An instrument for plotting scotomata.

Scotophobia. Abnormal dread of the dark.

Scotopia. Night vision.

Scotopic. Pertaining to vision in the dark.

Scrofula. An old term for tuberculosis of the lymphatic glands.

Scrofuloderma. Tuberculosis of the skin secondary to tuberculosis of the underlying lymph nodes, joints or bones.

Scrotum. The cutaneous pouch, containing the testes and the lower part of the spermatic cords, placed below the symphysis pubis and in front of the upper parts of the thighs.

Scruple. An apothecaries' weight of 20 grains.

Scurf. Dandruff.

Scurvy. A deficiency disease due to lack of ascorbic acid (vitamin C), and characterized by extravasations of blood in various parts of the body, particularly the skin and gums.

Scybalum. A mass of hard, inspissated faeces. (*Plural:* scybala.)

Seasickness. Nausea and/or vomiting induced by the movement of a ship at sea.

Sebaceous. Pertaining to sebum.

Seborrhoea. A disturbance of the skin caused by overaction of the sebaceous glands.

Sebum. The secretion of the sebaceous glands.

Secbutobarbitone. The B.P. Commission approved name for 5-ethyl-5-s-butylbarbituric acid. A hypnotic and sedative.

Secretagogue. Stimulating secretion. A substance that stimulates secretion.

Secretin. A hormone secreted by the duodenum when stimulated by chyme, which stimulates the production of pancreatic juice.

Secretinase. An enzyme that destroys secretin.

Secretion. The substance produced by a gland. The process whereby glands produce their products.

Secretor. An individual in whom the blood group factors are found, not only in erythrocytes, but also in all tissue fluids and secretions, including saliva.

Section. The act of cutting. A cutting or slice. **Caesarean section,** delivery of a foetus by surgical division of the uterus. **Frozen section,** a section cut from a frozen specimen. **Serial section,** one of a series of consecutive histological sections.

Secundi- (L *secundus:* second). Prefix meaning second.

Secundigravida. A woman pregnant for the second time.

Secundines. The afterbirth.

Secundipara. A woman who has had two children, not twins.

Sedative. A drug or agent that quietens the nervous system and helps to induce sleep.

Segment. A section or subdivision. **Bronchopulmonary segments,** the self-contained, functionally independent units of lung tissue. **Internodal segment,** the length of a nerve between two nodes of Ranvier. **Medullary segments,** irregular portions of nerve produced by incisures or funnel-shaped clefts. **Primitive segment of the embryo,** metamere. **Spinal segment,** the portion of the spinal cord to which a pair of nerves is attached. **Splenic segment,** the portion of the spleen supplied by one of the hilar branches of the splenic artery. **Uterine segment, lower,** the thinned-out lower portion of the uterus in pregnancy. **Uterine segment, upper,** the upper active section of the gravid uterus.

Selenium. A metallic element. Symbol Se. Atomic weight 78·96. Atomic number 34.

Selenium sulphide. B.P.C. 1968, Supplement 1971. SeS_2. A local application for the management of dandruff and seborrhoeic dermatitis of the scalp.

Sella turcica. The saddle-shaped hollow on the upper surface of the sphenoid bone which houses the hypophysis.

Semantics. The study of the meaning of words and symbols.

Semeiology. Symptomatology.

Semen. The thick whitish fluid carrying the spermatozoa.

Semi- (L *semis:* half). Prefix meaning one-half.

Semilunar. Crescentic.

Seminiferous. Producing or carrying semen.

Seminoma. The most common testicular cancer, derived from the seminiferous epithelium.

Semipermeable. Permeable to some molecules, but not to others.

Semolina. A preparation of wheat.

Senega. B.P.C. 1968. The dried root-stock and root of *Polygala senega* or *P. senega* var. *latifolia*. It is used, usually along with other expectorants, in the alleviation of the cough in chronic bronchitis.

Senescence. The state of growing old.

Senile. Pertaining to old age.

Senna fruit. B.P. 1968. The dried ripe fruits of *Cassia senna* (Alexandrian senna) and *C. angustifolia* (Tinnevelly senna pods). It is an anthraquinone purgative, now prescribed as an infusion. **Senna leaf,** B.P.C. 1968, the dried leaflets of the paripinnate leaves of *Cassia senna* and *C. angustifolia*. It has the same properties as senna fruit. **Senna tablets,** B.P. Addendum 1971, tablets containing the powdered pericarp of senna fruit.

Sensation. The feeling or impression created by stimulation of an afferent nerve. **Epicritic sensation,** the fine, discriminative type of cutaneous sensation. **Painful sensation,** the unpleasant sensation elicited by stimulation of specific end-organs. **Protopathic sensation,** the cruder variety of cutaneous sensation. **Tactile sensation,** the sensation induced by stimulation of the tactile corpuscles. **Thermal sensation,** the sensation of heat or cold induced by stimulation of specific end-organs.

Sense. The faculty of perceiving a stimulus.

Sensibility. The ability to appreciate sensation. **Cutaneous sensibility,** a sensation arising in the skin. **Deep sensibility,** sensation in the muscles, joints, tendons and deeper layers of the skin. **Exteroceptive sensibility,** sensation initiated on the surface of the body. **Gustatory sensibility,** sensation of taste. **Interoceptive sensibility,** sensations arising in the viscera. **Olfactory sensibility,** the sensation of smell. **Proprioceptive sensibility,** sensations arising from the muscles, tendons and joints.

Sensitization. The rendering of an individual, or bacteria, sensitive to a drug, protein or some other substance. Anaphylaxis.

Sensory. Pertaining to sensation.

Sensual. Pertaining to the bodily passions.

Sentient. Capable of feeling.

Sepsis. The condition characterized by the presence of micro-organisms.

Sept-, Septi- (L *septum:* seven). Prefixes signifying seven.

Septate. Possessing a septum.

Septic. Related to, or produced by, sepsis.

Septicaemia. The condition characterized by the presence of micro-organisms in the blood stream.

Septum. A partition or thin wall. (*Plural:* septa.) **Aortopulmonary septum, spiral,** the septum that divides the truncus arteriosus into the ascending aorta and the pulmonary trunk. **Atrioventricular septum,** the posterior part of the ventricular septum, that intervenes between the aortic vestibule of the left ventricle and the right atrium. **Bulbar septum, distal,** the septum that later becomes the semilunar valves. **Bulbar septum, proximal,** the septum that separates the bulbus cordis into pulmonary and aortic channels. **Femoral septum,** the condensed portion of extraperitoneal tissue that closes the femoral ring. **Interatrial septum,** the septum that separates the two atria. **Intermuscular septa,** the septa of fascia that separate adjacent groups of muscles. **Intermuscular septa, anterior and posterior crural,** septa of the fascia cruris on the lateral side of the leg, that are attached to the anterior and posterior borders of the fibula. **Nasal septum,** the cartilaginous, membranous and bony partition between the two nasal cavities. **Orbital septum,** a weak membranous sheet attached to the edge of the orbit where it is continuous with the periosteum. **Palmar septum, intermediate,** the septum between the flexor tendons of the index finger and the 2nd lumbrical muscle. **Palmar septum, lateral,** the septum that passes dorsally from the lateral border of the palmar aponeurosis to the palmar surface of the 1st metacarpal bone. **Palmar septum, medial,** the septum that passes dorsally from the medial border of the palmar aponeurosis to the palmar surface of the 5th metacarpal bone. **Septum pellucidum,** a thin vertical partition, consisting of two laminae separated by a cavity, that separates the two anterior horns of the lateral ventricles of the brain. **Septum of the scrotum,** the septum that divides the scrotal pouch into two cavities for the testes. **Spinal cord, posterior median septum of,** a septum of neuroglia that reaches more than half-way into the substance of the spinal cord from the posterior median sulcus. **Subarachnoid septum,** an interrupted sheet of fibrous tissue that connects the arachnoid to the pia mater opposite the posterior median sulcus. **Septum of tongue,** a median fibrous partition that extends throughout the length of the tongue. **Septum transversum,** the embryonic predecessor of the central tendon of the diaphragm and the connective tissue of the liver. **Urorectal septum,** the partition dividing the cloaca into a dorsal segment or rectum, and a ventral segment or urogenital sinus. **Ventricular septum,** the partition between the two ventricles of the heart.

Septuplet. One of seven offspring of a single gestation.

Sequel. A morbid consequence of a disease. (*Plural:* sequelae.)

Sequestration. The formation of a sequestrum. Isolation.

Sequestrum. A portion of dead or necrosed bone that has been separated from the surrounding healthy bone. (*Plural:* sequestra.)

Ser-, Sero- (L *serum:* whey). Prefixes indicating association with serum, or of a watery consistency.

Serofibrinous. Consisting of serum and fibrin.

Serology. The study of serum, with particular reference to immunity reactions.

Seropus. A mixture of serum and pus.

Serosa. A serous membrane.

Serosanguineous. Consisting of serum and blood.

Serositis. Inflammation of a serous membrane.

Serotherapy. The treatment of disease by the injection of specific serum or antitoxin.

Serotonin. 5-Hydroxytryptamine. A vasoconstrictor substance present in blood and derived from the enterochromaffin cells of the gastrointestinal tract.

Serotype. A type of micro-organism as defined by its antigenic reactions.

Serous. Pertaining to serum.

Serpiginous. Spreading in a creeping manner.

Serrated. Having a saw-like edge.

Serratus. Serrated.

Serum. The supernatant yellow fluid that forms when blood clots. (*Plural:* sera.)

Serum agar, a culture medium for bacteria consisting of 10 per cent animal serum in nutrient agar. **Serum albumin,** the major protein in blood (concentration of 4 to 5 grammes per cent). **Serum anaphylaxis,** the acute reaction of severe shock following the injection of serum into a sensitized individual. **Antibacterial serum,** a specially prepared serum containing substances that have a specific prophylactic or therapeutic action when injected into persons exposed to, or suffering from, a disease due to a prescribed bacterium that does not produce an exotoxin. There is one B.P. antibacterial serum: *Leptospira antiserum.* **Antilymphocyte serum,** a specially prepared serum which destroys lymphocytes, and is used as part of the immunosuppressive procedure in organ transplantation. **Antitoxic serum,** a specially prepared serum containing antitoxin that has a specific prophylactic or therapeutic action when injected into persons exposed to, or suffering from, a disease due to a prescribed toxin. There are 10 B.P. antitoxic sera: *Botulinum antitoxin*; *diphtheria antitoxin*; *gas-gangrene antitoxin* (*oedemtiens*); *gas-gangrene antitoxin* (*septicum*); *gas-gangrene antitoxin* (*welchii*); *mixed gas-gangrene antitoxin*; *scorpion venom antiserum*; *snake venom antiserum*; *staphylococcus antitoxin*; *tetanus antitoxin.* **Antiviral serum,** with the exception of rabies antiserum, a serum obtained from human convalescents who have recovered from a virus disease, which contains antibodies to the virus in question. There is one B.P. viral antiserum: *Rabies antiserum.* **Dried human serum,** B.P. 1968, a serum prepared by drying the pool of fluids separated from blood withdrawn from human subjects and allowed to clot in the absence of any anticoagulant. **Native serum,** natural serum as it is obtained from the blood of immunized animals before it has undergone any process of concentration or purification. **Serum globulin,** one of the plasma proteins (concentration of 2 to 3 grammes per cent). **Serum hepatitis,** the form of hepatitis in which the responsible virus is acquired from contaminated blood. **Iodinated (^{125}I) human serum albumin injection,** B.P. Addendum 1971, a sterile solution of human serum albumin which has been iodinated with iodine-125 and subsequently freed from iodide. It is used for various diagnostic procedures. **Iodinated (¹³¹I) human serum albumin injection,** B.P. 1968, a sterile solution of human serum albumin which has been iodinated with iodine-131 and subsequently freed from iodide. It is used for diagnostic and investigative purposes. **Serum reaction,** a reaction that occurs in a sensitized person following the injection of serum. **Serum sickness,** a syndrome of rash, pyrexia and joint pains occurring in a sensitized person following the injection of serum.

Sesame oil. B.P. 1968. The fixed oil expressed from the seeds of *Sesamum indicum.* It is used instead of olive oil in the preparation of liniments, plasters, ointments and soaps.

Sesamoid. Resembling a grain of sesame. **Sesamoid bone,** a rounded nodule of bone embedded in certain tendons, and usually related to articular surfaces.

Sesqui- (L *sesqui:* a half more). Prefix meaning one-and-a-half.

Sessile. Attached by a broad base.

Seton. A few strands or threads drawn through a skin wound to establish a fistula.

Sewage. Solid and liquid human excreta, waste water from dwelling-houses, trade wastes, surface or rain water, road washings.

Sex. The sum of those differences that distinguish male from female.

Sexology. The study of sex.

Sexti-, Sextu- (L *sextus:* six). Prefixes signifying six.

Sextigravida. A woman who is pregnant for the sixth time.

Sextipara. A woman who has given birth to six children in the same number of labours.

Sextuplet. One of six children resulting from one pregnancy.

Sheath. An enveloping structure. **Axillary sheath,** the fibrous sheath continuous above with the prevertebral layer of the deep cervical fascia that surrounds the front part of the axillary artery, the axillary vein and the brachial plexus. **Carotid sheath,** a condensation of the cervical fascia in which are embedded the common and internal carotid arteries, the internal jugular vein, the vagus nerve and the ansa cervicalis. **Dentinal sheath,** the thin homogeneous membrane that separates the two layers of calcified dentine around the lumen of the dentinal tubule. **Femoral sheath,**

the prolongation downwards of the fascia lining the abdomen, which encloses the first 3 or 4cm. of the femoral artery together with femoral vein. **Synovial sheaths,** sheaths that occur where tendons pass under ligamentous bands or through fascial slings or osseofibrous canals.

Shellac. A resinous substance formed by the scale insect, *Laccifer lacca,* which is used as an enteric coating for pills.

Shigella. A genus of the family Enterobacteriaceae, the members of which are the causative organisms of bacillary dysentery: *Shigella dysenteriae* and *S. sonnei.* (*Plural:* shigellae.)

Shigellosis. An infection with a member of the genus Shigella.

Shin. The sharp crest on the upper part of the anterior border of the shaft of the tibia.

Shingles. Herpes zoster.

Shock. A condition in which the vital capacity is profoundly lowered, often as a result of severe injury, and characterized by cold clammy skin, pallor, rapid pulse, and low blood pressure.

Shoulder. The joint formed by the upper end of the humerus and the scapula. **Drop shoulder,** drooping of one shoulder. **Frozen shoulder,** a painful stiffness of the shoulder of unknown origin.

Shunt. An alternative route. A diversion. An anastomosis.

Sial-, Sialo- (Gk *sialon:* saliva). Prefixes signifying relationship to saliva.

Sialadenitis. Inflammation of a salivary gland.

Sialic. Salivary.

Sialogogue. A substance that produces a profuse flow of saliva.

Sialography. Radiological examination of the salivary glands after the injection of a radio-opaque substance.

Sialolith. A salivary calculus.

Sialorrhoea. An excessive flow of saliva. Ptyalism.

Sibilant. Whistling or hissing.

Sibling. A brother or sister. Sib.

Sickling. The production of sickle-shaped erythrocytes.

Sickness. Illness. Nausea. **Air sickness,** sickness and/or vomiting induced by air travel. **Car sickness,** sickness and/or vomiting, induced by travelling in a motor car. **Morning sickness,** the nausea and/or vomiting that occurs in the early months of pregnancy. **Motion sickness,** travel sickness.

Radiation sickness, the nausea and/or vomiting induced by irradiation. **Sea sickness,** the nausea and/or vomiting induced on board ship. **Serum sickness,** the syndrome induced by the injection of serum in a sensitized person. **Sleeping sickness,** African trypanosomiasis. **Sleepy sickness,** encephalitis lethargica. **Travel sickness,** the nausea and/or vomiting induced by any form of travel.

Side-effect. An effect produced by a drug, or some other form of therapy, in addition to the derived or expected effect.

Sideraemia. An excess of plasma iron.

Sidero- (Gk *sideros:* iron). Prefix signifying relationship with iron.

Sideroblast. A normoblast containing granules of haemosiderin.

Siderocyte. An erythrocyte containing siderotic granules.

Sideropenia. A deficiency of plasma iron.

Siderophilin. Transferrin.

Siderosis. A form of pneumoconiosis due to the inhalation of iron oxide.

Siderotic. Pertaining to siderosis.

Sight. Vision. **Long sight,** hypermetropia. **Near sight,** myopia. **Short sight,** myopia.

Sigmoid. S-shaped. Pertaining to the sigmoid colon.

Sigmoid-, Sigmoido- (Gk *sigmoeidēs:* shaped like the letter S). Prefixes signifying s-shaped or related to the sigmoid colon.

Sigmoidoscope. A speculum for viewing the sigmoid colon.

Sign. An objective manifestation of disease, as opposed to symptom, which is a subjective manifestation of disease.

Silica. Silicon dioxide. SiO_2. A hard compound widely spread in nature as quartz, flint and sand.

Silicate. A salt of silicic acid.

Silico- (L *silex, silicis:* flint). Prefix indicating relationship to flint.

Silicon. A non-metallic element. Symbol Si. Atomic weight 28·09. Atomic number 14. It does not occur free in nature, but as silica and silicates.

Silicones. Polymers with a structure consisting of alternate atoms of silicon and oxygen, with organic groups, such as methyl and phenyl, attached to the silicon atoms. They are widely used as water repellents, barrier creams and antifoaming agents.

Silicosis, The form of pneumoconiosis due to the inhalation of silica-containing dusts.

Silver. A soft malleable metallic element. Symbol Ag. (L *argentum.*) Atomic weight, 107·88. Atomic number 47.

Silver nitrate. B.P. 1968. $AgNO_3$. A caustic astringent and bactericidal agent. **Toughened silver nitrate,** B.P. 1968, a mould prepared by fusing together 95 parts of silver nitrate and 5 parts of potassium nitrate.

Silver protein. B.P.C. 1968. A preparation produced by the interaction of a silver compound and gelatin in the presence of an alkali. It has antibacterial properties. **Mild silver protein,** B.P.C. 1968, a preparation produced by the interaction of denatured serum albumin, casein or other suitable protein with moist silver oxide.

Simuliidae. A family of flies of the order Diptera, known variously as black flies and buffalo flies.

Simulium. A genus of flies of the family Simuliidae. *S. damnosum* is the vector to man of onchocerciasis.

Sinapsis. Mustard.

Sinew. Tendon.

Singultus. Hiccup.

Sinister. Left.

Sinistral. On the left side. Showing preference for the left side.

Sinistro- (L *sinister:* left). Prefix meaning left or associated with the left side.

Sino-, Sinu- (L *sinus:* fold, hollow). Prefixes indicating association with a sinus.

Sinu-atrial. Pertaining to the sinus venosus and the right atrium.

Sinus. A hollow, cavity or channel. A fistula. (*Plural:* sinuses.) **Anal sinuses,** the small recesses above the anal valves. **Aortic sinuses,** the three small dilatations opposite the cusps of the aortic valve. **Carotid sinus,** the dilatation in the common carotid artery at its point of division. **Cavernous sinus,** one of the various sinuses of the dura mater, lying on the side of the body of the sphenoid bone. **Circular sinus,** the venous circle formed by the intercavernous and the cavernous sinuses. **Coronary sinus,** the wide venous channel in the coronary sulcus, into which most of the veins of the heart open. **Sinuses of the dura mater,** venous channels between the two layers of the dura mater, which drain the blood from the brain. **Sinus of the epididymis,** a recess of the tunica vaginalis lying between the body of the epididymis and the lateral surface of the testis. **Ethmoidal**

sinuses, 3 to 18 thin-walled cavities in the ethmoidal labyrinth, which open into the nasal cavity. **External jugular sinus,** the dilated part of the external jugular vein between its two pairs of valves. **Frontal sinuses,** 2 cavities situated behind the superciliary arches, between the outer and inner tables of the frontal bone, which drain into the middle meatus of the nose. **Intercavernous sinuses** (an anterior and a posterior), venous sinuses of the dura mater that connect the cavernous sinuses across the median plane. **Lactiferous sinuses,** dilatations in the lactiferous ducts which serve as reservoirs for the milk. **Laryngeal sinus,** a fusiform recess lying between the vestibular and vocal folds. **Lymph sinuses,** irregular spaces within lymph nodes for the passage of lymph. **Maxillary sinus,** the largest of the accessory air sinuses of the nose, situated in the body of the maxilla. **Paranasal sinuses,** the ethmoidal, frontal, maxillary and sphenoidal sinuses. **Petrosal sinus, inferior,** one of the venous sinuses of the dura mater, that drains the corresponding cavernous sinus into the internal jugular vein. **Petrosal sinus, superior,** one of the venous sinuses of the dura mater that drains the corresponding cavernous sinus into the transverse sinus. **Prostatic sinus,** a shallow depression in the male urethra on each side of the urethral crest, the floor of which is perforated by the orifices of the prostatic ducts. **Renal sinus,** the central recess of the kidney. **Sagittal sinus, inferior,** one of the venous sinuses of the dura mater, in the free margin of the falx cerebri. **Sagittal sinus, superior,** one of the venous sinuses of the dura mater, situated in the convex margin of the falx cerebri. **Sigmoid sinus,** one of the venous sinuses of the dura mater, which is directly continuous with the corresponding transverse sinus. **Sphenoidal sinus,** one of a pair of paranasal sinuses, situated in the body of the sphenoid bone behind the upper part of the nasal cavity. **Sphenoparietal sinus,** one of a pair of venous sinuses of the dura mater, on the under-surface of the upper wing of the sphenoid bone. **Straight sinus,** one of the venous sinuses of the dura mater situated in the line of junction of the falx cerebri with the tentorium cerebelli. **Sinus tarsi,** a bony canal in the articulation of the calcaneus and the talus. **Tonsillar sinus,** the triangular recess between the palatoglossal and palatopharyngeal arches, containing the palatine tonsils. **Transverse sinus,** one of a pair of venous sinuses of the dura mater, lying in the attached margin of the tentorium cerebelli. **Tympanic sinus,** a depression in the median wall of the tympanic cavity which indicates the position of the ampulla of the posterior semicircular canal. **Sinus venarum,** the posterolateral part of the right atrium, into which the inferior and superior venae cavae open. **Sinus venosus sclerae,** a canal in the substance of the sclera. **Venous sinuses of the dura mater,** venous channels which drain the blood from the brain.

Sinusitis. Inflammation of a sinus.

Sinusoid. The type of terminal blood vessel found in the red bone marrow, heart, liver, suprarenal and parathyroid glands, and carotid and coccygeal bodies. It is wider than a capillary, with very thin walls which contain many phagocytic cells.

Sinusoidal. Pertaining to a sinusoid, or a certain form of electric current.

Siphon. A doubly bent tube with one arm longer than other, used for removing fluids from a cavity by means of atmospheric pressure.

Siphonage. The removal of fluids by means of a siphon, particularly from the stomach.

Siphunculina. A genus of flies of the suborder Cyclonapha, some species of which are responsible for outbreaks of conjunctivitis in the Far East.

-sis (Gk -*sis:* suffix signifying a state or condition). Suffix signifying a state or condition. It is usually preceded by a vowel: e.g. esis, osis.

Sito- (Gk *sitos:* food). Prefix signifying relationship to food.

Situs. Site or position. (*Plural:* situs.) **Situs inversus,** transposition of a viscera: e.g. the heart.

Skatole. A decomposition product of tryptophan, which gives the characteristic unpleasant smell to faeces.

Skeleton. The bony framework of the body.

Skew. Squint.

Skia- (Gk *skia:* shadow). Prefix indicating relationship to shadows, particularly in radiology.

Skiagram. A roentgenogram. An x-ray film.

Skin. The membranous covering of the body, made up of epidermis and corium.

Skull. The skeleton of the head, consisting of 22 bones.

Sleep. A periodic resting condition of the body, marked by relative unconsciousness.

Sling. A piece of material, or a bandage, for the suspension of a part—usually the arm.

Slough. A separating, or separated, mass of necrosed tissue.

Smallpox. An acute infectious, highly contagious disease, due to a specific virus, and characterized by a papular→vesicular→pustular eruption. The incubation period is 8 to 17 days. Variola.

Smegma. The sebum, with a characteristic odour, secreted by the external genitalia. *Mycobacterium smegmatis* (Smegma bacillus), a commensal organism found in smegma.

Smell. Odour. The sensation produced by the olfactory apparatus. To perceive by means of the olfactory apparatus.

Snare. A wire loop used to remove polypi or small pedunculated tumours.

Sneeze. A sudden, noisy expulsion of air through the nose, designed to remove irritating material from the upper air passages.

Snore. The noise produced by vibrations of the soft palate during sleep.

Snow. A crystalline precipitation of frozen aqueous vapour. **Carbon dioxide snow,** a spray of frozen carbon dioxide used in the treatment of certain skin conditions.

Snuff. A powder inhaled through the nose.

Snuffles. The noisy respiration in children induced by persisting nasal discharge interfering with breathing.

Soap. A salt formed from metals, or other base-forming compounds, and fatty acids containing eight or more carbon atoms. **Soft soap,** B.P. 1968, a preparation made by the interaction of potassium or sodium hydroxide with a suitable vegetable oil or oils or with fatty acids derived therefrom.

Socket. A hollow or depression into which another part fits.

Soda. An alkaline sodium salt. **Baking soda,** sodium bicarbonate. **Caustic soda,** sodium hydroxide. **Washing soda,** sodium carbonate. **Soda water,** water charged with carbon dioxide.

Soda lime. B.P. 1968. A mixture of sodium hydroxide, or sodium hydroxide and potassium hydroxide, with calcium hydroxide. It is used to absorb carbon dioxide in closed-circuit anaesthetic apparatus.

Sodium. An alkaline metallic element. Symbol Na. (*L natrium.*) Atomic weight 22·991. Atomic number 11.

Sodium acetate. B.P. 1968. $CH_3.CO_2Na$, $3H_2O$. A source of sodium ions in preparing solutions for haemodialysis and intraperitoneal dialysis.

Sodium acetrizoate injection. B.P. 1968. A sterile solution in water for injections B.P. of sodium acetrizoate $(C_9H_5I_3NNaO_3)$, a radio-opaque substance.

Sodium acid citrate. B.P. 1968. $C_6H_6Na_2O_7,1\frac{1}{2}H_2O$. An anticoagulant used to prevent the clotting of blood intended for transfusion.

Sodium acid phosphate. B.P. 1968. NaH_2PO_4, 2HO. A saline purgative.

Sodium alginate. B.P.C. 1968. A suspending and emulsifying agent.

Sodium aminosalicylate, B.P. 1968. $C_7H_6NNaO_3,2H_2O$. An anti-tuberculosis agent, only used in conjunction with streptomycin, or isoniazed, or both.

Sodium anoxynaphthonate. The B.P. Commission approved name for a blue or bluish-black dye used as a diagnostic agent in determining blood and plasma volumes.

Sodium antimonylgluconate. B.P. 1968. A trivalent antimony derivative used in the treatment of schistosomiasis.

Sodium apolate. The B.P. Commission approved name for poly(sodium ethylenesulphate). An anticoagulant.

Sodium aurothiomalate. B.P. 1968. A gold preparation used in the treatment of rheumatoid arthritis.

Sodium benzoate. B.P. 1968. $C_7H_5NaO_2$. A preservative and a urinary antiseptic, which is also used as the basis of a liver function test.

Sodium bicarbonate. B.P. 1968. $NaHCO_3$. An antacid. **Sodium bicarbonate Injection,** B.P. 1968, a sterile solution of 1·4 per cent w/v of sodium bicarbonate in water for injections, B.P. **Compound sodium bicarbonate tablets,** B.P. 1968, tablets each containing 300mg. of sodium bicarbonate and 0·03ml. of peppermint oil. Soda mint tablets.

Sodium bromide. B.P. 1968. $NaBr$. A sedative.

Sodium calciumedetate. B.P. 1968. $C_{10}H_{12}CaN_2Na_2O_8,2H_2O$. A chelating agent used in the treatment of lead poisoning.

Sodium carbonate. B.P.C. 1968. $Na_2CO_3,10H_2O$. A salt used in the preparation of alkaline baths and of surgical chlorinated soda solution, **B.P.C. Anhydrous sodium carbonate,** B.P.C. 1968, $NaCO_3$. A preparation used as a water softener.

Sodium carboxymethylcellulose. B.P.C. 1968. A suspending agent, which is also used as a bulk laxative.

Sodium chloride. B.P. 1968. NaCl. Common salt. The major inorganic constituent of the body, playing a dominant role in maintaining the osmatic tension of the blood and tissues. **Sodium chloride and dextrose injection,** B.P. 1968, a sterile solution of 0·18 per cent of sodium chloride and 4·3 per cent of dextrose in water for injections, B.P. **Sodium chloride injection,** B.P. 1968, a sterile solution containing 0·9 per cent of sodium chloride in water for injections, B.P. Normal saline for injection.

Sodium chromate (^{51}Cr) solution. B.P. 1968. A sterile solution of sodium chromate (^{51}Cr) made isotonic with blood by addition of sodium chloride. A radioactive isotope used to label erythrocytes for investigational purposes.

Sodium citrate. B.P. 1968. $C_6H_5Na_3O_7$, $2H_2O$. A systemic alkalinizing substance, which has also anticoagulant properties.

Sodium cromoglycate. B.P. Addendum 1971. $C_{23}H_{14}Na_2O_{11}$. Used by inhalation in the treatment of asthma.

Sodium cyclamate. B.P. 1968. $C_6H_{12}N$ NaO_3S. A sweetening agent.

Sodium diatrizoate. B.P. 1968. $C_{11}H_8I_3$ $N_2NaO_4,4H_2O$. A radio-opaque substance.

Sodium dibunate. The B.P. Commission approved name for a cough suppressant.

Sodium diprotrizoate. The B.P. Commission approved name for a radio-opaque substance.

Sodium fluoride. B.P. 1968. NaF. A salt used in the prevention of dental caries.

Sodium fusidate. B.P. 1968. $C_{31}H_{47}$ NaO_6. The sodium salt of fusidic acid, an antimicrobial substance produced by certain strains of *Fusidium coccineum*. An antibiotic active against gram-positive micro-organisms, including penicillin-resistant staphylococci.

Sodium glucaldrate. The B.P. Commission approved name for a drug for the treatment of gastric hyperacidity.

Sodium glucaspaldrate. The B.P. Commission approved name for octasodium tetrakis(gluconato)bis(salicylato)-μ-diacetatodialuminate (III) hydrate. An analgesic.

Sodium hydroxide. B.P. 1968. NaOH. A powerful caustic.

Sodium iodide. B.P. 1968. NaI. A salt used for the prevention of simple goitre and as a preoperative medication in thyrotoxicosis. **Sodium iodide (^{131}I) injection,** B.P. 1968, a sterile solution containing sodium iodide (^{131}I), suitable for intravenous injection. It has the same action as **Sodium iodide (^{131}I) solution,** B.P. 1968, a preparation for oral use. It is used in the diagnosis and treatment of thyrotoxicosis and carcinoma of the thyroid. **Sodium iodide (^{125}I) solution,** B.P. Addendum 1969, a preparation used for the investigation of thyroid disease.

Sodium iodohippurate (^{131}I) injection. B.P. 1968. A sterile solution containing sodium-*o*-hippurate (^{131}I), which is used as a test of renal function.

Sodium iothalamate injection. B.P. 1968. A sterile solution of the sodium salt of iothalamic acid, which is used as a radio-opaque agent in angiography.

Sodium ipodate. The B.P. Commission approved name for sodium 3-(3-dimethylaminomethyenamino-2,4,6-tri-iodophenyl)propionate. A radio-opaque substance.

Sodium ironedate. The B.P. Commission approved name for an iron chelate of the monosodium salt of ethylenediamine-*NNN'N'*-tetra-acetic acid. A drug for the treatment of iron-deficiency anaemia.

Sodium lactate injection. B.P. 1968. A sterile solution containing sodium lactate prepared from 14ml. of lactic acid and 6·7G. of sodium hydroxide, in water for injections, B.P. to 1000ml. It is used intravenously in the treatment of diabetic coma. **Compound sodium lactate injection,** B.P. 1968, a sterile solution containing sodium lactate prepared from 2·4ml. of lactic acid and 1·15G. of sodium hydroxide, with sodium chloride, potassium chloride and calcium chloride in water for injections, B.P. to 1000ml. A preparation given orally to infants with gastroenteritis. Hartman's solution for injection.

Sodium lauryl sulphate. B.P. 1968. A mixture of the sodium salts of sulphated normal primary alcohols. It is an anionic emulsifying agent.

Sodium metabisulphite. B.P. 1968. $Na_2S_2O_5$. An antoxidant and reducing agent widely used in pharmaceutical preparations.

Sodium metrizoate. The B.P. Commission approved name for sodium 3-acetamido-2, 4, 6-tri-iodo-5-N-methylacetamidobenzoate. A radio-opaque substance.

Sodium nitrite. B.P.C. 1968. $NaNO_2$. A coronary vasodilator. **Sodium nitrite injection,** B.P.C. 1968, a sterile solution of 3G. of sodium nitrite in water for injections, B.P. to 100ml., used intravenously in the treatment of cyanide poisoning.

Sodium perborate. B.P.C. 1968. $NaBO_2$, H_2O_2,$3H_2O$. A preparation that readily releases oxygen in contact with oxidizable matter.

Sodium phosphate. B.P. 1968. Na_2HPO_4, $12H_2O$. A saline purgative. **Sodium phosphate (^{32}P) injection,** B.P. 1968, a sterile solution of sodium phosphate (^{32}P), given intravenously in the treatment of polycythaemia vera.

Sodium polymetaphosphate. B.P.C. 1968. A preparation which combines with calcium and magnesium ions to form soluble compounds, and is therefore used to prevent the precipitation of calcium and magnesium compounds from water.

Sodium potassium tartrate. B.P.C. 1968. $C_4H_4KNaO_6$,$4H_2O$. A saline purgative. Rochelle salt.

Sodium salicylate. B.P. 1968 $C_7H_5NaO_3$. An analgesic and antipyretic. The drug of choice in the treatment of acute rheumatism.

Sodium stibogluconate. B.P. 1968. A pentavalent antimony compound used in the treatment of leishmaniasis.

Sodium sulphate. B.P. 1968. Na_2SO_4, $10H_2O$. A saline purgative. Glauber's salt.

Sodium sulphite. B.P.C. 1968. Na_2SO_3, $7H_2O$. A preservative used in acidic solutions and syrups, its bacterial action being due to the sulphur dioxide liberated.

Sodium thiosulphate. B.P.C. 1968. $Na_2S_2O_3$,$5H_2O$. A salt used in conjunction with sodium nitrite in the treatment of cyanide poisoning.

Sodoku. Rat-bite fever caused by *Spirillum minus*.

Sodomy. Penetration of the anus by the penis.

Solapsone. B.P. 1968. $C_{30}H_{28}N_2Na_4O_{14}S_5$. A sulphone used in the treatment of leprosy.

Solarium. A room in which the inmates are exposed to natural or artificial sunlight.

Sole. The plantar surface of the foot.

Soleno- (Gk *sōten:* channel, gutter). Prefix signifying relationship to a pipe, meaning grooved or tubular.

Solipsism. The philosophical concept that the world consists merely of oneself and one's experiences.

Solute. The dissolved substance in a solution.

Solution. The incorporation of a solid, liquid, or gas, in a fluid substance to produce a homogeneous liquid. In pharmacopoeial terms, a liquid preparation containing one or more soluble ingredients, usually dissolved in water. **Colloidal solution,** a solution in which particles of colloid dimension are homogeneously distributed through a solvent. **Gramme-molecular solution,** a solution which contains the gramme-molecular weight of a reagent per litre. **Haemodialysis solutions,** B.P.C. 1968, aqueous solutions of electrolytes and dextrose approximating in composition to a normal extracellular body fluid. **Hyperbaric solution,** a solution of spinal anaesthetic with a specific gravity higher than that of cerebrospinal fluid. **Hypertonic solution,** a solution with an osmotic pressure higher than that of blood serum. **Hypotonic solution,** a solution with an osmotic pressure lower than that of blood serum. **Intraperitoneal dialysis solutions,** B.P.C. 1968, sterile aqueous solutions of electrolytes and dextrose approximating in composition to a normal extracellular body fluid. **Isotonic solution,** a solution with the same osmotic pressure as a standard: in medicine, usually blood serum. **Molar solution,** gramme-molecular solution. **Normal solution,** a solution which contains 1 gramme equivalent weight of the active substance per litre. **Normal saline solution,** a solution isotonic with body fluids, containing 0·9 per cent w/v of sodium chloride in distilled water. Sodium Chloride Solution, B.P.C. 1968. **Supersaturated solution,** a solution containing more of a solute than it will normally or permanently hold. There are 16 solutions in the *British Pharmacopoeia* 1968: Adrenaline solution; Aqueous iodine solution; Benzalkonium chloride solution; Calciferol solution; Calcium hydroxide solution; Chlorhexidine gluconate solution; Coal tar solution; Cresol and soap solution; Formaldehyde solution; Hydrogen peroxide solution; Morphine hydrochloride solution; Potassium hydroxide solution; Sodium chromate (^{51}Cr) solution; Sodium iodide (^{131}I) solution; Strong hydrogen peroxide solution; Weak iodine solution. There are 28 solutions in the *British Pharmaceutical Codex*, 1968: Aluminium acetate solution; Amaranth solution; Aromatic ammonia solution; Dilute ammonia solution; Strong ammonium acetate solution; Benzoic acid solution; Cetrimide solution; Strong cetrimide solution; Chlorinated lime and boric acid solution; Surgical chlorinated soda solution; Chloroxylenol solution; Strong coal tar solution; Ferric chloride solution; Strong ferric chloride solution; Green S and tartrazine solution; Haemolysis solutions; Intraperitoneal dialysis solutions; Dilute lead subacetate solution; Strong lead subacetate solution; Sterile strong noradrenaline solution; Ethereal soap solution; Sodium chloride solution; Sterile sodium citrate solution for bladder irrigation; Strong sodium hypochlorate solution; Dilute sodium hypochlorite solution; Sorbitol solution; Compound tartrazine solution; Tolu solution.

Solution-tablet. A compact product containing a medicament or a mixture of medicaments in compressed form, intended after solution in water to be used externally or on mucous surfaces. There are two solution-tablets in the *British Pharmaceutical Codex*, 1968: Buffered benzylpenicillin solution-tablets; Mouth-wash solution-tablets.

Solvent. The liquid that holds a solute to produce a solution.

Soma. The body as distinct from the mind.

Somat-, Somato- (Gk *soma:* body). Prefixes signifying relationship to the body.

Somatic. Pertaining to the framework of the body.

Somatomammotrophin. A hormone produced by the placenta that stimulates growth of the breasts: *Chorionic somatomamotrophin.*

Somatopleure. The embryonic body wall consisting of ectoderm and somatic mesoderm.

Somatotrophin. The growth hormone.

Somatotype. Body build.

Somite. One of the paired segments in the early embryo.

Somnambulism. Sleep-walking.

Somni- (L *somnus:* sleep). Prefix indicating association with sleep.

Somniloquence. Somniloquism. Sleep-talking.

Somnolence. Sleepiness.

Somnolent. Sleepy.

Somnolism. A hypnotic trance.

Soporific. Inducing sleep. A measure or drug that induces sleep.

Sorbic acid. B.P.C. 1968. $C_6H_8O_2$. A preservative with antibacterial and antifungal properties.

Sorbide nitrate. The B.P. Commission approved name for 1,4:3,6-dianhydrosorbitol dinitrate. A coronary vasodilator.

Sorbitan monolaurate, B.P.C. 1968. Sorbitan mono-oleate, B.P.C. 1968. Sorbitan monostearate, B P.C. 1968. Non-ionic surface-active agents used in the preparation of emulsions, creams, and ointments. Other members of the series to which approved names have been given by the B.P. Commission are: **Sorbitan monopalmitate; Sorbitan sesquioleate; Sorbitan trioleate;** and **Sorbitaln tristearate.**

Sorbitol, B.P. Addendum 1971. $C_6H_{14}O_6$. A preparation used for the intravenous administration of carbohydrate in parenteral feeding.

Sordes. The thick offensive material that collects on the lips, teeth and gums in people with prolonged low fevers.

Sore. An ulcer. **Bed sore,** decubitus ulcer. **Cold sore,** herpes labialis. **Hard sore,** syphilitic chancre. **Pressure sore,** decubitus ulcer. **Soft sore,** chancroid.

Souffle. A soft blowing sound heard on auscultation.

Sound. The sensation produced by stimulation of the auditory nerve by waves transmitted by the air or other media. A rod, usually curved, for examination of a body cavity. Healthy, whole.

Soya bean. The bean of *Glycine hispida,* a leguminous plant related to peas and beans. It has a high protein and fat content, and also contains calcium, iron and B vitamins.

Spa. A health resort with mineral springs.

Space. An area, region or cavity. **Cavernous spaces of the penis,** the blood-filled spaces in the body of the penis. **Corneal spaces,** stellate spaces in the substantia propria of the cornea. **Endolymphatic space,** the space containing the endolymphatic sac. **Epidural space,** the extradural space. **Episcleral space,** the space between the inner surface of the fascial sheath of the eyeball and the outer surface of the sclera. **Extradural space,** the space between the spinal dura mater and the periosteum and ligaments lining the vertebral canal. **Extraperitoneal space, left,** the extraperitoneal connective tissue round the left suprarenal gland and the upper pole of the left kidney. **Extraperitoneal space, right,** the space which lies between the two layers of the cornonary ligament, the bare area of the liver, and the diaphragm. **Fascial spaces of the palm,** middle palmar and thenar spaces. **Infracolic space, left,** the space below and behind the transverse colon and mesocolon and to the left of the mesentery. **Infracolic space, right,** the space below and behind the transverse colon and mesocolon and to the right side of the mesentery; it often contains the appendix. **Intercostal spaces,** the spaces between the ribs. **Intervillous space,** the space between the chorion and the shell of the trophoblast. **Palmar space, middle,** the space between the medial palmar septum and the intermediate septum. **Pelvirectal space,** the loose extraperitoneal connective tissue, above the levator ani. **Perianal space,** the space surrounding the anal canal below the white line. **Perichoroidal space,** the space that separates the sclera from the outer surface of the choroid. **Perilymphatic space,** the space between the membranous and bony labyrinth. **Perineal space, deep,** the space between the superior and inferior fasciae of the urogenital diaphragm. **Perineal space, superficial,** the space between the membranous layer of superficial fascia and the inferior fascia of the urogenital diaphragm. **Retrocardiac space,** posterior mediastinum. **Retromammary space,** the space between the breast and the underlying deep fascia. Submammary space. **Retropharyngeal space,** the space between the pharynx and prevertebral lamina. **Retrosternal space,** the anterior mediastinum. **Subarachnoid space,** the interval between the arachnoid and pia mater. **Subdural space,** the potential space between the dura mater and the arachnoid mater.

Subhepatic space, left, the omental bursa. **Subhepatic space, right,** hepatorenal pouch. **Submammary space,** retromammary space **Subphrenic space, left,** the space between the diaphragm, the anterior and superior surfaces of the left lobe of the liver, the anteroposterior surface of the stomach, and the diaphragmatic surface of the spleen. **Subphrenic space, right,** the space between the diaphragm and the anterior, superior and right lateral surfaces of the right lobe of the liver. **Supracolic space,** the space between the diaphragm above and the transverse colon and mesocolon below. **Suprasternal space,** the space between the two layers of the cervical fascia where they are attached to the manubrium sterni. **Thenar space,** the space between the lateral and the intermediate palmar septum. **Zonular spaces,** a series of sacculated spaces between the anterior and posterior fibres of the suspensory ligament of the lens.

Spasm. A sudden, involuntary muscular contraction. **Cadaveric spasm,** rigor mortis. **Carpopedal spasm,** spasm of the feet and hands, as occurs in tetany. **Clonic spasm,** alternating involuntary contraction and relaxation. **Tetanic spasm,** tonic spasm. **Tonic spasm,** persisting spasm without relaxation.

Spasmo- (Gk *spasmos:* spasm). Prefix indicating relationship to spasm.

Spasmodic. Occurring in spasms.

Spasmolytic. Checking spasms. An agent that relieves spasm.

Spasmophilia. The condition in which the motor nerves are unduly sensitive, resulting in a tendency for the individual to develop muscular spasm or convulsions.

Spasmophilic. Having a tendency to spasms.

Spasmus. Spasm. **Spasmus nutans,** rhythmic nodding of the head.

Spastic. Related to spasm. An individual affected by spasticity.

Spasticity. A state of increased tension of the muscles, accompanied by exaggerated reflexes and clonus.

Spatula. A flat, knife-like instrument used to spread plasters and ointments, and also for depressing the tongue.

Spay. To remove the ovaries.

Spearmint oil. B.P.C. 1968. A distillation from fresh flowering plants of *Mentha spicata* and *Mentha x cardiaca.* A flavouring agent and carminative.

Species. A biological division subordinate to a genus, and consisting of individuals possessing common characteristics which differentiate them from other groups. (*Plural:* species.)

Specific. Pertaining to a species. That which distinguishes a thing, whether it be a drug, a bacterium or a disease.

Specificity. The quality of being specific.

Spectacles. Framed or mounted lenses worn to assist vision.

Spectinomycin. The B.P. Commission approved name for an antibiotic produced by *Streptomyces spectabilis*.

Spectro- (L *spectrum:* appearance). Prefix indicating association with a spectrum.

Spectrograph. An instrument for recording spectra on a photographic plate.

Spectrometer. An instrument for measuring the refractive index of a translucent substance. A spectroscope for measuring the wave-lengths of any part of a spectrum.

Spectrophotometer. An apparatus for measuring the intensity of light transmitted by a given substance.

Spectroscope. An instrument for analysing the spectrum of a body.

Spectrum. The band of colours produced when white light is passed through a prism. The range of wavelengths of electromagnetic radiation. (*Plural:* spectra.)

Speculum. An instrument for dilating an orifice to allow for examination of the passage or cavity beyond. (*Plural:* specula.)

Speech. The production of sound in the form of words. Words spoken. **Oesophageal speech,** speech produced after laryngectomy using the oesophagus as an air reservoir. **Scanning speech,** slow, measured speech in which words are pronounced with accentuation of each syllable. **Slurred speech,** slovenly articulation, as in general paralysis of the insane. **Staccato speech,** jerky speech, as in multiple sclerosis.

Sperm-, Spermato-, Spermo- (Gk *spermatos:* seed). Prefixes signifying relationship to seed. particularly semen and spermatozoa.

Spermaceti, B.P.C. 1968. A solid wax derived from the oils recovered from the head, blubber and carcase of the sperm whale and the bottle-nosed whale. It is used in cold creams and ointments.

Spermateleosis. The complicated process of differentiation which a spermatid undergoes in conversion into a spermatozoon.

Spermatic. Pertaining to spermatozoa or semen.

Spermatid. The immediate precursor of the spermatozoon. It develops from the secondary spermatocyte by meiotic division.

Spermatocele. A cystic swelling of the epididymis.

Spermatocyte. The cell produced by a spermatogonium, and which in turn gives rise to spermatids.

Spermatogenesis. The process of forming spermatozoa.

Spermatogonium. The primordial male germ cell. (*Plural:* spermatogonia.)

Spermatorrhoea. Involuntary emission of semen without orgasm.

Spermatozoon. The mature male germ cell. (*Plural:* spermatozoa.)

Spermaturia. The presence of spermatozoa in the urine.

Spermicide. An agent, procedure or drug that kills spermatozoa.

Spheno- (Gk *sphēn:* wedge). Prefix signifying association with the sphenoid, or being wedge-shaped.

Sphenocephaly. Having a wedge-shaped head.

Sphenoid bone. The bone situated at the base of the skull, in front of the temporal bones and the basilar part of the occipital bone.

Sphenoidostomy. Surgical drainage of the sphenoid sinus.

Sphenomaxillary. Pertaining to the sphenoid bone and the maxilla.

Sphenopalatine. Pertaining to the sphenoid bone and the palate.

Sphero- (Gk *spheira:* a ball). Prefix meaning round or sphere-like.

Spherocyte. A small, spherical-shaped erythrocyte.

Spherocytosis. The presence of spherocytes in the circulating blood. **Hereditary spherocytosis,** a hereditary disease characterized by spherocytosis, increased fragility of the spherocytes, jaundice, anaemia, and splenomegaly.

Sphincter. An annular muscle that surrounds an orifice and keeps it closed. **Sphincter ani, externus,** the muscle that surrounds the whole length of the anal canal. **Sphincter ani, internus,** a thickened ring of the unstriped circular muscle coat of the rectum at the anorectal junction. **Sphincter choledochus,** the part of the sphincter of the hepatopancreatic ampulla surrounding the lower part of the bile duct. **Sphincter of the hepatopancreatic ampulla,** the thickened circular muscle around the lower part of the bile duct, the ampulla and the terminal part of the main pancreatic duct. The sphincter of Oddi. **Palatopharyngeal sphincter,** a band of muscle fibres which arises from the palatine aponeurosis, sweeps backwards lateral to the levator veli palatini, to blend with the inner surface of the superior constrictor muscle of the pharynx. **Sphincter pancreaticus,** the part of the sphincter of the hepatopancreatic ampulla that surrounds the terminal part of the pancreatic duct. **Sphincter pupillae,** the circular bundle of unstriped muscle running round the margin of the pupil of the eye. **Pyloric sphincter,** the muscular ring surrounding the pylorus. **Sphincter urethrae,** the ring of involuntary muscle controlling the neck of the bladder and the prostatic urethra in the male above the opening of the ejaculatory ducts. **Sphincter vesicae,** the ring of voluntary muscle surrounding the membranous urethra.

Sphincter- (Gk *sphinktēr:* a band). Prefix indicating association with a sphincter.

Sphincterectomy. Surgical excision of a sphincter.

Sphincterotomy. Surgical incision of a sphincter.

Sphygmo- (Gk *sphygmos:* pulse). Prefix signifying relationship to the pulse.

Sphygmograph. An instrument for recording the excursions of the arterial pulse.

Sphygmomanometer. An instrument for measuring the arterial blood pressure.

Spica. A figure-of-eight bandage.

Spicule. A sharp, needle-shaped body or protuberance.

Spike lavender oil. B.P.C. 1968. The oil obtained from the flowering herb *Lavandula latifolia.* It has the same action and uses as lavender oil.

Spina. The vertebral column. A sharp projection. (*Plural:* spinae.) **Spina bifida,** developmental defect of the spine, in which part of the central lamina of one or more vertebrae are missing with varying degrees of protrusion of the spinal cord and its meninges. **Spina bifida occulta,** such a defect without any protrusion or external evidence of the defect.

Spinal. Pertaining to the spine or vetrebral column.

Spindle. A fusiform structure. **Achromatic spindle,** the delicate achromatic fibrils to which the chromosomes become attached in metaphase. **Muscle spindle,** neuromuscular spindle. **Neuromuscular spindle,** the terminal of the sensory nerve in a muscle which is responsible for the initiation of proprioceptive impulses. **Neurotendinous spindle,** the equivalent in tendons of the neuromuscular spindle.

Spine. A short sharp projection. The vertebral column. Spina. **Iliac spine,** four projections of the ilium known, respectively, as the anterior inferior and superior iliac spines, and the posterior inferior and superior iliac spines. **Ischial spine,** a downward projection of the ischium, the margins of which give attachment to the sacrospinous ligament which separates the greater sciatic foramen from the lesser. **Nasal spine, anterior,** a prominent sharp projection which marks the meeting of the two maxillae in the lower boundary of the nasal aperture. **Nasal spine of frontal bone,** the sharp termination of the nasal part of the frontal bone. **Nasal spine, posterior,** the projection formed by the medial ends of the posterior borders of the two palatine bones, to which is attached the musculus uvulae. **Spine of the scapula,** the shelf-like projection on the dorsal surface of the scapula. **Sphenoidal spine,** a small pointing process of the wing of the sphenoid bone which forms the lateral wall of the sulcus for the auditory tube. **Suprameatal spine,** a small process projecting from the temporal bone above and behind the external acoustic meatus. **Trochlear spine,** a small projection in the orbit giving attachment to the pulley of the superior oblique muscle. **Vertebral spine,** the backward and downward projection from the junction of the laminae of the vertebrae which serves for the attachment of muscles and ligaments.

Spini-, Spino- (L *spina:* thorn). Prefixes indicating relationship to the spine.

Spinothalamic. Pertaining to the spinal cord and the thalamus.

Spiperone. The B.P. Commission approved name for 8-[3-(4-fluorobenzoyl) propyl]-1,3,8-triazaspiro[4,5] decan-4-one. A tranquillizer.

Spir-, Spiro- (Gk *speira:* coil). Prefixes meaning coil-shaped, spiral.

Spiral. Coiled. A coil-shaped structure. **Curschmann's spirals,** twisted masses of mucus present in the sputum in bronchial asthma.

Spiramycin. The B.P. Commission approved name for an antibiotic derived from *Streptomyces ambofaciens* which is used mainly in the treatment of infections with grampositive micro-organisms resistant to other antibiotics, and also toxoplasmosis.

Spiricidal. Capable of killing spirilla.

Spirilene. The B.P. Commission approved name for 8-[4-(4-fluorophenyl) pent - 3 - enyl] - 1- phenyl - 1,3,8-triazaspiro[4,5] decan-4-one. A tranquilizer.

Spirillaceae. A family of the order Pseudomonadales, the members of which are rigid, curved or spiral rods.

Spirillum. A genus of the family Spirillaceae, the members of which are non-flexuous spiral filaments. (*Plural:* spirilla.) **Spirillum minus**, the causative organism of rat-bite fever.

Spirit. An alcoholic or hydroalcoholic solution of a volatile substance. Any distilled liquid. **Absolute spirit**, dehydrated alcohol, B.P. 1968. **Industrial methylated spirit**, B.P. 1968, a mixture of 19 volumes of alcohol (95 per cent) with 1 volume of approved wood naphtha. **Rectified spirit**, 90 per cent alcohol. **Soap spirit**, B.P.C. 1968, soft soap 650 grammes; alcohol (90 per cent) to 1000ml. **Surgical spirit**, B.P.C. 1968, castor oil 25ml.; diethyl phthalate 20ml.; methyl salicylate 5ml.; industrial methylated spirit to 1000ml. **White spirit**, a turpentine substitute, consisting of petroleum fractions. There are eight spirits in the *British Pharmaceutical Codex* 1968: Aromatic ammonia spirit; Benzaldehyde spirit; Ether spirit; Lemon spirit: Compound orange spirit: Peppermint spirit; Soap spirit; Surgical spirit.

Spiro- (L *spirare:* to breath). Prefix signifying relationship to breathing.

Spirochaetales. An order of the class Schizomycetes, the members of which are flexuous, slender, spiral-shaped, motile by flexion of the cell body, and gram-negative.

Spirograph. An instrument for the graphic recording of the respiratory movements.

Spirometer. An instrument for measuring the capacity of the lungs.

Spironolactone. B.P. 1968. $C_{24}H_{32}O_4S$. A diuretic by virtue of being an aldosterone inhibitor.

Splanch-, Splancho- (Gk *splanchnos:* viscus). Prefixes indicating association with the viscera.

Splanchnic. Pertaining to the viscera.

Splanchnology. The study of the viscera.

Splanchnopleure, The splanchnic layer, together with the underlying entoderm, of the primitive embryonic gut.

Spleen. An abdominal organ, averaging 150G. in weight in the adult, in the left hypochondriac region, with its long axis in the line of the 10th rib. In the foetus it is one of the main centres of blood formation. After birth it normally produces lymphocytes and monocytes, but in certain pathological states it produces erythrocytes and myeloid cells. It has also an important phagocytic function. **Accessory spleens**, small encapsulated nodules of splenic tissue, often present in the abdomen, particularly in the neighbourhood of the spleen.

Splen-, Spleno- (Gk *splēn:* spleen). Prefixes indicating association with the spleen.

Splenectomy. Surgical excision of the spleen.

Splenitis. Inflammation of the spleen.

Splenium. A bandage or bandage-like structure. The thickened, rounded posterior extremity of the corpus callosum.

Splenocolic. Pertaining to the spleen and the colon.

Splenodynia. Pain in the spleen.

Splenomegaly. Enlargement of the spleen.

Splenorenal. Pertaining to the spleen and the kidney.

Splenosis. Implantation and growth of splenic tissue in the peritoneal cavity.

Splint. A support for a wounded or injured part.

Spodo- (Gk *spodos:* ashes). Prefix signifying relationship to waste matter.

Spondyl-, Spondylo- (Gk *spondylos:* vertebra). Prefixes indicating association with a vertebra or the spinal column.

Spondylitis. Arthritis of the spine. **Ankylosing spondylitis,** a diffuse arthritis of the spine, usually in young men, and resulting in stiffness often leading to ankylosis of the spine. Poker spine.

Spondylolisthesis. Forward displacement of a vertebra on the one below it, usually the 5th lumbar vertebra on the sacrum.

Spondylomalacia. Softening of vertebrae.

Spondylosis. A degenerative lesion of the spine leading as a rule to ankylosis.

Spondylosyndesis. Operative ankylosis of two or more vertebrae.

Sponge. The elastic fibrous skeleton of various species of marine organisms of the order Porifora, used mainly as an absorbent. **Absorbable gelatin sponge,** B.P.C. 1968, a sterile, absorbable, water-soluble gelatin-base sponge, which is used as a haemostatic. **Gauze sponge,** a pad of gauze used for mopping up.

Spongio- (Gk *spongia:* sponge). Prefix meaning sponge-like.

Spongioblast. The primitive neuroglial cell that gives rise to astrocytes and oligodendrocytes.

Spongioblastoma. A glioma derived from spongioblasts.

Spor-, Sporo- (Gk *sporos:* seed). Prefixes indicating association with spores or seeds.

Sporadic. Scattered. Occasional. Not epidemic.

Sporangiospore. A spore produced within a sporangium, as by the class of fungi known as Phycomycetes.

Sporangium. The swollen spore case at the ends of aerial hyphae, within which spores develop. (*Plural:* sporangia.)

Spore. The reproductive cell of one of the lower organisms or higher plants.

Sporicide. An agent that kills spores.

Sporocyst. A cyst or sac containing spores.

Sporogony. Reproduction by means of spores.

Sporothrix. A genus of dimorphic fungi, organisms existing in nature in filamentous form but which become converted to a yeast or other unicellular structure within host tissues into which they are introduced.

Sporotrichosis. A chronic infection with *Sporothrix schenkii,* giving rise to subcutaneous nodules.

Sporozoa. A class of the phyllum Protozoa, the members of which have no means of locomotion, and reproduce in alternate generations by schizogony and sporogony.

Sporozoite. The product of schizogony. The form in which the malaria plasmodium is introduced into the human body by an infected mosquito.

Sporulation. The production or formation of spores.

Spot. A small, circumscribed area. **Blind spot,** the optic disc. **Germinal spot,** the nucleolus of the ovum. **Koplik's spots,** the small red spots with a bluish-white centre which appear in the buccal mucous membrane in the early stages of measles. **Milky spots,** aggregations of macrophages that occur in the subserous connective tissue of the pericardium, peritoneum and pleura. **Rose spots,** the faint pinkish spots that appear transitorily on the abdomen and thigh in typhoid fever.

Sprain. Injury, usually of a joint, without dislocation, and resulting in tearing or rupture of ligaments with accompanying effusion.

Spray. A preparation of medicaments in aqueous, alcoholic or glycerin-containing media intended to be applied by means of an atomizer.

Sprue. A disease of uncertain origin, due to intestinal malabsorption, and characterized by steatorrhoea, dyspepsia, glossitis and loss of weight.

Spud. A flattened, bevelled surgical blade. An instrument used for removing foreign bodies, as from the cornea.

Spur. An outgrowth, usually of bone.

Sputum. Material from the respiratory passages which is ejected by means of expectoration. (*Plural:* sputa.)

Squalene. A hydrocarbon which is converted into cholesterol by enzymes in the liver.

Squama. A flattened scale or plate. Squame. (*Plural:* squamae.)

Squamo- (L *squama:* scale). Prefix signifying relationship to the squamous portion of the occipital or temporal bones, or to scales.

Squamous. Scale-like. Scaly.

Squill, B.P.C. 1968. The bulb of *Urginea maritima.* The glycosides of squill have a weak digitalis-like action on the heart. It is a reflex expectorant.

Squint. Strabismus.

Stain. A dye used in histology and microbiology. A mark or discoloration. To discolour or colour. **Gram's stain,** the basis for one of the most important diagnostic methods of identification in bacteriology, bacteria being classified as gram-positive or gram-negative, depending on whether or not they resist decolorization with alcohol or aniline oil after staining with a pararosaniline dye and subsequently with iodine.

Stalk. A slender, connecting structure. **Connecting stalk,** a mass of primary mesoderm which connects the tail end of the embryonic area with the chorion. **Optic stalk,** the proximal part of the primitive eye.

Stammering. A disturbance of speech characterized by hesitancy due to difficulty in pronouncing certain syllables, and resulting in their being repeated over and over again. Stuttering.

Stannate. A salt of stannic acid.

Stannic. Containing tin in its tetravalent form.

Stannosis. The form of benign pneumoconiosis caused by the inhalation of fumes of stannous (tin) oxide.

Stannous. Containing tin in its divalent form.

Stannum. Tin.

Stanolone. The B.P. Commission approved name for an anabolic steroid.

Stanozolol. The B.P. Commission approved name for an anabolic steroid.

Stapedectomy. Surgical excision of the stapes.

Stapes. One of the three auditory ossicles, the base of which is attached to the circumference of the fenestra vestibuli. (*Plural:* stapedes.)

Staphyl-, Staphylo- (Gk *staphylē:* bunch of grapes). Prefixes signifying resemblance to bunch of grapes.

Staphylococcus. A genus of the family Micrococcaceae, the members of which are gram-positive cocci growing in clusters. They are classified mainly on the basis of coagulase production. *Staphylococcus aureus,* the main pathogenic member of the genus responsible for a range of infections. *Staphylococcus albus,* a relatively non-pathogenic commensal on human skin.

Staphyloma. A bulging or protrusion of the cornea or sclera due to inflammatory softening.

Starch. B.P. 1968. Polysaccharide granules obtained from the grains of maize, rice, or wheat, or the tubers of the potato. It is an absorbent, and is used in dusting powders, mucilages and ointments to protect or soothe the skin.

Stasis. Stagnation. The slowing down or stoppage of flow of a fluid.

Static. At rest. Stationary. In equilibrium.

Statistics. The study of quantitative data affected by a multiplicity of causes. **Vital statistics,** the branch of statistics that deals with data concerning human beings. Biostatistics.

Stearate. A salt of stearic acid.

Stearic acid. B.P.C. 1968. A mixture of acids, chiefly stearic and palmitic acids. It is used as a lubricant in making compressed tablets, as an enteric coating for pills and tablets, and as a basis for vanishing creams.

Stearo-, Steato- (Gk *stear, steatos:* fat). Prefixes indicating association with fat.

Steatopyga, Steatopygia. Excessive fatness of the buttocks.

Steatorrhoea. The presence of excess fat in the stools.

Stegomyia. A subgenus of the genus Aedes.

Stellate. Shaped like a star.

Stellectomy. Surgical excision of the stellate ganglion.

Stem. Pedicle or stalk. **Brain stem,** the midbrain, pons and medulla oblongata.

Steno- (Gk *stenos:* narrow). Prefix meaning narrow or narrowing.

Stenocephaly. Excessive narrowness of the head.

Stenopaeic. Having a narrow slit. Applied to optical devices with a narrow slit.

Stenosis. Constriction or narrowing of a channel, duct, or opening.

Stenostomia. Abnormal narrowness of the mouth.

Steradian. The solid angle which, having its vertex in the centre of a sphere, cuts off an area of the surface of the sphere equal to that of a square having sides of length equal to the radius of the sphere.

Sterco- (L *stercus:* dung). Prefix indicating relationship to faeces.

Stercobilin. The chief pigment of the faeces, giving them their brown colour.

Stercobilinogen. The precursor of stercobilin.

Stercoraceous. Faecal.

Stercula. B.P.C. 1968. The gum obtained from various species of Sterculia. It is used as a substitute for tragacanth in lozenges, pastes and denture-fixative powders.

Stereo- (Gk *stereos:* solid). Prefix signifying being solid or having three dimensions.

Stereochemistry. The study of the space relationships of atoms in a molecule.

Stereocilium. A large, non-motile process found on the epithelial cells of the epididymis and the columnar cells lining the central canal of the spinal cord. (*Plural:* stereocilia.)

Stereognosis. The ability to be able to recognize an object by touch.

Stereoisomer. A molecule having the same number and kind of atoms as another, but grouped differently.

Stereopsis. Stereoscopic vision.

Stereoscope. An instrument which combines the images of two similar pictures so as to give an impression of depth, or three dimensions.

Stereoscopic. Giving the impression of depth and solidity.

Stereotropism. Growth or movement upwards or away from a solid body or a rigid surface.

Sterile. Infertile. Free from micro-organisms.

Sterilization. The process of rendering an individual infertile, or incapable of producing progeny. Castration. The destruction of all micro-organisms.

Sterilizer. An apparatus for the destruction of micro-organisms in the process of rendering material sterile.

Sternebra. One of the original four segments which constitute the sternum. (*Plural:* sternebrae.)

Sterno- (Gk *sternon:* chest). Prefix signifying relationship to the sternum.

Sternocleidomastoid. Relating to the sternum, clavicle and mastoid process.

Sternocostal. Relating to the sternum and the ribs.

Sternodymus. Conjoint twins united at the sternum.

Sternohyoid. Relating to the sternum and the hyoid bone.

Sternotomy. An incision through the sternum.

Sternum. The long (average length 17cm.) flat bone forming the median portion of the anterior wall of the thorax. The breast bone. (*Plural:* sterna.)

Sternutary. A substance that provokes sneezing.

Sternutation. Sneezing.

Steroid. One of a group of substances which have a wide range of biological activities. They have one feature in common in that they all contain the nucleus known as the perhydro*cyclo*pentenophenanthrene ring system. They include the sex hormones, the hormones of the adrenal cortex, and the bile acids.

Sterol. A steroid alcohol. Cholesterol is the best known.

Stertor. Noisy breathing.

Steth-, Stetho- (Gk *stethos:* chest). Prefixes indicating relationship to the chest.

Stethograph. An instrument for recording movements of the chest.

Stethoscope. An instrument for listening to sounds produced in the body, particularly those from the heart and lungs.

Sthenia. A state of strength and vigour.

Sthenic. Being in a state of sthenia.

Stibamine glucoside. The B.P. Com-

mission approved name for sodium 4-glucosylaminophenylstibonate. A drug for the treatment of leishmaniasis.

Stibium. Antimony.

Stibocaptate. The B.P. Commission approved name for antimony (III) sodium *meso*-2,3-dimercaptosuccinate. A drug for the treatment of schistosomiasis.

Stibophen. B.P. 1968. $C_{12}H_4Na_5O_{16}S_4$ Sb, $7H_2O$. A drug used in the treatment of schistosomiasis.

Stigma. A mark or blemish. A peculiarity of a given condition which is diagnostic. (*Plural:* stigmata.)

Stilbamidine. The B.P. Commission approved name for 4,4′-diamidinostilbene. A drug for the treatment of trypansomiasis.

Stilbazium iodide. The B.P. Commission approved name for 1-ethyl-2,6-di -[4 -(pyrrolidin -1- yl)styryl]pyridinium iodide. An anthelmintic.

Stilboestrol. B.P. 1968. $C_{18}H_{20}O_2$. An oestrogen which is active when taken by mouth.

Stilet. Stylet.

Stillbirth. The birth of a viable foetus (i.e. after the 28th week of pregnancy) in which pulmonary respiration does not occur and there is no other sign of life.

Sting. The acute burning sensation produced by the bite of an insect or snake or contact with a venomous plant, or by some other toxic substance. The organ that produces a sting.

Stippling. A spotted appearance.

Stitch. A sharp pain, usually at the left costal margin, and often evoked by exercise. A suture.

Stoichiometry. The mathematics of chemistry.

Stoma. A minute opening or pore. (*Plural:* stomata.)

Stoma-, Stomato- (Gk *stoma, stomatos:* mouth). Prefixes signifying association with the mouth.

Stomach. The most dilated part of the digestive tube, with a mean adult capacity of around 1500ml., and situated between the end of the oesophagus and the beginning of the small intestine.

Stomatitis. Inflammation of the mucous membrane of the mouth.

Stomatology. The study of the mouth and its diseases.

Stomodeum. The primitive mouth.

Stomoxys. A genus of muscid flies which includes *Stomoxy calcitrans*, the stable fly.

-stomy (Gk *stomoun:* to provide with an opening). Suffix signifying the surgical formation of an opening in an organ.

Stone. A calculus or concretion. A unit of weight avoirdupois equal to 14 pounds (6·35kg.)

Stool. An evacuation of the bowels. Stools, faeces.

Storax, prepared. B.P.C. 1968. The purified balsam obtained from the trunk of *Liquidambar orientalis*. It is a constituent of compound benzoin tincture and benzoin inhalation.

Strabismus. The condition in which the visual axes assume a position relative to each other different from that conforming to physiological conditions. Squint. Alternating strabismus, the condition in which the squint changes from one eye to the other. Apparent strabismus, the appearance of a squint that may be due to configuration of the palpebral fissure, or divergence between the visual axis and the optic axis. Concomitant strabismus, squint in which the visual axes, although abnormally directed, retain their abnormal relation to each other in all movements of the eyes. Congenital strabismus, squint present at birth. Convergent strabismus, the form of concomitant strabismus, in which the deviating eye looks inwards towards the nose. Divergent strabismus, the form of concomitant strabismus, in which the deviating eye looks outwards. Kinetic strabismus, squint due to irregular or spasmodic activity of individual muscles or groups of muscles. Latent strabismus, heterophoria. Paralytic strabismus, squint due to paralysis of one or more of the ocular muscles. Periodic strabismus, concomitant strabismus which occurs only at intervals. Unilateral strabismus, the condition in which one eye habitually fixes and the other squints.

Stramonium. B.P. 1968. The dried leaves and flowering tops of *Datura stramonium*. It has a belladonna-like action by virtue of the fact that it contains hyoscyamine and atropine.

Strangulation. Asphyxiation by means of compression of the air passages. Constriction of a part resulting in arrest of the circulation: e.g. as may occur in a hernia.

Strangury. Painful difficult passage of urine.

Stratum. A layer. (*Plural:* strata.) Stratum basale of the skin, the deeper

layer of the germinative zone of the skin. Stratum basale of the uterus, the layer of the decidua next to the uterine muscle. Stratum cinereum, a cap-like layer of grey matter in the superior colliculus. Stratum compactum, the layer of the decidua next to the free surface. Stratum corneum, the most superficial layer of the skin. Fibrous stratum, the intermediate layer of the tympanic membrane. Stratum germinativum, the deeper of the two embryonic strata of the skin. Stratum granulosum of the ovary, the outer layer of cells surrounding the ovary. Stratum granulosum of the skin, the innermost layer of the horny zone. Stratum intermedium, the layer of fine elastic fibres connecting the two laminae of the choroid. Stratum lemnisci, the innermost layer of the superior colliculus. Stratum lucidum, the intermediate layer of the horny zone of the skin. Stratum opticum of the retina, the layer of nerve fibres in the retina. Stratum opticum of the superior colliculus, the layer containing large multipolar nerve cells separated by fine nerve fibres derived from the retina and lateral geniculate body. Stratum spinosum of skin, the outer layer of the germinative zone. Stratum spongiosum of the decidua, the intermediate layer of the decidua. Stratum zonale of the superior colliculus, a thin layer of white fibres derived from the occipital cortex. Stratum zonale of the thalamus, the layer of white matter covering the superior surface.

Streak. A line or stripe. Primitive streak, a localized opacity which appears in the embryonic area in the 3rd week of development, the cells of which retain their pluripotency and continue to differentiate rapidly.

Strept-, Strepto- (Gk *streptos:* twisted). Prefixes meaning twisted.

Streptobacillus. A genus of the family Bacteroidaceae. *Streptobacillus moniliformis*, the causative organism of a proportion of cases of rat-bite fever.

Streptococcus. A genus of the family Lactobacillaceae, the members of which are gram-positive, spherical or oval cells arranged in pairs or chains of varying lengths. (*Plural:* streptococci.) Streptococcus pyogenes, Group A streptococcus, which is the principal etiological agent in tonsillitis and scarlet fever, and is also causally related to acute rheumatism and acute glomerulonephritis. Streptococcus viri-

dans, the commonest cause of subacute bacterial endocarditis, but also occurs as a common commensal in the mouth. **Streptococcus faecalis**, a commensal in the intestine which not infrequently invades the urinary tract.

Streptodornase. An enzyme obtained from cultures of various strains of haemolytic ˹streptococci, and capable of catalysing the depolymerization of polymerized deoxyribonucleoproteins.

Streptoduocin. The B.P. Commission approved name for a mixture of equal parts of dihydrostreptomycin sulphate and streptomycin sulphate. An antibiotic.

Streptokinase. An enzyme obtained from cultures of various strains of haemolytic streptococci, and capable of changing plasminogen into plasmin.

Streptolysin. A haemolysin produced by streptococci.

Streptomyces. A genus of the family Streptomycetaecae, the members of which consist of vegetative mycelia not fragmenting into short forms. *Streptomyces griseus*, the source of streptomycin.

Streptomycetaceae. A family of the order Actinomycetales, the members of which are filamentous, branching cells, which grow as a mycelium but do not fragment.

Streptomycin sulphate. B.P. 1968. The sulphate of an antimicrobial base produced by certain strains of *Streptomyces griseus* or by any other means. It has a wide antibacterial spectrum, including both gram-positive and gram-negative organisms, but its main value is its action against *Mycobacterium tuberculosis*. It is also active against *Escherichia coli*, and *Klebsiella pneumoniae*.

Streptonicozid. The B.P. Commission approved name for a compound formed by interaction of a suitable streptomycin salt and isoniazid, for the treatment of tuberculosis.

Stretcher. A sheet of canvas slung between two poles, each with two handles, giving two handles fore, and two handles aft, for the transport of the injured, sick or wounded.

Stria. A streak or stripe. (*Plural: striae.*) **Stria atrophica**, one of the white bands on the lower abdomen and thighs induced by mechanical stretching of the skin such as occurs in pregnancy. **Longitudinal striae, lateral and medial,** two fine longitudinal

bundles of fibres in the indusium griseum, the thin layer of grey substance that covers the trunk of the corpus callosum. **Striae medullares of the 4th ventricle,** external arcuate fibres which course across the floor of the 4th ventricle. Their precise functions and connexions are not known. **Stria medullares thalami,** a small bundle of white fibres on the medial surface of the thalamus. **Olfactory stria,** the lateral root of the olfactory tract. **Stria terminalis,** a small collection of myelinated nerve fibres which issues from the posterior end of the amygdaloid body and acts as a pathway for the association of the olfactory and autonomic systems. **Stria vascularis,** a collection of blood-vessels in the cochlear duct. **Visual stria,** a band of white matter in the visuosensory cortex formed by intracortical connecting fibres.

Stricture. Narrowing of a duct, passage or orifice.

Stridor. The harsh, high-pitched inspiratory sound produced characteristically by partial laryngeal obstruction.

Stridulous. Related to stridor.

Strigeata. The suborder of the class Trematoda which includes the superfamily Schistosomatoidea.

Stroboscope. An instrument for studying the successive phases of a periodic motion by means of periodically interrupted light.

Stroke. A synonym in popular parlance for apoplexy.

Stroma. The framework of an organ.

Stromuhr. An instrument for measuring the velocity of blood flow.

Strongyloides. A superfamily of nematodes, which includes hookworms, but not the genus Strongyloides.

Strongyloides. A genus of nematodes. *Strongyloides stercoralis*, the member of the genus that commonly affects man, especially in Brazil, Burma and Thailand.

Strongyloidiasis. Infestation with *Strongyloides stercoralis*.

Strontium. A metallic element. Symbol Sr. Atomic weight 87·63. Atomic number 38. It is one of the alkaline series and similar to calcium in chemical properties.

Strophulus. A papular eruption in infants. Red gum.

Struma. Scrofula. Goitre.

Strychnine hydrochloride. B.P.C. 1968. $C_{21}H_{23}ClN_2O_2,2H_2O$. The hydrochloride of the alkaloid strychnine, which is obtained from the seeds of *Strychnos nux-vomica*. It stimulates all parts of the nervous system.

Stupe. A hot fomentation on which turpentine has been sprinkled.

Stupor. A state of lowered consciousness. Reduced responsiveness.

Stuttering. Stammering.

Stye. A suppurative inflammation of one of the hair follicles of the eyelids. Hordoleum.

Styl-, Stylo- (Gk *stylos:* pillar). Prefixes signifying resemblance to a stake, pillar, or pole.

Stylet. A fine probe, particularly one used to keep the lumen of a needle or catheter patent. Stilet.

Styloglossal. Pertaining to the styloid process and the tongue.

Stylohyoid. Pertaining to the styloid process and the hyoid bone.

Styloid. Peg-shaped.

Stylomastoid. Pertaining to the styloid and mastoid processes of the temporal bone.

Stylus. A stylet.

Styptic. Astringent. A local application that arrests haemorrhage.

Styramate. The B.P. Commission approved name for β-hydroxyphenethyl carbamate. A skeletal muscle relaxant.

Sub- (L *sub:* under). Prefix meaning beneath, near, less than normal.

Subacromial. Beneath the acromion.

Subapical. Below the apex.

Subarachnoid. Beneath the arachnoid.

Subchloride. The chloride of a series that contains the smallest proportion of chloride.

Subclavian. Beneath the clavicle.

Subclinical. Referring to the stage of a disease before symptoms or signs appear.

Subconjunctival. Beneath the conjunctiva.

Subconscious. Partially conscious. The part of the mind, of the activities of which the individual is not conscious.

Subcostal. Beneath a rib.

Subcutaneous. Beneath the skin. Hypodermic.

Subcuticular. Beneath the epidermis.

Subdural. Beneath the dura mater.

Subinvolution. Incomplete involution.

Subjective. Perceived by the individual but not by the observer.

Sublimation. The process of converting a solid into a vapour and then condensing it. The process of converting the sexual drive into sociably acceptable channels.

Sublingual. Underneath the tongue.

Subluxation. Partial dislocation.

Submammary. Beneath the breast.

Submandibular. Below the mandible.

Submaxilla. The mandible.

Submental. Under the chin.

Submicroscopic. Too small to be visible under a light microscope.

Submucosa. The layer of tissue beneath mucous membrane.

Subnormal. Below normal.

Suboccipital. Beneath the occiput.

Suborbital. Beneath the orbit.

Subphrenic. Below the diaphragm.

Subscapular. Beneath the scapula.

Subscleral. Beneath the sclera.

Substance. Material. Matter. **British Chemical Reference Substance,** a sample which has been purified as far as is practicable and economically feasible, any remaining impurities having been identified and a limit set on their presence. **Cement substance,** the substance, chemically similar to the ground substance of connective tissue, that unites epithelial cells. **Ground substance,** the matrix of connective tissue. **Intercellular substance,** the ground substance and fibres surrounding the connective tissue cells. **Perforated substance, anterior,** the part of the rhinencephalon that lies in the angle between the optic tract and the uncus. **Perforated substance, posterior,** a small area of greyish substance on the floor of the 3rd ventricle.

Substantia. Substance. **Substantia ferruginea,** a patch of deeply pigmented cells in the locus coeruleus of the rhomboid fossa. **Substantia gelatinosa centralis,** a band of gelatinous substance encircling the central canal of the spinal cord. **Substantia gelatinosa of the medulla oblongata,** an upward continuation of the apex of the posterior grey column of the spinal cord. **Substantia gelatinosa of the spinal cord,** a v-shaped mass of translucent nervous tissue which caps the apex of the posterior column. **Substantia nigra,** a lamina of deeply pigmented grey matter in the midbrain that divides the cerebral peduncles into a ventral part, the crus cerebri, and a dorsal part, the tegmentum. It is part of the extrapyramidal system. **Substantia propria,** the fibrous transparent layer of the cornea.

Substernal. Deep to the sternum.

Substrate. The compound acted upon by an enzyme.

Subsultus. Convulsive twitching of the muscles.

Subtertian. The term applied to the intermittent fever in malignant tertian malaria. **Subtertian malaria,** malignant tertian malaria.

Subthalamic. Below the thalamus.

Subungual. Underneath a nail.

Succedaneum. A substitute. **Caput succedaneum,** the temporary swelling on the presenting part of the skull in the new-born infant.

Succinate. A salt of succinic acid. **Succinate dehydrogenase,** the flavoprotein that dehydrogenates succinic acid.

Succinylsulphathiazole. B.P. 1968. $C_{13}H_{13}N_3O_5S_2.H_2O$. A sulphonamide which is poorly absorbed from the gastro-intestinal tract, and is therefore used in the treatment of bacillary dysentery, and to reduce the bacterial content of the colon.

Succus. Juice. **Succus entericus,** intestinal juice.

Succussion. The method of eliciting the presence of fluid and gas in a cavity by shaking the patient and thus eliciting splashing.

Suckle. To nurse at the breast.

Sucralox. The B.P. Commission approved name for a polymerized complex of sucrose and aluminium hydroxide. A drug for the treatment of gastric hyperacidity.

Sucrase. The enzyme in the intestinal juice that hydrolyses sucrose to glucose and fructose.

Sucrose. $C_{12}H_{22}O_{11}$. A disaccharide present in certain plants. On hydrolysis it yields one molecule of glucose and one of fructose. Cane sugar. Beet sugar. **Sucrose,** B.P. 1968, obtained from the juice of sugar-cane or of sugar-beet.

Sucrosuria. The presence of sucrose in urine.

Sudamen. A small vesicle due to retention of sweat in a sweat follicle. (*Plural:* sudamina.)

Sudor. Sweat.

Sudorific. An agent that induces sweating. Inducing sweating. Diaphoretic.

Suet. The abdominal fat of ruminants.

Suffocation. Interference with the entry of air into the lungs.

Suffusion. An extravasation. Reddening of the surface.

Sugar. A sweet carbohydrate. If it contains an aldehyde group it is known as an *aldose*. If it contains a ketone grouping it is known as a ketose. The simplest sugars are known as *monosaccharides:* glucose, galactose, fructose (laevulose). When two monosaccharides condense together with the elimination of water a disaccharide is formed: sucrose, maltose, lactose. *Polysaccharide* is formed by the condensation of a large number of monosaccharides: starch, glycogen, cellulose. **Sugar of lead,** lead acetate.

Suicide. The act of taking one's own life. One who kills himself.

Sulcus. A groove or furrow. (*Plural:* sulci.) **Basilar sulcus,** a shallow furrow in the anterior surface of the pons that lodges the basilar artery. **Sulcus calcanei,** a groove on the medial side of the calcaneus. **Calcarine fissure,** a horizontal fissure on the medial surface of the cerebral hemisphere, running from the occipital pole. **Callosal sulcus,** a sulcus on the medial aspect of the cerebral hemisphere, separating the cingulate gyrus from the corpus callosum. **Carotid sulcus,** a broad groove in the sphenoid bone that lodges the internal carotid artery and the cavernous sinus. **Central sulcus,** a deep fissure on the superolateral surface of the cerebral hemisphere that separates the frontal from the parietal lobe. **Sulcus centralis insulae,** a sulcus that divides the insula into an anterior and a posterior part. **Sulcus chiasmatis,** a transverse groove in the body of the sphenoid, which leads to the optic canal. **Cingulate sulcus,** a sulcus on the medial surface of the cerebral hemisphere, running round the corpus callosum. **Circular sulcus** a sulcus that almost completely surrounds the insula. **Collateral sulcus,** a sulcus that starts near the occipital pole and runs parallel to the calcarine sulcus, from which it is separated by the lingual gyrus. **Coronary sulcus,** the external demarcation between the atria and ventricles of the heart. **Fimbriodentate sulcus,** the sulcus which separates the dentate gyrus from the fimbria of the hippocampus. **Frontal sulci, inferior and superior,** two sulci which run forwards and downwards, parallel to each other, from the upper part of the precentral sulcus. **Sulcus habenulae,** a sulcus that separates the trigonum habenulae from the upper surface of the thalamus. **Hippocampal sulcus,** a sulcus that sometimes intervenes between the dentate gyrus and the parahippocampal gyrus. **Hypothalamic sulcus,** an often ill-defined curved groove that separates the anterior two-thirds of the thalamus from the hypothalamus. **Intertuber-**

cular sulcus, the sulcus that separates the two tubercles of the humerus and lodges the tendon of the long head of the biceps. **Intraparietal sulcus,** a sulcus on the lateral aspect of the parietal lobe. **Lateral sulcus,** a deep cleft in the inferior and lateral surfaces of the cerebral hemisphere. **Sulcus limitans,** the lateral boundary of the medial eminence of the rhomboid fossa. **Lunate sulcus,** a sulcus just in front of the occipital lobe that forms the posterior boundary of the gyrus descendens. **Malleolar sulcus,** the sulcus in the temporal bone that lodges the anterior process of the malleus, the chorda tympani nerve and the anterior tympanic artery. **Medial sulcus of the cerebral peduncle,** the sulcus from which the roots of the oculomotor nerve emerge. **Median sulcus of 4th ventricle,** the sulcus that divides the rhomboid fossa into symmetrical halves. **Median sulcus, anterolateral, of the medulla oblongata,** the furrow from which the fibres of the hypoglossal nerve emerge. **Median sulcus, posterior, of the medulla oblongata,** a narrow groove continuous below with the posterior median sulcus of the spinal cord. **Median sulcus, posterolateral, of the medulla oblongata,** the sulcus to the bottom of which are attached the accessory, vagus, and glossopharyngeal nerves. **Median sulcus, posterior, of the spinal cord,** a very shallow sulcus. **Median sulcus, posterointermedius, of the spinal cord,** a longitudinal furrow in the cervical and upper thoracic regions which marks the position of a septum that divides the posterior funiculus into the fasciculus gracilis and the fasciculus cuneatus. **Median sulcus, posterolateral, of the spinal cord,** the vertical furrow to which the dorsal nerve roots are attached. **Occipitotemporal sulcus,** a sulcus that runs parallel to the collateral sulcus. **Olfactory sulcus,** an anteroposterior sulcus in the inferior surface of the cerebral hemisphere, underlying the olfactory bulb and tract. **Orbital sulci,** irregular H-shaped sulci in the inferior surface of the cerebral hemisphere. **Parieto-occipital sulcus,** a deep sulcus on the posterior part of the medial surface of the cerebral hemisphere. **Polar sulci,** two curved sulci in occipital lobe that enclose semilunar extensions of the striate area. **Postcentral sulcus,** a sulcus on the lateral aspect of the parietal lobe. **Postero-**

lateral sulcus, a sulcus on the inferior surface of the cerebellum that separates the uvula from the nodule. **Preauricular sulcus,** a roughened groove on the pelvic surface of the ilium, which gives attachment to the lower fibres of the ventral sacro-iliac ligament, and is better developed in the female than the male. **Precentral sulcus,** a sulcus on the superolateral surface of the frontal lobe, which is separated from the central sulcus by the precentral gyrus. **Rhinal sulcus,** the sulcus on the inferior surface of the cerebral hemisphere that separates the temporal bone from the uncus. **Sagittal sulcus,** the sulcus in the median plane of the internal surface of the skull cap that lodges the sagittal sinus. **Sulcus sclerae,** a slight furrow at the junction of the cornea and sclera. **Sigmoid sulcus,** the sulcus on the lateral wall of the posterior cranial fossa, which lies behind the mastoid antrum and contains the sigmoid sinus. **Sulcus spiralis internus,** a C-shaped concavity in the wall of the duct of the cochlea. **Sulcus tali,** a deep groove in the plantar surface of the talus. **Temporal sulci,** two sulci on the lateral surface of the temporal lobe. **Sulcus terminalis of the heart,** a shallow groove on the outer surface of the lateral wall of the right atrium. **Sulcus terminalis of the tongue,** a V-shaped furrow at the base of the tongue. **Sulcus of the transverse sinus,** a wide groove on each side of the internal aspect of the occipital bone. **Sulcus tubae,** the furrow between the greater wing of the sphenoid bone and the petrous portion of the temporal bone that lodges the cartilaginous part of the auditory tube. **Tympanic sulcus,** the narrow groove in which the circumference of the tympanic membrane is attached. **Sulcus valleculae,** the sulcus on the inferior surface of the cerebellar hemisphere that surrounds the vermis.

Sulfadoxine. The B.P. Commission approved name for 4-(4-aminobenzenesulphonamido) - 5, 6 - dimethoxypyrimidine. A sulphonamide.

Sulfametopyrazine. The B.P. Commission approved name for 2-(4-amino-benzenesulphonamido) - 3 - methoxypyrazine. A long-acting sulphonamide.

Sulphacetamide sodium. B.P. 1968. $C_8H_9N_2NaO_3S,H_2O$. A sulphonamide used chiefly for local application in infections and injuries of the conjunctiva.

Sulphadiazine. B.P. 1968. $C_{10}H_{10}N_4$ O_2S. A sulphonamide. **Sulphadiazine sodium,** B.P. 1968, the sodium derivative of sulphadiazine for intravenous or intramuscular use.

Sulphadimethoxine. B.P. 1968. $C_{12}H_{14}$ N_4O_4S. A long-acting sulphonamide.

Sulphadimidine. B.P. 1968. $C_{12}H_{14}N_4$ O_2S. A widely used sulphonamide. **Sulphadimidine sodium.** B.P. 1968, a preparation for intramuscular or intravenous use.

Sulphaethidole. The B.P. Commission approved name for 5-(4-aminobenzene-sulphonamido)-2-ethyl-1,3,4-thiadiazole. A sulphonamide which is rapidly absorbed, and only a small proportion of which is acetylated.

Sulphafurazole. B.P. 1968. $C_{11}H_{13}N_3$ O_3S. A sulphonamide with a relatively high solubility in urine.

Sulphaguanidine. B.P.C. 1968. C_7H_{10} N_4O_2S,H_2O. A poorly absorbed sulphonamide used in the treatment of local intestinal infections.

Sulphaloxic acid. The B.P. Commission approved name for 2-[4-(hydroxy-methylureidosulphonyl) phenylcarbamoyl]-benzoic acid. A sulphonamide.

Sulphamethizole. B.P. 1968. $C_9H_{10}N_4$ O_2S_2. A sulphonamide largely used for the treatment of coliform infections of the urinary tract.

Sulphamethoxazole. B.P. Addendum 1971. $C_{10}H_{11}N_3O_3S$. A sulphonamide.

Sulphamethoxydiazine. B.P. 1968. $C_{11}H_{12}N_4O_3S$. A rapidly absorbed, slowly excreted sulphonamide.

Sulphamethoxypyridazine. B.P. 1968. $C_{11}H_{12}N_4O_3S$. A sulphonamide with an exceptionally slow rate of excretion.

Sulphamoprine. The B.P. Commission approved name for 2-(4-aminobenzenesulphonamido)-4,6-dimethoxy-pyrimidine. A long-acting sulphonamide.

Sulphamoxole. The B.P. Commission approved name for 2-(4-aminobenzenesulphonamido)-4,5-dimethyloxazole. A long-acting sulphonamide.

Sulphan blue. The B.P. Commission approved name for the sodium salt of 4,4'-di(diethylamino)-4'',6''-disulpho-triphenylmethanol anhydride. A dye used in the investigation of the cardiovascular system.

Sulphanilamide. B.P.C. 1968. $C_6H_8N_2$ O_2S. The first of the widely used sulphonamides. Now largely used, when used at all, for the treatment of haemolytic streptococcal infections.

Sulphaphenazole. B.P. 1968. $C_{15}H_{14}N_4$ O_2S. A sulphonamide.

Sulphaproxyline. The B.P. Commission approved name for N^1-(4-isopropoxy-benzoyl)-4-aminobenzenesulphonamide. A sulphonamide which is rapidly absorbed and slowly excreted.

Sulphapyridine. B.P. 1968. $C_{11}H_{11}N_3$ O_2S. One of the earlier sulphonamides, which is seldom used now, except for cases of dermatitis herpetiformis which do not respond to dapsone.

Sulphasalazine. The B.P. Commission approved name for 4-hydroxy-4'-(2-pyridylsulphamoyl) azobenzene-3-carboxylic acid. A sulphonamide with a special affinity for connective tissue.

Sulphasomidine. The B.P. Commission approved name for 4-(4-aminobenzenesulphonamido)-2,6-dimethylpyri-midine. A sulphonamide which is rapidly absorbed and excreted.

Sulphasomizole. The B.P. Commission approved name for 5-(4-aminoben-zenesulphonamido)-3-methylisothia-zole. A sulphonamide with a relatively long duration of action.

Sulphate. A salt of sulphuric acid.

Sulphathiazole. B.P.C. 1968. $C_9H_9N_3$ O_2S_2. The only sulphonamide that has any effect in staphylococcal infections.

Sulphathiourea. The B.P. Commission approved name for 4-aminobenzene-sulphonylthiourea. A sulphonamide which is used topically.

Sulphatolamide. The B.P. Commission approved name for 4-aminobenzene-sulphonylthiourea salt of 4-sulpha-moylbenzylamine. A sulphonamide.

Sulphaurea. The B.P. Commission approved name for 4-aminobenzene-sulphonylurea. A sulphonamide which is rapidly absorbed and excreted.

Sulphide. A compound of sulphur with an element or basic radical.

Sulphinpyrazone. B.P. 1968. $C_{23}H_{20}N_2$ O_3S. A uricosuric agent.

Sulphite. A salt of sulphurous acid.

Sulpho- (L *sulfur:* brimstone). Prefix indicating association with divalent sulphur, or the sulphonamide group.

Sulphobromophthalein sodium. B.P. 1968. $C_{20}H_8Br_4Na_2O_{10}S_2$. A dye used as a liver function test.

Sulphomyxin sodium. B.P. 1968. A mixture of sulphomethylated poly-myxin B and sodium bisulphite. Administered by intramuscular injection it has the same actions as polymyxin, but less toxic. **Sulpho-myxin injection,** B.P. 1968, a sterile solution of sulphomyxin sodium in water for injections, B.P., which should be used within 48 hours of preparation and stored during this period at a temperature between 2° and 10°C.

Sulphonamide. A drug having the grouping $-SO_2NH_2$.

Sulphone. A compound of SO_2 attached to one or more hydrocarbons. Several sulphones are proving useful in the treatment of leprosy.

Sulphonic acid. An organic acid containing the $-SO_2OH$ or SO_3H group.

Sulphonylureas. A group of sulphonamide derivatives that have a hypoglycaemic action. They include carbutamide, chlorpropamide, and tolbutamide.

Sulphur. A non-metallic element. Symbol S. Atomic weight 32·066. Atomic number 16. **Precipitated sulphur, B.P. 1968,** a preparation obtained by adding hydrochloric acid to a solution prepared by boiling sulphur and calcium oxide with water. A mild antiseptic and parasiticide, and mild laxative. **Sulphur ointment, B.P. 1968,** an ointment containing 10 per cent of precipitated sulphur in simple ointment, **B.P. Sublimed sulphur, B.P.C. 1968,** a preparation obtained by sublimation of native sulphur, or from sulphides, or as a by-product of the refining of crude petroleum. Flowers of sulphur.

Sulphurated. Sulphuretted. Sulphurated potash, B.P.C. 1968, a mixture of potassium polysulphides and other potassium compounds. Used as a peeling agent in acne.

Sulphuretted. Combined, or treated, with sulphur.

Sulphuric acid. H_2SO_4. A powerful corrosive. **Dilute sulphuric acid, B.P.C. 1968,** 104 grammes of sulphuric acid and 896 grammes of purified water, **B.P.** A stomachic.

Sulphurous. A tetravalent compound of sulphur. Derived from sulphur dioxide. Containing sulphur.

Sulphurous acid. H_2SO_3. A strong disinfectant with a pungent odour.

Sulphydryl. The monovalent radical $-SH$.

Sulthiame. B.P. 1968. $C_{10}H_{14}N_2O_4S_2$. An anticonvulsant, particularly useful in psychomotor epilepsy.

Sunburn. The effect of the sun's rays on the skin, ranging from tanning to redness and severe dermatitis.

Sunstroke. A form of heatstroke due to over-exposure to sunlight.

Super- (L *super:* above). Prefix meaning over, excess, above.

Superciliary. Referring to the eyebrow.

Superfecundation. The fertilization of two or more ova, resulting from the same period of ovulation, by separate acts of coitus.

Superfoetation. The fertilization of two or more ova from different ovulation periods, separated by weeks or even months.

Superinvolution. The term used to describe excessive reduction in the size of the uterus after pregnancy.

Supernatant. Floating. The term used to describe the fluid left when a precipitate has settled.

Superphosphate. An acid phosphate.

Supersaturation. The state of containing solute above the saturation point.

Supersonic. Having a speed greater than that of sound. Ultrasonic.

Supination. The movement of the forearm, whereby the radius lies lateral, and parallel, to the humerus.

Supinator. A muscle that induces supination.

Supine. In the state of supination. Lying on the back, face upwards.

Suppository. A solid body suitably shaped for rectal administration, and usually containing medicaments. (*Plural:* suppositories.) There are eight suppositories in the *British Pharmaceutical Codex*, 1968: Aminophylline suppositories; Bismuth subgallate suppositories; Compound bismuth subgallate suppositories; Cinchocaine suppositories; Hamamelis suppositories; Hamamelis and zinc suppositories; Hydrocortisone suppositories; Morphine suppositories.

Suppuration. The formation of pus.

Supra- (L *supra:* above). Prefix meaning over or above.

Supraclavicular. Above the clavicle.

Suprahyoid. Above the hyoid bone.

Supranuclear. Situated above a nucleus or on the cortical side of a nucleus.

Supra-orbital. Above the orbit.

Suprapubic. Above the pubic arch.

Suprarenal. Above the kidney. Pertaining to the suprarenal gland.

Suprascapular. Above, or situated in the upper part of, the scapula.

Suprasellar. Above the sella turcica.

Suprasternal. Above the sternum.

Supratrochlear. Above a trochlea, particularly the trochlea of the humerus.

Supraventricular. Above the ventricle, particularly in relation to the ventricles of the heart.

Sural. Pertaining to the calf of the leg.

Suramin. B.P. 1968. $C_{51}H_{34}N_6Na_6O_{23}S_6$.

An intravenous trypanocide. **Suramin injection,** B.P. 1968, a sterile solution of suramin in water for injections, B.P., prepared immediately before use.

Surfactant. A surface-active agent.

Surgery. The branch of medicine that has to do with the operative treatment of disease.

Surrogate. A substitute.

Suspension. A dispersion of solid particles throughout a liquid medium. Temporary cessation. A method of treatment, either by fixation of an organ, or by traction.

Suspensory. Supporting.

Sustenaculum. A support. (*Plural: sustenacula.*) **Sustenaculum tali,** a projection from the medial surface of the calcaneus that supports the talus.

Suture. A fibrous joint found only in the skull, in which the margins of the bones articulate with one another, but with no appreciable motion, and are separated from each other by a thin layer of fibrous tissue: the sutural ligament. The material by which the two edges of a wound or incision are kept in apposition. The process of uniting edges of a wound or incision. **Coronal suture,** the suture between the posterior edge of the frontal bone and the anterior borders of the parietal bones. **Cruciform suture,** the suture between the palatine processes of the maxillae and the horizontal plates of the palatine bones. **Denticulate suture,** a suture in which the margins present a series of tooth-like processes which widen towards their free ends. **Fronto-ethmoidal suture,** the suture joining the crista galli and alae of the cribriform plate of the ethmoid bone to the nasal spine and anterior border of the ethmoidal notch of the frontal bone. **Frontolacrimal suture,** the suture between the anterior part of the medial border of the orbital plate of the frontal bone and the upper border of the lacrimal bone. **Frontomaxillary suture,** the suture between the nasal part of the frontal bone and the frontal process of the maxilla. **Frontonasal suture,** the suture between the nasal bone and the frontal process of the maxilla. **Frontozygomatic suture,** the suture between the zygomatic process of the frontal bone and the frontal process of the zygomatic bone. **Intermaxillary suture,** the intermaxillary stretch of the cruciform suture. **Internasal suture,** the suture between the nasal bones. **Interpalatine suture,** the interpalatine stretch of the cruciform suture. **Lacromaxillary suture,** the suture between the anterior border of the lacrimal bone and the frontal process of the maxilla. **Lambdoid suture,** the suture between the parietal bones and the occipital bone. **Lens sutures,** faint sutural lines which radiate from the poles to the equator of the lens of the eye. **Limbous suture,** a suture in which one bone overlaps another and the overlapping edges are ridged or serrated. **Nasomaxillary suture,** the suture between the nasal bone and the frontal process of the maxilla. **Occipitomastoid suture,** the suture between the occipital bone and the mastoid part of the temporal bone. **Palatomaxillary suture,** the suture between the orbital process of the palatine bone and the orbital portion of the maxilla. **Parietomastoid suture,** the suture between the parietal bone and the mastoid process of the temporal bone. **Petro-occipital suture,** the suture between the petrous portion of the temporal bone and the occipital bone. **Petrosquamosal suture,** the suture between the petrous and squamosal parts of the temporal bone. **Plane suture,** a suture which consists of the simple apposition of contiguous rough surfaces. **Sagittal suture,** the suture between the interlocking upper borders of the two parietal bones. **Serrate suture,** a suture in which the bony margins have saw-like edges. **Spheno-ethmoidal suture,** the suture between the sphenoid bone and the cribriform plate of the ethmoid bone. **Sphenozygomatic suture,** the suture between the sphenoid bone and the zygomatic bone. **Tympanomastoid suture,** the suture between the tympanic plate and the mastoid process. **Vomero-ethmoidal suture,** the suture between the vomer and the perpendicular plate of the ethmoid bone. **Wedge-and-groove suture,** schindylesis. **Zygomaticomaxillary suture,** the suture between the zygomatic bone and the maxilla. **Zygomatic temporal suture,** the suture between the zygomatic bone and the temporal bone.

Suxamethonium bromide, B.P. 1968. $C_{14}H_{30}Br_2N_2O_4,2H_2O$. A short-acting relaxant of voluntary muscle. **Suxamethonium bromide injection,** B.P. 1968, a sterile solution of suxamethonium bromide prepared immediately before use by dissolving the sterile contents of a sealed container in water for injections, B.P.

Suxamethonium chloride, B.P. 1968, $C_{14}H_{30}Cl_2N_2O_4,2H_2O$. A short-acting relaxant of voluntary muscle. Like the bromide it is given intravenously. **Suxamethonium chloride injection, B.P. 1968,** a sterile solution of suxamethonium chloride in water for injections, B.P.

Suxethonium bromide. The B.P. Commission approved name for bis-2-dimethylaminoethyl succinate bisethobromide. A neuromuscular blocking agent.

Swab. An absorbent pad for mopping up cavities or wounds, or for applying medications locally. A sterilized swab on the end of a stick or wire for taking specimens, as from the tonsils, for bacteriological examination.

Swallowing. The process of the passage of solids or liquids from the mouth to the stomach.

Sweat. A watery fluid of variable composition, but always hypotonic with respect to blood plasma, secreted by the sweat glands. To secrete sweat. Perspiration. **Night sweats,** the excessive sweating that occurs at night in some diseases.

Sweetbread. The lungs, thymus, pancreas, or testes.

Swelling. A prominence. An enlargement. **Calabar swellings,** the transient swellings that characterize infections with loa loa. **Cloudy swelling,** a degenerative change in cells characterized by swelling and granulation of the cytoplasm.

Sycosis. An infection of the superficial parts of the hair follicles by *Staphylococcus aureus*. **Sycosis barbae,** sycosis of the beard area. **Sycosis nuchae,** a chronic staphylococcal infection of the back of the neck in men.

Symbiosis. Living together in mutual tolerance or to mutual advantage.

Symblepharon. The condition of adhesion of the eyelid to the eyeball.

Symmelia. Fusion of the legs and feet.

Symmetry. Equality of paired parts.

Sympathectomy. Surgical excision of part of the sympathetic nervous system.

Sympathetic. Pertaining to the sympathetic nervous system. Exhibiting sympathy.

Sympathoblast. The embryonic precursor of the sympathetic nerve cell.

Sympatholytic. Antagonistic to the action of the sympathetic nervous system.

Sympathomimetic. Producing the same effect as stimulation of the sympathetic nervous system.

Sympathy. Mutual understanding. The mutual relationship between different parts of the body, whereby a change in one may induce a change in the other: e.g. the two eyes.

Symphysiotomy. Division of the symphysis pubis, to facilitate passage of the foetus during labour.

Symphysis. A cartilaginous joint in which the opposed bone surfaces are covered with hyaline cartilage and are connected to each other by a flattened disc of fibrocartilage. (*Plural:* sympheses.) **Symphysis menti,** the line of fusion of the two halves of the mandible. **Symphysis pubis,** the cartilaginous joint formed by the meeting of the two pubic bones in the midline.

Sympodia. Fusion of the two feet.

Symptom. A manifestation of disease as felt and described by the patient, as opposed to a sign which is a manifestation of disease apparent to the observer.

Syn- (Gk *syn:* with). Prefix meaning with, together, association. It is converted to sym- before b, p, ph, and m.

Synapse. The meeting place of two neurones, where their surface membranes are very close together, but there is no cytoplasmic continuity between them.

Synarthrosis. A fixed joint.

Syncephalus. Conjoined twins with a single head.

Synchilia. Congenital fusion of the lips.

Synchisis. Fluidity of the vitreous.

Synchondrosis. A cartilaginous joint in which the cartilage is hyaline in character and temporary in nature, being ultimately replaced by bone.

Synchroton. A machine for generating high-speed electrons and protons.

Syncope. Sudden transient loss of consciousness due to an inadequate supply of blood to the brain.

Syncytiotrophoblast. The outer layer of the trophoblast, in which no cell outlines can be distinguished.

Syncytium. A continuous multinucleated mass of protoplasm with no evidence, or only traces, of cell walls.

Syndactyly. Webbing or fusion of the fingers and/or toes.

Syndesmo- (Gk *syndesmos:* band or ligament). Prefix signifying relationship to connective tissue, particularly ligaments.

Syndesmology. The study of the articular system or joints.

Syndesmosis. A joint in which the opposed bony surfaces are connected by an interosseous ligament.

Syndrome. A collection of symptoms and signs that occur together so often as to provide a recognizable clinical entity. Symptom-complex. Current practice is to discourage the use of syndromes in favour of disease entities.

Synechia. Adhesion, particularly between the iris and the cornea or lens. (*Plural:* synechiae.)

Syneresis. The contraction of a gel, whereby some of the dispersed fluid is squeezed out, as in the clotting of blood.

Synergy. Combined or cooperative action.

Synkinesis. Involuntary movement accompanying voluntary movement.

Synoptophore. An instrument for the measurement of the angle of deviation in strabismus.

Synostosis. Bony ankylosis.

Synovectomy. Surgical excision of synovial membrane.

Synovia. The viscous fluid in joints secreted by the synovial membrane.

Synovioma. A tumour derived from synovial membrane.

Synovitis. Inflammation of synovial membrane.

Synovium. A synovial membrane.

Syphilid. A cutaneous manifestation of syphilis.

Syphilis. An infectious venereal disease caused by *Treponema pallidum*.

Syphilomania. A morbid dread of syphilis.

Syringe. An instrument for injecting fluids into the body.

Syringo- (Gk *syrinx:* pipe, cleft). Prefix indicating association with a tube or fistula.

Syringobulbia. Syringomyelia which has spread upwards into the medulla oblongata.

Syringocystadenoma papilliferum. An adenoma of the apocrine ducts that occurs as a yellowish papilliferous lesion with crusting on the scalp.

Syringoma. A pinhead, yellowish soft nodule which develops in and around the eyelids, on the chest and abdomen in women. (*Plural:* syringomata.) It is an adenoma of the sweat glands.

Syringomyelia. A chronic and slowly progressive disease of the spinal cord, characterized by cavitation and gliosis in the spinal cord, with wasting of the upper limbs, spastic paresis of the lower limbs, and sensory loss.

Syrosingopine. The B.P. Commission approved name for methyl *O*-(4-ethoxycarbonyloxy-3,5 -dimethoxybenzoyl)reserpate. A hypotensive agent.

Syrup. A concentrated aqueous solution of sucrose, or other sugars, to which medicaments or flavourings may be added. **Syrup, B.P.** 1968, a preparation containing 667 grammes of sucrose in purified water sufficient to produce 1000 grammes (i.e. 66·7 per cent w/w of sucrose. **Tolu syrup,** B.P. 1968, a preparation of 1 in 80 tolu balsam, used to flavour cough mixtures. The *British Pharmaceutical Codex*, 1968 contains 13 syrups: Black currant syrup; Chloral syrup; Codeine phosphate syrup; Compound ferrous sulphate syrup; Ferrous phosphate, quinine and strychnine syrup; Compound fig syrup; Ginger syrup; Invert syrup; Lemon syrup; Orange syrup; Raspberry syrup; Squill syrup; Wild cherry syrup.

System. A method of classification. A set of interconnected parts. **Autonomic nervous system,** that part of the nervous system which controls the activity of those parts of the body not under voluntary control. It is made up of the parasympathetic and the sympathetic nervous systems. **Cardiovascular system,** the heart and blood vessels. **Central nervous system,** the spinal cord, medulla oblongata, pons, cerebellum, midbrain, and cerebrum. **Chromaffin system,** the medulla of the suprarenal glands, the paraganglia, the para-aortic bodies, and small masses of chromaffin cells scattered throughout the body. Their distinguishing feature is that all contain chromaffin cells, which secrete adrenaline and noradrenaline. **Conducting system of the heart,** the sinu-atrial node, the atrioventricular node and bundle and its two limbs, together with the subendocardial plexuses of Purkinje fibres in the ventricles. **Digestive system,** all the organs which are concerned in the mastication swallowing and digestion of food and in the elimination from the body of the unabsorbed and unabsorbable constituents. **Extrapyramidal nervous system,** the various pathways for impulses which unconsciously modify the activities of the pyramidal system: (i) a system of grey matter involving the cerebral cortex, corpus striatum and numerous nuclear masses in the reticular formation in the brain stem; (ii) olivospinal tracts; (iii) medial longitudinal bundles; (iv) tectobulbar and tectospinal tracts; (v) vestibulo-spinal tracts; (vi) cerebellum; (vii) reflex pathways. **Haemopoietic system,** the tissues concerned with the production of blood, including the bone marrow, lymph nodes and the spleen. **Haversian system,** a unit of compact bone, consisting of a central canal surrounded by concentric lamellae of bony tissue. **Lymphatic system,** the lymph capillaries, lymph nodes, and collections of lymphoid tissue situated in the walls of the alimentary tract and in the spleen and thymus. **Motor nervous system,** the cortico-spinal (pyramidal), corticonuclear and extrapyramidal fibres which control the voluntary motor activity of the body. **Parasympathetic nervous system,** the smaller subdivision. of the autonomic nervous system The visceral efferent component has a limited origin from the cranial and sacral ends of the central nervous system, but a wide distribution. The afferent reflex afferent fibres are concerned in the normal reflex control of the viscera. Others are concerned with organic visceral sensation: e.g. hunger, sexual sensations. Others carry visceral pain fibres. **Peripheral nervous system,** the efferent, or centripetal, fibres which connect the sensory end-organs to the central nervous system, and the efferent, or centrifugal, fibres which connect the central nervous system to the effector apparatus. **Portal system of veins,** all the veins which drain the blood from the abdominal part of the digestive tube (with the exception of the lower part of the anal canal) and from the spleen, pancreas and gall-bladder. **Pyramidal nervous system,** the axis cylinder processes of the large pyramidal cells of the motor area of the cortex, which, as the corticospinal fibres, descend to the pyramid of the medulla oblongata where some of them cross over to the opposite side and descend in the spinal cord as the lateral corticospinal tract, while the remainder descend in the same side of the spinal cord as the anterior corticospinal tract. **Respiratory system,** the two lungs, the nasal cavities, the pharynx, the larynx, and the trachea and its divisions. **Sensory nervous system,** fibres conveying interoceptive sensitivity from the viscera, proprioceptive sensibility from the muscles, tendons and joints, exteroceptive sensibility from the surface of the body. **Skeletal system,** the skeleton. **Somatic nervous system,** the afferent and efferent neurones concerned with the innervation of the skin, skeletal muscles and their tendons, joints and associated connective tissues. **Splanchnic nervous system,** the afferent and efferent neurones concerned with the innervation of the viscera, glands and blood vessels. **Sympathetic nervous system,** the larger subdivision of the autonomic nervous system, which includes the two ganglionated sympathetic trunks, their branches, plexuses and subsidiary ganglia. **Urogenital system,** the urinary organs (kidneys, ureters, urinary bladder, and urethra), and the genital organs (testes, epididymes, deferent ducts, seminal vesicles, ejaculatory ducts, penis, prostate and bulbo-urethral glands in the male; ovaries, uterine tubes, uterus, vagina, labia majora and minora, pudendi, clitoris, bulb of the vestibule and the greater vestibular glands in the female). **Visceral nervous system,** splanchnic nervous system.

Systole. The contraction, or period of contraction, of the heart.

T

Tabanidae. A family of the suborder Brachycera, flies with a worldwide distribution, and popularly known as horse flies, gad flies, and clegs. It includes the genus Chrysops.

Tabanus. A genus of biting flies of the family Tabanidae.

Tabardillo. The name given to murine typhus in Mexico.

Tabes. A wasting disease. **Tabes dorsalis,** a form of neurosyphilis, characterized by ataxia and sensory disturbances resulting from involvement of the posterior columns of the spinal cord. Locomotor ataxia. **Tabes mesenterica,** tuberculosis of the mesenteric lymphatic glands.

Tablet. A compact product containing a medicament or a mixture of medicaments in a moulded or compressed form.

Taboparesis. The condition in which the manifestations of tabes dorsalis and general paralysis of the insane are combined in whole or in part.

Tache. A spot or mark. **Tache cérébrale,** a bright red line of congestion produced when the finger nail is drawn across the patient's skin in certain cerebral diseases, including meningitis.

Tachy- (Gk *tachys:* swift). Prefix meaning rapid.

Tachycardia. Rapid action of the heart. **Paroxysmal tachycardia,** bouts of tachycardia that begin and end suddenly. They may be atrial, nodal, or ventricular, depending upon their site of origin in the heart. **Sinus tachycardia,** simple tachycardia, originating like the normal heart beat, in the sinu-atrial node.

Tachylalia. Rapid speaking.

Tachyphagia. Rapid eating.

Tachyphylaxis. Rapid production of immunity.

Tachypnoea. Rapid breathing.

Tacrine. The B.P. Commission approved name for 9-amino-1,2,3,4-tetrahydroacridine. A central nervous system stimulant.

Tactile. Pertaining to the sense of touch.

Taenia. A genus of tapeworms. *Taenia saginata,* the beef tapeworm, acquired by eating inadequately cooked infested beef. *Taenia solium,* the pork tapeworm acquired by eating measly pork. *Taenia taeniaformis,* a tapeworm that infects cats.

Taenia. A band. (*Plural:* taeniae.) **Taeniae coli,** three bands of longitudinal muscle fibres in the large intestine. **Taenia fornicis,** the free medial edge of the fimbria of the hippocampus. **Taenia of the 4th ventricle,** a narrow white ridge on each side of the floor of the 4th ventricle. **Taenia libera,** one of the taenia coli. **Taenia mesocolica,** one of the taenia coli. **Taenia omentalis,** one of the taenia coli. **Taenia pontis,** a thin white band on the surface of the crus cerebri. **Taenia thalami,** the sharp angle between the medial and superior surfaces of the thalamus.

Taeniafuge. A procedure that expels tapeworms.

Taeniasis. Infestation with tapeworms.

Taenicide. A drug or measure that kills tapeworms.

Taeniidae. A family of the Cestode order that includes the following genera that affect man: Taenia, Multiceps, and Echinococcus.

Tail. The caudal extremity. A slender appendage. **Tail of the caudate nucleus,** the posterior end of the caudate nucleus. **Tail of the dentate gyrus,** the transverse portion of the gyrus. **Tail of the embryo,** the caudal end of the embryo which appears during the 3rd week and begins to disappear during the 7th or 8th week. **Tail of the epididymis,** the lower pointed end of the epididymis. **Tail of the mammary gland,** the upward, lateral prolongation of the superolateral part of the breast. **Tail of the pancreas,** the narrow left extremity of the gland which lies in contact with the spleen.

Talc, purified. B.P. 1968. A purified native magnesium silicate. Talc. Purified French chalk. A dusting powder.

Talipes. Club-foot. A congenital

deformity of the foot, in which the foot is permanently twisted out of shape. **Talipes calcaneovalgus,** the form in which the heel is drawn upwards and the sole everted outwards. **Talipes calcaneus,** the form in which the individual walks on the heel alone. **Talipes equinovarus,** the form in which the heel is drawn upwards and the sole is inverted. **Talipes equinus,** the form in which the heel is drawn upwards and the individual walks on the toes. **Talipes valgus,** the form in which the foot is elevated and the individual walks on the inside of the foot. **Talipes varus,** the form in which the foot is inverted and the individual walks on the outside of the foot.

Talo- (L *talus:* ankle). Prefix signifying association with the talus.

Taloximine. The B.P. Commission approved name for 4-(2-dimethylaminoethoxy)-1,2-dihydro-1-hydroxyiminophthalazine. A respiratory stimulant.

Talus. The bone which forms the principal connecting link between the foot and the bones of the leg. Placed above the calcaneus it articulates with the tibia and fibula to form the ankle joint.

Tambour. A cylinder with a drum-like membrane stretched over the open end, and incorporated into various instruments as a means of recording variations of pressure.

Tampon. A pack or plug made of cotton or some comparable material and used as a plug: e.g. in the nose or vagina.

Tamponade. The insertion of a tampon. **Cardiac tamponade,** the symptoms and signs of cardiac distress induced by compression of the heart by a rapidly increasing amount of fluid in the pericardial cavity.

Tan. The brownish coloration of the skin induced by exposure to sun, wind, or artificial ultraviolet light.

Tannate. A salt or ester of tannic acid.

Tannic acid. B.P. 1968. Prepared from oak galls. Tannin. An astringent.

Tannin. Tannic acid.

Tantalum. A non-corrosive metallic element. Symbol Ta. Atomic weight 180·95. Atomic number 73. Being non-corrosive and malleable, it is used as an implant: e.g. for repairing defects in the skull.

Tapetum. A layer or membrane.

Tapeworm. A member of the class Cestoda. There are five orders of tapeworms, but only two affect man: Pseudophyllidea, and Cyclophyllidea. It is an intestinal parasite consisting of a chain of segments and a scolex, or head.

Taphophobia. A morbid dread of being buried alive.

Tapioca. A preparation of cassava, from which most of the protein has been removed, and therefore consisting almost entirely of starch.

Tapotement. A movement in massage, consisting of striking with the side of the curved hand.

Tapping. Paracentesis. The removal of fluid from a cavity by means of a trocar and cannula. A series of sudden slight blows in massage.

Tar. B.P. 1968. The bituminous liquid obtained from the wood of the Scots pine *Pinus sylvestris* and other trees of the family Pinaceae. Stockholm tar. An antipruritic used in the treatment of certain chronic skin diseases such as psoriasis. **Prepared coal tar,** B.P. 1968, obtained by heating commercial tar. It has the same uses as tar.

Tarantula. A spider. A term usually restricted to biting spiders, which may or may not be venomous.

Taraxacum. A species of plants which includes the dandelion (*Taraxacum officinale*).

Tars-, Tarso- (Gk *tarsos:* a broad flat surface). Prefixes indicating relationship to the edge of the eyelid or the instep of the foot.

Tarsal. Pertaining to the tarsus of the eyelid or the foot.

Tarsalgia. Pain in the tarsus of the foot.

Tarsectomy. Surgical excision of the tarsus of the foot or of the eye.

Tarsitis. Inflammation of the tarsus of the eyelid or of the foot.

Tarsorrhaphy. Suturing together the eyelids to provide protection for the cornea.

Tarsus. (i) The seven short bones which compose the skeleton of the posterior half of the foot: talus, calcaneus, medial cuneiform, intermediate cuneiform, lateral cuneiform, cuboid, and navicular. (ii) The thin elongated plate of fibrous tissue in the eyelid. (*Plural:* tarsi.)

Tartar. A deposition on the teeth of the organic constituents of saliva, along with calcium and magnesium salts and food particles. **Cream of tartar,** potassium acid tartrate.

Tartaric acid. B.P. 1968. $C_4H_6O_6$. A saline purgative and constituent of effervescing powders and granules and cooling drinks.

Tartrate. A salt or ester of tartaric acid.

Tasikinesia. Inability to keep still.

Taste. The sensation produced by appropriate stimulation of the taste receptors, or taste buds, which are situated mainly on the peripheral parts of the dorsum of the tongue.

Tattooing. Indelible colouring of the skin.

Taurocholate. A salt or ester of taurocholic acid.

Taurocholic acid. $C_{26}H_{45}NSO_7$. One of the organic acids in bile.

Taurolin. The B.P. Commission approved name for 4,4′-methylenedi (tetrahydro-1, 2, 4-thiadiazine-1-dioxide). An antibacterial agent.

Tauto- (Gk *tauto:* the same). Prefix meaning the same.

Taxis. Reduction of a hernia by means of manipulation.

Taxonomy. The classification of plants and animals.

Tea. The dried leaves of *Thea sinensis*, the principal constituents of which are caffeine and tannin. The infusion made from tea. **Beef tea,** an infusion of lean beef.

Tears. The secretion of the lacrimal glands.

Teat. A nipple.

Technetium. A radioactive element. Symbol Tc. Atomic weight 99. Atomic number 43.

Teclothiazide. The B.P. Commission approved name for 6-chloro-3,4-dihydro-3-trichloromethyl-1,2,4-benzothiadiazine-7-sulphonamide 1,1-dioxide. A diuretic.

Tectospinal. Pertaining to the tectum of the midbrain and the spinal cord.

Tectum. A roof, or covering. **Tectum of the midbrain,** the colliculi.

Tegmen. A roof or covering. (*Plural:* tegmina.) **Tegmen tympani,** a thin lamella of bone that forms the roof of the tympanic cavity.

Tegmentum. A roof or covering. (*Plural:* tegmenta.) **Tegmentum of mesencephalon,** the dorsal part of the cerebral peduncle with the exception of the colliculi.

Teichopsia. The zig-zag coloured lines seen during a migrainous attack. Fortification spectra.

Tel-, Tele-, Telo- (Gk *tēle:* far off; *telos:* end). Prefixes signifying distance or end.

Tela. A web, or web-like structure. (*Plural:* telae.) **Tela choroidea,** a double layer of pia mater containing the highly vascular fringes forming the choroid plexus, present in the 3rd and 4th ventricles of the brain.

Telangiectasia. The condition characterized by the presence of telangiectases. **Hereditary haemorrhagic telangiectasia,** a hereditary disease characterized by recurrent bleeding from multiple telangiectases. **Multiple familial haemorrhagic telangiectasia,** a condition characterized by the presence of multiple telangiectases and haemangiomas in the skin and mucous membrane.

Telangiectasis. A dilatation of capillaries and/or arterioles. (*Plural:* telangiectases.)

Telangiitis. Inflammation of the capillaries.

Telemetry. The process of measuring at a distance.

Telencephalon. The cerebral hemispheres, with their commissures and cavities, the anterior parts of the hypothalamus and the 3rd ventricle.

Telepathy. Extrasensory perception of the thought processes of others.

Teleradiography. Radiography of the body with the x-ray tube $6\frac{1}{2}$ to 7 feet (200 to 215cm.) from the body.

Tellurate. A salt of telluric acid.

Telluric. Pertaining to the soil or to tellurium.

Tellurite. A salt of tellurous acid.

Tellurium. A semi-metallic element. Symbol Te. Atomic weight 127·60. Atomic number 52.

Telodendron. The terminal filament of an axon. (*Plural:* telodendria.)

Telophase. The final phase of mitosis.

Temazepam. The B.P. Commission approved name for 7-chloro-3-hydroxy-1-methyl-5-phenyl-1*H*-1, 4-benzodiazepin-2(3*H*)-one. A tranquillizer.

Temperature. The degree of heat of a body as measured by a thermometer. **Absolute temperature,** the temperature reckoned from absolute zero ($-273\cdot16°C$) **Axillary temperature,** body temperature as recorded in the axilla. **Body temperature,** the internal temperature of the body. **Critical temperature,** the temperature below which a gas can be reduced to a liquid by pressure. **Dry-bulb temperature,** the temperature of the air as recorded by a thermometer, the bulb of which has been kept dry. **Mouth temperature,** body temperature as recorded in the mouth. **Normal temperature,** body temperature of a healthy individual at rest (98·4°F;

37°C) **Rectal temperature,** internal temperature of the body as recorded in the rectum. **Wet-bulb temperature,** the temperature of the air as recorded on a thermometer, the bulb of which has been kept moist.

Template. A mould or cast.

Temple. The upper part of the side of the head above the zygoma and anterior to the ear.

Temporal. Pertaining to the temple or to time. **Temporal bone,** a bone situated at the side and base of the skull, consisting of squamous, petromastoid and tympanic parts and the styloid process.

Temporo- (L *tempus, tempora:* time). Prefix signifying relationship to the temple or to the temporal lobe of the brain.

Tenaculum. A hook-like surgical instrument for picking up or holding parts such as a blood vessel. (*Plural:* tenacula.)

Tendinitis. Inflammation of a tendon.

Tendon. The tough, whitish, almost inextensible cord consisting of numerous parallel fascicles of collagen fibres, by which a muscle is attached to a bone or other structure. **Tendo calcaneus,** the thickest, strongest tendon in the body, which fixes the gastrocnemius and soleus to the calcaneus. **Central tendon of the diaphragm,** a trefoil-shaped tendon situated near the centre of the vault of the diaphragm. **Conjoint tendon of the internal oblique and transversus,** a tendon mainly formed by the lower part of the aponeurosis of the transversus, which descends behind the superficial inguinal ring.

Tendovaginitis. Tenosynovitis.

Tenesmus. Ineffectual, painful straining at stool.

Teno-, Tenonto- (Gk *tenōn, tenontos:* tendon). Prefixes signifying relationship to a tendon.

Tenorraphy. The operation for suturing together the ends of a ruptured tendon.

Tenosynovitis. Inflammation of a tendon.

Tenotomy. Surgical incision of a tendon.

Tensor. A muscle that stretches or tenses. (*Plural:* tensores.)

Tent. A plug for dilating a narrow opening. A covering.

Tentorium. A tent. (*Plural:* tentoria.) **Tentorium cerebelli,** a crescentic arched lamina of dura mater that covers the cerebellum and supports the occipital lobes of the cerebrum.

Ter- (L *ter:* three). Prefix meaning three or thrice.

Tera-, Terato- (Gk *teras, teratos:* monster). Prefixes signifying relationship to a monster.

Teratogenesis, Teratogeny. The production of physical defects in the foetus.

Teratology. The study of the embryonic development of malformations.

Teratoma. A tumour consisting of multiple tissues foreign to the part from which it arises. (*Plural:* teratomata.)

Teratophobia. Morbid fear of giving birth to a monster. Abnormal aversion to deformity.

Teratospermia. Abnormality of spermatozoa.

Terbium. A metallic element. Symbol Tb. Atomic weight 158·93. Atomic number 65.

Terbutaline. The B.P. Commission approved name for 1-(3,5-dihydroxyphenyl)-2-(t-butylamino)ethanol. A bronchodilator.

Terebene. A colourless fluid with a smell like fresh pine sawdust, prepared by the action of sulphuric acid on turpentine, and used as a deodorant and as an inhalation in bronchitis and nasal catarrh.

Teres. Round and elongated. A muscle that is round and elongated. (*Plural:* teretes.)

Tergum. The back.

Terpene. Any unsaturated hydrocarbon of the formula $C_{10}H_{16}$, derived from essential oils and resins.

Terpineol. B.P.C. 1968. $C_{10}H_{18}O$. An antiseptic with solvent properties.

Terpin hydrate. B.P.C. 1968. $C_{10}H_{20}O_2$, H_2O. An inhibitor of cough and sputum.

Tertian. Recurring every third day.

Tertigravida. A woman pregnant for the third time.

Tertipara. A woman who has had three pregnancies resulting in three live children.

Tesla. The unit of magnetic flux density, being 1 weber per square metre of circuit area.

Testalgia. Pain in the testes.

Testicle. Testis.

Testicular. Pertaining to a testis.

Testis. The male gonad. (*Plural:* testes.) The two testes, each, on average, 4 to 5cm. long, 2·5cm in breadth and 3cm. in depth, and weighing 10 to 14 grammes, are suspended in the scrotum by the spermatic cords.

Test meal. A test of gastric function.

Augmented histamine test meal, the analysis of gastric secretion collected before and after the administration of histamine. Insulin test meal, the analysis of gastric secretion after the administration of insulin. Tubeless test meal, a method of gastric analysis dependent upon the liberation of quinine from either a quinine salt or a quinine-resin complex by free gastric hydrochloric acid.

Testosterone. B.P. 1968. $C_{19}H_{28}O_2$. The androgenic hormone formed in the interstitial cells of the testes, which controls the development and maintenance of the male gonads and secondary sex characteristics. Testosterone implants, B.P. 1968, sterile cylinders containing 100mg. of testosterone, implanted subcutaneously in order to achieve prolonged action. Testosterone phenylpropionate, B.P. 1968, $C_{28}H_{36}O_3$, a preparation with an action similar to that of testosterone but more potent and longer acting. It is given subcutaneously or intramuscularly. Testosterone propionate, B.P. 1968, $C_{22}H_{32}O_3$, a preparation with an action similar to that of testosterone, but inactive by mouth. It is given intramuscularly.

Test-tube. A tube of thin glass, closed at one end, and used in chemical analysis.

Tetanic. Pertaining to, or of the nature of, tetanus. Inducing tetanus.

Tetano- (Gk *tanos:* convulsive tension). Prefix indicating relationship to tetanus.

Tetanolysin. The haemolytic exotoxin of *Clostridium tetani.*

Tetanospasmin. The neurotoxin in *Clostridium tetani* responsible for the convulsions of tetanus.

Tetanus. An infectious disease of the central nervous system caused by *Clostridium tetani,* and characterized by paroxysms of muscle spasm superimposed on an increased muscular rigidity. The spasm is most marked in the masseter muscles. Hence the alternative name of lockjaw. A sustained tonic spasm of a muscle. Tetanus antitoxin, B.P. 1968, a preparation from native serum containing the antitoxic globulins or their derivatives that have the specific power of neutralizing the toxin formed by *Cl. tetani.* Tetanus vaccine, B.P.C. 1968, vaccine prepared from tetanus toxin produced by the growth of *Cl. tetani.* It is available as *Tetanus vaccine in simple solutions; Alum pre-*cipitated tetanus vaccine; Purified toxoid aluminium phosphate; Purified toxoid alumiuium hydroxide. Tetanus and pertussis vaccine, B.P. 1968, a mixture of tetanus vaccine in simple solution and pertussis vaccine.

Tetany. A disease characterized by intermittent fibrillary twitchings and spasm of muscle, usually caused by a fall in the ionic calcium of the blood, and which may result from alkalosis, parathyroid hypofunction, or vitamin D deficiency.

Tetr-, Tetra- (Gk *tetra:* four). Prefixes meaning four.

Tetrabenazine. The B.P. Commission approved name for 1,3,4,6,7,11b-hexahydro-3-isobutyl-9,10-dimethoxy-benzo[α] quinolizin-2-one. A tranquillizer.

Tetrachloride. A chloride which contains four atoms of chlorine.

Tetrachloroethylene. B.P. 1968 $CCl_2:CCl_2$. A drug used in the treatment of hookworm.

Tetracosactrin, The B.P. Commission approved name for a synthetic corticotrophin.

Tetracycline. B.P.C. 1968. $C_{22}H_{24}N_2O_8$. A hydrated form of tetracycline hydrochloride, which is used in the preparation of oral liquid preparations of the antibiotic. Tetracycline hydrochloride, B.P. 1968, $C_{22}H_{25}CEN_2O_8$, an antibiotic that may be obtained from chlortetracycline or oxytetracycline, or by the growth of certain strains of *Streptomyces aureofaciens.* It is one of the broad-spectrum antibiotics effective, orally as well as parenterally, against a wide range of bacteria, both gram-positive and gram-negative. Tetracycline phosphate complex, the B.P. Commission approved name for a complex of tetracycline and sodium metaphosphate which is better absorbed orally than tetracycline.

Tetrad. An element with a valency of four.

Tetradactyly. Having four digits on a hand or foot.

Tetrahydrozoline. The B.P. Commission approved name for 2-(1,2,3,4-tetrahydro-1-naphthyl)-2-imidazoline. A vasoconstrictor.

Tetralogy. A collection of four. Tetralogy of Fallot, the congenital heart condition characterized by pulmonary stenosis, interventricular septal defect, overriding of the interventricular septum by the aorta, right ventricular hypertrophy.

Tetrascelus. A foetal monster with four legs.

Tetravalent. Having a valency of four.

Thalamencephalon. The thalamus, metathalamus and epithalamus. The interbrain.

Thalamo- (Gk *thalamos:* chamber). Prefix signifying relationship to a chamber, particularly the thalamus.

Thalamolenticular. Pertaining to the thalamus and the lenticular nucleus.

Thalamomammillary. Pertaining to the thalamus and the mammillary bodies.

Thalamotomy. Surgical destruction of circumscribed areas in the thalamus, performed for the amelioration of certain psychotic conditions.

Thalamus. A large ovoid mass of grey matter on each side of the 3rd ventricle, which acts as an important sensory relay station. (*Plural:* thalami.)

Thalass- (Gk *thalassa:* the sea). Prefix signifying relationship to the sea.

Thalassaemia. A haemolytic anaemia found typically in Mediterranean peoples due to a dominant Mendelian inherited abnormality of haemoglobin caused by abnormalities of globin production.

Thalassophobia. Morbid fear of the sea.

Thalassotherapy. Treatment by sea bathing, sea voyages or residence by the sea.

Thalidomide. The B.P. Commission approved name for 2-phthalimidoglutarimide. A sedative that was withdrawn from use because of the high incidence of deformed foetuses it produced when given to pregnant women.

Thallium. A metallic element. Symbol Tl. Atomic weight 204·39. Atomic number 81. Its salts are highly toxic.

Thanato- (Gk *thanatos:* death). Prefix signifying association with death.

Thanatology. The study of death.

Thanatophobia. Abnormally morbid dread of death.

Thea. Tea.

Thebacon. The B.P. Commission approved name for a narcotic analgesic and cough suppressant.

Thebaine. $C_{19}H_{21}NO_3$. One of the alkaloids in opium.

Theca. A sheath. (*Plural:* thecae). **Theca folliculi,** the sheath formed round the follicle by the stromal cells of the cortex of the ovary.

Thenalidine. The B.P. Commission approved name for an antihistaminic.

Thenar. The fleshy mass at the base of the thumb. **Thenar eminence.** Pertaining to the palm.

Thenium closylate. The B.P. Commission approved name for dimethyl-(2-phenoxyethyl)-2-thenylammonium. An anthelmintic.

Thenyldiamine. The B.P. Commission approved name for $N'N'$-dimethyl-N -2 -pyridyl -N -3 -thenylethylenediamine. An antihistaminic.

Theo- (Gk *theos:* a god). Prefix signifying association with god.

Theobroma, prepared. B.P.C. 1968. The roasted seed of *Theobroma cacao,* used as a chocolate base for tablets. **Theobroma oil,** B.P. 1968, the solid fat expressed from the roasted seeds of *Theobroma cacao.* It is used for the preparation of bougies, pessaries and suppositories.

Theobromine. B.P.C. 1968. $C_7H_8N_4O_2$. An alkaloid contained in the seeds of *Theobroma cacao,* which has an action on the kidneys like that of caffeine, but no stimulant action on the central nervous system.

Theodrenaline. The B.P. Commission approved name for $7\text{-}[2\text{-}(3,4,\beta\text{-}trihydroxyphenethylamino})$ ethyl] theophylline. An analeptic.

Theomania. Religious insanity.

Theophylline. B.P. 1968. $C_7H_8N_4O_2$. An alkaloid isomeric with theobromine, which has a diuretic action and is a relaxant of involuntary muscle. **Theophylline hydrate,** B.P. 1968, $C_7H_8N_4O_2,H_2O$. The monohydrate of theophylline, with the same action.

Theotherapy. The treatment of disease by prayer and religious exercises.

Therapeutics. That branch of medicine concerned with treatment.

Therapy. Treatment.

Therm. A unit of heat energy equivalent to 100,000 British Thermal Units. A British Thermal Unit (B.T.U.) is the amount of heat necessary to raise 1 pound of water 10°F.

Therm-, Thermo- (Gk *thermē:* heat). Prefixes signifying relationship to heat.

Thermalgia. A burning pain or sensation.

Thermoalgesia. Excessive sensitivity to heat.

Thermoanaesthesia. Loss of sensibility to heat.

Thermocoagulation. The process of inducing destruction of tissues, such as tumours, by means of coagulation of the tissues by high-frequency currents.

Thermocouple. An instrument for

recording slight changes of temperature.

Thermodynamics. The branch of science concerned with the study of heat and its relationship to other forms of energy.

Thermogenesis. The production of heat.

Thermograph. An instrument for recording changes in temperature. The instrument used in thermography.

Thermography. The method whereby the patterns of emissions of infra-red radiation by the skin are converted into electric signals which are recorded on an oscilloscope, and used as a diagnostic measure, particularly in cancer of the breast.

Thermolabile. Subject to alteration by heat.

Thermometer. An instrument for measuring temperature. **Air thermometer,** a thermometer in which air is the expansible substance. **Alcohol thermometer,** a thermometer in which the indicator is alcohol. **Centigrade thermometer,** a thermometer calibrated in the Centigrade scale, in which the boiling point of water is 100°, and the freezing point is 0°. **Clinical thermometer,** the thermometer used for recording body temperature. **Fahrenheit thermometer,** a thermometer calibrated in the Fahrenheit scale, in which the boiling point of water is 212°, and the freezing point is 32°. **Katathermometer,** see Katathermometer. **Maximum and minimum thermometer,** a thermometer which records the maximum and minimum temperature in a given period. **Mercury thermometer,** a thermometer in which mercury is the indicator. **Reaumur thermometer,** a thermometer calibrated in the Reaumur scale, in which the boiling point of water is 80° and the freezing point 0°.

Thermophilic. Preferring heat. Thriving in heat.

Thermophore. An appliance for the local application of heat which retains heat for several hours.

Thermopile. An instrument for measuring radiant heat.

Thermoreceptor. A nerve ending sensitive to heat.

Thermoscope. An instrument for indicating slight differences of temperature.

Thermostabile. Not subject to alteration by heat.

Thermostat. An apparatus for the automatic controlling of temperature.

Thermotaxis. The reaction of an organism to heat as judged by its movement to, or away from, it.

Thiabendazole. B.P.C. 1968, Supplement 1971. $C_{10}H_7N_3S$. An anthelmintic.

Thiacetazone. B.P.C. 1968, Supplement 1971. $C_{10}H_{12}N_4OS$. An anti-tuberculosis drug, and anti-leprosy drug.

Thiaemia. The presence of excessive sulphur in the blood.

Thialbarbitone. The B.P. Commission approved name for 5-allyl-5-(cyclohex-2-enyl)-2-thiobarbituric acid. A short-acting barbiturate used as a basal anaesthetic for the production of general anaesthesia of short duration.

Thiambutosine. B.P. 1968. $C_{19}H_{25}N_3OS$. An oral preparation for the treatment of leprosy.

Thiamine hydrochloride, B.P. 1968. $C_{12}H_{18}Cl_2N_4OS$. Vitamin B_1. Widely distributed in foods, the richest sources being whole grains, pulses, yeast and pork, it plays an essential role in carbohydrate metabolism. The major deficiency disease is beri-beri.

Thiazesim. The B.P. Commission approved name for 5-(2-dimethylaminoethyl)-2,3-dihydro-2-phenyl-1,5-benzothiazepin-4-one. An anti-depressant.

Thiazole. An organic heterocyclic compound bound upon a ring consisting of a sulphur atom, a nitrogen atom and three CH rings.

Thiethylperazine. The B.P. Commission approved name for 2-ethylthio-10-[3-(4-methylpiperazin-1-yl)propyl]-phenothiazine. A central nervous system depressant.

Thigh. The portion of the lower limb between the hip and the knee.

Thio- (Gk *theion:* sulphur). Prefix indicating association with sulphur.

Thio-acid. An organic acid in which sulphur replaces one or more of the oxygen atoms.

Thiocarlide. The B.P. Commission approved name for NN'-di-(4-isopentyloxyphenyl) thiourea. An anti-tuberculosis drug.

Thiochrome. The yellow pigment of yeast which fluoresces, and is an oxidation product of thiamine.

Thiol. The univalent radical — SH. An organic compound containing the — SH radical.

Thiomersal. B.P. 1968. $C_9H_9HgNaO_2S$. An antiseptic, fungicide, and preservative.

Thiomesterone. The B.P. Commission approved name for 1α,7-bis(acetyl-thio)-17β-hydroxy-17α-methylandrost-4-en-3-one. An anabolic steroid.

Thionic. Pertaining to sulphur.

Thionine. A purple stain used in microscopy.

Thiopentone sodium. B.P. 1968. $C_{11}H_{17}N_2NaO_2S$. A short-acting barbiturate administered intravenously for the induction of general anaesthesia, or for the induction of general anaesthesia for a short period.

Thiophilic. Having an affinity for sulphur.

Thiopropazate hydrochloride. B.P.C. 1968. $C_{23}H_{30}Cl_3N_3O_2S$. A tranquillizer.

Thioproperazine. The B.P. Commission approved name for 2-dimethylsulpha-moyl-10-[3-(4-methylpiperazin-1-yl)-propyl] phenothiazine. A tranquillizer and anti-emetic.

Thioridazine hydrochloride. B.P. 1968. $C_{21}H_{27}ClN_2S_2$. A tranquillizer.

Thiosulphate. A salt of thiosulphuric acid ($H_2S_2O_3$).

Thiotepa. B.P. Addendum 1969. $C_6H_{12}N_3PS$. A cytotoxic agent used in the treatment of neoplastic disease.

Thiothixene. The B.P. Commission approved name for NN-dimethyl-9-[3-(4-methylpiperazin-1-yl)-propylidene] thioxanthen-2-sulphonamide. A tranquillizer.

Thioxolone. The B.P. Commission approved name for 6-hydroxy-1,3-benzoxathiol-2-one. A keratolytic agent.

Thirst. The sensation, characterized by dryness of the mouth and throat in the initial stages, induced by lack of water.

Thixotropy. The property of certain gels of becoming liquid on being shaken, and returning to the gel form on standing.

Thonzylamine. The B.P. Commission approved name for N-4-methoxyben-zyl-$N'N'$-dimethyl-N-pyrimidin-2-yl-ethylenediamine. An antihistaminic.

Thorac-, Thoraco- (Gk *thōrax, thōrakos:* chest). Prefixes signifying relationship to the chest.

Thoracectomy. Resection of part of a rib.

Thoracic. Pertaining to the chest.

Thoraco-abdominal. Pertaining to the thorax and the abdomen.

Thoraco-acromial. Pertaining to the thorax and the acromion.

Thoracocentesis. Withdrawal of fluid from the pleural cavity.

Thoracodidymus. Conjoined twins united at the thorax.

Thoracodynia. Pain in the chest. Pleurodynia.

Thoracolumbar. Pertaining to the thoracic and lumbar portions of the spine.

Thoracopagus. Conjoined twins united at the sternum.

Thoracoplasty. The surgical procedure of removing a varying number of ribs in order to induce collapse of the underlying lung.

Thoracoscope. An endoscope for examining the pleural cavity.

Thoracotomy. Surgical incision of the thoracic wall.

Thorax. The portion of the trunk between the neck and the diaphragm. (*Plural:* thoraces.) The chest. It is bounded behind by the 12 thoracic vertebrae and the posterior part of the ribs, laterally by the ribs, and anteriorly by the sternum, anterior ends of the ribs and the costal cartilages. The *inlet* is bounded by the 1st thoracic vertebra behind, the superior border of the manubrium sterni anteriorly and the 1st ribs laterally. The *outlet* is bounded by the 12th thoracic vertebra posteriorly, by the 11th and 12th ribs laterally, and the cartilages of the 7th-10th ribs anteriorly, and is closed by the diaphragm.

Thorium. A radioactive metal. Symbol Th. Atomic weight 232·05. Atomic number 90.

Thorium-X. A naturally occurring isotope of radium.

Thoron. A thorium emanation.

Threadworm. *Enterobius vermicularis.*

Threonine. α-Amino-β-hydroxy-butyric acid. One of the essential amino-acids.

Threpsology. The science of nutrition.

Threshold. The minimal level at which a stimulus takes effect. The critical level above which a substance is excreted or absorbed. The entrance to a canal or duct.

Thrill. A vibration felt on placing the hand or finger-tips on the body.

-thrix (Gk *thrix:* hair). Suffix signifying relationship to hair.

Throat. An ill-defined term, referring variously to the front of the neck, the fauces, the pharynx, and even the larynx.

Throm-, Thrombo- (Gk *thrombos:* clot). Prefixes indicating relationship with a clot.

Thrombasthenia. A rare congenital, haemorrhagic condition characterized by platelets that are normal in number but which can neither aggregate nor produce normal clot retraction.

Thrombectomy. Surgical excision of a thrombus.

Thrombin. An enzyme which can clot many hundred times its own weight of fibrinogen. Its precursor is pro-thrombin which is present in circulating blood and is converted to thrombin in the presence of calcium ions and thromboplastin.

Thrombo-angiitis obliterans. A disease of unknown etiology characterized by inflammation and thrombosis of the arteries and veins, particularly of the lower limbs. It occurs predominantly in male smokers.

Thrombocyte. Platelet.

Thrombocythaemia. An excess of platelets in the blood. **Haemorrhagic thrombocythaemia,** a haemorrhagic disease in adults in which there is a chronic elevation of the platelets, often to over 1 million per c.mm.

Thrombocytopenia. A reduction in the number of platelets in the blood. **Essential thrombocytopenia,** idiopathic thrombocytopenic purpura.

Thrombocytopenic. Characterized by a deficiency of platelets.

Thrombocytopoiesis. The process of formation of thrombocytes.

Thrombocytosis. An abnormally large number of platelets in the blood.

Thromboelastograph. An instrument for studying the rigidity of the blood during coagulation.

Thrombo-embolism. The formation of an embolus from a thrombus.

Thrombokinase. Thromboplastin.

Thrombolysis. Dissolution of a thrombus.

Thrombolytic. Inducing dissolution of a thrombus.

Thrombophlebitis. Inflammation of a vein combined with thrombus formation. **Thrombophlebitis migrans,** recurrent thrombotic episodes in the superficial and deep veins, especially of the extremities.

Thromboplastin. One of several factors present in the tissues and in the blood which, in the right form, and in the presence of calcium ions, converts prothrombin to thrombin and thereby initiates the clotting of blood. Thrombokinase.

Thrombosis. The formation of a solid mass in the circulation from the constituents of the blood.

Thrombus. A clot forming in a blood vessel or heart, and consisting of aggregated platelets and fibrin in which red and white blood cells are entrapped.

Thrush. Infection of the mucosa of the oropharynx with *Candida albicans.*

Thulium A rare metallic element. Symbol Tm. Atomic weight 168·94. Atomic number 69.

Thumb. The first digit on the radial side of the hand. It has only two phalanges.

Thurfyl nicotinate. The B.P. Commission approved name for tetrahydrofurfuryl nicotinate. A topical vasodilator.

Thymectomy. Surgical excision of the thymus.

-thymia (Gk *thymos:* mind). Suffix indicating association with mind.

Thymic. Pertaining to the thymus. **Thymic alymphoplasia,** the condition in which the thymus is absent or rudimentary. Thymic dysplasia. **Thymic aplasia,** absence of the thymus and the parathyroid glands.

Thymidine. The deoxyriboside of thymine, which can satisfy the metabolic requirements of *Lactobacillus lactis* and other organisms for vitamin B_{12}.

Thymine. 5-Methyl uracil.A pyrimidine base which is a constituent of deoxyribonucleic acid, and can replace folic acid as a growth factor for *Lactobacillus casei.*

Thymitis. Inflammation of the thymus.

Thymo- (Gk *thymos:* mind, thymus). Prefix indicating association with either the mind or the thymus.

Thymocyte. The lymphocyte of the thymus.

Thymol. B.P. 1968. $C_{10}H_{14}O$. It may be obtained by synthesis or from the volatile oils of *Thymus vulgaris, Monarda punctata,* or *Trachyspermum ammi.* An antiseptic and preservative.

Thymoma. A primary tumour of the thymus.

Thymosin. A lymphocytopoietic factor produced by the thymus.

Thymoxamine. The B.P. Commission approved name for 4-(2-dimethyl-aminoethoxy) -5 -isopropyl -2 -methylphenyl acetate. A peripheral vasodilator.

Thymus. A gland lying in the anterior and superior medistina of the thorax, which continues to grow until puberty, and then gradually atrophies. Its precise role is still uncertain, but it appears to play an important part in immunogenesis.

Thyro- (Gk *thyreoeidēs:* shield-shaped). Prefix indicating relationship to the thyroid gland.

Thyro-arytenoid. Pertaining to the thyroid gland and arytenoid cartilages.

Thyrocalcitonin. A hormone secreted

by the thyroid gland which helps to control the metabolism of calcium.

Thyrocele. A goitre.

Thyroglobulin. The characteristic iodine-containing protein in the colloid of the thyroid gland.

Thyroglossal. Pertaining to, or connecting, the thyroid gland and the tongue.

Thyrohyoid. Pertaining to the thyroid gland or cartilage and the hyoid bone.

Thyroid. The thyroid gland. (*See* Gland.)

Thyroid. B.P. 1968. Dried, powdered, defatted thyroid gland (*See* Gland) of the ox, sheep or pig, diluted with lactose to the required strength. It has the same action and uses, given orally, as thyroxine sodium. Also known as thyroid extract.

Thyroidectomy. Surgical excision of the thyroid gland.

Thyroiditis. Inflammation of the thyroid gland. **Hashimoto's thyroiditis,** an auto-immune disease characterized by chronic inflammatory changes in the thyroid gland resulting in enlargement of the gland and the development of hypothyroidism.

Thyrotoxicosis. The toxic condition induced by overaction of the thyroid gland, and characterized by nervousness, palpitations, tachycardia, loss of weight, excessive sweating and exophthalmos. Hyperthyroidism.

Thyrotrophic. Affecting the thyroid gland.

Thyrotrophin. The B.P. Commission approved name for the thyrotrophic hormone of the adenohypophysis, which is responsible for controlling the thyroid gland. Thyroid stimulating hormone. TSH.

Thyroxine sodium. B.P. 1968. $C_{15}H_{10}I_4$ $NNaO_4,5H_2O$. A synthetic iodine-containing compound possessing the physiological properties of thyroid (thyroid extract) and used in the treatment of hypothyroid states.

Tibia. The medial and larger of the two bones in the leg. (*Plural:* tibiae.)

Tibio- (L *tibia:* shinbone). Prefix indicating relationship to the tibia.

Tibiofibular. Pertaining to the tibia and fibula.

Tic. A repetitive twitching. **Tic douloureux,** trigeminal neuralgia.

Tick. A blood-sucking arachnoid of the super-family Ixodoidea, many of which are responsible for the transmission of disease to man and lower orders of animals.

Tiemonium iodide. The B.P. Commission approved name for an antispasmodic and anticholinergic.

Tigloidine. The B.P. Commission approved name for tiglylpseudotropeine. A drug for the treatment of parkinsonism.

Tiletamine. The B.P. Commission approved name for 2-ethylamino-2-(2-thienyl)cyclohexanone. An anticonvulsant and anaesthetic.

Time. A period during which a certain action takes place. **Bleeding time,** the time during which a stab puncture of the ear keeps bleeding or oozing. **Circulation time,** the time it takes for the circulating blood to pass through a given section of the vascular system. **Clotting time,** the time it takes for a drop of blood to coagulate under controlled conditions. **Coagulation time,** clotting time. **Forced expiratory time,** the shortest duration of expiration after a forced inspiration. **Prothrombin time,** the length of time taken for plasma to clot in the presence of an excess of thromboplastin and calcium ions.

Tin. A metallic element. Symbol Sn (L *stannum*). Atomic weight 118·70. Atomic number 50.

Tincture. An alcoholic liquid containing the active principle of a vegetable drug in comparatively low concentration. It is commonly prepared by maceration or percolation, but may be obtained by dilution of the corresponding liquid extract.

Tinea. Ringworm. A fungal infection of the skin or its appendages. **Tinea barbae,** ringworm of the beard. **Tinea capitis,** ringworm of the scalp. **Tinea circinata,** an annular form of ringworm of the body. **Tinea glabrosa,** ringworm of the glabrous skin. **Tinea pedis,** ringworm of the feet. **Tinea unguicum,** ringworm of the nails. **Tinea versicolor,** pityriasis versicolor.

Tinidazole. The B.P. Commission approved name for ethyl 2-(2-methyl-5-nitroimidazol-1-yl)ethyl sulphone. An anti-trichomonal agent.

Tinnitus. Subjective noises in the ear.

Tintometer. A colorimeter.

Tissue. A conglomeration of similar cells and their intercellular substance. **Adipose tissue,** connective tissue containing an abundance of fat cells. Fatty tissue. **Angioblastic tissue,** the embryonic tissue from which the blood corpuscles and blood vessels develop. **Areolar tissue,** the loose connective tissue, whose main function is to bind parts together. **Connective tissue,** tissue derived from the mesenchyme, consisting of cells embedded in a matrix or ground substance, whose main function is that of binding together or supporting functionally active structures. **Elastic yellow tissue,** a connective tissue in which yellow elastic fibres have developed to the practical exclusion of the other elements. **Epithelial tissue,** epithelium. **Epitheliolymphoid tissue,** the collections of lymphoid tissue situated in the walls of the alimentary tract. **Erectile tissue,** tissue containing large venous spaces connecting directly with arteries, as in the penis. **Fibro-areolar tissue,** tissue which has a higher proportion of collagenous fibres than are commonly present in areolar tissue. **Fibrous white tissue,** tissue, in which white fibres predominate, and which develops in response to tensile strains in situations in which strength is needed without rigidity or extensibility, as in ligaments and tendons. **Mucoid tissue,** a foetal type of connective tissue found chiefly as a stage in the development of connective tissue from mesenchyme, as in the umbilical cord, and consisting of a matrix largely composed of mucosubstances, in which are embedded nucleated cells with branching and anastomosing processes. **Muscular tissue,** tissue composed of bundles of reddish fibres endowed with the property of contractility. **Nervous tissue,** the tissue, consisting predominantly of neurones and neuroglia, of which the central nervous system and the peripheral nerves are composed. **Osteogenic tissue,** the layer of soft tissue in young bone separating the periosteum from the bone, and containing the osteoblasts by which ossification is achieved. **Reticular tissue,** a network of reticular fibres and reticular cells, found extensively in the body, forming the internal framework of many organs, including the liver, lungs, and kidneys. **Retiform tissue,** the tissue which supports and holds together the constituents of the intestinal villi. **Sclerous tissue,** the skeletal tissue of the body, consisting of bone and cartilage. **Sympathochromaffin tissue,** the tissue from which the sympathetic ganglia are formed. It contains masses of chromaffin cells, and includes the medulla of the suprarenal glands, the paraganglia, the para-aortic bodies,

and small masses of chromaffin cells scattered throughout the body. **Trabecular tissue,** loose connective tissue present in the subarachnoid space, and the sclera of the eye.

Titanium. A tough metallic element. Symbol Ti. Atomic weight 47·90. Atomic number 22.

Titanium dioxide. B.P.C. 1968. TiO_2. A preparation used in the treatment of dermatoses with exudation and pruritus. An ingredient of face powders.

Titration. Volumetric chemical analysis by means of standard solutions of known strength.

Titre. The amount of one substance which is equivalent to a stated amount of another. **Agglutination titre,** the highest dilution of a serum that will produce clumping of the relevant micro-organisms.

Titubant. A person who reels or staggers.

Tobacco. The dried leaf of *Nicotiana tabacum,* the chief constituent of which is nicotine.

Toco-, Toko- (Gk *tokos:* childbirth). Prefixes indicating association with childbirth.

Tocopherol. Vitamin E. It occurs in small amounts in most vegetables, in dairy produce and in meat. Wheatgerm oil is the richest source. There is no sound evidence that a deficiency syndrome occurs in man.

Toe. A digit of the foot. **Hammer toe,** a deformed toe in which the proximal interphalangeal joint is hyperflexed.

Tolazamide. The B.P. Commission approved name for 1,1-hexamethylene-4 - toluene - p - sulphonylsemicarbazide. An oral hypoglycaemic agent.

Tolazoline hydrochloride. B.P. 1968. $C_{10}H_{13}ClN_2$. A peripheral vasodilator.

Tolbutamide. B.P. 1968. $C_{12}H_{18}N_2O_3S$. An oral hypoglycaemic sulphonylurea.

Tolnaftate. B.P. Addendum 1969. $C_{19}H_{17}NOS$. A topical fungicide.

Tolpentamide. The B.P. Commission approved name for N-cyclopentyl-N'-toluene-p-sulphonylurea. A hypoglycaemic agent.

Tolpronine. The B.P. Commission. approved name for 1-(1, 2, 3, 6-tetra-hydro-1-pyridyl)-3-o-tobyloxypropan-2-ol. An analgesic.

Tolpropamine. The B.P. Commission approved name for NN-dimethyl-3-phenyl-3-p-topylpropylamine. An antipruritic.

Tolu balsam. B.P. 1968. A solid or semisolid balsam obtained by incision from the trunk of *Myroxylon balsamum*. In the form of Tolu syrup B.P. 1968 it is used to flavour cough mixtures.

Toluene. C_7H_8. Toluole. A highly inflammable distillation product of coal tar, used as a solvent.

Toluidine blue. A blue dye used in microscopy. **Toluidine blue O**, tolonium chloride. $C_{15}H_{16}ClN_3S$. An antidote to heparin.

Tolycaine. The B.P. Commission approved name for methyl 2-diethylaminoacetamido-*m*-toluate. A local anaesthetic.

Tomato. The fruit of *Lycopersicum esculentum*. A relatively rich source of vitamin C.

-tome (Gk *tomē:* a cutting). Suffix indicating an instrument for cutting, or a segment.

Tomo- (Gk *tomē:* a cutting). Prefix indicating relationship to a cutting.

Tomography. Sectional or body-section radiography. A technique whereby the shadow of a given plane can be clarified by a relative displacement of all other planes which are consequently blurred.

Tomotocia. Caesarean section.

-tomy (Gk *tomē:* a cutting). Suffix signifying a cutting operation.

Tone. The basic tension of resting muscle. The quality of a sound. Tonus.

Tongue. The muscular organ associated with the functions of speech, swallowing and taste which lies partly in the mouth and partly in the pharynx. The root of the tongue is attached to the hyoid bone and the mandible. **Black hairy tongue,** a tongue with elongated black or brown papillae, often due to a fungal infection. **Furred tongue,** a tongue coated with debris, a sign of indigestion, pyrexia, mouth-breathing, or dehydration. **Geographical tongue,** a tongue with areas of superficial desquamation, giving a map-like appearance; of no pathological significance. **Magenta tongue,** a purplish red discoloration, suggestive of riboflavine deficiency. **Parrot tongue,** the dried atrophied tongue seen in continued low fevers. **Raw-beef tongue,** the bright-red tongue seen in some cases of anaemia. **Strawberry tongue,** the white tongue with swollen red papillae, seen in scarlet fever. **Tongue-tie,** congenital shortening of the frenulum.

Tonic. In a state of continuous tension. Something that increases tone. A

conventional generic term for a medicinal preparation that by some means appears to increase an individual's sense of well-being.

Tono- (Gk *tonos:* tension). Prefix indicating association with tension or tone.

Tonofibril. A fine fibril which traverses the protoplasmic bridges that connect the cells in the stratum spinosum of the epidermis.

Tonography. The recording of intraocular pressure.

Tonometer. An instrument for measuring tension, particularly intra-ocular tension.

Tonsil. A rounded mass. When used alone, and particularly in the plural, it can be assumed to refer to the palatine tonsil. **Cerebellar tonsil,** a circumscribed portion of the cerebellum on its inferior aspect adjoining the uvula. **Lingual tonsil,** nodules of lymphoid tissue in the pharyngeal part of the tongue. **Palatine tonsils,** two masses of lymphoid tissue situated in the lateral walls of the oral part of the pharynx, in the triangular recess between the diverging palatoglossal and palatopharyngeal arches. **Pharyngeal tonsil,** a collection of lymphoid tissue, best developed in children, in the roof and posterior part of the pharynx. **Tubal tonsil,** the lateral projection of the pharyngeal tonsil behind the pharyngeal opening of the auditory tube.

Tonsillitis. Inflammation of a tonsil, particularly the palatine tonsil.

Tonsillolith. A concretion in a tonsil.

Tonus. The slight degree of continuing tension present in muscle, and which is manifest in the resistance to stretching shown by healthy muscle.

Tooth. One of the bone-like structures in the jaws used in mastication, and which also aid in articulation. Each consists of a projecting *crown*, a *root* embedded in the maxilla or mandible, and a *neck* which is the constriction between the crown and the root. Each tooth consists of a soft interior, the *pulp*. This is surrounded by the *dentine* which forms the bulk of the tooth. Covering the crown is the *enamel*, and covering the root is the *cement*. (*Plural:* teeth.) **Auditory teeth,** a row of tooth-like projections on the limbus laminae spiralis. **Bicuspid teeth,** premolar teeth. **Canine teeth,** four in number, two in each jaw, placed distal to the corresponding lateral incisor. **Deciduous teeth,** 20 in number, the first of the two sets of teeth, which is temporary, erupting during the first and second years. **Eye teeth,** the upper canine teeth. **Impacted tooth,** a tooth so badly set in the jaw that it cannot erupt spontaneously. **Incisor teeth,** eight in number, forming the four front teeth in each dental arch. **Milk teeth,** deciduous teeth. **Molar teeth,** twelve in number, six in each dental arch, three being placed distal to each second premolar tooth. **Mottled teeth,** teeth with discoloured enamel, usually due to the drinking in childhood of water with a high fluoride content. **Permanent teeth,** 32 in number, the second of the two sets of teeth, which begin to erupt and replace the deciduous teeth about the sixth year and, with the possible exception of the wisdom tooth, have all erupted by the 25th year. **Premolar teeth,** eight in number, four in each dental arch, situated distal to the canine teeth. **Supernumerary tooth,** a tooth additional to the normal dentition. **Wisdom tooth,** the 3rd molar tooth, which does not usually erupt until after the 21st year, and may not erupt or develop at all.

Toothache. Pain in or about a tooth.

Topagnosis. Loss of touch localization.

Topectomy. Surgical exision of an area of cerebral cortex for the alleviation of mental disorder.

Tophaceous. Pertaining to a tophus.

Tophus. A deposit of sodium biurate which develops in the cartilage of the ear and around the joints in gout. (*Plural:* tophi.)

Topo- (Gk *topos:* place). Prefix signifying place.

Topography. Regional anatomy.

Tormina. Intestinal colic.

Torpor. A state of bodily and mental inactivity.

Torque. A rotatory force. The rotation of a tooth around its long axis.

Torsion. Twisting.

Torso. The trunk.

Torticollis. Spasmodic contraction of the muscles of the neck, particularly the sternocleidomastoid muscle, resulting in drawing of the head to one side. Wry-neck.

Toruloma. The primary lesion in cryptococcosis.

Torulosis. Cryptococcosis.

Totipotent. The term applied to a cell, such as the fertilized ovum, which is capable of giving rise to a complete embryo.

Touch. The tactile sense, whereby we become conversant with our surroundings by contact. Palpation.

Tourniquet. An instrument for the temporary arrest of haemorrhage by pressure on the bleeding blood vessel.

Tow. Firm coarse hemp, flax or jute, which is hygroscopic and is used as a surgical dressing.

Toxaemia. The condition evoked by the presence of bacterial toxins in the circulating blood.

Toxalbumin. An albumin with toxic properties.

Toxic. Pertaining to a toxin. Poisonous.

Toxicity. The state of being toxic or poisonous.

Toxico- (Gk *toxikon:* poison). Prefix meaning poisonous or relationship to poisoning.

Toxicology. The study of poisons.

Toxin. A poisonous substance. **Bacterial toxin,** a product of bacteria that is injurious to the tissues and in virtue of which disease processes result from bacterial infection.

Toxocara. A genus of nematodes. **Toxocara canis,** the dog ascarid. **Toxocara cati,** the cat ascarid.

Toxocariasis. The condition induced by infestation with *Toxocara canis* or *cati*, and characterized by granulomatous swellings in various parts of the body, including the eye, pneumonitis and eosinophilia.

Toxoid. A toxin which has been detoxified without losing its antigenic potency.

Toxoplasma. A genus of protozoon parasites. *Toxoplasma gondii* infects man.

Toxoplasmosis. The disease induced in man by infestation with *Toxoplasma gondii*. The most serious form is the congenital form in which the foetus is infected via the mother, and may be born with hydrocephalus or may develop chorioretinitis.

Trabecula. A strut or beam. (*Plural:* trabeculae.) **Trabeculae of bone,** the meshwork of superimposed lamellae of bony tissue in spongy bone laid down in such a way as to enable them to withstand the stresses to which they are subject. **Trabeculae carneae,** muscular ridges on the inner aspect of the cavities of the heart. **Trabeculae of lymph nodes,** collagen fibres which extend from the capsule into the interior of the node, where they become continuous with the reticulum. **Trabeculae of the penis,** the fibromuscular bands that divide the corpora cavernosa into cavernous spaces. **Septomarginal trabecula,** a muscular band that conveys the right limb of the atrioventricular bundle. Moderator band. **Trabeculae of the spleen,** fibroelastic bands that constitute the framework of the spleen.

Trache-, Tracheo- (Gk *trachys:* rough). Prefixes signifying relationship to the trachea.

Trachea. A cartilaginous and membranous tube about 10cm. long, continued downwards from the lower end of the larynx. In the cadaver it stretches from the level of the 6th cervical vertebra to that of the upper border of the 5th thoracic vertebra, where it divides into the two bronchi.

Tracheitis. Inflammation of the trachea.

Trachelo- (Gk *trachēlos:* neck). Prefix signifying association with the neck.

Tracheostomy. The surgical procedure of making an opening into the trachea for the insertion of a tube to maintain respiration.

Tracheotomy. The making of an opening in the trachea.

Trachoma. A severe form of kerato-conjunctivitis, highly prevalent in the East, Middle East, Africa and parts of South America, due to infection with a virus of the psittacosis group.

Tract. A tract. A bundle of nerve fibres. A nervous pathway in the brain or spine. A series of associated parts. **Afferent tract,** sensory tract. **Alimentary tract,** the passage from the mouth to the anus. Alimentary canal. Digestive tract. **Ascending tract,** sensory tract. **Biliary tract,** the hepatic ducts, gall-bladder, cystic duct and common bile duct. **Corticonuclear tract,** nerve fibres running from the cerebral cortex to the motor nuclei of the cranial nerves. **Corticopontine tract,** nerve fibres running from the cerebral cortex to the nuclei pontis. **Corticospinal tract,** the major motor pathway in the spinal cord that connects the cerebral cortex with the motor cells in the spinal cord. It was long known as the pyramidal tract. It is divided into an anterior and a lateral corticospinal tract. The latter is the old crossed pyramidal tract. **Dentato-rubrothalamic tract,** afferent fibres from the cerebellum and red nucleus to the intermediate thalamic nucleus. **Descending tract,** motor tract. Efferent tract. **Digestive tract,** alimentary tract. **Dorsolateral tract,** a small strand of nerve fibres situated between the top of the posterior grey column and the surface of the spinal cord, close to

the dorsal roots, and concerned with pain and thermal sensation. **Efferent tract,** motor tract. **Exteroceptive tracts,** nerve tracts concerned with conveying exteroceptive impulses. **Extrapyramidal tracts,** pathways for impulses which unconsciously modify the activities of the pyramidal system. **Fastigiovestibular tract,** nerve fibres that connect the nucleus fastigii with the vestibular nuclei. **Gastro-intestinal tract,** the stomach and intestines. **Genito-urinary tract,** the urinary and genital organs. **Iliotibial tract,** the strong band of fascia lata on the lateral aspect of the thigh that extends from the iliac crest to the lateral condyle of the tibia. **Intersegmental tracts, anterior,** one of the three sets of tracts in the anterior funiculus. **Intersegmental tracts, lateral,** one of the three sets of tracts in the lateral funiculus. **Intersegmental tracts, posterior,** one of the three sets of tracts in the posterior funiculus. **Intestinal tract,** the intestines. **Mamillotegmental tract,** nerve fibres which connect the medial nucleus with the tegmentum. **Mamillothalamic tract,** nerve fibres which connect the medial nucleus with the anterior nucleus of the thalamus. **Mesencephalic tract of the trigeminal nerve,** nerve fibres that convey proprioceptive impulses from the muscles of mastication. **Motor tract,** a tract that conveys impulses regulating movement. Descending tract. Efferent tract. **Olfactory tract,** the nerve fibres that connect the olfactory bulb to the cerebral hemispheres. **Olivocerebellar tract,** nerves that pass from the olivary nucleus to the inferior cerebellar peduncle of the opposite side. **Olivospinal tract,** one of the descending pathways of the extrapyramidal system. **Optic tract,** a bundle of nerve fibres that runs from the optic chiasma to the lateral geniculate body. **Proprioceptive tracts,** nerve tracts concerned with conveying proprioceptive impulses. **Pyramidal tract,** corticospinal tract. **Respiratory tract,** the nasal cavities, the pharynx, the larynx, the trachea and the lungs. **Reticulospinal tract,** nerve fibres that arise in the reticular formation of the brain stem and synapse with internuncial and motor cells in the anterior grey column. **Rubroreticular tract,** nerve fibres that pass from the red nucleus to the olivary nucleus. **Rubrospinal tract,** nerve fibres that arise in the red nucleus, decussate and synapse with cells in the anterior grey column in the thoracic region. **Semilunar tract,** a comma-shaped tract in the posterior funiculus. **Sensory tract,** a tract that conveys impulses originating peripherally. Ascending tract. Afferent tract. **Septomarginal tract,** intersegmental fibres in the posterior funiculus. **Tractus solitarius,** a tract in the medulla oblongata that receives gustatory fibres from the vii, ix and x cranial nerves. **Spinal tract of the trigeminal nerve,** a descending tract of the trigeminal nerve that carries pain and temperature impulses from the face. **Spinocerebellar tract, anterior,** a tract which lies in front of the posterior spinocerebellar tract and runs from the lumbar region to the cerebellum. **Spinocerebellar tract, posterior,** a band of nerve fibres in the lateral funiculus that runs from the lumbar region to the cerebellum. **Spino-olivary tract,** nerve fibres running from all levels of the spinal cord to the olivary nucleus. **Spinotectal tract,** nerve fibres, closely related topographically to the anterior spinocerebellar and spinothalamic tracts, which arise in the posterior grey column and end in the superior colliculus of the tectum on the opposite side. **Spinothalamic tract, anterior,** an ascending tract in the anterior funiculus subserving tactile sensation. **Spinothalamic tract, lateral,** an ascending tract in the lateral funiculus, conveying pain and temperature sense to the thalamus. **Tractus spiralis foraminosus,** a series of openings in the cochlear area of the internal auditory meatus for transmission of branches of the cochlear nerve. **Tectobulbar tract,** nerve fibres that run from the superior colliculi to the pontine nuclei and the motor nuclei of the cranial nerves concerned with the innervation of the orbital muscles. **Tectocerebellar tract,** nerve fibres in the superior cerebellar peduncle for the passage of visual, and possibly auditory, impulses to the cerebellum. **Tectospinal tract,** nerve fibres that run from the superior colliculi and descend in the anterior column of the opposite side. **Urinary tract,** the ureter, bladder and urethra. **Urogenital tract,** the genito-urinary tract. **Uveal tract,** the vascular coat of the eye, consisting of the chorioid, ciliary body, and iris. **Vestibulospinal tract,** nerve fibres that bring the anterior column cells under the control of the vestibular nuclei of the

same side, and serve as an efferent pathway for equilibratory control.
Traction. The act of drawing or pulling. **Axis traction,** traction in the line of the birth canal applied by forceps to the oncoming foetus in parturition. **Skeletal traction,** traction applied to a long bone by means of pins.
Tractotomy. Surgical section of a nerve tract.
Tractus. Tract.
Tragacanth. B.P. 1968. The dried gummy exudation obtained by incision from species of *Astragalus*. It forms viscous solutions or gels with water, and is used as a suspending agent.
Tragus. The small curved flap that projects backwards over the external acoustic meatus.
Tramazoline. The B.P. Commission approved name for 2-(5,6,7,8-tetrahydro-1-naphthylamino)-2-imidazoline. A sympathomimetic.
Trance. A state of diminished consciousness up to the stage of profound sleep, from which it may be difficult to arouse the individual. It may be a manifestation of catalepsy, or induced by hypnosis, or be a hysterical manifestation.
Tranexamic acid. The B.P. Commission approved name for *trans*-4-aminomethylcyclohexanecarboxylic acid. A drug that inhibits plasminogen activation and so reduces fibrinolysis.
Tranquillizer. A term applied to a drug that induces a state of tranquillity.
Trans- (L *trans:* through). Prefix meaning through, across, beyond.
Transaldolase. The enzyme responsible for the transaldolation reaction in carbohydrate metabolism, whereby a dihydroxyacetone residue is transferred.
Transamidination. A reaction in the synthesis of creatine in which an amidine group is transferred in the reaction between arginine and glycine.
Transaminase. An enzyme that catalyses the transfer of an amino group from an amino-acid to a keto-acid. Aminotransferase.
Transamination. The process whereby an amino group is transferred from a donor amino-acid to a recipient keto-acid under the influence of a transaminase, the donor amino-acid thus becoming a keto-acid and the recipient keto-acid an amino-acid.
Transcription. The process, whereby the genetic message is transferred from DNA to messenger RNA which

carries it to the ribosomes in which it is translated into the 20-letter language of the amino-acids in the proteins.

Transduction. The transfer of genetic attributes from one micro-organism to another by means of bacteriophage.

Transferase. An enzyme that catalyses the transfer of a group of atoms from one molecule to another.

Transferrin. A β-globulin in the serum that takes up iron after it has been absorbed, and acts as a transport protein conveying iron between tissues without itself being metabolized.

Transfusion. The introduction of fluid directly into the circulation. This may be blood, blood substitutes, normal saline, or other solutions. **Blood transfusion,** the transfusion of blood. **Drip transfusion,** the administration of the transferred fluid very slowly, drip by drip. **Exchange transfusion,** the method of treating severe cases of haemolytic disease of the newborn by replacing the whole of the baby's blood with Rh-negative blood of the correct blood group for the baby. Exsanguination transfusion.

Transient. A consonant, like p, b, t, d, which is so short that it gives no sensation of pitch.

Transillumination. The passage of light through the tissues for the purpose of examining a part.

Transketolase. An enzyme that transfers a ketol residue in the pentose phosphate pathway, one of the alternative methods whereby glucose is oxidized to carbon dioxide and water.

Translation. The process which culminates in the synthesis of protein, whereby following transcription the RNA intermediary transports the genetic information to the protein-synthesizing centres of the cell where the information is translated from the linear sequence of codons in the RNA into a linear sequence of amino-acids which are concurrently polymerized into protein.

Transmethylation. The transfer of a methyl group from one compound to another.

Transpiration. The passage of watery vapour through the skin. Insensible perspiration.

Transplacental. Across or through the placenta.

Transplantation. The process of transferring tissue from one site to another, or organs or tissue from one individual another.

Transposition. Change of position. Displacement of an organ to the opposite side.

Transudate. A morbid accumulation of fluid due to a hydrostatic imbalance between the intravascular and extravascular compartments of the body, despite normal vascular permeability.

Transudation. The passage of a fluid with its dissolved salts through a membrane.

Transurethral. Through the urethra.

Transvesical. Through the bladder.

Transvestitism. The psychosexual abnormality characterized by the compulsion to dress in the clothes of the opposite sex to achieve sexual satisfaction.

Tranylcypromine sulphate. B.P. 1968. $C_{18}H_{24}N_2,O_4S$. A monoamine-oxidase inhibitor used in the treatment of depressive states.

Trapezium bone. The most lateral bone in the distal row of bones in the carpus.

Trapezoid bone. The small bone in the distal row of bones in the carpus, which lies between the trapezium and the capitate.

Trauma. Injury or wound (*Plural:* traumata.)

Traumato- (Gk *trauma, traumatos:* wound). Prefix signifying relationship to trauma.

Traumatology. The branch of surgery concerned with trauma and its management.

Treacle. A brown thick syrup, one of the by-products of the manufacture of crystallized sugar.

Treatment. The means employed in the management and care of patients.

Trematoda. The class of the phylum Platyhelminths. Also known as flukes.

Tremor. Involuntary rhythmic quivering or trembling. **Intention tremor,** a tremor which is initiated or enhanced in voluntary movement.

Trephine. A surgical instrument for removing a circular disc—usually of bone from the skull. To use a trephine.

Trephone. A hypothetical wound hormone said to be responsible for healing.

Treponema. A genus of the family Treponemataceae. The members are slender, flexuous spirals 4 to 16μ in length and 0·1 to 0·6μ thick. *Treponema calligyrum,* a non-pathogenic organism, morphologically resembling *Tr. pallidum,* found in the secretions of the genitalia. *Treponema carateum,* the causative organism of pinta. *Treponema genitalis*, a commensal in the genital mucosa, morphologically similar to *Tr. pallidum. Treponema macrodentium*, an organism found in the mouth. *Treponema microdentium*, an organism that flourishes in carious teeth. *Treponema mucosum*, an organism similar to *Tr. microdentium*, that produces a mucin-like substance. *Treponema pallidum*, the causative organism of syphilis. *Treponema pertenue*, the causative organism of yaws.

Treponema. An organism belonging to the genus Treponema. (*Plural:* treponemata.)

Treponemataceae. A family of the order Spirochaetales. It contains three genera: Borrelia, Leptospira, and Treponema.

Treponematosis. The group of diseases caused by treponemata.

Tretamine. B.P.C. 1968. $C_9H_{12}N_6$. A cytotoxic drug used in the treatment of lymphadenoma and chronic leukaemia.

Trethinium tosylate. The B.P. Commission approved name for 2-ethyl-1,2,3,4-tetrahydro-2-methylisoquinolinium toluene-*p*-sulphonate. A hypotensive agent.

Tri- (Gk *treis:* three). Prefix meaning three or thrice.

Triacetate. An acetate that contains three acetate radicals.

Triacetyloleandomycin. B.P.C. 1968. $C_{41}H_{67}NO_{15}$. The triacetyl ester of oleandomycin, an antibiotic produced by *Streptomyces antibioticus*, which is orally active against the same microorganisms as oleandomycin.

Triad. A group of three comparable objects or elements.

Triamcinolone. B.P.C. 1968. $C_{21}H_{27}FO_6$. A corticosteroid with the same action as cortisone acetate but virtually no sodium-retaining effect. It is active by mouth. **Triamcinolone acetonide**, B.P. 1968. $C_{24}H_{31}FO_6$. a corticosteroid with the same action topically as hydrocortisone, but more potent.

Triamterine, B.P. 1968. $C_{12}H_{11}N_7$. A diuretic which antagonizes the effects of aldosterone.

Triangle. A geometrical three-sided figure. A three-sided object or area. **Trigone. Anterior triangle of the neck,** one of the two triangular areas into which the sternocleidomastoid muscle divides the neck. Its boundaries are: in front, the median line of the neck;

above, the base of the mandible and a line continuing this from the angle of the mandible to the sternocleidomastoid; behind, the anterior border of the sternocleidomastoid. **Triangle of auscultation,** the triangle formed by the trapezius, the latissimus dorsi, and the medial border of the scapula. **Carotid triangle,** the triangle in the neck bounded by the sternocleidomastoid, the superior belly of the omohyoid, and above by the stylohyoid and the posterior belly of the digastric. **Digastric triangle,** the triangle in the neck bounded above by the base of the mandible and a line drawn from its angle to the mastoid process, below and behind by the posterior belly of the digastric and the stylohyoid, below and in front by the anterior belly of the digastric. **Femoral triangle,** the triangle corresponding to the depression seen immediately below the fold of the groin, and bounded laterally by the medial margin of the sartorius, medially by the medial margin of the adductor longus, and above by the inguinal ligament. **Hypoglossal triangle,** a triangular area in the floor of the rhomboid fossa that corresponds with the nucleus of the hypoglossal nerve and the nucleus intercalatus. **Inguinal triangle,** the triangle through which a direct inguinal hernia protrudes, bounded by the medial half of the inguinal ligament, the lower part of the lateral border of the rectus abdominalis, and the inferior epigastric artery. **Lumbar triangle,** a small triangular area in the back bounded by the lateral margin of the latissimus dorsi, the posterior border of the external oblique, and the iliac crest. **Muscular triangle,** the triangle bounded in front by the median line of the neck from the hyoid bone to the sternum, behind and below by the anterior margin of the sternocleidomastoid, behind and above by the superior belly of the omohyoid. **Posterior angle of the neck,** the triangle bounded in front by the sternocleidomastoid, behind by the anterior margin of the trapezius, and below by the middle third of the clavicle. **Occipital triangle,** the triangle bounded in front by the sternocleidomastoid, behind by the trapezius, and below by the omohyoid. **Submental triangle,** the triangle lying between the anterior bellys of the digastric, with the body of the hyoid bone as its base. **Suboccipital triangle,** the triangle bounded by the rectus capitis posterior major, the obliquus capitis superior, and the obliquus capitus inferior. **Supraclavicular triangle,** the triangle bounded by the inferior belly of the omohyoid, the clavicle, and the lower part of the posterior border of the sternocleidomastoid. **Suprameatal triangle,** the triangle bounded by the supramastoid crest, the postero-superior margin of the orifice of the external acoustic meatus, and behind by a vertical line drawn as a tangent to the curve of the posterior margin of the meatal orifice. **Vagal triangle,** an area in the rhomboid fossa between the hypoglossal triangle and the vestibular area, which overlies the dorsal nucleus of the vagus nerve.

Triatoma. A genus of blood-sucking bugs of the family Reduviidae. Known also as kissing bugs, assassin bugs, and cone nose bugs. Predominantly found in America, their major medical significance is as the transmitters of *Tryponosoma cruzi.*

Triaziquone. The B.P. Commission approved name for tri(aziridin-1-yl)-1, 4-benzoquinone. An anti-neoplastic agent.

Tricephalus. A three-headed monster.

Trich-, Tricho- (Gk *thrix, trichos:* hair). Prefixes signifying relationship to hair, or hair-like.

Trichiasis. Distortion of the eyelashes so that they are directed backwards and rub against the cornea.

Trichinella. A genus of the class Aphasmidia of nematodes or round-worms. *Trichinella spiralis,* the causative organism of trichiniasis (trichinosis).

Trichiniasis. The disease caused by *Trichinella spiralis,* usually acquired by eating raw or undercooked pork (measly pork) infested with encysted larvae of *T. spiralis,* and characterized by muscular pains, peri-orbital oedema, eosinophilia and pyrexia. Trichinosis.

Trichinosis. Trichiniasis.

Trichloracetic acid. B.P. 1968. $C_2HCl_3O_2$. A caustic.

Trichloride. A chloride containing three chlorine atoms.

Trichloroethylene, B.P. 1968. CHCl: CCl_2. A general anaesthetic, widely used to induce analgesia in childbirth.

Trichlorofluoromethane. B.P.C. 1968. CCl_3F. A refrigerant and aerosol propellent.

Trichobezoar. A hairball in the stomach.

Trichobilharzia ocellata. A schistosome

responsible for cercarial or schistosomal dermatitis.

Trichoepithelioma. A tumour, usually benign, which occurs on the face and scalp in the form of multiple skin-coloured nodules.

Trichoglossia. Hairy tongue.

Trichology. The study of hair.

Trichomonacide. An agent or drug that destroys trichomonads.

Trichomonad. A member of the genus Trichomonas.

Trichomonas. A genus of flagellate protozoa, which are pear-shaped, flagellae and have an undulating membrane. *Trichomonas hominis,* a trichomonad found in the gut in man, and sometimes associated with diarrhoea. *Trichomonas tenax,* a commensal in the mouth. *Trichomonas vaginalis,* a common cause of vaginitis.

Trichomoniasis. Infestation with *Trichomonas vaginalis,* usually manifested by vaginitis in women and urethritis in men.

Trichonocardiosis. Infestation of the hair with *Nocardia tenuis,* which produces reddish concretions. **Trichonocardiosis axillaris,** infestation of the hair of the axilla with *Nocardia tenuis.*

Trichophyton. A genus of *Fungi imperfecti.* They are dermatophytic fungi which are responsible for various forms of ringworm. The main members of the genus causing ringworm in man are *T. mentagrophytes, T. rubrum, T. verrucosum.*

Trichorrhexis. Brittleness of the hair.

Trichorrhoea. Falling out of hair.

Trichosporon. A genus of fungi that infests the hair.

Trichostrongylus. A genus of nematodes which are parasites in herbivorous animals and only rarely affect man.

Trichotlliomania. Nervous or obsessional pulling out of the hair.

Trichromatic. Relating to three colours. Able to distinguish the three primary colours: red, green, and blue.

Trichuriasis. A worldwide disease, especially in the tropics, due to ingestion of the eggs of *Trichuris trichiura,* the whipworm.

Trichuris. A genus of nematodes. *Trichuris trichiura,* the whipworm, responsible for causing trichuriasis.

Triclofenol piperazine. The B.P. Commission approved name for piperazine di-(2,4,5-trichlorophenoxide). An anthelmintic.

Triclofos sodium. B.P. 1968. $C_2H_3Cl_3$ NaO_4P. A sedative and hypnotic.

Tricresol. Cresol. B.P. 1968.

Tricuspid. Having three cusps. **Tricuspid valve,** the right atrioventricular valve.

Tric virus (or agent). The name sometimes given to the organisms responsible for trachoma and inclusion conjunctivitis.

Tricyclamol chloride. B.P. 1968. $C_{20}H_{32}ClNO$. An anticholinergic drug.

Tridactyl. Having three fingers or toes.

Tridihexethyl chloride. The B.P. Commission approved name for an anticholinergic agent.

Triethanolamine. B.P.C. 1968. A variable mixture of bases, which is used as an emulsifying agent.

Triethylene glycol. $C_6H_{14}O_4$. A solvent of nitrocellulose, resins and oils. It is also used as an air disinfectant and in anti-freeze solutions.

Trifluoperazine hydrochloride. B.P. 1968. $C_{21}H_{26}Cl_3F_3N_3S$. A tranquillizer.

Trifluperidol. The B.P. Commission approved name for 1-[3-(4-fluoro-benzoyl)propyl]-4-(3-trifluoromethyl-phenyl)piperidin-4-ol. A neuroleptic.

Trifocal. Having three foci. **Trifocal lenses,** ophthalmic lenses in which the upper part contains the distant correction, the middle part the intermediate, and the lower part the near correction.

Trigeminal. Triple. **Trigeminal nerve,** the 5th cranial nerve.

Trigeminy. The state of occurring in threes.

Triglyceride. A combination of glycerol with three molecules of a fatty acid.

Trigone. Triangle. **Trigone of the bladder,** a small triangular area immediately above and behind the internal orifice of the urethra, in which the mucous membrane is smooth and firmly bound to the muscular coat. **Collateral trigone,** the floor of the lateral ventricle between the posterior and inferior horns. **Trigonum fibrosum dextrum,** a tough mass of tissue between the aortic arterial ring and atrioventricular rings. **Trigonum fibrosum sinistrum,** a mass of fibrous tissue between the left side of the aortic arterial ring and the front of the left atrioventricular ring. **Trigonum habenulae,** a triangular area in the epithalamus, which contains the habenular nucleus. **Olfactory trigone,** the expanded posterior end of the olfactory tract.

Trigonitis. Inflammation of the trigone of the urinary bladder.

Trigono- (Gk *trigonos:* three-cornered). Prefix meaning triangular.

Trigonocephaly. A cranial deformity characterized by a triangular configuration of the skull.

Triiodothyronine. A derivative of thyronine which possesses all the biological properties of thyroxine and is more potent.

Trilocular. Having three cells or chambers.

Trimeperidine. The B.P. Commission approved name for 1,2,5-trimethyl-4-phenyl-4-piperidyl propionate. A narcotic analgesic.

Trimeprazine tartrate. B.P.C. 1968. $C_{40}H_{50}N_4O_6S_2$. An antihistaminic with a relatively powerful antipruritic action.

Trimetaphan camsylate. B.P. 1968. $C_{32}H_{40}N_2O_5S_2$. A ganglion-blocking agent with an action of short duration, used mainly for inducing controlled hypotension during neurosurgery.

Trimetazidine. The B.P. Commission approved name for 1-(2,3,4-trimethyloxybenzyl)piperazine. A vasodilator.

Trimethidinium methosulphate. The B.P. Commission approved name for (+)-3-(3-dimethylaminopropyl)-1,8,8-trimethyl-3-azabicyclo[3.2.1]octanedi-(methylmethosulphate). A hypotensive agent.

Trimethoprim. B.P. Addendum 1971. $C_{14}H_{18}N_4O_3$. An antibacterial agent.

Trimipramine maleate. B.P. Addendum 1971. $C_{24}H_{30}N_2O_4$. An anti-depressant.

Trimustine. The B.P. Commission approved name for tri-(2-chloroethyl) amine. An antineoplastic agent of the nitrogen mustard series.

Trinitrin. Glyceryl trinitrate.

Trinitroglycerin. Glyceryl trinitrate.

Trinitrophenol. $C_6H_3N_3O_7$. Picric acid. An antiseptic.

Triolein. Glyceryl ester of oleic acid. A liquid, unsaturated fat.

Triose. A monosaccharide containing three carbon atoms in the molecule.

Trioxide. A compound containing three atoms of oxygen.

Triparanol. The B.P. Commission approved name for 2-(4-chlorophenyl)-1-(4-diethylaminoethoxyphenyl)-1-*p*-tolylethanol. A blood cholesterol lowering agent.

Tripe. The stomach and intestine of the ox.

Tripelennamine. The B.P. Commission approved name for *N*-benzyl-*N'N'*-

dimethyl-*N*-2-pyridylethylenediamine. An antihistaminic.

Tripeptide. A polypeptide containing three amino-acids.

Triplet. One of three individuals produced at the same birth.

Triploid. Possessing three times the haploid number of chromosomes in the cell nucleus.

Triprolidine hydrochloride. B.P. 1968. $C_{19}H_{23},ClN_2,2H_2O$. An antihistaminic

Triquetral. Three-cornered.

Triquetral bone. The bone in the proximal row of the carpus, situated between the lunate and pisiform bones.

Triradiate. Radiating in three directions.

Trisaccharide. A carbohydrate containing three monosaccharide units.

Trismus. Lockjaw. Inability to open the mouth, as in tetanus.

Trisodium edetate injection. B.P. 1968. A chelating agent given by intravenous infusion in the treatment of hypercalcaemia, and also used topically in the treatment of calcified corneal opacities.

Trisomy. The presence of an extra chromosome, resulting in man in the cell containing 47 chromosomes.

Tritanopia. Blue-blindness. Inability to distinguish blue from green.

Tritiation. The process of introducing tritium into a molecule.

Tritium. An isotope of hydrogen. H_3.

Trituration. The process of reducing to a fine powder.

Trivalent. Having a valency of three.

Trocar. An instrument provided with a sharp, three-sided point, fitted inside a tube or cannula, and used for puncturing cavities of the body in which fluid has accumulated.

Trochanter. One of two bony prominences on the upper end of the femur. **Greater trochanter,** a large quadrangular eminence at the upper part of the junction of the neck of the femur with the shaft, the lateral surface of which is palpable in the living subject. **Lesser trochanter,** a conical eminence which projects medially and backwards from the shaft of the femur at its junction with the lower and posterior part of the neck.

Troche. A lozenge.

Trochlea. A pulley. **Trochlea of the humerus,** a pulley-shaped surface at the lower end of the humerus that articulates with the trochlear notch of the ulna. **Peroneal trochlea,** a small elevation on the anterior part of the lateral surface of the calcaneus. **Trochlea of the superior oblique muscle,** a fibrocartilaginous ring on the medial side of the roof of the orbit, through which the tendon of the superior oblique muscle passes.

Trochlear nerve. The 4th cranial nerve.

Troglotrematoidea. A super-family of flukes, which includes the genus Paragonimus.

Trolnitrate phosphate. The B.P. Commission approved name for triethanolamine $OO'O''$-trinitrate diorthophosphate. A vasodilator.

Trombicula. A genus of mites, which includes harvest mites and the mites responsible for the transmission of scrub typhus (*Trombicula akamushi* and *T. deliensis*).

Trometamol. The B.P. Commission approved name for 2-amino-2-hydroxymethylpropane-1,3-diol. A drug for the treatment of gastric hyperacidity.

Troph-, Tropho- (Gk *trophē:* nutrition). Prefixes signifying relationship to nutrition or food.

Trophic. Pertaining to nutrition.

-trophic, -trophin (Gk *trophikos:* nourishing). Suffixes meaning nourishing or indicating a relationship to nutrition.

Trophoblast. The outer, ectodermal layer of the blastocyst, concerned with the embedding and attachment of the zygote.

Trophozoite. The precursor of the schizont in the development of the malarial plasmodium.

-trophy (Gk *trophē:* nourishment). Suffix indicating association with nutrition or food.

-tropic (Gk *tropikos:* turning). Suffix indicating a turning.

Tropicamide. The B.P. Commission approved name for *N*-ethyl-*N*-(4-pyridylmethyl)tropamide. An anticholinergic agent.

Tropigline. The B.P. Commission approved name for tiglyltropeine. A drug for the treatment of parkinsonism.

Tropism. The involuntary movement of living cells or organisms towards or away from an external stimulus.

-tropism (Gk *tropē:* turn). Suffix signifying an affinity for, or a tendency to turn.

Tropocollagen. The fundamental unit of collagen.

Troxerutin. The B.P. Commission approved name for 7,3′,4′-tri-

[*O*-(2-hydroxyethyl)]rutin. A drug used in the treatment of venous disorders.

Troxidone. B.P. 1968. $C_6H_9NO_3$. An anticonvulsant used in the treatment of petit mal.

Troxonium tosylate. The B.P. Commission approved name for triethyl-2-(3,4,5-trimethoxybenzoyloxy)-ethyl-ammonium toluene-*p*-sulphonate. A hypotensive agent.

Troxypyrrolium tosylate. The B.P. Commission approved name for *N*-ethyl-*N*-2-(3,4,5-trimethoxybenzoyloxy)-ethylpyrrolidinium toluene-*p*-sulphonate. A hypotensive agent.

Truncus. Trunk. (*Plural:* trunci.) **Truncus arteriosus,** the embryonic arterial trunk of the heart, which later becomes the ascending aorta and the pulmonary trunk.

Trunk. The torso. The body without head or limbs. A main blood vessel, nerve or lymphatic vessel. **Trunks of the brachial plexus,** three trunks consisting of a *lower trunk* formed by the 8th cervical and 1st thoracic nerves; a *middle trunk* formed by the 7th cervical nerve; an *upper trunk* formed by the 5th and 6th cervical nerves. **Coeliac trunk,** a wide short artery that arises from the aorta just below the diaphragm and divides into three branches: *left gastric, hepatic,* and *splenic*. **Trunk of the corpus callosum,** the part lying between the genu and the splenium. **Costocervical trunk,** the artery that arises from the subclavian artery and divides into the superior intercostal and deep cervical arteries. **Linguofacial trunk,** the common trunk whereby the facial and lingual arteries sometimes arise from the external carotid artery. **Lumbosacral trunk,** a trunk formed by part of the ventral ramus of the 4th lumbar nerve and the ventral ramus of the 5th lumbar nerve which joins the sacral plexus. **Lymphatic trunks,** the series of lymphatic vessels that feed into the right lymphatic duct, the thoracic duct and the cisterna chyli. **Pulmonary trunk,** the main arterial exitus from the right ventricle which, dividing into the left and the right pulmonary artery, carries deoxygenated blood from the heart to the lungs. **Sympathetic trunks,** two ganglionated nerves on either side of the vertebral column which extend from the base of the skull to the coccyx. **Thyrocervical trunk,** a short wide trunk that arises from the first part of the sub-

clavian artery and divides into three branches: *inferior thyroid, suprascapular,* and *transverse cervical*. **Vagal trunks,** two trunks that arise from the oesophageal plexus and descend into the abdomen in front of, and behind, the oesophagus, respectively.

Truss. An instrument for supporting a hernia and preventing the egress of organs in the affected cavity.

Trypanocide. An agent or drug that kills trypanosomes.

Trypanosoma. A genus of the class Mastigophora, members of which have an elongated, sinuous, fusiform structure, with a longitudinal undulating membrane, and a flagellum at each end, which renders it motile. Three species are pathogenic to man: *Tryponosoma cruzi* which causes American (Brazilian) trypansomiasis (Chaga's disease), *T. gambiense* and *T. rhodesiense,* which cause African sleeping sickness.

Trypanosomiasis. The condition caused by infection with trypanosomes. **African trypansomiasis,** sleeping sickness, caused by *T. gambiense* and *T. rhodesiense,* which are transmitted by the bite of infected Glossina (tsetse) flies. It is restricted to Africa and is characterized by glandular swellings, hepatomegaly and splenomegaly, leading up to involvement of the central nervous system with the characteristic drowsiness. **American trypansomiasis,** Chaga's disease, caused by *T. cruzi,* which is transmitted by bugs belonging to the family Triatomedae. It tends to involve the heart more than the central nervous system. The acute form occurs mainly in children.

Tryparsamide. B.P. 1968. $C_8H_{10}AsN_2NaO_4,\frac{1}{2}H_2O$. A drug used parenterally, usually intravenously, in the treatment of trypansomiasis.

Trypsin. The chief proteolytic enzyme in pancreatic juice.

Trypsinogen. The inactive precursor of trypsin in the pancreatic juice. It is converted into trypsin under the influence of enteropeptidase (enterokinase) secreted by the duodenal mucosa.

Tryptophan. α-Amino-β-indole-propionic acid. One of the essential amino-acids.

Tsetse. A fly of the genus Glossina, responsible for the transmission of trypanosomes in Africa.

Tuaminoheptane. The B.P. Commission

approved name for 1-methylhexyl-amine. A vasoconstrictor.

Tube. An elongated hollow structure. A pipe. **Auditory tube,** the tube through which the tympanic cavity communicates with the nasal part of the pharynx. The eustachian tube. **Capillary tube,** a tube with a minute lumen. **Digestive tube,** alimentary canal. **Drainage tube,** a tube, usually made of rubber, inserted into an operation wound to facilitate drainage. **Duodenal tube,** a thin, flexible, rubber tube used to obtain samples of duodenal or gastric contents. **Eustachian tube,** auditory tube. **Fallopian tube,** uterine tube. **Neural tube,** the embryonic predecessor of the brain and spinal cord. **Southey's tube,** a small cannula inserted subcutaneously for the drainage of subcutaneous oedema. **Stomach tube,** a tube for the withdrawal of the contents of the stomach as a diagnostic or therapeutic procedure. **T-tube,** a self-retaining drainage tube in the shape of a T. **Test tube,** a thin-walled glass tube closed at one end, used in the laboratory. **Uterine tube,** one of two tubes, one end of which opens into the uterus, the other into the peritoneal cavity close to the ovary for the transport of ova to the uterus. Fallopian tube. **X-ray tube,** a tube for the production of x-rays for radiological examination.

Tuber. A swelling or protuberance. Tuberosity. **Tuber cinereum,** a sheet of grey matter, forming part of the hypothalamus, and situated between the mamillary bodies behind and the optic chiasma in front.

Tubercle. A nodule. The basic lesion of tuberculosis. **Adductor tubercle,** a small projection on the medial condyle of the lower end of the femur, which gives attachment to the tendon of the adductor magnus. **Tubercles of the atlas, anterior** and **posterior,** small bony prominences on the anterior and posterior arches, respectively, of the 1st cervical vertebra. **Auditory tubercle,** a swelling in the lateral recess of the 4th ventricle produced by the underlying dorsal cochlear nucleus and cochlear part of the vestibulocochlear nerve. **Auricular tubercle,** a small tubercle on the helix of the external ear. **Calcaneal tubercle, anterior,** a prominence on the distal part of the plantar surface of the calcaneus. **Carotid tubercle,** the anterior tubercle of the transverse process of the 6th cervical vertebra. **Conoid tubercle,** a

tubercle in the lateral third of the clavicle, to which is attached the conoid part of the coracoclavicular ligament. **Cuneate tubercle,** the swelling on the fasciculus cuneatus in the medulla oblongata. **Tubercle of the epiglottis,** the backward projection of the lower part of the epiglottis. **Genial tubercle,** a small irregular elevation on the posterior surface of the symphysis menti. **Genital tubercle,** the surface elevation at the cranial end of the cloacal membrane that lengthens to form the phallus. **Gracile tubercle,** the swelling on the fasciculus gracilis in the medulla oblongata. **Tubercle of the humerus, greater,** the lateral part of the upper end of the humerus. **Tubercle of the humerus, lesser,** a prominence on the anterior aspect of the humerus immediately beyond the anatomical neck. **Iliac tubercle,** a prominent projection on the iliac crest behind and above the anterior superior spine. **Infraglenoid tubercle,** a roughened triangular area at the upper end of the lateral border of the scapula. **Intercondylar tubercles of the tibia, lateral and medial,** two elevations on the upper surface of the tibia, or the medial border of the lateral condyle and the lateral border of the medial condyle, respectively. **Jugular tubercle,** a rounded elevation on the posterior cranial fossa which marks the condylar part of the occipital bone. **Marginal tubercle of the zygomatic,** a small, rounded projection in the bone a little below the fronto-zygomatic suture. **Mental tubercle,** the two elevations caused by the central depression of the mental protuberance at the point of the chin. **Obturator tubercle, anterior,** the anterior end of the inferior border of the superior ramus of the pubis. **Obturator tubercle, posterior,** a tubercle on the anterior border of the acetabular notch. **Pharyngeal tubercle,** a small elevation in front of the foramen magnum on the inferior surface of the occipital bone that gives attachment to the fibrous raphe of the pharynx. **Tubercle of the philtrum,** a slight prominence at the lower end of the philtrum of the lips. **Postglenoid tubercle,** a small downward projection from the posterior root of the zygoma. **Pterygoid tubercle,** a small projection that lies immediately below the posterior opening of the pterygoid canal. **Pubic tubercle,** the lateral extremity of the pubic crest. **Quadrate tubercle,** a rounded elevation on the intertrochanteric crest of the femur. **Radius, dorsal tubercle of,** an elevation on the posterior surface of the radius. **Tubercle of the rib,** a prominence on the outer surface of the posterior part of the rib at the junction of the neck with the shaft, the articular portion of which articulates with the transverse process of the numerically corresponding vertebra. **Sacrum, articular tubercles of,** a row of four small tubercles on either side of the mid-line. **Sacrum, spinous tubercles of,** four (sometimes three) elevations in the median sacral crest. **Sacrum, transverse tubercles of,** the tips of the fused transverse processes of the sacrum. **Scalene tubercle,** a small projection on the upper surface of the 1st rib, to which the scalenus anterior is attached. **Tubercle of the scaphoid bone,** a rounded elevation on the distal part of the palmar surface. **Serratus anterior, tubercle for,** a tubercle on the external surface of the 2nd rib. **Supraglenoid tubercle,** a small roughened area immediately above the glenoid cavity. **Talus, tubercles of,** a lateral and a medial tubercle on the posterior surface. **Teeth, tubercles of,** the two elevations on the crowns of the premolar teeth, and the three, four, or five on the crowns of the molar teeth. **Thyroid tubercle, inferior,** the prominence on the lower border of the lamina of the thyroid cartilage. **Thyroid tubercle, superior,** the prominence situated in front of the root of the superior horn of the thyroid cartilage. **Tubercle of the trapezium,** a prominence on the palmar surface. **Tubercle of the root of the zygoma,** a small tubercle where the anterior root of the zygoma springs from the zygomatic process.

Tubercular. Pertaining to tubercles (not tuberculosis).

Tuberculid, tuberculide. A lesion of the skin due to tuberculous toxins or to allergy to *Mycobacterium tuberculosis*.

Tuberculin. The name originally given by Koch to a preparation derived from *Mycobacterium tuberculosis*, and intended for the treatment and diagnosis of tuberculosis. **Old tuberculin,** B.P. 1968, the heat-concentrated filtrate from a fluid medium on which the human or bovine type of *Myco. tuberculosis* has been grown. It contains 100,000 units per ml. **Tuberculin purified protein derivative, B.P. 1968,** Tuberculin P.P.D., prepared by the fractional precipitation of a fluid

synthetic medium on which *Myco. tuberculosis* has been grown and from which the mycobacteria have been removed by filtration. It is supplied as a liquid containing 100,000 units per ml., and as a powder containing 40,000 units per mg.

Tuberculoid, Resembling tuberculosis.

Tuberculoma. A circumscribed tuberculous lesion.

Tuberculosis. The disease caused by infection with *Mycobacterium tuberculosis*.

Tuberculous. Pertaining to tuberculosis.

Tuberculum. A nodule or small eminence. (*Plural:* tubercula.) **Tuberculum cinereum,** a swelling in the lower part of the posterior region of the medulla oblongata. **Tuberculum sellae,** a median elevation on the anterior slope of the sella turcica.

Tuberose. Tuberous. **Tuberose sclerosis,** a condition, usually hereditary, characterized by multiple cutaneous tumours of the face, mental deficiency, and epilepsy.

Tuberosity. A swelling or protuberance. **Calcaneal tuberosity,** a protuberance on the plantar surface of the calcaneus, which has a lateral and a medial process. **Tuberosity of the cuboid bone,** an enlargement of the lateral end of the ridge on the plantar aspect of the cuboid. **Deltoid tuberosity,** a V-shaped roughened area on the anterolateral surface of the shaft of the humerus. **Frontal tuberosity,** the rounded elevation on the frontal bone above the superciliary arch. **Gluteal tuberosity,** a roughened ridge on the upper third of the shaft of the femur. **Ischial tuberosity,** the large, roughened impression which marks the lower part of the dorsal surface and the inferior extremity of the body of the ischium. **Maxillary tuberosity,** a small rounded eminence on the infratemporal surface of the maxilla. **Tuberosity of the 5th metatarsal,** a rough eminence on the lateral aspect of the base. **Tuberosity of the navicular,** a prominent projection on the medial surface. **Omental tuberosity of the liver,** a rounded ridge on the inferior surface of the liver, which occupies the concavity of the lesser curvature of the stomach and is in contact with the lesser omentum. **Omental tuberosity of the pancreas,** a process that projects from the right end of the superior border of the pancreas. **Parietal tuberosity,** a slight elevation near the centre of the parietal bone. **Phalangeal tuberosity,** a rough elevation on the palmar surface of the distal phalanxes of the fingers and toes. **Tuberosity of the radius,** an elevation below the medial part of the neck. **Tuberosity of the tibia,** a low eminence at the upper end of the anterior border of the shaft. **Tuberosity of the ulna,** a roughened prominence below the radial notch.

Tuberous. Nodular. Lumpy.

Tubo- (L *tubus:* tube). Prefix signifying association with a tube.

Tubocurarine chloride. B.P. 1968. $C_{38}H_{44}Cl_2N_2O_6,5H_2O$. The chloride of an alkaloid, $(+)$-tubocurarine, obtained from the stems of *Chondodendron tomentosum*, and possessing the specific biological activity of curare of paralysing voluntary muscle by antagonizing acetylcholine. Arrow poison.

Tubo-ovarian. Pertaining to the uterine tube and the ovary.

Tubotympanic. Pertaining to the auditory tube and the tympanic membrane.

Tubular. Pertaining to a tubule. Shaped like a tube.

Tubule. A small tube. **Collecting tubule,** the uriniferous tubule which carries the urine from a number of renal tubules to a terminal duct of Bellini. **Convoluted tubule, proximal,** the part of the renal tubule that links the glomerular capsule with the descending limb of the loop of Henle. **Convoluted tubule, distal,** the part of the renal tubule that links the ascending limb of the loop of Henle with the junctional tubule. **Dentinal tubule,** one of the minute tubules in dentine. **Junctional tubule,** the part of the renal tubule that links the distal convoluted tubule with a collecting tubule. **Renal tubule,** the part of a uriniferous tubule concerned with the selective resorption of substances from the glomerular filtrate until it attains the composition of urine. It links a renal corpuscle with a collecting tubule. **Seminiferous tubules, convoluted,** the tubules in the testis in which spermatozoa are formed. **Seminiferous tubules, straight,** the 20 to 30 tubules in the testis that connect the convoluted seminiferous tubules with the efferent ductules. **Uriniferous tubule,** one of the tortuous, closely packed tubules in the kidney, consisting of a nephron and a collecting tubule.

Tug. Pull. **Tracheal tug,** the downward pulsating movement of the trachea induced by an aneurysm of the arch of the aorta.

Tularaemia. An infectious disease of rodents due to *Pasteurella tularensis,* transmitted to man by ticks, and presenting a clinical picture comparable to that of plague.

Tumefaction. Swelling.

Tumescence. The process of swelling. Tumefaction.

Tumid. Swollen.

Tumour. 'An abnormal mass of tissue, the growth of which exceeds, and is uncoordinated with, that of the normal tissues, and persists in the same excessive manner after cessation of the stimuli which evoked the change' (Willis). A tumour may be *benign* (or *innocent*): that is, show no tendency to invade the surrounding tissues or to metastasize; or it may be *malignant*: that is, invade the surrounding tissues and metastasize. A tumour may also be classified according to the tissue of origin: e.g. epithelium, connective tissue, and the like.

Tunga. A genus of 'combless' fleas. *Tunga penetrans,* the jigger flea, prevalent in tropical Africa and America, which burrows beneath the skin of man.

Tungsten. A hard chemical element. Symbol W (*wolfram*). Atomic weight $183 \cdot 86$. Atomic number 74.

Tunica. A tunic or covering. (*Plural:* tunicae.) **Tunica adventitia,** the external fibrous coat of the arteries and veins. **Tunica albuginea of the ovary,** the condensation of connective tissue in the ovary immediately beneath the germinal epithelium. **Tunica albuginea of the penis,** the fibrous coat of the corpus spongiosum penis. **Tunica albuginea of the testis,** the fibrous covering of the testis. **Tunica externa of the ovarian follicle,** the outer fibrous layer of the theca folliculi. **Tunica interna of the ovarian follicle,** the inner layer of the theca folliculi which becomes the thecal gland as the follicle develops. **Tunica intima,** the innermost endothelial layer of the arteries and veins. **Tunica media,** the middle coat of arteries and veins composed predominantly of elastic and muscle fibres. **Tunica propria,** the middle layer of the walls of the utricle, saccule and semicircular ducts. **Tunica vaginalis,** the outermost of the three coats of the testis. **Tunica vasculosa,** the innermost of the three coats of the testis.

Tunnel. A corridor or canal. **Carpal tunnel,** the space between the carpus and the flexor retinaculum, through which passes the flexor tendons and median nerve to the hand. **Tunnel of Corti,** the triangular space between the basilar membrane and the rods of Corti in the spiral organ.

Turbidimeter. An instrument for measuring the degree of turbidity.

Turgescence. Swelling.

Turgor. The state of being swollen.

Turpentine. The oleoresin obtained as an exudate from various species of *Pinus.* **Turpentine oil,** B.P. 1968, the oil distilled from the oleoresin obtained from various species of *Pinus.* A counter-irritant and rubefacient. **Turpentine liniment,** B.P. 1968, a preparation containing 65 per cent of turpentine oil, with soft soap and camphor.

Turricephaly. An abnormality of the skull produced by precocious union of the fronto-parietal suture. Tower skull.

Tussive. Pertaining to a cough.

Twin. One of two offspring born as the result of one pregnancy. **Binovular twins,** twins developed from two ova. **Conjoined twins,** twins whose bodies are joined to a varying degree. **Dizygotic twins,** binovular twins. **Identical twins,** monozygotic twins. **Monozygotic twins,** twins developed from the same ovum. **Siamese twins,** conjoined twins. **Uniovular twins,** monozygotic twins.

Tybamate. The B.P. Commission approved name for 2-methyl-2-propyltrimethylene butylcarbamate carbamate. A tranquillizer.

Tyformin. The B.P. Commission approved name for 4-guanidinobutyramide. An oral hypoglycaemic agent.

Tylosis. A congenital hyperkeratosis of the palms and soles. Keratosis palmaris et plantaris.

Tyloxapol. The B.P. Commission approved name for oxyethylated t-octylphenol formaldehyde polymer. A surface-active agent.

Tymazoline. The B.P. Commission approved name for 2-thymyloxymethyl-2-imidazoline. A vasoconstrictor.

Tympan-, Tympano- (Gk *tympanon:* drum). Prefixes meaning drum-like or related to the tympanic cavity.

Tympanectomy. Surgical excision of the tympanic membrane.

Tympanic. Pertaining to the tympanum. Resonant.

Tympanites. Distension of the abdomen due to the accumulation of gas in the intestines or in the peritoneal cavity.

Tympanitic. Pertaining to tympanites. Bell-like or resonant.

Tympanoplasty. Surgical reconstruction of the middle ear.

Tympanosclerosis. Thickening of the tympanic membrane.

Tympanotomy. Surgical incision of the tympanic membrane.

Typhlitis. Inflammation of the caecum.

Typho-, Typh- (Gk *typhos:* delusion). Prefixes signifying relationship to typhoid or typhus fevers.

Typhoid fever, An acute infectious fever due to *Salmonella typhi,* and characterized by a continued fever, abdominal symptoms, splenomegaly and rose spots. Enteric fever. **Typhoid vaccine.** B.P. Addendum 1969, a sterile suspension of *S. typhi* (1000 million) in the volume stated on the label as the dose. **Typhoid-paratyphoid A and B vaccine,** B.P. 1968, T.A.B. vaccine, a sterile suspension of *Salmonella typhi* (1000 million), *S. paratyphi A* (500 or 750 million), and *S. paratyphi B* (500 or 750 million) in 1ml. **Typhoid-paratyphoid A, B, and C vaccine,** B.P. 1968, T.A.B.C. vaccine, a sterile suspension of *S. typhi* (1000 million), *S. paratyphi A* (500 or 750 million), *S. paratyphi B* (500 or 750 million), and *S. paratyphi C* (500 or 750 million). **Typhoid-paratyphoid A and B and cholera vaccine,** B.P. 1968, T.A.B. and cholera vaccine, a sterile suspension of T.A.B. vaccine, to which has been added 8000 million *Vibrio cholerae* per ml. **Typhoid-paratyphoid A and B and tetanus vaccine,** B.P. 1968, T.A.B. and tetanus vaccine, a mixture of a sterile suspension of *S. typhi* (500 or 1000 million), *S. paratyphi A* (250 or 500 million), *S. paratyphi B* (250 or 500 million) and 0·9ml. of tetanus vaccine in simple solution, in 1ml.

Typhus. One of a group of related infections caused by Rickettsiae. **Flea-borne typhus:** murine endemic typhus, caused by *Rickettsia mooseri.* **Louse-borne typhus:** epidemic typhus caused by *R. prowazekii*; recrudescent typhus (Brill's disease) caused by *R. prowazekii*; trench fever caused by *R. quintana.* **Mite-borne typhus:** scrub typhus (Tsutsugamushi fever) caused by *R. tsutsugamushi*; rickettsialpox caused by *R. akari.* **Tick-borne typhus:** Mediterranean fever (fièvre boutonneuse) caused by *R. conorii*; Rocky mountain spotted fever caused by

R. ricketsii; South African tick bite fever caused by *R. ricketsii var. pijperi.* **Typhus vaccine,** B.P. 1968, a sterile suspension of epidemic and murine typhus rickettsiae which have been killed.

Tyramine. A pressor amine produced in the large intestine by decarboxylation of tyrosine. It is present in certain cheeses, ergot and decayed animal tissue. It is a precursor of adrenaline.

Tyro-, Tyr- (Gk *tyros:* cheese). Prefixes signifying relationship to cheese.

Tyrosinase. The enzyme which catalyses the first step in the conversion of tyrosine to melanin.

Tyrosine. α-Amino-β-*p*-hydroxyphenyl-propionic acid. An amino-acid.

Tyrosinosis. One of the inborn errors of metabolism, due to faulty metabolism of tyrosine, resulting in the excretion of large amounts of tyrosine in the urine.

Tyrothricin. The B.P. Commission approved name for an antibiotic derived from *Bacillus brevis* Dubos, which is used as a local preparation. It has the same antibacterial spectrum as gramicidin.

U

Ulcer. A breach on the surface of the skin or a mucous surface, with a necrotic or inflammatory base. **Anastomotic ulcer,** a peptic ulcer which develops at the site of the anastomosis between the stomach and the small intestine following gastro-enterostomy. **Aphthous ulcer,** a small, shallow ulcer in the mucous membrane of the mouth and pharynx. **Callous ulcer,** a chronic ulcer with indurated edges which show no tendency to heal—usually on the leg. **Catarrhal ulcer,** a superficial corneal ulcer near the limbus, especially in old people. **Chrome ulcer,** the ulceration induced in the nasal septum and the skin by chromium poisoning. **Decubital ulcer,** bedsore. **Dendritic ulcer,** a branching ulcer of the cornea which occurs as a complication of herpes of the cornea. **Duodenal ulcer,** a peptic ulcer occurring in the duodenum. **Gastric ulcer,** a peptic ulcer occurring in the stomach. **Gastrojejunal ulcer,** anastomotic ulcer. **Hypopyon ulcer,** a corneal ulcer with pus in the anterior chamber. **Jejunal ulcer,** anastomotic ulcer. **Junctiona ulcer,** anastomotic ulcer. **Peptic ulcer,** an ulcer due in part at least to erosion of the gastric juice, and occurring in the oesophagus, stomach, duodenum, or jejunum. **Perforating ulcer,** an ulcer perforating through the entire wall of a viscus. A deep, painless, persistent ulcer on the sole of the foot which may occur in diabetes mellitus and tabes dorsalis as well as other conditions in which there is sensory loss. **Phlyctenular ulcer,** a small, superficial corneal ulcer of allergic origin. **Rodent ulcer,** a painless, ulcerating basal-cell carcinoma, most commonly on the upper part of the face, which spreads locally but does not metastasize. **Serpiginous ulcer,** a creeping ulcer which heals in one part and spreads in another. **Snail-track ulcer,** a long, narrow, rapidly spreading ulcer, most common in the fauces, leaving a track behind it, in secondary syphilis. **Stercoral ulcer,** an ulcer in the colon due to the pressure of impacted faeces. **Stomal ulcer,** anastomotic ulcer. **Varicose ulcer,** a chronic ulcer of the skin, most common in the leg, resulting from chronic varicose veins.

Ulcus. Ulcer. (*Plural:* ulcera.)

Ule-, Ulo- (Gk *oulē:* scar). Prefixes indicating relationship to a scar. (Gk *oulon:* gum). Prefixes signifying relationship to the gums.

Ulitis. Inflammation of the gums.

Ulna. The medial bone of the forearm. (*Plural:* ulnae.)

Ultra- (L *ultra:* beyond). Prefix meaning in excess or beyond.

Ultracentrifuge. A high-speed centrifuge which can develop a centrifugal field sufficient to spin down particles as small as 10Å.

Ultrafiltration. Filtration under pressure through collodion membranes with pores of known diameter, to separate viruses or collodion particles of a given size.

Ultramicroscope. A microscope utilizing refracted light for the visualization of objects too small to be seen by direct light in the ordinary microscope.

Ultrasonic. Pertaining to sound waves in the frequency above 15 to 20 kilocycles per second: that is, above the audible range of sound. These frequencies are used as a method of treatment, and also as a diagnostic procedure, particularly in pregnancy.

Ultraviolet. Beyond the violet end of the spectrum. **Ultraviolet rays,** those between the violet and the roentgen rays: i.e. with wave-lengths between 1800 and 3900Å. They have powerful actinic and biochemical properties.

Umbilicated. With depressed areas like the umbilicus.

Umbilicus. The depression near the centre of the abdominal wall which marks the site of attachment of the umbilical cord in the foetus.

Umbo. The point of greatest convexity of the handle of the malleus, which produces a convexity in the tympanic membrane.

Unction. Ointment. The application of an ointment.

Uncus. The hook-like, anterior end of the parahippocampal gyrus.

Undecenoic acid. B.P. 1968. $C_{11}H_{20}O_2$. A fungicide used topically for the prophylaxis and treatment of superficial dermatophytoses, and for moniliasis and mycotic infections of the vulva and vagina.

Undine. A small glass flask used for irrigating the eye.

Undulant. Wave-like.

Ungual. Pertaining to the nails.

Unguentum. Ointment. (*Plural:* unguenta.)

Uni- (L *unus:* one). Prefix meaning one.

Unicellular. Composed of one cell.

Unidirectional. Moving in one direction.

Unilateral. One-sided.

Unilocular. Having a single cavity.

Union. A joining together. **Bony union,** repair of a fracture of a bone by the laying down of new bone. **False union,** healing of a fracture by scar tissue. **Primary union,** immediate healing of a wound without complications. Healing by first intention.

Uniovular. Arising from a single ovum.

Unit. The term applied to a quantity recognized as a standard for measurement. A single item. **Board of Trade Unit** (BTU), the work done when 1 kilowatt is maintained for one hour. Kilowatt hour. **British Thermal Unit** (Btu), the amount of heat required to raise the temperature of 1 pound of water at its maximum density through 1°F. **Centimetre-Gramme-Second Unit** (CGS), any unit in the centimetre-gramme-second system. **International System Unit** (SI), any unit in the newly rationalized system of metric units that is coming into international use in replacement of the CGS system. **Intensive Care Unit,** a unit in a hospital for the specialized care of dangerously ill patients such as those in shock after severe operations, or patients with severe myocardial infarctions. **International Unit** (IU), a unit as defined and adopted by the World Health Organization for the standardization of drugs and biologicals. **King Unit,** the quantity of phosphatase which, acting on an excess of disodium phenylphosphate at pH 9 for 30 minutes, liberates 1mg. of phenol. **Mache Unit,** the unit of measure of radium emanation. **Motor Unit,** the unit of motor activity, being an effector neurone and the muscle fibres supplied by it.

Univalent. Having the combining power of one atom of hydrogen.

Urachus. A fibrous cord stretching between the apex of the bladder and the umbilicus, the remains of the obliterated allantoic stalk.

Uracil. A pyrimidine derivative present in ribonucleic acid.

Uraemia. The terminal stage of renal failure.

Uramustine. The B.P. Commission approved name for 5-di-(2-chloroethyl)aminouracil. An antineoplastic agent.

Uranism. Homosexuality.

Uranium. A radioactive metallic element. Symbol U. Atomic weight 238·03. Atomic number 92.

Urano- (Gk *ouranos:* roof of the mouth). Prefix signifying relationship to the palate.

Uranyl. A salt of uranium, in which the group UO_2 takes the place of the metallic radical.

Urate. A salt of uric acid.

Urea. Carbamide. $CO(NH_2)_2$. A crystalline substance soluble in water and alcohol, which is the end-product of protein metabolism, being formed in the liver and excreted in the urine. It is also used as a diuretic, and as a test of renal function.

Urease. The enzyme that catalyses the conversion of urea into ammonium carbonate.

Urecchysis. Extravasation of urine into the tissues.

Ureide. A compound of urea and an acid radical.

Ureometer. An instrument for measuring the amount of urea in urine. Ureameter.

Ureter. The tube conveying urine from the kidney to the bladder. It measures 25 to 30cm. in length.

Ureter-, Uretero- (Gk *ourētēr:* the duct that conveys the urine from the kidney to the bladder). Prefixes indicating association with the ureters.

Ureterectomy. Surgical excision of a ureter.

Ureteric. Pertaining to the ureter.

Ureterocele. Dilatation of the lower end of a ureter. The inclusion of a ureter in a hernial sac.

Ureterocolic. Pertaining to a ureter and the colon.

Uretero-enterostomy. The surgical formation of an anastomosis between a ureter and the intestine.

Ureterolith. A calculus in a ureter.

Ureterolithotomy. Removal of a calculus from a ureter.

Ureteronephrectomy. Surgical removal of a kidney with its ureter.

Ureteroplasty. Plastic repair of a ureter: as for stricture.

Ureteropyelonephritis. Inflammation of a ureter and the pelvis of the associated kidney.

Ureterosigmoidoscopy. Surgical establishment of an anastomosis between a ureter and the sigmoid colon.

Ureterostomy. The establishment of an external opening into a ureter.

Ureterotomy. Surgical incision into a ureter.

Ureterovaginal. Pertaining to a ureter and the vagina.

Ureterovesical. Pertaining to a ureter and the bladder.

Urethr-, Urethro- (Gk *ourēthra:* urethra). Prefixes signifying association with the urethra.

Urethra. The canal that connects the internal urethral orifice of the urinary bladder with the external urethral orifice—at the end of the penis in the male, in front of the opening of the vagina in the female.

Urethritis. Inflammation of the urethra.

Urethrocele. A prolapse of the female urethra.

Urethrorrhagia. Haemorrhage from the urethra.

Urethrorrhaphy. Repair of the urethra.

Urethrorrhoea. Discharge from the urethra.

Urethroscope. An instrument for examining the urethra under illumination.

Urethrostomy. The surgical establishment of a permanent opening into the membranous urethra from the perineum.

Urethrotomy. Surgical division of a stricture.

-uretic. (Gk *ourētikos:* ureter). Suffix indicating relationship to the urine or having a diuretic action.

-uria (Gk *ouron:* urine + *ia:* state). Suffix signifying a characteristic, or constituent, of urine.

Uric acid. $C_5H_4N_4O_3$. The end product of purine metabolism in man. Human blood normally contains 2·0 to 3·5mg. per 100ml.

Uricacidaemia. An excess of uric acid in the blood.

Uricaciduria. An excess of uric acid in the urine.

Uricase. An enzyme present in most mammals, apart from man and other primates, that catalyses the conversion of uric acid to allantoin.

Uridine. The nucleoside containing uracil.

Urin-, Urino- (Gk *ouron:* urine). Prefixes indicating association with urine.

Urinal. A receptacle, or place, for micturition.

Urinanalysis. Analysis of the urine.

Urination. The act of voiding urine. Micturition.

Urine. The fluid excreted by the kidneys.

Uro-, Ur- (Gk *ouron:* urine). Prefixes indicating relationship to urine.

Urobilin. The pigment to which urobilinogen is converted when urine is exposed to air.

Urobilinogen. A pigment derived from bilirubin, which is excreted in small amounts in the urine in health. It is identical with stercobilinogen.

Urobilinuria. The presence of an excess of urobilin in the urine.

Urocele. Distension of the scrotum with extravasated urine.

Urochesia. Passage of urine through the anus.

Urochrome. The pigment to which the yellow colour of urine is mainly due.

Urodynia. Pain on micturition.

Uroerythrin. A pigment in urine which gives the red colour to deposits of urates.

Urogenital. Pertaining to the urinary and genital apparatus.

Urography. Radiological examination of the urinary tract.

Urokinase. An enzyme in urine which acts as an activator of plasminogen, converting it to plasmin.

Urolith. A urinary calculus.

Urology. The study of the genito-urinary tract.

Uropepsinogen. One of two pepsinogens in the urine.

Uroporphyrin. A porphyrin occurring in the urine.

Uroporphyrinogen. A precursor of uroporphyrin.

Urticaria. An eruption characterized by the development of weals similar to those caused by the sting of a nettle. Hence the alternative name of nettle rash. The weals wax and wane and itch intensely.

Uter-, Utero- (L *uterus:* uterus) Prefixes indicating relationship to the uterus.

Uterocervical. Pertaining to the body and the cervix of the uterus.

Utero-ovarian. Pertaining to the uterus and the ovaries.

Uteropelvic. Pertaining to the uterus and the pelvis.

349

UVULITIS

Uterosacral. Pertaining to the uterus and the sacrum.

Uterovesical. Pertaining to the uterus and the urinary bladder.

Uterus. The hollow muscular organ situated in the pelvis behind the bladder and in front of the rectum, in which the impregnated ovum develops. The virgin uterus measures about 7·5cm. in length, 5cm. in breadth at its upper part, and 2·5cm. in thickness. It consists of a body and a cervix. (*Plural:* uteri.) **Bicornuate uterus,** a uterus that is more or less divided into two cavities; the cervix may be double or single. **Uterus didelphys,** double uterus. **Double uterus,** the presence of two distinct uteri lying side by side, the result of complete lack of fusion of the Müllerian ducts. **Infantile uterus,** a uterus in which the cervix is long in proportion to the body, and the body is thin-walled and small. **Septate uterus,** a uterus in which a septum divides the cavity into two. **Unicornuate uteris,** a uterus which has only one fully developed horn.

Utricle. A small sac. **Utricle of the ear,** the larger of the two vestibular sacs in the membranous labyrinth. **Prostatic utricle,** a cul-de-sac in the prostatic portion of the urethra.

Uvea. Uveal tract.

Uveitis. Inflammation of the uveal tract.

Uveoparotid. Pertaining to the uveal tract and the parotid gland.

Uveoparotitis. A bilateral affection characterized by simultaneous uveitis and parotitis. Uveoparotid fever. It is a form of sarcoidosis.

Uveoscleral. Pertaining to the uveal tract and the sclera.

Uvula. A fleshy pendent mass. **Uvula of the cerebellum,** the portion of the inferior surface of the cerebellum lying between the pyramid and the nodule. **Uvula of the palate,** the small conical process hanging from the middle of the lower border of the soft palate. **Uvula of the urinary bladder,** the slight elevation immediately behind the internal urethral orifice in the middle-aged male.

Uvulectomy. Surgical excision of the uvula.

Uvulitis. Inflammation of the uvula.

V

Vaccinate. To administer vaccine in order to induce immunity against a given organism or organisms.

Vaccination. The term originally introduced to denote the process of inoculating the lymph from a cowpox lesion as a means of inducing immunity against smallpox. It is now used to denote the administration of attenuated or dead cultures of any organism to induce immunity.

Vaccine. A preparation of antigenic material administered to induce a specific immunity to infection by the organism from which the antigenic material has been prepared. **Autogenous vaccine,** a vaccine prepared from organisms isolated from the individual to be vaccinated. **Bacillus Calmette-Guérin vaccine,** B.P. 1968, a suspension of living cells of an authentic strain of the tubercle bacillus of Calmette and Guérin. B.C.G. vaccine. **Bacillus Calmette-Guérin vaccine, percutaneous,** B.P. 1968, a suspension of living cells of an authentic strain of the tubercle bacillus of Calmette and Guérin with a higher viable bacterial count than Bacillus Calmette-Guérin vaccine. **Bacterial vaccine,** a vaccine made from bacteria. **Cholera vaccine,** B.P. 1968, a sterile suspension of suitable strains of *Vibrio cholerae*, containing not less than 8000 million *V. cholerae* per millilitre. **Cholera vaccine, mixed,** B.P. Addendum 1969, a mixture of cholera vaccine and el tor vaccine, containing not less than 4000 million *V. cholerae* and not less than 4000 million *V. cholerae* biotype *el tor* in 1 ml. **Diphtheria vaccine,** B.P. 1968, a vaccine prepared from diphtheria toxin produced by the growth of *Corynebacterium diphtheriae*. It occurs in the following forms: *Formol toxoid, Alum precipitated toxoid, Purified toxoid aluminium phosphate, Purified toxoid aluminium hydroxide, Toxoid-antitoxin floccules*. **Diphtheria and pertussis vaccine,** B.P. 1968, a mixture of diphtheria vaccine formol toxoid and] pertussis vaccine. **Diphtheria and tetanus vaccine,** B.P. 1968, a mixture of diphtheria vaccine, formol toxoid and tetanus vaccine in simple solution, or of the constituent toxoids absorbed on to aluminium hydroxide or phosphate. **Diphtheria, tetanus, and pertussis vaccine,** B.P. 1968, a mixture of diphtheria formol toxoid vaccine, tetanus vaccine in simple solution, and pertussis vaccine. **Diphtheria, tetanus, pertussis, and poliomyelitis vaccine,** B.P. 1968, a mixture of diphtheria formol toxoid vaccine, tetanus vaccine in simple solution, pertussis vaccine, and poliomyelitis vaccine (inactivated). **Diphtheria, tetanus, and poliomyelitis vaccine,** B.P. 1968, a mixture of diphtheria formol toxoid vaccine, tetanus vaccine in simple solution and poliomyelitis vaccine (inactivated). **El tor vaccine,** B.P. Addendum 1969, a sterile suspension of not less than 8000 million *V. cholerae* biotype *el tor* in 1 ml. **Influenza vaccine** B.P. 1968, an aqueous suspension of a suitable strain or strains of influenza virus, so inactivated that they are non-infective but retain their antigenic properties. **Measles vaccine (inactivated),** B.P. 1968, an aqueous suspension of a suitable measles virus inactivated so that it is non-infective but retains its antigenic properties. **Measles vaccine (live attenuated),** B.P. 1968, an aqueous suspension of an approved strain of live attenuated measles virus, grown in cultures of chick embryo cells. **Mixed vaccines,** mixture of two or more simple vaccines. **Pertussis vaccine,** B.P. 1968, a sterile suspension of killed *Bordetella pertussis*. **Plague vaccine,** B.P. 1968, a sterile suspension of suitable strains of *Pasteurella pestis*, containing 3000 million *P. pestis* per millilitre. **Poliomyelitis vaccine (inactivated),** B.P. 1968, an aqueous suspension of suitable strains of poliomyelitis virus, types 1, 2 and 3, grown in cultures of monkey kidney tissue and inactivated by a suitable method. **Poliomyelitis vaccine (oral),** B.P. 1968, an aqueous suspension of suitable, live, attenuated strains of poliomyelitis virus, types 1, 2, or 3, grown in cultures of monkey kidney tissue. **Rabies vaccine,** B.P. 1968, a suspension of a suitable killed rabies virus in uncontaminated brain tissue derived from animals previously infected intracerebrally with rabies virus. **Rubella vaccine (live attenuated),** B.P. addendum, 1971, an aqueous suspension of a suitable live attenuated strain of rubella virus grown in suitable cell cultures. **Smallpox vaccine,** B.P. 1968, a preparation of vaccinial material obtained from the lesions produced on the skin of living mammals, or in the membranes of the chick embryo, or in cultures of suitable tissue, by the inoculation of vaccinia virus. **Tetanus vaccine,** B.P. 1968, a vaccine prepared from tetanus toxin produced by the growth of *Clostridium tetani.* It occurs in the following forms: *Tetanus vaccine in simple solution, Alum precipitated tetanus vaccine, Purified toxoid aluminium hydroxide, Purified toxoid aluminium phosphate.* **Tetanus and pertussis vaccine,** B.P. 1968, a mixture of tetanus vaccine in simple solution and pertussis vaccine. **Typhoid vaccine,** B.P. Addendum 1969, a sterile suspension of 1000 million *S. typhi* in the volume stated on the label as the dose. **Typhoid-paratyphoid vaccines,** sterile mixed suspensions of *Salmonella typhi* and *Salmonella paratyphi.* **Typhoid-paratyphoid A and B vaccine,** B.P. 1968, 1000 million *S. typhi,* 500 or 750 million *S. paratyphi A,* and 500 or 750 million *S. paratyphi B.* in 1ml. **T.A.B. Vaccine. Typhoid-paratyphoid A, B, and C vaccine,** B.P. 1968, 1000 million *S. typhi,* and 500 or 750 million each of *S. paratyphi A., S. paratyphi B.,* and *S. paratyphi C* in 1ml. **T.A.B.C.** vaccine. **Typhoid-paratyphoid A and B and cholera vaccine,** B.P. 1968, 1000 million *S. typhi,* 500 or 750 million of both *S. paratyphi A* and *S. paratyphi B,* and 8000 million cholera vibrios in 1ml. **typhoid-paratyphoid A and B and tetanus vaccine,** B.P. 1968, 500 or 1000 million *S. typhi,* 250 or 500 million of both *S. paratyphi A* and *S. paratyphi B,* and 0·9 ml. of tetanus vaccine in simple solution, in 1ml. **Typhus vaccine,** B.P. 1968, a sterile suspension of epidemic and murine typhus rickettsiae which have been killed.

Viral vaccine, a vaccine made from viruses. **Yellow fever vaccine,** B.P. 1968, an aqueous suspension of chick-embryo tissue containing the attenuated but antigenic strain of yellow fever virus known as 17D.

Vaccinia. The infectious condition induced in man by smallpox vaccination. **Generalized vaccinia,** a widespread vesicular eruption following smallpox vaccination. **Progressive vaccinia,** a rare and lethal complication of primary smallpox vaccination, characterized by massive necrotic lesions. Vaccinia gangrenosa.

Vaccinoid. Resembling vaccinia.

Vacuole. A small space.

Vacuum. A space exhausted of gas or air.

Vagal. Pertaining to the vagus nerve.

Vagin-, Vagino- (L *vagina:* sheath, vagina). Prefixes indicating association with the vagina.

Vagina. A sheath. The canal which extends from the vestibule to the uterus.

Vaginismus. Painful spasm of the vagina on attempted coitus.

Vaginitis. Inflammation of the vagina.

Vaginoplasty. A plastic operation on the vagina.

Vaginoscope. A vaginal speculum.

Vagitus. The cry of an infant.

Vago- (L *vagus:* wandering). Prefix indicating association with the vagus nerve.

Vagotomy. Surgical division of the vagus nerve.

Vagotonia. A somewhat nebulous condition characterized by over-action or irritability of the vagus nerve or parasympathetic nervous system.

Vagovagal. Pertaining to the state induced when the afferent and efferent fibres of the vagus are both stimulated.

Vagus. The 10th cranial nerve. (*Plural:* vagi.)

Valency. The combining power of one atom or radical.

Valetudinarian. An invalid.

Valgus. Bent or displaced outwards. **Hallux valgus,** displacement of the big toe laterally. **Pes valgus,** outward distortion of the foot. **Talipes valgus,** pes valgus.

Valine. α-Amino-isovaleric acid. One of the essential amino-acids.

Vallecula. A depression or furrow. (*Plural:* valleculae.) **Vallecula of the cerebellum,** the deep hollow that separates the two cerebellar hemispheres inferiorly. **Vallecula of the**

larynx, the depression on each side of the median glossoepiglottic fold.

Valve. A device to prevent reflux. **Anal valves,** small, crescentic, valve-like folds that link the lower ends of the anal columns. **Aortic valve,** the three semilunar cusps which surround the orifice of the aorta and prevent reflux of blood into the left ventricle. **Atrioventricular valves,** the mitral and tricuspid valves. **Coronary sinus, valve of,** a thin semicircular valve that guards the opening of the coronary sinus into the right atrium. **Ileocaecal valve,** the valve that covers the opening of the ileum into the caecum. **Lymphatic valves,** the semilunar folds of intima, usually occurring in pairs, that prevent reflux of lymph in the lymph vessels. **Mitral valve,** the bicuspid left atrioventricular valve that guards the orifice between the left atrium and left ventricle. **Pulmonary valve,** the three semilunar cusps attached to the wall of the pulmonary trunk at its junction with the right ventricle which prevent reflux from the trunk into the ventricle. **Spiral valve,** the series of 5 to 12 crescentic folds of mucous membrane in the cystic duct. **Tricuspid valve,** the tricuspid right atrioventricular valve that guards the opening between the right atrium and right ventricle. **Venous valves,** semilunar reduplications of the inner coat, strengthened by connective tissue and elastic fibres, and covered by endothelium, found throughout the venous system to prevent reflux of blood.

Valvotomy. Surgical operation for widening a stenosed valve.

Valvule. A small valve or cusp.

Valvulitis. Inflammation of a valve.

Vanadium. A rare metallic element. Symbol V. Atomic weight 50·95. Atomic number 23.

Vancomycin hydrochloride. B.P. 1968. An antibiotic produced by the growth of certain strains of *Streptomyces orientalis,* which is active against gram-positive cocci.

Vanilla. The cured, full-grown, unripe fruit of *Vanilla planifolia,* used as a flavouring agent.

Vanillin, B.P.C. 1968. $C_8H_8O_3$. A flavouring agent obtained from *Vanilla planifolia* and other species of vanilla.

Vaporizer. An instrument for producing a fine, vaporized spray for inhalation. An atomizer.

Vapour. A gaseous phase of matter which is solid or liquid at ordinary temperature.

Varicectomy. Surgical excision of a varicose vein or varix.

Varicella. Chickenpox.

Varicocele. Varicosity of the testicular veins.

Varicoid. Resembling a varix.

Varicose. Of the nature of a varix. Dilated and tortuous.

Variola. Smallpox.

Variolar. Pertaining to smallpox.

Varioloid. A term applied to the mild form of smallpox that sometimes occurs in individuals who have been vaccinated.

Varix. An enlarged and tortuous vein, artery, or lymphatic channel—usually the first of these.

Varus. Inversion. **Talipes varus,** inversions of the foot.

Vas-, Vaso- (L *vas:* vessel). Prefixes signifying relationship with the blood-vessels.

Vas. A duct or channel, more particularly a blood vessel. (*Plural:* vasa.) **Vasa vasorum,** the nutrient blood vessels of the arteries and veins.

Vascular. Relating to, or containing, blood vessels.

Vascularization. The formation or development of blood vessels.

Vasculitis. Inflammation of a blood vessel.

Vasculo- (L *vasculum:* a small vessel). Prefix signifying relationship to blood vessels.

Vasectomy. Surgical excision of the whole, or part, of the ductus deferens.

Vasoactive. Exerting an action on blood vessels.

Vasoconstriction. Narrowing of the lumen of a blood vessel.

Vasodepression. Damping down of vasomotor activity.

Vasodilatation. Widening of the lumen of a blood vessel.

Vasoligation. Ligation of the ductus deferens.

Vasomotion. The term applied to the spontaneously occurring periodic relaxation and constriction of the thoroughfare channel and its precapillaries, which connect the arterioles with the venules.

Vasomotor. Concerned with, or pertaining to, the control of blood vessels, whether vasoconstriction or vasodilatation.

Vasoparesis. Paresis of the vasomotor nerves.

Vasopressin injection. B.P. 1968. A sterile aqueous solution containing the pressor and antidiuretic principles of the posterior lobe of the pituitary. It is used in the treatment of diabetes insipidus.

Vasopressor. Producing vasoconstriction and a rise in blood pressure.

Vasospasm. Spasmodic vasoconstriction.

Vasotomy. Surgical incision into, or division of, the ductus deferens.

Vasovagal. Pertaining to blood vessels and the vagus nerve. **Vasovagal attack,** a paroxysmal syndrome characterized by precordial discomfort, dyspnoea, and fatigue without loss of consciousness. **Vasovagal syncope,** fainting.

Vastus. Vast.

Vector. A carrier. A quantity that has both magnitude and direction.

Vectorcardiography. The study of the spatial orientation of the electrical forces of the heart.

Vegan. An extreme vegetarian who does not even take milk, butter, cheese or eggs.

Vegetable. A plant used as a food. Pertaining to plants as distinguished from animals and minerals.

Vegetarian. One who does not eat meat.

Vegetation. A plant-like growth, such as the organized clots that form on the heart valves in subacute bacterial endocarditis. The process of growth in plants.

Vegetative. Concerned with growth and nutrition, living without will or effort, like a vegetable.

Veillonella. A genus of gram-negative cocci which grow as commensals in the mouth and alimentary tract of man and animals.

Vein. A blood vessel conveying blood from the capillary bed towards the heart. **Venae comitantes,** veins accompanying arteries. **Deep veins,** veins usually enclosed in the same connective-tissue sheaths with the arteries. **Emissary veins,** veins which pass through apertures in the cranial wall and establish communications between the venous sinuses inside the skull and the veins external to it. **Pulmonary veins,** the only veins which contain oxygenated blood which they return from the lungs to the heart. **Superficial veins,** veins that lie in the superficial fascia and are very variable in their disposition. **Systemic veins,** the veins that return venous blood to the heart, as opposed to the pulmonary veins. **Varicose veins,** veins that are abnormally dilated and tortuous. **Vortex veins,** the ciliary veins as seen on the outer surface of the choroid.

Velamen. Velum. (*Plural:* velamina.)

Velamentum. Velum. (*Plural:* velamenta.)

Vellus. The fine hair that covers the body up to puberty.

Velum. Veil or covering. (*Plural:* vella.)

Vena. Vein. (*Plural:* venae.)

Vene- (L *vena:* vein). Prefix indicating association with veins. (L *venenum:* venom). Prefix indicating association with venom.

Venepuncture. Puncture of a vein.

Venereal. Relating to, or propagated by, sexual intercourse.

Venereology. The branch of medicine concerned with venereal disease.

Venesection. The withdrawal of blood by puncture of a vein.

Veno- (L *vena:* vein). Prefix signifying relationship with veins.

Venography. Visualization of the veins by radiography, with or without the injection of radio-opaque substances.

Venom. Poison, particularly that secreted by snakes and the like. **Snake venom antiserum,** B.P.C. 1968, native serum, or a preparation from native serum, containing the antitoxic globulins, or their derivatives, that have the power of neutralizing the venom of one or more kinds of snakes.

Venomotor. Causing veins to dilate or constrict.

Veno-occlusive. Pertaining to occlusion or obstruction of veins. **Veno-occlusive disease of the liver,** an acute type of hepatic vein occlusion, predominantly in children, due to plant toxins imbibed in bush tea, which occurs in Jamaica, India and Africa.

Venosclerosis. Thickening of the walls of the veins. Phlebosclerosis.

Venospasm. Spasm of the veins.

Venter. Belly.

Ventilation. The process of change of air. The exchange of air in the lungs. **Maximum voluntary ventilation,** maximum amount of air that can be breathed by a voluntary effort in one minute. Maximum breathing capacity.

Ventouse. A cupping glass. Now being used in obstetrics as a means of facilitating the birth of the child. Vacuum extractor.

Ventr-, Ventro- (L *venter:* belly). Prefixes signifying association with the belly, or the front of the body.

Ventral. Relating to the front of the body or limbs. Relating to the belly.

Ventricle. A small cavity. **Ventricles of the brain,** 4 cavities in the interior of the brain: 2 lateral ventricles, a 3rd and a 4th ventricle. **Fourth ventricle,** a tent-shaped space in front of the cerebellum and behind the pons and upper part of the medulla oblongata. It is continuous superiorly through the cerebral aqueduct with the 3rd ventricle, and inferiorly with the central canal of the medulla oblongata. **Lateral ventricles,** irregular cavities in the lower and medial parts of the cerebral hemispheres, one on each side of the median plane, which communicate with the 3rd ventricle. **Third ventricle,** a median cleft between the two thalami, which communicates behind with the 4th ventricle and in front with the lateral ventricles. **Ventricles of the heart,** a left and a right ventricle. **Left ventricle,** the cardiac cavity that receives arterial blood from the left atrium and pumps it into the systemic circulation through the aorta. **Right ventricle,** the cardiac cavity that receives venous blood through the venae cavae and pumps it into the lungs through the pulmonary arteries. **Terminal ventricle,** the fusiform dilatation in the lower part of the conus medullaris.

Ventriculitis. Inflammation of the ventricles of the brain.

Ventriculo- (L *ventriculus:* diminutive of *venter:* belly). Prefix signifying relationship to a ventricle.

Ventriculoatriostomy. The surgical procedure of establishing a passage between a cerebral ventricle and the right atrium, as a palliative means of treating hydrocephalus.

Ventriculocisternosty. The surgical procedure of establishing a passage between the ventricles of the brain and the subarachnoid space.

Ventriculography. Radiography of the cerebral ventricles by means of the injection of a radio-opaque substance or air. Radiography of the ventricles of the heart, after injection of a radio-opaque substance.

Ventriculoscopy. Direct examination of the ventricles of the brain by means of the insertion of a special endoscope (or ventriculoscope).

Ventriculostomy. Surgical establishment of an opening between the 3rd ventricle and the subarachnoid space.

Ventrofixation. The suturing of an abdominal organ to give it support.

Venule. A small vein.

Verapamil. The B.P. Commission approved name for a coronary dilator.

Verazide. The B.P. Commission approved name for an anti-tuberculosis drug.

Verbigeration. The constant repetition of meaningless sentences and words.

Verdigris. A green deposit upon copper due to the formation of cupric salts. A basic copper acetate.

Vermicide. An anthelmintic. An agent or drug that kills worms.

Vermiculation. Worm-like movement.

Vermiform. Shaped like a worm.

Vermifuge. An agent that expels intestinal worms.

Vermis. A worm-like structure. **Vermis of the cerebellum,** the narrow median strip that joins the two cerebellar hemispheres.

Vernier. A finely graduated scale auxiliary to a cruder scale, to allow fine measurements to be made.

Vernix. Varnish. **Vernix caseosa,** the desquamated epidermis mixed with sebaceous secretion, with which the skin is covered during the last three months of foetal life.

Verruca. Wart. (*Plural:* verrucae.)

Verrucous. Warty. Covered with warts. Verruose.

Verruga peruana. The form of bartonellosis characterized by multiple miliary haemangiomas.

Versicolour. Variegated.

Version. The procedure whereby an unfavourable lie or presentation, of the foetus in utero is changed. **Bipolar version,** turning performed by insertion of the fingers into the dilated cervix. **External version,** turning of the foetus by bimanual abdominal manipulation. **Internal version,** turning of the foetus with one hand inside the uterine cavity and the other on the abdominal wall. **Podalic version,** when the breech is made to present.

Vertebr-, Vertebro- (L *vertebra* from *vertere*: to turn). Prefixes indicating association with the vertebral column.

Vertebra. One of the bones forming the spinal column, firmly connected to one another but capable of a limited amount of movement on one another. (*Plural:* vertebrae.) **Cervical vertebrae,** the upper 7 vertebrae. The 1st is known as the *atlas* because it supports the globe of the head. The 2nd is known as the *axis*, as it provides the pivot upon which the atlas, with the skull, rotates. **Coccygeal vertebrae,** the four fused rudimentary vertebrae which constitute the coccyx. **Fixed vertebrae,** the coccygeal and sacral vertebrae, so called because they are fused into the coccyx and sacrum, respectively.

Lumbar vertebrae, the 5 vertebrae in the lumbar region between the thoracic vertebrae and the sacrum. **Movable vertebrae,** the cervical, thoracic and lumbar vertebrae, all of which are separate bones. **Sacral vertebrae,** the 5 vertebrae which are fused to form the sacrum. **Thoracic vertebrae,** the 12 vertebrae which constitute the spinal column between the cervical and lumbar vertebrae.

Vertebrata. The division of the animal kingdom consisting of all those animals with a spinal column: mammals, birds, reptiles and fishes.

Vertex. The crown or summit. (*Plural:* vertices.)

Vertiginous. Relating to, or affected with, vertigo.

Vertigo. Consciousness of disordered orientation of the body in space.

Vesic-, Vesico- (L *vesica:* bladder). Prefixes indicating association with a bladder or blister.

Vesica. A bladder. (*Plural:* vesicae.)

Vesical. Pertaining to a bladder.

Vesicant. An agent that induces blistering.

Vesication. The production of blisters.

Vesicle. A small bladder or sac. A small blister formed by circumscribed elevation of the epidermis by serous fluid. **Amnio-embryonic vesicle,** the early amnion. **Seminal vesicle,** one of two sacculated pouches placed between the base of the bladder and the rectum, a straight narrow duct from which joins with the corresponding deferent duct to form the ejaculatory duct.

Vesicosigmoidostomy. The surgical formation of a communication between the urinary bladder and the sigmoid colon.

Vesicoureteric. Pertaining to the urinary bladder and the ureter.

Vesicula. Vesicle. (*Plural:* vesiculae.)

Vesicular. Pertaining to a vesicle. Containing vesicles. **Vesicular breathing,** breath sounds produced in the air vesicles of the lungs.

Vesiculated. Made up of, or containing, vesicles.

Vesiculectomy. Surgical excision of a vesicle, usually a seminal vesicle.

Vesiculitis. Inflammation of a vesicle.

Vesiculography. Contrast radiography of the seminal vesicles.

Vesiculopapular. Consisting of vesicles and papules, as of a skin eruption.

Vesiculopustular. Consisting of vesicles and pustules, as of a skin eruption.

Vestibule. An antechamber. **Aortic**

vestibule, the portion of the left ventricle immediately below the aortic orifice. **Vestibule of the bony labyrinth,** the central part of the bony labyrinth, situated medial to the tympanic cavity, behind the cochlea and in front of the semicircular canals. **Vestibule of the larynx,** the part between the laryngeal inlet and the level of the vestibular folds. **Vestibule of the mouth,** the slit-like space bounded externally by the lips and cheeks, internally by the gums and teeth. **Vestibule of the nose,** a slight dilatation just inside the aperture of the nostril. **Vestibule of the omental bursa,** the narrow passage lying to the left of the epiploic foramen, below the caudate process of the liver and above the superior part of the duodenum. **Vestibule of the vagina,** the cleft between the labia minora.

Vestige. A rudimentary structure. A remnant. A trace.

Viable. Capable of living.

Vial. Phial.

Vibration. Oscillation. A to-and-fro movement.

Vibrator. An instrument used for vibratory massage.

Vibrio. A genus of the family Spirillaceae, consisting of short, nonflexuous, curved, motile, gram-negative rods. *Vibrio cholerae,* the causative organism of cholera. *El tor vibrio,* a variant of the cholera vibrio.

Vibrissa. One of the coarse hairs growing in the vestibule of the nose. (*Plural:* vibrissae.)

Vicarious. Acting as a substitute.

Vidarabine. The B.P. Commission approved name for 9-β-D-arabinofuranosyladenine. An antiviral agent.

Vidiocystography. A method of investigation of the lower genito-urinary tract, whereby the bladder, bladder neck and urethra can be viewed on a screen during the act of micturition.

Villus. A minute, elongated projection. (*Plural:* villi.) **Arachnoid villus,** a diverticulum of the arachnoid space penetrating into the interstices of the dura mater. **Chorionic villus,** one of the vascular processes of the chorion, some of which enter into the formation of the placenta. **Intestinal villus,** one of the highly vascular processes that project from the mucous membrane of the small intestine.

Vinbarbitone. The B.P. Commission approved name for 5-ethyl-5-(1-methylbut-1-enyl)barbituric acid. A hypnotic and sedative.

Vinblastine sulphate. B.P. Addendum 1971. The sulphate of an alkaloid obtained from *Vinca rosea*. A cytotoxic agent used in the treatment of neoplastic disease.

Vincristine. The B.P. Commission approved name for an alkaloid extracted from *Vinca rosea*, which is an antineoplastic agent.

Vinculum. A band or ligament. (*Plural:* vincula.) **Vincula tendinum,** triangular, thread-like bands of synovial membrane that connect the flexor tendons of the fingers and toes to the dorsal part of the enclosing synovial sheath.

Vinegar. Impure, dilute acetic acid. A solution of the active principle of a drug in diluted acetic acid. **Squill vinegar,** B.P.C. 1968, a preparation containing 100 grammes of bruised squill in 1 litre of dilute acetic acid.

Vinum. Wine. A pharmaceutical preparation similar to a tincture, but using wine as the menstruum.

Vinylbitone. The B.P. Commission approved name for 5-(1-methylbutyl)-5-vinylbarbituric acid. A hypnotic and sedative.

Vinyl ether. B.P. 1968. C_4H_6O. A volatile general anaesthetic used in minor surgical procedures of short duration.

Viomycin sulphate. B.P. 1968. The sulphate of an antimicrobial base produced by certain strains of *Streptomyces griseus* var. *purpureus*, which is active against *Mycobacterium tuberculosis*.

Viper. A poisonous snake of the genus Vipera. *Vipera berus*, the only poisonous snake in Great Britain. The adder.

Viraemia. The presence of viruses in the blood stream.

Virgin. A woman who has never had sexual intercourse.

Virginiamycin. The B.P. Commission approved name for an antibiotic produced by *Streptomyces virginiae*, which is active against gram-positive microorganisms.

Virilism. Masculinity. The development of masculine tracts in the female.

Virilization. The response to excessive androgen of the androgen-sensitive structures of the female, such as the clitoris, sexual hair follicles, and larynx.

Virology. The study of viruses and virus diseases.

Virus. An infective agent which is so small that it can pass through filters that retain bacteria, can grow only in living cells, and contains only one kind of nucleic acid (deoxyribonucleic acid [DNA], or ribonucleic acid [RNA]) contained within a protein coat. Viruses are divided into eight main groups: **Adenoviruses, Arborviruses, Herpesviruses, Myxoviruses, Papovaviruses, Picornaviruses, Poxviruses, Reoviruses.**

Visceral. Pertaining to a viscus.

Viscero- (L *viscus, viscera:* internal organ). Prefix indicating relationship to the organs (viscera) of the body.

Visceroptosis. A falling down of the abdominal viscera. Splanchnoptosis.

Viscid. Sticky. Adherent.

Viscus. One of the organs enclosed within the thorax, abdomen or pelvis. (*Plural:* viscera.)

Viscosity. The resistance to flow or alteration of shape as a result of molecular cohesion. The quality of being viscid.

Vision. The faculty of seeing. Sight. Dreams or foresight. **Binocular vision,** the successful fusion of the retinal images from the two eyes into one. **Colour vision,** the ability to differentiate colours. **Coloured vision,** chromatopsia. **Dichromatic vision,** the form of colour blindness in which only two of the three primary colours are recognized. **Double vision,** diplopia. **Field of vision,** the area over which objects are visible simultaneously without movement of the eyes. **Night vision,** scotopic vision. **Peripheral vision,** vision recorded on the periphery of the retina away from the macula. **Phototopic vision,** vision in bright illumination, involving the cones. **Red vision,** erythropsia. **Scotopic vision,** vision in the dark or low illumination, involving the rods. Night vision. **Stereoscopic vision,** vision in depth. **Tube vision,** marked contraction of the fields of vision so that it is restricted to a narrow area round the fixation point.

Viprynium embonate. B.P. 1968. $C_{75}H_{70}N_6O_6$. A dye used in the treatment of threadworm infestation.

Visnadine. The B.P. Commission approved name for a coronary vasodilator.

Vitamin. An organic substance present in minute amounts in natural foodstuffs, which is essential for normal nutrition. **Vitamin A,** a fat-soluble vitamin found in foods of animal origin. Its precursor, carotene, is found chiefly in green vegetables. Halibut-liver oil is the richest source.

Deficiency leads to xerophthalmia, night blindness, skin eruptions and defective development of the teeth. Chemically there are two forms of vitamin A: retinol (vitamin A$_1$) and dehydroretinol (vitamin A$_2$). **Vitamin B complex,** a conglomeration of water-soluble vitamins which has now been split up into: thiamine (B$_1$), cyanocobalamin (B$_{12}$), folic acid, nicotinic acid, pantothenic acid, pyridoxine, and riboflavine. **Vitamin C,** ascorbic acid. The anti-scorbutic vitamin, found predominantly in fruits and vegetables. **Vitamin D$_2$** the anti-rachitic vitamin. Calciferol, B.P. (ergocalciferol). Fish-liver oils are the richest source. **Vitamin E,** tocophenol. **Vitamin K,** phytomenadione. **Vitamins capsules,** B.P.C. 1968, capsules each containing ascorbic acid 15mg., nicotinamide 7·5mg., thiamine hydrochloride 1mg.; riboflavine 0·5 mg.; vitamin-A activity 2,500 units; vitamin D 300 units. **Vitamins A and D capsules,** B.P.C. 1968, capsules, each containing 4500 units of vitamin-A activity and 450 units of vitamin D.

Vitamin A ester concentrate. B.P. 1968. An ester, or a mixture of esters, of retinol in arachis, or other suitable vegetable, oil, which contains in 1 gramme not less than 485,000 units of vitamin-A activity.

Vitelline. Resembling, or pertaining to, the yolk of an egg.

Vitellus. The yolk of an egg.

Vitiligo. A condition characterized by white patches of skin. Leucoderma.

Vitrella. A thin-walled glass capsule containing a volatile medicament, such as amyl nitrite, protected by a wrapping of fabric or other suitable material, and intended for use by crushing the glass and inhaling the vapour of the medicament.

Vitreous. Glass-like. The inert, jelly-like structure which occupies about four-fifths of the eyeball, hollowed in front for the reception of the lens. Vitreous body. Vitreous humour.

Vitriol. Sulphuric acid. Oil of vitriol. Blue vitriol, copper suphate. Green vitriol, ferrous sulphate. White vitriol, zinc sulphate.

Vivi- (L *vivus:* alive). Prefix meaning alive, or relationship to life.

Viviparous. Giving birth to living young, as apposed to oviparous.

Vivisection. The use of living animals for research purposes.

Vocal. Pertaining to the voice.

Voice. The sound produced by the passage of air through the vocal cords.

Volar. Pertaining to the palm of the hand or the sole of the foot.

Volatile. Tendency to evaporate rapidly.

Volatilize. To convert into vapour.

Volition. The exercise of the will.

Volsella. Forceps with hooked blades.

Volt. The unit of electric potential. The difference of electrical potential between 2 points of a conducting wire carrying a constant current of 1 ampere when the power dissipated between these two points is equal to 1 watt.

Volume. The space which a substance fills. Cubic capacity. **Blood volume,** the total or circulating blood volume, being the volume of whole blood in the body. Normally this is around 5 to 6 litres, equivalent to 3 to 3·5 litres per square metre of body surface, or 75 to 85ml. per kg. body weight. **Expiratory reserve volume,** the volume of air that can be expelled by a maximum expiration following a normal expiration (ERV). **Forced expiratory volume,** the volume of air expired between two stated time intervals during estimation of the forced [vital capacity (FEV). **Inspiratory reserve volume,** the maximum volume of air that can be inhaled after a normal inspiration (IRV). **Maximum voluntary ventilation,** the maximum volume of air that can be breathed by a voluntary effort in one minute (MVV). **Mean corpuscular volume,** mean or average volume of a single red cell expressed in cubic microns:

$$\frac{\text{Volume of packed cells in ml. per 1000 ml. blood}}{\text{Red cells in millions per c. mm.}}$$

Also known as mean red cell volume (MCV). The normal is 78 to 94 cubic microns. **Packed cell volume,** the volume occupied by the red cells contained in 100ml. of blood after packing by centrifugalization at an appropriate speed for an appropriate time, and expressed as a percentage (PCV). The normal is 42 to 47ml. per cent. **Residual volume,** the volume of air remaining in the lungs after a maximum [expiration (RV). **Stroke volume,** the volume of blood expelled from the left ventricle per beat. **Tidal volume,** the air shifted in one respiratory cycle (TV).

Volvulus. A twisting of the bowel on itself, resulting in obstruction.

Vomer. A thin, flat, quadrilateral bone which forms the posterior and inferior part of the septum of the nose.

Vomica. A cavity, especially in the lung. (*Plural:* vomicae.)

Vomit. To bring up the contents of the stomach. The material thus brought up.

Vomiting. The forceful expulsion of the contents of the stomach through the mouth. **Central vomiting,** vomiting induced by increased intracranial pressure. **Cerebral vomiting,** central vomiting. **Cyclical vomiting,** vomiting recurring at intervals. **Faecal vomiting,** vomiting in which the vomitus includes intestinal contents, and diagnostic of intestinal obstruction. **Vomiting of pregnancy,** the vomiting liable to occur in the early months of pregnancy. **Projectile vomiting,** vomiting in which the vomitus is shot out at high speed, as occurs in infants with congenital pyloric stenosis.

Vomitus. The material expelled in the process of vomiting.

Voyeur. One who indulges in voyeurism. A peeping Tom.

Voyeurism. Sexual gratification achieved from viewing the genital organs of others or sexual intercourse.

Vulv-, Vulvo- (L *vulva:* a covering). Prefixes indicating relationship to the vulva.

Vulva. The external genital organs of the female, comprising the mons pubis, the labia majora and minora, the clitoris, the vestibule of the vagina, the bulb of the vestibule and the greater vestibular glands. The pudendum.

Vulvectomy. Surgical excision of the vulva.

Vulvitis. Inflammation of the vulva.

Vulvovaginitis. Inflammation of the vulva and vagina.

W

Wafer. A cachet made of thin circular discs of flour and water, to contain powders.

Waist. The portion of the body between the costal margin and the pelvis.

Walnut. The seed of *Juglans regia*. One of the edible nuts.

Warble. A fly of the genus Hypoderma.

Warfarin sodium. B.P. 1968. $C_{19}H_{15}NaO_4$. An oral anticoagulant.

Wart. Verruca.

Wash. A lotion. An aqueous solution for external use. **Mouth-wash,** an aqueous solution, in a concentrated form, of substances with antiseptic, local analgesic, or astringent properties. There are two in the *British Pharmaceutical Index*, 1968; Sodium chloride mouth-wash, compound; Zinc sulphate and zinc chloride mouth-wash.

Wasp. A member of the order Hymenoptera, with a poisonous sting.

Water. H_2O. A clear, odourless, tasteless fluid freezing at 0°C (32°F) and boiling at 100°C (212°F). **Aromatic waters,** solutions, usually saturated, of volatile oil or other aromatic substances in water, mainly used for their flavouring properties as vehicles for the internal administration of medicaments. There are three in the *British Pharmacopoiea*, 1968: Chloroform water; Peppermint water; and Peppermint water, concentrated. There are six in the *British Pharmaceutical Codex*, 1968: Anise water, concentrated; Camphor water; Caraway water, concentrated; Chloroform water, double-strength; Cinnamon water, concentrated; Dill water, concentrated. **Distilled water,** Purified water, B.P. **Hard water,** water containing salts of calcium and magnesium in excess. **Heavy water,** water in which the hydrogen has been replaced by heavy hydrogen or deuterium. **Lime water,** Calcium hydroxide solution B.P. **Purified water,** B.P. 1968, water prepared from suitable potable water by distillation or by treatment with ion-exchange materials. Distilled water. It is unsuitable for making parenteral injections. **Soft water,** water low in salts of calcium and magnesium. **Water for injections,** B.P. 1968, sterilized distilled water free from pyrogens. Used for the making of parenteral injections.

Waterbrash. The regurgitation into the mouth of sour acid fluid from the stomach. Pyrosis.

Water-glass. A solution of sodium or potassium silicate.

Watt. The unit of power. It equals 1 joule per second.

Wave. An advancing series of alternating elevations and depressions. **Alpha waves,** waves in the electroencephalogram which have a frequency of 8 to 13 per second. **Anacrotic wave,** a notch in the upstroke of the pulse wave in aortic stenosis. Anadicrotic wave. **Beta waves,** waves in the electroencephalogram which have a frequency of 18 to 30 per second. **Delta waves,** waves in the electroencephalogram which have a frequency of 0·5 to 3 per second. **Dicrotic wave,** the positive pressure wave following the dicrotic notch on the downward stroke of the pulse wave. **Electrocardiographic waves,** the waves in the electrocardiogram: P, Q, R, S, T, U. **Electroencephalographic waves,** the waves in the electroencephalogram: alpha, beta, delta. **Electromagnetic waves,** the entire series of ethereal waves, all of which move with the velocity of light, but vary in wave-length from 10 million (10^7) to 10^{-11} cm. **ff waves,** the small, rapid, wholly irregular waves seen in the electrocardiogram in atrial fibrillation. **Hertzian waves,** the electromagnetic waves of relatively long wave-length used in radio and television. **Light waves,** the electromagnetic waves to which the retina is sensitive. **P wave,** the deflexion in the electrocardiogram representing atrial depolarization. **Peristaltic wave,** the wave of alternating contraction and relaxation in the small intestine responsible for the onward movement of the contents. **Pulse wave,** the pressure wave induced in the arteries by the passage of blood from the left ventricle into the aorta. **Q wave,** the initial downward deflexion of the QRS complex in the electrocardiogram, which represents ventricular depolarization. **R wave,** the first upward deflexion of the QRS complex in the electrocardiogram, which represents ventricular depolarization. **S wave,** the downward deflexion following R of the QRS complex in the electrocardiogram, which represents ventricular depolarization. **Sound waves,** the vibrations produced by a sounding body to which the ear is sensitive. **T wave,** the deflection in the electrocardiogram representing ventricular repolarization. **U wave,** a wave following the T wave in the electrocardiogram, of doubtful pathogenesis. **Ultrasonic waves,** waves of such frequency that the human ear is unable to hear them. **Ultraviolet waves,** electromagnetic waves beyond the violet end of the spectrum, which have powerful actinic and chemical properties.

Wave-length. The distance between two points in the identical phase of a wave cycle: i.e. from crest to crest.

Wax. An ester of a high-molecular-weight, monohydric alcohol, and a high-molecular-weight fatty acid: e.g. spermaceti. **Cetomacrogol emulsifying wax,** B.P.C. 1968, an emulsifying agent for producing oil-in-water creams. **Cetrimide emulsifying wax,** B.P.C. 1968, an emulsifying agent for producing water-in-oil creams. **Ear wax,** cerumen. **Emulsifying wax,** B.P. 1968, an emulsifying agent for producing oil-in-water creams. **Horsley's wax,** a preparation of 10 per cent of phenol in a mixture of olive oil and yellow beeswax, used to control haemorrhage in bone in cranial surgery. **Paraffin wax,** Hard paraffin, B.P.

Weal. A well-defined, slightly raised, flat lesion with reddened margins, caused by the release of histamine. A manifestation of nettlerash, or the sting of a nettle or insect.

Wean. To discontinue breast feeding.

Web. A membrane. The fold of skin joining the proximal aspects of the fingers and toes.

Weber. The magnetic flux which, linking a circuit of one turn, produces

in it an electromotive force of 1 volt as it is reduced to zero at a uniform rate in 1 second.

Weep. To shed tears. To exude fluid slowly.

Weight. The force with which a body is attracted to the earth by gravity. A standardized item, usually of metal, for weighing objects in a balance. **Atomic weight,** the weight of an atom of a substance as compared with an atom of oxygen which is taken as 16. **Equivalent weight,** the weight of an element which can replace, or combine with, a unit weight of hydrogen. **Gramme molecular weight,** the molecular weight of a substance expressed in grammes. **Molecular weight,** the sum of the weights of the atoms composing a molecule.

Wen. A sebaceous cyst.

Wheat. The grain of *Triticum vulgare,* the major cereal consumed in the English-speaking world. The germ and scutellum are relatively rich in the vitamin B complex.

Wheeze. To breathe noisily and with difficulty. The sound produced by obstructed breathing, usually of a whistling character.

Whelk. An edible mollusc which contains rather more protein (15 per cent) than fish.

Whey. The fluid that separates from clotted milk. Its nutritive value is low.

Whipworm. *Trichuris trichiura.*

Whisky. The alcoholic spirit distilled from malted grain (rye or maize in North America).

Whites. Leucorrhoea.

Whitlow. Infection of the pulp of the finger quick. Paronychia.

Whoop. The crowing inspiration of whooping-cough.

Whooping-cough. One of the commonest infectious diseases of childhood, due to infection of the respiratory tract with *Bordetella pertussis,* and characterized by a cough terminating in a typical whoop. Hence its name. Pertussis.

Windpipe. The trachea.

Wine. The fermented juice of the grape or other fruits. A weak tincture.

Wintergreen. Gaultheria.

Witch hazel. Hamamelis.

Womb. The uterus.

Wool. The hair or fleece of sheep and similar animals. **Wool alcohols,** B.P.C. 1968, an emulsifying agent for water-in-oil emulsions, obtained by treating wool fat with alkali. **Wool alcohols ointment,** B.P. 1968, a preparation containing 6 per cent of wool alcohols, with hard, soft, and liquid paraffins. **Wool fat,** B.P. 1968, the purified, anhydrous, fat-like substance obtained from the wool of sheep. Used to make emollient cream- and in the preparation of water-in-oil emulsions. **Hydrous wool fat,** B.P. 1968, a preparation containing 70 per cent of wool fat. Lanolin.

Wormwood. Absinthium. The fresh or dried leaves and flowering tops of *Artemisia absinthum.* The toxic factor in absinthe.

Wound. A sudden breach in the tissues of the body produced by physical means. **Contused wound,** a wound with broken edges produced by a blunt instrument. **Entry wound,** a wound made by a missile on entering the body. **Lacerated wound,** a wound in which the tissues are torn. **Penetrating wound,** a wound which enters into one of the cavities of the body. **Perforating wound,** a wound in which the causative agent has passed right through the body, causing both an entry and an exit wound. **Puncture wound,** a wound made by a pointed instrument. **Sucking wound,** open pneumothrax. A chest wound in which air is aspirated into the pleural cavity.

Wrist. Carpus. The part of the upper limb between the forearm and the hand.

Wrist-drop. Paralysis of the extensor muscles of the hand and fingers.

Wry-neck. Torticollis.

Wuchereria. A genus of filarial worms of the phylum Nematoda (class Phasmidia; superfamily Filaroidea), which occur in all warm climates. *Wuchereria bancrofti,* the most important and widespread of the genus, spread as a rule by *Culex fatigans,* resulting in lymphangitis and lymphadenitis in the acute stage, and elephantiasis in the chronic stage. *Wuchereria malayi,* a species found in Indonesia, India, Malaysia, Ceylon and the Far East, and transmitted by certain species of Mansonia and Anopheles.

X

Xanthelasma. Plaques of xanthomas in the eyelids, most commonly in elderly women.

Xanthine. $C_5H_5N_4O_2$. A naturally occurring purine derivative. **Xanthine oxidase,** an enzyme in the liver that oxidizes hypoxanthine to xanthine, and xanthine to uric acid.

Xanthinol nicotinate. The B.P. Commission approved name for 7- (2-hydroxy-3-[N-(2-hydroxyethyl)methylamino]-propyl) theophylline nicotinate. A vasodilator.

Xanthinuria. A rare metabolic disorder, due in part at least to the absence of xanthine oxidase in the liver, and characterized by the presence of excess xanthine in the urine, often accompanied by xanthine calculi. The presence of excess xanthine in the urine.

Xantho- (Gk *xanthos:* yellow). Prefix meaning yellow.

Xanthochromia. Yellowish discoloration.

Xanthocillin. The B.P. Commision approved name for antibiotics derived from the mycelium of *Penicillium notatum*.

Xanthoma. A small yellow-orange focal accumulation of fat-laden macrophages found in the skin. **Xanthoma diabeticorum,** the transitory, itchy yellow-orange papules, associated with hypercholesterolaemia, which occur in some patients with diabetes mellitus. **Xanthoma disseminatum,** a rare condition in which xanthomas are present in the skin and in the mucous membrane of the mouth, larynx and bronchi. **Juvenile xanthoma,** the occurrence of a few yellowish skin nodules in the first year or so of life, which disappear spontaneously. **Xanthoma palpebranum,** xanthelasma. **Xanthoma planum,** the form of xanthomatosis characterized by the presence of yellow streaks in the folds of the palms and soles. **Xanthoma tuberosum,** a familial form of xanthomatosis associated with hypercholesterolaemia, and characterized by the presence of yellow nodules on the extensor aspects of the larger joints.

Xanthomatosis. The state characterized by the appearance of xanthomas. It may be primary or secondary, often associated with hypercholesterolaemia, but sometimes merely a degenerative process.

Xanthophyll. One of the groups of yellow pigments known as lipochromes or carotenoids.

Xanthopsia. Yellow vision.

Xeno- (Gk *xenos:* stranger). Prefix meaning strange or foreign.

Xenodiagnosis. The method of diagnosing *Trypanosoma cruzi* infections by allowing the vector bug, *Panstrongylus megistus*, to feed on suspected cases, and recovering the trypanosome from the bug's droppings.

Xenograft. Heterograft.

Xenon. A gaseous element present in minute proportion in the atmosphere. Symbol Xe. Atomic weight 131·30. Atomic number 54.

Xenophobia. Morbid dread of meeting strangers or foreigners.

Xenopsylla. A genus of fleas. *Xenopsylla cheopis*, the rat flea, the transmitter of bubonic plague and of some cases of murine typhus.

Xenopus. A genus of South African toad used in a pregnancy diagnosis test.

Xenysalate. The B.P. Commission approved name for 2-diethylaminoethyl 3-phenylsalicylate. A preparation for the treatment of seborrhoea.

Xero- (Gk *xeros:* dry). Prefix meaning dry or relationship to dryness.

Xeroderma. A hereditary condition characterized by dryness of the skin, with branny scaling on the extensor aspects of the limbs and body. **Xeroderma pigmentosum,** a congenital condition, in which there is an inborn susceptibility to sunlight.

Xerophthalmia. A dry, lustreless condition of the conjunctiva due either to local infection or lack of vitamin A. Xerosis.

Xerosis. Abnormal dryness, as of the eye or skin.

Xerostomia. Dryness of the mouth due to inadequate salivary secretion.

Xiph-, Xiphi-, Xipho- (Gk *xiphos:* sword). Prefixes signifying relationship with the xiphoid process.

Xiphicostal. Pertaining to the xiphoid process and the costal cartilages.

Xiphisternum. The xiphoid process.

Xiphoid. Shaped like a sword. **Xiphoid process,** the lowest of the three sections of the sternum.

X-rays. Electromagnetic radiations of short wave-length, characterized by their ability to penetrate solid opaque matter and to produce ionization. The x-rays used in diagnostic radiography are produced by accelerating electrons in an electron field between two electrodes maintained at high potential difference, not less than 40 kVp.

Xyl-, Xylo- (Gk *xylon:* wood). Prefixes indicating relationship to wood.

Xylamidine tosylate. The B.P. Commission approved name for N-2-(3-methoxyphenoxy)propyl - m-tolylacetamidine. An antiserotonin agent.

Xylene. $C_6H_4(CH_3)_2$. Dimethylbenzene. Used as a solvent and clarifier in microbiology. Xylol.

Xylol. Xylene.

Xylometazoline. The B.P. Commission approved name for 2-(4-t-butyl-2,6-dimethylbenzyl)-2-imidazoline. A vasoconstrictor.

Xylose. A pentose. Wood sugar. **Xylose excretion test,** a test of intestinal function, in which the fasting patient is given 25 grammes of D-xylose, and a five-hour specimen of urine is then collected.

Xylulose. A pentose excreted in the urine in pentosuria.

Y

Yawn. An involuntary opening of the mouth accompanied by marked widening of the pharynx, a deep inspiration, and facial and limb-stretching gestures.

Yaws. A contagious disease caused by *Treponema pertenue* and transmitted by direct human-to-human contact. It is characterized by a typical skin eruption of raspberry-like excrescences (yaws). The incidence is virtually limited to humid tropical areas.

Yeast. The name applied to various species of Saccharomyces, particularly *Saccharomyces cerevisiae*. It is a rich source of some members of the vitimin B complex. **Commercial yeast extract,** prepared from washed cells of brewers' or bakers' yeast. **Dried yeast,** B.P.C. 1968, unicellular fungi of the family saccharomycetaceae, which have been dried by a process which avoids decomposition of the vitamins present. Each gramme contains 0·1 to 0·2 mg. of thiamine, 0·3 to 0·6mg. of nicotinic acid and 0·04 to 0·06mg. of ribflavine.

Yellow fever. An acute febrile infectious disease caused by the yellow fever virus which is transmitted by mosquitos, mainly *Aëdes aegypti*. It is endemic in Africa south of the Sahara and north of Rhodesia, and in Central and South America.

-yl (Gk *hylē:* substance). Suffix signifying a radical in chemistry.

Yoghurt. Sour milk that has been curdled with organisms of the genus Lactobacillus after having been sterilized.

Yolk. The nutritive part of the egg or ovum.

Ytterbium. A metallic element. Symbol Yb. Atomic weight 173·04. Atomic number 70.

Yttrium. A rare metallic element. Symbol Y. Atomic weight 88·92. Atomic number 39.

Z

Zein. The principal protein of maize. It is lacking in lysine and contains very little trytophan.

Zero. Nought. **Absolute zero,** the lowest possible temperature: 0 on the Kelvin scale; $-273 \cdot 16°C$.

Zinc. A metallic element. Symbol Zn. Atomic weight $65 \cdot 38$. Atomic number 30.

Zinc chloride. B.P.C. 1968. $ZnCl_2$. A powerful caustic and astringent.

Zinc oxide. B.P. 1968. ZnO. A mild astringent and soothing constituent of dusting powders, ointments and lotions. **Compound zinc paste,** B.P. 1968, a preparation containing 25 per cent each of starch and zinc oxide in white soft paraffin. **Zinc and castor oil ointment,** B.P. 1968, a preparation containing $7 \cdot 5$ per cent of zinc oxide and 50 per cent w/w of castor oil. **Zinc and salicylic acid paste,** B.P. 1968, a preparation containing 24 per cent each of starch and zinc oxide and 2 per cent of salicylic acid in white soft paraffin, Lassar's paste. **Zinc cream,** B.P. 1968, a preparation containing 32 per cent of zinc oxide. **Zinc ointment,** B.P. 1968, a preparation containing 15 per cent of zinc oxide in simple ointment, B.P.

Zinc stearate. B.P.C. 1968. A soothing and protective application in the treatment of inflammation of the skin.

Zinc sulphate. B.P. 1968. $ZnSO_4$, $7H_2O$. Used as an astringent lotion. Very occasionally as an emetic.

Zinc undecenoate. B.P. 1968. ($C_{10} H_{19}$. $CO_2)_2Zn$. A topical fungicide. **Zinc undeconoate ointment,** B.P. 1968, a preparation containing 20 per cent of zince undecenoate and 5 per cent of undecenoic acid in Emulsifying ointment, B.P. Zinc undecylenate ointment.

Zirconium. A metallic element. Symbol Zr. Atomic number 40. Atomic weight $91 \cdot 22$.

Zona. A belt or girdle. A zone. (*Plural:* zonae.) Herpes zoster. **Zona arcuata,** the thin inner part of the basilar membrane of the cochlea that supports the spiral organ. **Zona cornea,** the outer layer of the skin, consisting of the stratum corneum, the stratum lucidum, and the stratum granulosum. **Zona fasciculata,** the middle zone of the cortex of the suprarenal gland. **Zona germinativa,** the outer zone of the epidermis, consisting of the stratum spinosum and the stratum basale. **Zona glomerulosa,** the outer zone of the cortex of the suprarenal gland. **Zona incerta,** a narrow layer that separates the subthalamic nucleus from the thalamus. **Zona orbicularis,** the ring round the neck of the femur formed by the circular fibres of the fibrous capsule of the hip joint. **Zona pectinata,** the outer part of the basilar membrane of the cochlea. **Zona pellucida,** the transparent membrane [surrounding the ovum. **Zona reticularis,** the innermost zone of the cortex of the suprarenal gland. **Zona striata,** zona pellucida.

Zone. A belt or girdle. **Horny zone,** the outer layer of the epidermis, consisting of the stratum corneum, the stratum lucidum and the stratum granulosum. **Predentine zone,** a clear layer seen in young teeth lying between the odontoblasts and the fully formed dentine. **Transitional zone,** the stretch of the anal canal from the pectinate line to the white line.

Zonular. Pertaining to a zonule. **Zonular fibres,** the fibres which constitute the suspensory ligament of the lens.

Zonule. A small band. **Ciliary zonule,** a thickening of the vitreous membrane, one layer of which forms the suspensory ligament of the lens.

Zonulolysis. Dissolution of the ciliary zonule by means of enzymes.

Zoo- (Gk *zoon:* animal). Prefix indicating relationship to animals.

Zoolagnia. Sexual attraction towards animals.

Zoomastigophora. The class of protozoa that contains the family Trypanosomatidae.

Zoonosis. An animal disease that is

transmissible to man. (*Plural:* zoonoses.)

Zoophilic. Having a preference for animals as opposed to man.

Zoopsia. Hallucinations of seeing animals.

Zoospore. A motile spore.

Zoster. Herpes zoster.

Zoxazolamine. The B.P. Commission approved name for 2-amino-5-chlorobenzoxazole. A muscle relaxant.

Zwitterion. A dipolar ion.

Zygoma. The zygomatic process of the temporal bone.

Zygomycetes. A group of phygomycetes.

Zygospore. A spore formed by the conjugation of two other spores.

Zygote. The fertilized ovum.

Zygotene. The second stage of the prophase of the first meiotic division of the sex cells, during maturation, in which genetically homologous chromosomes are attracted to each other and lie side-by-side.

Zymo- (Gk *zymē:* ferment). Prefix indicating relationship to an enzyme or fermentation.

Zymogen. The inactive precursor of an enzyme.

Zymology. The study of fermentation.

Zymolysis. Fermentation. Zymosis.

Zymotic. Relating to the infectious diseases.

Appendixes

Appendix I—Tables

Appendix II—Weights and Measures

APPENDIX I—TABLES

Table of Arteries

Name	Origin	Branches	Distribution
Alveolar, inferior	Maxillary	Mylohyoid, incisor, mental, lingual	Mylohyoid muscle, buccal mucous membrane, lower teeth, mandible, gums
Alveolar, superior anterior	Infraorbital		Upper incisor and canine teeth, maxillary sinus
Alveolar, superior posterior	Maxillary		Molar and premolar teeth, maxillary sinus, gums
Aorta (see Aorta)			
Appendicular	Ileocolic		Appendix
Arcuate of foot	Dorsalis pedis	2nd, 3rd and 4th dorsal metatarsal	Dorsal metatarsal portion of foot
Arcuate of kidney	Interlobar	Interlobular	Glomeruli
Auricular, deep	Maxillary		Tympanic membrane, temporomandibular joint
Axillary	Subclavian	Superior thoracic, thoraco-acromial, lateral thoracic, subscapular, circumflex scapular, anterior and posterior and circumflex humeral	Muscles and skin of shoulder, upper limb and chest, breast, shoulder joint

Basilar	Junction of two vertebral arteries	Pontine, labyrinthine, anterior inferior cerebellar, superior cerebellar, posterior cerebellar	Pons, internal ear, cerebellum, pineal body, temporal and occipital lobes of cerebrum
Brachial	Axillary	Profunda brachii, superior and inferior ulnar collateral, radial, ulnar	Shoulder, arm, forearm and hand
Brachiocephalic (innominate)	Aorta	Right common carotid, right subclavian	Right side of head and neck, right shoulder girdle and arm
Bronchial	Descending aorta		Bronchi and bronchioles, alveolar tissue of lungs
Buccal	Maxillary		Buccinator, mouth
Carotid, common	Right from brachiocephalic, left from arch of aorta	External and internal carotid	Head and neck
Carotid, external	Common carotid	Superior thyroid, ascending pharyngeal, lingual, facial, occipital, posterior auricular, superficial temporal, maxillary	Front of neck, face and scalp, side of head, ear, dura mater
Carotid, internal	Common carotid	Caroticotympanic, pterygoid, cavernous, hypophyseal, ophthalmic, anterior and middle cerebral, posterior communicating anterior, choroidal	Greater part of cerebral hemisphere, the eye, forehead and nose

Table of Arteries—*continued*

Name	Origin	Branches	Distribution
Central artery of retina	Ophthalmic		Retina
Cerebellar, inferior anterior	Basilar		Cerebellum
Cerebellar, inferior posterior	Vertebral		Medulla oblongata, choroid plexus of 4th ventricle
Cerebellar, superior	Basilar		Cerebellum, pons, pineal body, tela choroidea of 3rd ventricle
Cerebral, anterior	Internal carotid	Central and cortical	Corpus callosum, septum lucidum, putamen, caudate nucleus, frontal lobe, cingulate gyrus precentral gyrus, the precuneus
Cerebral, middle	Internal carotid	Central and cortical	The internal capsule, lentiform nucleus, caudate nucleus, frontal lobe, postcentral gyrus, parietal lobule, temporal lobe
Cerebral, posterior	Basilar	Central and cortical	Thalamus, globus pallidus, lateral geniculate body, choroid plexuses of 3rd and lateral ventricles, cerebral peduncle, pineal, quadrigeminal and medial geniculate bodies
Cervical, ascending	Inferior thyroid		Muscles of the neck, spinal cord, vertebrae
Cervical, deep	Costocervical trunk		Muscles of neck
Cervical, transverse	Thyrocervical trunk	Superficial, deep	Trapezius, rhomboids, latissimus dorsi, cervical lymph nodes
Choroidal	Internal carotid		Lateral geniculate body, choroidal plexus of lateral ventricle, globus pallidus, optic tract, hippocampus, posterior limb of internal capsule

Ciliary, anterior	Ophthalmic	Iris, conjunctiva
Ciliary, long posterior	Ophthalmic	Ciliary muscle, iris
Ciliary, short posterior	Ophthalmic	Choroid coat and ciliary processes
Circumflex, femoral, lateral	Profunda femoris	Muscles of thigh
Circumflex, femoral, medial	Profunda femoris	Thigh muscles, neck and head of femur
Circumflex, humeral, anterior	Axillary	Head of humerus, shoulder joint, muscles of shoulder
Circumflex, humeral, posterior	Axillary	Shoulder joint, deltoid, teres major and minor, long and lateral heads of triceps
Circumflex, iliac, deep	External iliac	Psoas, iliacus, sartorius, external and internal abdominal oblique, transverse abdominal muscles
Circumflex, iliac, superficial	Femoral	Skin and superficial fascia of thigh and abdomen, inguinal lymph nodes
Circumflex, scapular	Subscapular	Subscapularis, deltoid, long head of triceps
Coeliac	Abdominal aorta	Left gastric, hepatic, splenic — Oesophagus, stomach, liver, gall-bladder, duodenum, pancreas, greater omentum, spleen
Colic, left	Inferior mesenteric	Transverse and descending colon
Colic, middle	Superior mesenteric	Transverse colon
Colic, right	Superior mesenteric	Ascending colon and right colic flexure

Table of Arteries—*continued*

Name	Origin	Branches	Distribution
Coronary, left	Left posterior aortic sinus	Interventricular	Left atrium, both ventricles
Coronary, right	Anterior aortic sinus	Posterior interventricular	Right atrium, both ventricles
Costocervical	Subclavian	Superior intercostal, deep cervical	1st and 2nd intercostal spaces, muscles of neck, spinal cord
Cystic	Hepatic		Gall-bladder
Digital, common palmar (3)	Superficial palmar arch		Fingers
Dorsalis pedis	Anterior tibial	Tarsal, 1st dorsal metatarsal arcuate	Foot, toes, dorsum of foot
Epigastric, inferior	External iliac	Cremasteric, pubic	Skin and muscles of abdominal wall, cremaster, spermatic cord (or round ligament)
Epigastric, superficial	Femoral		Skin of lower abdominal wall, superficial inguinal lymph nodes
Epigastric, superior	Internal thoracic		Upper abdominal wall, rectus abdominis diaphragm
Ethmoidal, anterior	Ophthalmic		Dura mater, nose
Ethmoidal, posterior	Ophthalmic		Dura mater, nose
Facial	External carotid	Ascending palatine, tonsillar, submental, inferior and superior labial, lateral nasal	Tissues of the face, muscles of facial expression, tonsil, submandibular gland, soft palate

Artery	Origin	Branches	Distribution
Femoral	External iliac	Superficial epigastric, superficial circumflex iliac, superficial external pudendal, deep external pudendal, arteria profunda femoris, descending genicular	Skin of lower abdomen, external genitalia, inguinal lymph nodes, muscles of thigh, femur, knee joint
Gastric, left	Coeliac trunk	Oesophageal	Lesser curvature and cardia of stomach, lower end of oesophagus
Gastric, right	Common hepatic		Upper parts of anterior and posterior walls of stomach
Gastroduodenal	Hepatic	Right gastroepiploic, superior pancreaticoduodenal	Pylorus, duodenum, pancreas, common bile duct, greater omentum
Gastroepiploic, left	Splenic	Omental	Greater curvature of stomach, greater omentum
Gastroepiploic, right	Gastroduodenal		Stomach, duodenum, greater omentum
Gluteal, inferior	Internal iliac		Buttock and back of thigh and coccyx
Gluteal, superior	Internal iliac		Muscles of hip and buttocks
Hepatic	Coeliac trunk	Right gastric, gastroduodenal, cystic	Stomach, pancreas, gall-bladder, liver, greater omentum
Ileocolic	Superior mesenteric	Appendicular, ileal	Ascending colon, caecum, appendix, ilium
Iliac, common	Abdominal aorta	External and internal iliac	Psoas major, peritoneum, pelvic viscera, external genitalia, gluteal region, lower limb

Table of Arteries—*continued*

Name	Origin	Branches	Distribution
Iliac, external	Common iliac	Inferior epigastric, deep circumflex iliac	Cremaster, abdominal muscles, peritoneum, skin of lower abdominal wall, spermatic cord
Iliac, internal	Common iliac	Superior and inferior vesical, middle rectal, uterine, obturator, internal pudendal, inferior gluteal, iliolumbar, lateral sacral, superior gluteal	Pelvic wall and viscera, external genitalia, gluteal region, medial portion of thigh
Iliolumbar	Internal iliac	Lumbar, iliac	Cauda equina, iliacus, psoas major, quadratus lumborum
Infraorbital	Maxillary	Orbital, anterior superior alveolar	Rectus inferior, inferior oblique, lacrimal sac, upper incisor and canine teeth, maxillary sinus
Intercostal, anterior	Internal thoracic		Upper six intercostals, pectorals, the breast
Intercostal, posterior	Thoracic aorta	Lateral cutaneous, mammary, right bronchial	Muscles of the back, pectorals, serratus anterior, breast
Interosseous, anterior	Common interosseous		Radius, ulna, deep extensor muscles of forearm
Interosseous, common	Ulnar		Deep muscles of forearm, radius, ulna, median nerve
Interosseous, posterior	Common interosseous		Muscles on back of forearm
Labyrinthine	Anterior inferior cerebellar (or basilar)		Internal ear

Lacrimal	Ophthalmic	Lacrimal gland, eyelids, conjunctiva
Lingual	External carotid	Suprahyoid, dorsal lingual, sublingual	Tongue and floor of mouth
Lumbar	Abdominal aorta	Dorsal, spinal	Muscles and skin of back, vertebrae and vertebral canal
Malleolar, lateral, anterior	Anterior tibial		Lateral side of ankle
Malleolar, medial, anterior	Anterior tibial		Medial side of ankle
Masseteric	Maxillary		Masseter
Maxillary	External carotid	Deep auricular, anterior tympanic, middle meningeal, inferior alveolar, deep temporal, pterygoid, masseteric, buccal, posterior superior alveolar, greater palatine, pharyngeal, sphenopalatine	Upper and lower jaws, muscles of mastication, palate, nose, dura mater
Meningeal, middle	Maxillary		Trigeminal ganglion, facial and trigeminal nerves, tympanic cavity, tensor tympani
Mesenteric, inferior	Abdominal aorta	Left colic, sigmoid, superior rectal	Left third of transverse colon, descending and sigmoid colon, rectum
Mesenteric, superior	Abdominal aorta	Inferior pancreaticoduodenal, jejunal, ileal	Whole of small intestine except superior part of duodenum, caecum, ascending and most of transverse colon
Metacarpal, dorsal	Radial		Adjacent sides of thumb and index finger
Metacarpal palmar (3)	Deep palmar arch		Lumbricals, interossei, metacarpals

Table of Arteries—*continued*

Name	Origin	Branches	Distribution
Metatarsal, dorsal (3)	Arcuate		Adjacent sides of 2nd, 3rd, 4th and 5th toes
Metatarsal, dorsal, first	Dorsalis pedis		Medial border of great toe and adjoining sides of great and 2nd toe
Metatarsal, plantar (4)	Plantar arch		Adjacent sides of 2nd, 3rd, 4th and 5th toes
Metatarsal, plantar, first	Lateral plantar, dorsalis pedis		Medial side of great toe
Musculophrenic	Internal thoracic		Muscles of lower thorax and abdomen, pericardium
Obturator	Internal iliac	Iliac, vesical, pubic	Pelvic muscles, hip joint
Occipital	External carotid	Sternocleidomastoid, mastoid, auricular, meningeal	Mastoid, dura mater, auricle, muscles of neck and scalp
Ophthalmic	Internal carotid	Central artery of retina, lacrimal, ciliary, long posterior ciliary, short posterior ciliary, anterior ciliary, supraorbital, posterior ethmoid, anterior ethmoid, meningeal, medial palpebral, supratrochlear, dorsal nasal	Contents of the orbit, lacrimal sac, forehead, dorsum of nose, meatus of nose, frontal sinus and ethmoidal sinus
Ovarian	Abdominal aorta		Ovary, uterus, uterine tube, round ligament, skin of labium majoris and groin
Palatine, ascending	Facial		Soft palate, tonsil, auditory tube

Artery	Branch of	Branches	Distribution
Palatine, greater	Maxillary		Soft palate, tonsil, gums, palatine glands, roof of mouth
Palpebral, lateral	Lacrimal		Conjunctiva
Palpebral, medial (2)	Ophthalmic		Eyelids, nasolacrimal duct
Pancreaticoduodenal, inferior	Superior mesenteric		Duodenum, head of pancreas
Pancreaticoduodenal, superior	Gastroduodenal		Duodenum, head of pancreas
Peroneal	Posterior tibial		Deep calf muscle, soleus, fibula
Pharyngeal, ascending	External carotid	Pharyngeal, tympanic, meningeal	Constrictor muscles, stylopharyngeus, soft palate, tonsils, auditory tube, tympanic cavity, dura mater, hypoglossal and vagus nerves
Phrenic, inferior (2)	Aorta		Diaphragm
Plantar, lateral	Posterior tibial		Sole of foot, toes, heel and lateral side of foot
Plantar, medial	Posterior tibial		Abductor hallucis, flexor digitorium brevis, skin on medial aspect of sole of foot
Popliteal	Femoral	Anterior and posterior tibial	Knee and calf
Profunda brachii	Brachial	Radial collateral, superior and inferior ulnar collateral	Deltoid, triceps, humerus, coracobrachialis
Profunda femoris	Femoral	Lateral and medial circumflex femoral	Adductor, extensor and hamstring muscles, hip joint, femur
Pudendal, external, deep	Femoral		Skin of scrotum and perineum, labium majus, pectineus, adductor longus

Table of Arteries—*continued*

Name	*Origin*	*Branches*	*Distribution*
Pudendal, external, superficial	Femoral		Skin of lower abdominal wall, penis, scrotum, labium majus
Pudendal, internal	Internal iliac	Dorsal and deep arteries of the penis, inferior rectal, perineal, artery of the penis, posterior labial, deep and dorsal arteries of the clitoris	External genitalia, muscles in the pelvis and of the gluteal region
Pulmonary	Right ventricle	Right, left	Lungs
Radial	Brachial	Radial recurrent, palmar carpal, superficial palmar, dorsal carpal, first dorsal metacarpal, arteria princeps pollicis, arteria radialis indicis, palmar metacarpal (3)	Forearm, wrist, hand
Rectal, inferior	Internal pudendal		Anal canal, skin and muscles of anal region, skin of buttock
Rectal, middle	Internal iliac		Rectum, seminal vesicles, prostate
Rectal, superior	Inferior mesenteric		Rectum
Renal	Abdominal aorta		Kidney, suprarenal gland, ureter
Sacral, lateral (2)	Internal iliac		Sacral vertebrae, dorsum of sacrum
Sacral, median	Abdominal aorta		Coccygeal body, rectum, sacral foramina
Scapular, circumflex	Subscapular	Infrascapular	Subscapularis, deltoid, triceps

Artery	Source	Branches	Distribution
Sigmoid (2 or 3)	Inferior mesenteric		Descending and sigmoid colon
Sphenopalatine	Maxillary	Posterior lateral nasal, posterior septal	Nose, frontal, maxillary, ethmoidal, and sphenoidal sinuses
Spinal, anterior	Vertebral		Anterior spinal cord and its coverings
Spinal, posterior	Posterior inferior cerebellar		Posterior spinal cord and its coverings
Splenic	Coeliac trunk	Pancreatic, short gastric, left gastroepiploic	Pancreas, stomach, spleen, greater omentum
Sternocleidomastoid	Occipital		Sternocleidomastoid
Stylomastoid	Posterior auricular		Tympanic cavity, mastoid, semicircular canals
Subclavian	Right from brachiocephalic trunk, left from arch of aorta	Vertebral, internal thoracic, thyrocervical trunk, costo-cervical trunk	Muscles of neck and upper limb, brain and meninges, pleura, pericardium, bronchi, breast, peritoneum
Subcostal	Thoracic aorta		Quadratus lumborum, transversus abdominis, oblique internus abdominis, lumbar vertebrae
Sublingual	Lingual		Sublingual gland, mylohyoid and adjacent muscle, mucous membrane of mouth and gums
Submental	Facial		Mylohyoid and adjacent muscles, chin, gums
Subscapular	Axillary	Circumflex scapular	Muscles around the shoulder, scapula, shoulder joint

Table of Arteries—*continued*

Name	Origin	Branches	Distribution
Supraorbital	Ophthalmic		Skin, muscles and pericranium of forehead, rectus superior, levator palpebrae, frontal bone
Suprarenal, inferior	Renal		Suprarenal gland
Suprarenal, middle	Abdominal aorta		Suprarenal gland
Suprarenal, superior	Inferior		Suprarenal gland
Suprascapular	Thyrocervical trunk	Suprasternal, acromial	Shoulder joints, clavicle, scapula, and surrounding muscles
Tarsal (2)	Dorsalis pedis		Extensor digitorum brevis, tarsus
Temporal, deep (2)	Maxillary		Temporalis, skull
Temporal, middle	Superficial temporal		Temporalis
Temporal, superficial	External carotid	Transverse facial, anterior auricular, zygomatico-orbital, middle temporal, frontal, parietal	Parotid gland, masseter, temporomandibular joint, auricle, external meatus, orbicularis oculi, temporalis, frontal bone
Testicular	Abdominal aorta		Testis, cremaster
Thoracic, internal	Subclavian	Musculophrenic, superior epigastric, pericardiacophrenic, mediastinal, pericardial, sternal, anterior intercostal	Pleura, pericardium, diaphragm, anterior mediastinum, thymus, transversus thoracis-sternum, intercostals, pectoral muscles, breast, rectus abdominis
Thoraco-acromial	Axillary	Pectoral, acromial, clavicular, deltoid	Pectorals, breast, deltoid, sternoclavicular joint, subclavius

Artery	Branch of	Branches	Distribution
Thyrocervical trunk	Subclavian	Inferior thyroid, suprascapular, transverse cervical	Muscles of neck, scapular region and upper back, cervical spinal cord and vertebrae, larynx, trachea, oesophagus, thyroid, pharynx
Thyroid, inferior	Thyrocervical trunk	Ascending cervical, inferior laryngeal, tracheal, oesophageal, glandular	Muscles of the neck, cervical vertebrae and cord, trachea, oesophagus, thyroid, parathyroid
Thyroid, superior	External carotid	Infrahyoid, sternocleidomastoid, superior laryngeal, cricothyroid	Thyroid, larynx, hyoid muscles
Tibial, anterior	Popliteal	Posterior tibial recurrent, anterior tibial recurrent, anterior medial malleolar, anterior lateral malleolar	Leg, ankle, foot
Tibial, posterior	Popliteal	Medial and lateral plantar, circumflex fibular, peroneal	Leg, foot, heel
Tonsillar	Facial		Tonsil, base of tongue
Ulnar	Brachial	Anterior ulnar recurrent, posterior ulnar recurrent, common interosseous, anterior interosseous, posterior interosseous, palmar carpal, dorsal carpal, superficial palmar arch	Forearm, wrist, arm, hand
Uterine	Internal iliac		Uterus, part of vagina

Table of Arteries—*continued*

Name	Origin	Branches	Distribution
Vaginal	Internal iliac		Vagina, fundus of bladder, rectum
Vertebral	Subclavian	Posterior and anterior spinal, posterior inferior cerebellar, basilar	Muscles of neck, cerebellum, medulla oblongata
Vesical, inferior	Internal iliac		Bladder, prostate, seminal vesicles, ureter
Vesical, superior	Internal iliac		Bladder, ureter

Table of Muscles

Name	Origin	Insertion	Innervation	Action
Abductor digiti minimi (foot)	Lateral and medial tubercles of calcaneus; plantar aponeurosis	Lateral side of base of proximal phalanx of 5th toe	Lateral plantar nerve	Abducts little toe
Abductor digiti minimi (hand)	Pisiform bone; tendon of flexor carpi ulnaris	Ulnar side of base of proximal phalanx of little finger	Deep branch of ulnar nerve	Abducts little finger
Abductor hallucis	Medial tubercle of calcaneus; plantar aponeurosis	Medial side of base of proximal phalanx of great toe	Medial plantar nerve	Abducts and flexes great toe
Abductor pollicis brevis	Flexor retinaculum; tubercles of scaphoid bone and trapezium	Radial side of base of proximal phalanx of thumb	Lateral terminal branch of median nerve	Abducts and flexes thumb
Abductor pollicis longus	Lateral part of posterior surface of shaft of tibia	Radial side of bone of 1st metacarpal bone	Posterior interosseous nerve	Abducts and extends thumb
Adductor brevis	Inferior ramus of pubis	Femur along line from lesser trochanter to linea aspera; upper part of linea aspera	Obturator nerve	Adducts thigh
Adductor hallucis	Oblique head: bases of 2nd, 3rd and 4th metatarsal bones. Transverse head: plantar metatarsophalangeal ligaments of 3rd, 4th, 5th toes; deep transverse metatarsal ligaments	Lateral side of base of proximal phalanx of great toe	Deep branch of lateral plantar nerve	Adducts great toe
Adductor longus	Front of the pubis	Linea aspera of femur	Anterior division of obturator nerve	Adducts thigh

Tables of Muscles—*continued*

Name	*Origin*	*Insertion*	*Innervation*	*Action*
Adductor magnus	Inferior ramus of pubis; ramus of ischium; ischial tuberosity	Gluteal tuberosity of femur; linea aspera of femur	Obturator nerve; tibial portion of sciatic nerve	Adducts thigh
Adductor pollicis	Oblique head: capitate bone; bases of 2nd and 3rd metacarpal bones. Transverse head: palmar surface of 3rd metacarpal bone	Ulnar side of base of proximal phalanx of thumb	Deep branch of ulnar nerve	Approximates thumb to palm of hand
Anconeus	Posterior surface of lateral epicondyle of humerus	Lateral side of olecranon	Radial nerve	Extends elbow joint
Antitragicus	Outer part of antitragus	Tail of helix	Facial nerve	Vestigial
Arrectores pilorum	Corium	Hair follicle	Sympathetic	Erect hairs
Aryepiglottic	Back of muscular process of arytenoid cartilage	Apex of opposite arytenoid cartilage	Recurrent laryngeal nerve	Sphincter of inlet of larynx
Arytenoid, transverse	Back of muscular process and lateral border of arytenoid cartilage	Corresponding parts of opposite arytenoid cartilage	Recurrent laryngeal nerve	Closes opening of glottis
Auricularis, anterior	Epicranial aponeurosis	Spine of helix	Temporal branches of facial nerve	Draws auricle forwards and upwards
Auricularis, posterior	Mastoid	Ponticulus	Posterior auricular branch of facial nerve	Draws auricle backwards
Auricularis, superior	Epicranial aponeurosis	Cranial surface of auricle	Temporal branches of facial nerve	Raises auricle

Muscle	Origin	Insertion	Nerve supply	Action
Biceps brachii	Short head: apex of coracoid process Long head: Supraglenoid tubercle of glenoid cavity	Tubercle of radius; deep fascia of forearm	Musculocutaneous nerve	Flexes and supinates forearm
Biceps femoris	Long head: ischial tuberosity. Short head: linea aspera of femur	Head of fibula; fibular collateral ligament; lateral condyle of tibia	Sciatic nerve	Flexes knee joint
Brachialis	Front of humerus	Tuberosity of ulna; coronoid process	Musculocutaneous nerve	Flexes elbow joint
Brachioradialis	Lateral supracondylar ridge of humerus	Lower end of radius	Radial nerve	Flexes elbow joint
Buccinator	Outer surfaces of alveolar processes of maxilla and mandible; pterygomandibular raphe	Orbicularis oris muscle	Buccal branches of facial nerve	Compresses the cheeks
Bulbospongiosus	Median raphe of perineum; perineal body	Fascia of perineum and penis (or clitoris)	Perineal branch of pudendal nerve	Constricts penis in male, vagina in female
Chondroglossus	Hyoid bone	Muscles of tongue	Hypoglossal nerve	Depresses tongue
Ciliaris	Scleral spur	Ciliary processes	Parasympathetic	Accommodation of eye
Coccygeus	Spine of ischium	Coccyx; sacrum	4th–5th sacral nerves	Pulls coccyx forwards
Constrictor pharyngis inferior	Cricoid cartilage; thyroid cartilage	Median raphe of posterior pharyngeal wall	Pharyngeal plexus	Constricts pharynx
Constrictor pharyngis medius	Hyoid bone; stylohyoid ligament	Posterior median fibrous raphe	Pharyngeal plexus	Constricts pharynx

Table of Muscles—*continued*

Name	Origin	Insertion	Innervation	Action
Constrictor pharyngis superior	Pterygoid hamulus; pterygomandibular raphe; mandible	Median raphe of pharynx; pharyngeal tubercle of occiput	Pharyngeal plexus	Constricts pharynx
Coracobrachialis	Coracoid process	Medial border of humerus	Musculocutaneous nerve	Draws arms forwards and medially
Corrugator supercilii	Medial end of superciliary arch	Skin of forehead	Temporal branches of facial nerve	Draws eyebrows medially and downwards
Cremaster	Inguinal ligament	Pubic tubercle	Genital branch of genitofemoral nerve	Pulls testes up
Cricoarytenoid, lateral	Arch of cricoid cartilage	Arytenoid cartilage	Recurrent laryngeal nerve	Approximates vocal folds
Cricoarytenoid, posterior	Posterior surface of cricoid cartilage	Arytenoid cartilage	Recurrent laryngeal nerve	Separates vocal folds
Cricothyroid	Cricoid cartilage	Thyroid cartilage	External laryngeal nerve	Tenses vocal folds
Deltoid	Clavicle; acromion; spine of scapula	Deltoid tuberosity of humerus	Axillary nerve	Abducts, flexes and extends humerus
Depressor anguli oris	Mandible	Angles of mouth	Mandibular marginal branch of facial nerve	Draws angle of mouth downwards and laterally
Depressor labii inferioris	Mandible	Skin of lower lip	Mandibular marginal branch of facial nerve	Draws lips downwards
Depressor septi	Maxilla	Nasal septum	Upper buccal branches of facial nerve	Widens nasal aperture

Muscle	Origin	Central tendon	Nerve	Action
Diaphragm	Xiphoid process; lower 6 costal cartilages; lumbar vertebrae	Central tendon	Phrenic nerve	Principal muscle of inspiration
Digastric	Anterior belly: inner surface of mandible. Posterior belly: mastoid notch of temporal bone	Hyoid bone	Mylohyoid branch of inferior alveolar nerve; facial nerve	Depresses mandible; raises hyoid
Erector spinae	Median sacral crest; spines of the lumbar, and 11th and 12th thoracic vertebrae; supraspinous ligament; iliac crest; lateral sacral crest	Ribs and vertebrae	The spinal nerves	Maintenance of posture
Extensor carpi radialis brevis	Lateral epicondyle of humerus	Base of 2nd and 3rd metacarpal bones	Posterior interosseous nerve	Extends wrist
Extensor carpi radialis longus	Humerus	Base of 2nd metacarpal bone	Radial nerve	Extends wrist
Extensor carpi ulnaris	Lateral epicondyle of humerus	Base of 5th metacarpal bone	Posterior interosseous nerve	Extends wrist
Extensor digiti minimi	Common extensor tendon	Extensor aponeurosis of 5th finger	Posterior interosseous nerve	Extends little finger
Extensor digitorum	Lateral epicondyle of humerus	Extensor expansion of 4 medial fingers	Posterior interosseous nerve	Extends fingers
Extensor digitorum brevis	Calcaneus	Extensor tendons of 4 medial toes	Lateral terminal branch of deep peroneal nerve	Extends phalanges of 4 medial toes
Extensor digitorum longus	Lateral condyle of tibia; medial surface of fibula; interosseous membrane	Extensor tendons of 4 lateral toes	Deep peroneal nerve	Extends toes

Table of Muscles—_continued_

Name	Origin	Insertion	Innervation	Action
Extensor hallucis brevis	Calcaneus	Base of proximal phalanx of great toe	Lateral terminal branch of deep peroneal nerve	Extends great toe
Extensor hallucis longus	Fibula; interosseous membrane	Base of terminal phalanx of great toe	Deep peroneal nerve	Extends great toe; dorsiflexes foot
Extensor indicis	Ulna	Tendon of extensor digitorum to index finger	Posterior interosseous nerve	Extends index finger and wrist
Extensor pollicis brevis	Radius	Base of proximal phalanx of thumb	Posterior interosseous nerve	Extends thumb
Extensor pollicis longus	Ulna	Base of distal phalanx of thumb	Posterior interosseous nerve	Extends distal phalanx of thumb
Flexor carpi radialis	Medial epicondyle of humerus	Base of 2nd and 3rd metacarpal bones	Median nerve	Flexes wrist
Flexor carpi ulnaris	Medial epicondyle, and upper two-thirds, of ulna	Pisiform; hamate; 5th metacarpal bone	Ulnar nerve	Flexes wrist
Flexor digiti minimi brevis (foot)	Base of 5th metacarpal bone	Proximal phalanx of 5th toe	Superficial branch of lateral plantar nerve	Flexes little toe
Flexor digiti minimi brevis (hand)	Hamate bone; flexor retinaculum	Proximal phalanx of little finger	Deep branch of ulnar nerve	Flexes little finger
Flexor digitorum accessorius	Calcaneus; long plantar ligament	Fibrous connexion between flexores hallucis longus and digitorum longus	Lateral plantar nerve	Assists in flexion of toes

Flexor digitorum brevis	Medial tubercle of calcaneus; plantar aponeurosis	Middle phalanx of each of 4 lateral toes	Medial plantar nerve	Flexes toes
Flexor digitorum longus	Tibia	Distal phalanx of each of 4 lateral toes	Tibial nerve	Flexes toes
Flexor digitorum profundus	Ulna	Base of distal phalanx of each finger	Ulnar nerve; anterior interosseous branch of median nerve	Flexes fingers
Flexor digitorum superficialis	Medial epicondyle of humerus; coronoid process of ulna; radius	Middle phalanx of each finger	Median nerve	Flexes fingers and wrist
Flexor hallucis brevis	Cuboid; lateral cuneiform; tendon of tibialis posterior	Proximal phalanx of great toe	Medial plantar nerve	Flexes great toe
Flexor hallucis longus	Fibula; interosseous membrane	Base of distal phalanx of great toe	Tibial nerve	Flexes great toe
Flexor pollicis brevis	Flexor retinaculum; trapezium; trapezoid and capitate bones	Base of proximal phalanx of thumb	Median and ulnar nerves	Flexes thumb
Flexor pollicis longus	Radius; interosseous membrane	Base of distal phalanx of thumb	Anterior interosseous branch of median nerve	Flexes thumb
Gastrocnemius	Condyles of femur	Tendo calcaneus	Tibial nerve	Plantar flexes ankle
Gemellus, inferior	Ischial tuberosity	Greater trochanter of femur	Nerve to quadratus femoris	Rotates thigh laterally
Gemellus, superior	Spine of ischium	Greater trochanter of femur	Nerve to obturator internus	Rotates thigh laterally

Table of Muscles—*continued*

Name	Origin	Insertion	Innervation	Action
Genioglossus	Upper genial tubercle on mandible	Hyoid bone; tongue	Hypoglossal nerve	Protrudes and depresses tongue
Geniohyoid	Symphysis menti	Hyoid bone	Hypoglossal nerve	Raises hyoid
Gluteus maximus	Ilium; aponeurosis of erector spinae; sacrum; coccyx	Fascia lata; gluteal tuberosity of femur	Inferior gluteal nerve	Flexes hip
Gluteus medius	Ilium	Greater trochanter of femur	Superior gluteal nerve	Abducts thigh
Gluteus minimus	Ilium	Greater trochanter of femur	Superior gluteal nerve	Abducts thigh
Gracilis	Pubis; ischium	Tibia	Obturator nerve	Flexes leg
Helicis major	Spine of helix	Front of helix	Facial nerve	Vestigial
Helicis minor	Spine of helix	Crux of helix	Facial nerve	Vestigial
Hyoglossus	Hyoid bone	Tongue	Hypoglossal nerve	Depresses tongue
Iliacus	Iliac fossa; sacrum	Tendon of psoas major; lesser trochanter of femur	Femoral nerve	Flexes thigh
Iliococcygeus	Ischial spine	Coccyx		Part of levator ani
Iliocostalis cervicis	Angles of 3rd, 4th, 5th, 6th ribs	Posterior tubercles of transverse processes of 4th, 5th, 6th cervical vertebrae	Dorsal rami of lower cervical nerves	Extends vertebral column; bends it to one side
Iliocostalis lumborum	Iliac crest; lumbar vertebrae; sacrum; lumbodorsal fascia	Inferior border of angle of lower 6 or 7 ribs	Dorsal rami of upper lumbar nerves	Extends vetebral column; bends it to one side

Muscle	Origin	Insertion	Nerve supply	Action
Iliocostalis thoracis	Upper border of angle of lower 6 ribs	Upper border of angle of upper 6 ribs; back of transverse process of 7th cervical vertebra	Dorsal rami of thoracic nerves	Extends vertebral column; bends it to one side
Infraspinatus	Infraspinous fossa of scapula	Greater tubercle of humerus	Suprascapular nerve	Stabilizes, and laterally rotates humerus
Intercostales externi (11 pairs)	Lower border of one rib	Upper border of rib below	Intercostal nerves	Muscles of inspiration
Intercostales interni (11 pairs)	Floor of costal groove of one rib and corresponding costal cartilage	Upper border of rib below	Intercostal nerves	Muscles of expiration
Intercostales intimi (11 pairs)	Inner surfaces of two adjoining ribs as for intercostales interni	Inner surfaces of two adjoining ribs as for intercostales	Intercostal nerves	Muscles of expiration
Interossei dorsal (4) (of foot)	By two heads from sides of adjacent metatarsal bones	Medial side of 2nd toe; lateral side of 2nd, 3rd, 4th toes	Deep branch of lateral plantar nerve	Abduct toes
Interossei dorsal (4) (of hand)	By two heads from sides of adjacent metacarpal bones	Bone of proximal phalanx of 2nd, 3rd, 4th fingers	Deep branch of ulnar nerve	Abduct fingers
Interossei, palmar (4)	Metacarpal bone of one finger	Appropriate side of dorsal digital expansion	Deep branch of ulnar nerve	Adduct fingers
Interossei, plantar (3)	Base and medial side of shaft of 3rd, 4th, 5th metatarsal bones	Medial side of base of proximal phalanges of same toes	Deep branch of lateral plantar nerve	Adduct toes
Interspinales (12 pairs)	Apex of spine of vertebra	Apex of spine of vertebra below	Dorsal rami of spinal nerves	Extend vertebral column
Intertransversarii	Transverse process of vertebra	Transverse process of vertebra	Anterior rami of spinal nerves	Lateral movement of vertebral column

Table of Muscles—*continued*

Name	Origin	Insertion	Innervation	Action
Ischiocavernosus	Ischium	Crus penis (clitoridis)	Perineal branch of pudendal nerve	Erection of penis (clitoris)
Latissimus dorsi	Spines of lower six thoracic vertebrae; thoracolumbar fascia; crest of illium; three or four lower ribs	Humerus	Thoracodorsal nerve	Adduction, extension and medial rotation of humerus; pulling the trunk upwards
Levator anguli oris	Canine fossa	Angle of the mouth	Facial nerve	Raises angle of mouth
Levator ani	Inner surface of pelvis; obturator fascia	Perineal body; coccyx; corresponding fibres from opposite side	4th sacral nerve; pudendal nerve	Supports pelvic viscera
Levatores costarum (12 pairs)	Transverse processes of 7th cervical, and upper 11 thoracic, vertebrae	Upper edge and outer surface of rib below	Dorsal rami of thoracic nerves	Raise ribs
Levator labii superioris	Lower margin of orbital opening	Upper lip	Facial nerve	Raises and everts upper lip
Levator palpebrae superioris	Lesser wing of sphenoid bone	Upper eyelid; superior tarsus	Oculomotor nerve	Raises upper eyelid
Levator scapulae	Transverse processes of upper cervical vertebrae	Medial border of scapula	3rd, 4th, 5th cervical nerves	Aids in various movements of scapula
Levator veli palatini	Petrous part of temporal bone; auditory tube	Palatine aponeurosis	Accessory nerve	Raises soft palate
Longissimus capitis	Transverse processes of upper 4 or 5 thoracic vertebrae; articular processes of lower 3 or 4 cervical vertebrae	Mastoid process	Dorsal rami of lower cervical nerves	Extends head; turns face to same side

Muscle	Origin	Insertion	Nerve supply	Action
Longissimus cervicis	Transverse processes of upper 4 or 5 thoracic vertebrae	Transverse processes of 2nd to 6th cervical vertebrae	Dorsal rami of thoracic nerves	Bends vertebral column backwards and laterally
Longissimus thoracis	Transverse processes of lumbar vertebrae	Transverse processes of thoracic vertebrae; lower 9 or 10 ribs	Dorsal rami of lumbar nerves	Bends vertebral column backwards and laterally
Longitudinalis inferior linguae	Hyoid bone; root of tongue	Apex of tongue	Hypoglossal nerve	Shortens tongue and turns tip downwards
Longitudinalis superior linguae	Submucosa and septum of tongue	Edge of tongue	Hypoglossal nerve	Shortens tongue and turns tip upwards
Longus capitis	Transverse processes of 3rd to 6th cervical vertebrae	Occipital bone	Ventral rami of C. 1, 2, 3	Flexes the head
Longus colli	Inferior oblique portion: bodies of first 2 or 3 thoracic vertebrae. Superior oblique portion: transverse processes of 3rd, 4th, 5th cervical vertebrae. Vertical portion: bodies of upper 3 thoracic and lower 3 cervical vertebrae	Transverse processes of 5th and 6th cervical vertebrae / Anterior arch of atlas / Bodies of 2nd, 3rd, 4th cervical vertebrae	Ventral rami of C. 2, 3, 4, 5, 6	Bends cervical vertebral column forwards and laterally
Lumbricales (of foot) (4)	Tendons of flexor digitorum longus	Dorsal surfaces of proximal phalanges of 4 lateral toes	Medial plantar nerve; deep branch of lateral plantar nerve	Flex proximal phalanges

Table of Muscles—continued

Name	Origin	Insertion	Innervation	Action
Lumbricales (of hand) (4)	Tendons of flexor digitorum profundus	Base of proximal phalanges of 4 lateral toes; dorsal digital expansion of extensor digitorum	Median nerve; deep terminal branch of ulnar nerve	Flex digits at metacarpophalangeal joints
Masseter	Superficial layer: zygomatic process of maxilla; zygomatic arch. Middle layer: zygomatic arch. Deep layer: zygomatic arch	Angle, and ramus, of mandible. Ramus of mandible. Ramus of mandible; coronoid process	Mandibular nerve	Elevates mandible
Mentalis	Mandible	Chin	Facial nerve	Raises and protrudes lower lip
Multifidus	Back of sacrum; aponeurosis of erector spinae; posterior, superior iliac spine; mamillary processes of lumbar vertebrae; transverse processes of thoracic vertebrae; articular processes of lower 4 cervical vertebrae	Spine of vertebrae above	Dorsal rami of spinal nerves	Postural muscles
Mylohyoid	Mandible	Hyoid bone	Inferior alveolar nerve	Raises floor of mouth
Nasalis	Alar part: maxilla. Transverse part: maxilla	Ala nasi. Aponeurosis of opposite nasalis	Facial nerve. Facial nerve	Widens nostril. Compresses nasal aperture

Obliquus auriculae	Eminentia conchae	Eminentia triangularis	Facial nerve	One of intrinsic muscles of external ear
Obliquus capitis, inferior	Axis vertebra	Transverse process of atlas	Dorsal ramus of C.1.	Turns face to same side
Obliquus capitis, superior	Transverse process of atlas	Occipital bone	Dorsal ramus of C.1	Bends head back and to same side
Obliquus externus abdominis	Inferior border of lower 8 ribs	Iliac crest; linea alba	Ventral rami of lower 6 thoracic nerves	Compresses abdominal viscera
Obliquus internus abdominis	Inguinal ligament; iliac crest	Crest of pubis; pecten pubis; linea alba; cartilages of 7th, 8th, and 9th ribs	Ventral rami of lower 6 thoracic nerves	Compresses abdominal viscera; flexes and rotates vertebral column
Obliquus oculi, inferior	Orbital surface of maxilla	Sclera	Oculomotor nerve	Rotates eyeball laterally
Obturator externus	Pubis; ischium; obturator membrane	Trochanteric fossa of femur	Obturator nerve	Lateral rotator of thigh
Obturator internus	Inner surface of pelvis; obturator foramen	Greater trochanter of femur	L.5, S.1	Lateral rotator of thigh
Omohyoid	Upper border of scapula	Hyoid bone	Ansa; ansa cervicalis	Depresses hyoid bone
Opponens digiti minimi	Hamate bone	5th metacarpal bone	Deep branch of ulnar nerve	Draws 5th metacarpal bone forwards and laterally rotates it
Opponens pollicis	Trapezium	Metacarpal bone of thumb	Median nerve	Flexes metacarpal bone of thumb

Table of Muscles—*continued*

Name	Origin	Insertions	Innervation	Action
Orbicularis oculi	Lacrimal portion: lacrimal bone.	Lateral palpebral raphe	Temporal and zygomatic branches of facial nerve	Sphincter muscle of the eyelids
	Orbital portion: frontal bone; frontal process of maxilla.	Eyebrow		
	Palpebral portion: medial palpebral ligament	Lateral palpebral raphe		
Orbicularis oris	Complex muscle surrounding the mouth		Facial nerve	Sphincter muscle of mouth
Palatoglossus	Palatine aponeurosis	Side of the tongue	Accessory nerve	Pulls up root of tongue
Palatopharyngeus	Soft and bony palate	Posterior border of thyroid cartilage	Accessory nerve	Shortens pharynx
Palmaris brevis	Palmar aponeurosis	Ulnar border of hand	Ulnar nerve	Deepens hollow of hand
Palmaris longus	Medial epicondyle of humerus	Palmar aponeurosis	Median nerve	Flexes wrist
Pectineus	Pecten pubis	Femur	Femoral nerve	Adducts and flexes thigh
Pectoralis major	Clavicle; sternum; cartilages of true ribs; aponeurosis of obliquus externus	Intertubercular sulcus of humerus	Lateral and medial pectoral nerves	Adduction and medial rotation of arm
Pectoralis minor	2nd–5th ribs	Coracoid process	Lateral and medial pectoral nerves	Draws shoulder downwards

Peroneus brevis	Fibula	Base of 5th metatarsal bone	Superficial peroneal nerve	Everts foot
Peroneus longus	Fibula	Base of 1st metatarsal bone; medial cuneiform	Superficial peroneal nerve	Plantar flexes and everts foot
Peroneus tertius	Fibula	Base of 5th metatarsal bone	Deep peroneal nerve	Dorsiflexes foot
Piriformis	Sacrum; ilium	Greater trochanter of femur	L.5, S.1, S.2	Rotates thigh laterally
Plantaris	Femur	Calcaneus	Tibial nerve	Accessory to gastrocnemius
Platysma	Fascia covering pectoralis major and deltoid	Mandible	Facial nerve	Depresses jaw; wrinkles skin of neck
Popliteus	Lateral condyle of femur; arcuate popliteal ligament	Tibia	Tibial nerve	Rotates tibia medially
Procerus	Nasal bone	Skin of forehead	Facial nerve	Draws eyebrows down
Pronator quadratus	Ulna	Radius	Median nerve	Pronates forearm
Pronator teres	Humeral head: medial epicondyle of humerus. Ulnar head: coronoid process of ulna	Radius	Median nerve	Pronates arm and hand
Psoas major	Lumbar vertebrae	Lesser trochanter of femur	Ventral rami of L.1, 2, 3	Flexes thigh
Psoas minor	12th thoracic and 1st lumbar vertebrae	Pecten pubis	L.1	Weak flexor of trunk

Table of Muscles—*continued*

Name	Origin	Insertion	Innervation	Action
Pterygoid lateralis	Lower head: lateral pterygoid plate. Upper head: greater wing of sphenoid bone	Neck of the mandible; temporomandibular articulation	Mandibular nerve	Opens mouth
Pterygoid medialis	Lateral pterygoid plate; palatine bone	Mandible	Mandibular nerve	Raises mandible
Pyramidalis	Pubis	Linea alba	Subcostal nerve	Tenses abdominal wall
Quadratus femoris	Ischial tuberosity	Trochanteric crest of femur	L.5, S.1	Lateral rotator of thigh
Quadratus lumborum	Iliolumbar ligament; iliac crest	Last rib; upper 4 lumbar vertebrae	Ventral rami of T.12; L.1, 2, 3	Flexes trunk laterally
Quadriceps femoris	Subdivided into rectus femoris, vastus intermedius, vastus lateralis, vastus medialis			Extends leg
Rectus abdominis	Crest of pubis; symphysis pubis	Cartilages of 5th, 6th, 7th ribs	Ventral rami of T.7–12	Supports abdominal wall; flexes lumbar vertebrae
Rectus capitis anterior	Atlas	Occipital bone	Ventral rami of C.1, 2	Flexes head
Rectus capitis lateralis	Atlas	Occipital bone	Ventral rami of C.1, 2	Bends head to same side
Rectus capitis posterior major	Spine of axis vertebrae	Occipital bone	Dorsal ramus of C.1	Extends head; turns face to same side
Rectus capitis posterior minor	Atlas	Occipital bone	Dorsal ramus of C.1	Extends head

Muscle	Origin	Insertion	Nerve supply	Action
Rectus of eyeball (4)	Common tendinous ring	Sclera	Inferior, medialis, superior: oculomotor nerve. Lateralis: abducent nerve	Inferior: depresses, adducts and laterally rotates eyeball. Lateralis: abducts eyeball. Medialis: adducts, eyeball. Superior: elevates, adducts and medially rotates eyeball
Rectus femoris	Anterior, inferior iliac spine; rim of acetabulum	Base of patella	Femoral nerve	Extends leg; flexes thigh
Rhomboideus major	Spines of 2nd, 3rd, 4th, 5th thoracic vertebrae	Medial border of scapula	Dorsal scapular nerve	Fixes scapula
Rhomboideus minor	Spines of 7th cervical and 1st thoracic vertebrae; ligamentum nuchae	Spine of scapula	Dorsal scapular nerve	Fixes scapula
Risorius	Parotid fascia	Angle of mouth	Facial nerve	Retracts angle of mouth
Rotatores cervicis	Irregular and variable muscle bundles with similar attachments to rotatores thoracis		Dorsal rami of spinal nerves	Rotation of spine
Rotatores lumborum	Irregular and vapiable muscle bundles with similar attachments to rotatores thoracis		Dorsal rami of spinal nerves	Rotation of spine
Rotatores thoracis	Upper and posterior part of transverse process of one vertebra	Lower border and lateral surface of lamina of verterba next above	Dorsal rami of spinal nerves	Rotation of spine
Salpingopharyngeus	Cartilage of auditory tube	Palatopharyngeus	Pharyngeal plexus	Raises lateral wall of pharynx
Sartorius	Anterior superior iliac spine	Tibia	Femoral nerve	Flexes leg and thigh

Table of Muscles—continued

Name	Origin	Insertion	Innervation	Action
Scalenus anterior	Transverse processes of 3rd–6th cervical vertebrae	Scalene tubercle on 1st rib	Ventral rami of C.4-6	Bends cervical vertebrae laterally; raises 1st rib
Scalenus medius	Transverse processes of axis and lower 5 cervical vertebrae	Upper surface of 1st rib	Ventral rami of cervical nerves	As for scalenus anterior
Scalenus posterior	Transverse processes of 4th–6th cervical vertebrae	Outer surface of 2nd rib	Ventral rami of C.5-7	Bends cervical vertebrae laterally; raises 1st and 2nd ribs
Semimembranosus	Ischial tuberosity	Medial condyle and median margin of tibia; lateral condyle of femur	Sciatic nerve	Flexes leg; extends thigh
Semispinalis capitis	Upper 6 or 7 thoracic vertebrae; 4th–7th cervical vertebrae	Occipital bone	Dorsal rami of cervical and thoracic nerves	Extends head
Semispinalis cervicis	Upper 5 or 6 thoracic vertebrae	Cervical spines from axis to 5th	Dorsal rami of cervical nerves	Extends and rotates vertebral column
Semispinalis thoracis	6th–10th thoracic vertebrae	Spines of upper 4 thoracic and lower 2 cervical vertebrae	Dorsal rami of cervical and thoracic nerves	Extends and rotates vertebral column
Semitendinosus	Ischial tuberosity	Tibia	Sciatic nerve	Flexes leg; extends thigh
Serratus anterior	Upper 8 or 9 ribs	Scapula	Long thoracic nerve	Draws scapula forwards
Serratus posterior inferior	Lower 2 thoracic, and upper 2 lumbar, vertebrae; supraspinous ligament	Lower 4 ribs	Ventral rami of T.9-12	Draws lower ribs downwards

Muscle	Origin	Insertion	Nerve supply	Action
Serratus posterior superior	Ligamentum nuchae; 7th cervical, and upper 2 or 3 thoracic, vertebrae; supraspinous ligament	2nd–5th ribs	2nd–5th intercostal nerves	Raises ribs
Soleus	Fibula; tibia	Tendo calcaneus	Tibial nerve	Plantar flexes foot
Spinalis capitis	Blended with semispinalis capitis		Dorsal rami of lower cervical, and thoracic, nerves	Extends vertebral column
Spinalis cervicis	Ligamentum nuchae; 7th cervical and 1st and 2nd thoracic vertebrae	Spine of axis vertebrae	Dorsal rami of thoracic nerves	Extends vertebral column
Spinalis thoracis	11th and 12th thoracic, and 1st and 2nd lumbar, vertebrae	Upper 4 to 8 thoracic vertebrae	Dorsal rami of thoracic nerves	Extends vertebral column
Splenius capitis	Ligamentum nuchae; 7th cervical, and upper 3 or 4 thoracic vertebrae	Mastoid process; occiput	Dorsal rami of middle cervical nerves	Draws head backwards and rotates it
Splenius cervicis	3rd–6th thoracic vertebrae	Upper 2 or 3 cervical vertebrae	Dorsal rami of lower cervical nerves	Extends and rotates head
Stapedius	Pyramidal eminence of tympanic cavity	Stapes	Facial nerve	Dampens movements of stapes
Sternocleidomastoid	Lateral head: clavicle. Medial head: manubrium sterni	Mastoid process; superior nuchal line of occipital bone	Accessory and 2nd cervical nerves	Tilts head to shoulder of same side: rotates head
Sternohyoid	Clavicle; posterior sternoclavicular ligament; manubrium	Hyoid bone	Ansa cervicalis	Depresses hyoid bone
Sternothyroid	Manubrium sterni; 1st rib	Thyroid cartilage	Ansa cervicalis	Depresses larynx
Styloglossus	Styloid process	Tongue	Hypoglossal nerve	Raises and retracts tongue

Table of Muscles—continued

Name	Origin	Insertion	Innervation	Action
Stylohyoid	Styloid process	Hyoid bone	Facial nerve	Raises and retracts hyoid
Stylopharyngeus	Styloid process	Thyroid cartilage; wall of pharynx	Glossopharyngeal nerve	Raises and dilates pharynx
Subclavius	1st rib	Clavicle	C.5, 6	Depresses lateral end of clavicle
Subcostales	Inner surface of one rib	Inner surface of 2nd or 3rd rib below	Intercostal nerve	Depress ribs
Subscapularis	Subscapular fossa	Lesser tubercle of humerus	Subscapular nerves	Rotates arm laterally
Supinator	Lateral epicondyle of humerus	Radius	Posterior interosseous nerve	Supinates forearm
Supraspinatus	Supraspinous fossa of scapula	Greater tubercle of humerus	Suprascapular nerve	Abducts arm
Temporalis	Temporal fossa and fascia	Coronoid process and ramus of mandible	Mandibular nerve	Raises mandible
Tensor fasciae latae	Iliac crest	Iliotibial tract of fascia lata	Superior gluteal nerve	Tightens fascia lata
Tensor tympani	Cartilaginous portion of auditory tube; sphenoid bone	Handle of malleus	Mandibular nerve	Tenses tympanic membrane
Tensor veli palatini	Scaphoid fossa; ptyerygoid process; sphenoid bone	Palatine aponeurosis and bone	Mandibular nerve	Tenses and depresses soft palate
Teres major	Scapula	Intertubercular fossa of humerus	Lower subscapular nerve	Adducts arms

Teres minor	Scapula	Humerus	Axillary nerve	Rotates arm laterally
Thyroarytenoid	Thyroid cartilage; cricothyroid ligament	Arytenoid cartilage	Recurrent laryngeal nerve	Shortens and relaxes vocal ligaments
Thyroepiglottic	Thyroid cartilage	Epiglottis	Recurrent laryngeal nerve	Widens larynx
Thyrohyoid	Thyroid cartilage	Hyoid bone	Hypoglossal nerve	Lowers hyoid
Tibialis anterior	Lateral condyle and shaft of tibia; interosseous membrane	Medial cuneiform bone; 1st metatarsal	Deep peroneal nerve	Dorsiflexes and inverts foot
Tibialis posterior	Crural interosseous membrane; tibia; fibula	Metatarsal bones except talus; base of 2nd, 3rd, 4th metatarsal bones	Tibial nerves	Inverts foot
Tragicus	An intrinsic muscle of the external ear			
Transversospinalis	Composite name for: semispinalis capitis, cervicis, thoracis; rotatores cervicis, thoracis, lumborum; multifidus			
Transversus abdominis	Inguinal ligament; iliac crest; thoracolumbar fascia; lower 6 costal cartilages	Crest and pecten of pubis; linea alba	Ventral rami of T.6-12, L.1	Compresses abdominal viscera
Transversus auriculae	Eminentia conchae	Eminentiae scaphae	Facial nerve	Retracts helix
Transversus linguae	Median fibrous septum of tongue	Side of tongue	Hypoglossal nerve	Narrows and elongates tongue
Transversus perinei profundus	Ramus of ischium	Perineal body	Perineal branch of pudendal nerve	Steadies perineal body

Table of Muscles—continued

Name	Origin	Insertion	Innervation	Action
Transversus perinei superficialis	Ischial tuberosity	Perineal body	Perineal branch of pudendal nerve	Fixes perineal body
Transversus thoracis	Sternum; xiphoid process; costal cartilages of lower 3 or 4 true ribs	Lower borders and inner surfaces of costal cartilages of 2nd–6th ribs	Intercostal nerves	Depresses costal cartilages
Trapezius	Occipital bone; ligamentum nuchae; spines of 7th cervical and all thoracic vertebrae	Clavicle; acromion; spine of scapula	Accessory nerve	Controls movements of scapula
Triceps	Lateral head: posterior surface of humerus. Long head: infraglenoid tubercle of scapula. Medial head: posterior surface of humerus	Olecranon of ulna	Radial nerve	Extends forearm
Vastus intermedius	Anterior and lateral surfaces of femur	Quadriceps femoris tendon; patella	Femoral nerve	Extends leg
Vastus lateralis	Lateral aspect of femur	Quadriceps femoris tendon; patella	Femoral nerve	Extends leg
Vastus medialis	Medial aspect of femur	Quadriceps femoris tendon; patella	Femoral nerve	Extends leg
Verticalis linguae	Upper surface of tongue	Lower surface of tongue	Hypoglossal nerve	Changes shape of tongue
Zygomaticus major	Zygomatic bone	Angle of mouth	Facial nerve	Draws angle of mouth upwards
Zygomaticus minor	Zygomatic bone	Upper lip	Facial nerve	Raises upper lip

Table of Nerves

Name	Origin	Components	Branches	Distribution
Abducent (6th cranial)	Floor of 4th ventricle	Motor		Lateral rectus muscle of eyeball
Accessory (11th cranial)	Cranial root: side of medulla oblongata. Spinal root: upper 5 cervical segments of spinal cord	Motor Parasympathetic Motor	Thoracic and abdominal viscera	Laryngeal and pharyngeal muscles Sternocleidomastoid; trapezius
Alveolar, inferior	Mandibular nerve	Motor Sensory	Mylohyoid nerve Mental and incisive nerves	Mylohyoid; anterior belly of digastric muscle. Lower teeth; skin of lower lips and chin
Alveolar, superior, anterior	Infraorbital	Sensory	Nasal and terminal	Incisor and canine teeth; nasal mucous membrane
Alveolar, superior, middle	Infraorbital	Sensory		Upper premolar teeth
Alveolar, superior, posterior	Maxillary	Sensory		Molar teeth; upper gum
Auricular, anterior (2)	Auriculotemporal	Sensory		Skin of helix and tragus
Auricular, great	2nd, 3rd cervical nerves	Sensory	Anterior Posterior	Skin of face Skin over mastoid process and ear
Auricular, posterior	Facial	Motor	Auricular Occipital	Intrinsic muscles of auricle Occipital belly of occipitofrontalis

Table of Nerves—continued

Name	Origin	Components	Branches	Distribution
Auriculotemporal	Mandibular	Sensory Secretomotor	Anterior auricular, articular, parotid, branches to auditory meatus, superficial temporal	Skin of tragus, helix, auditory meatus, and temple; tympanic membrane; temporomandibular joint; parotid gland
Axillary	5th, 6th cervical nerves (brachial plexus)	Motor Sensory	Anterior Posterior	Deltoid and skin covering it Teres minor; skin covering deltoid and long head of triceps
Cardiac	A series of parasympathetic cardio-inhibitory nerves from the vagus; and a series of sympathetic accelerator and augmentor nerves from the superior, middle and inferior cervical ganglia, which are known as the superior, middle and inferior Cardiac nerves, respectively			
Cardiotympanic, inferior and superior	Carotid plexus of sympathetic	Sympathetic	Tympanic plexus	Tympanic membrane; auditory tube
Carotid, internal	Superior cervical ganglion	Sympathetic	Lateral and medial	Carotid plexus
Cavernous, greater and lesser	Prostatic plexus	Sympathetic		Erectile tissue of penis
Cervical	8 pairs of nerves that arise from cervical segments of the spinal cord and divide into dorsal and ventral rami. The dorsal rami innervate muscles. The ventral rami of the upper 4 pairs unite to form the *cervical plexus*. Those of the lower 4, with the ventral ramus of the 1st thoracic nerve, unite to form the *brachial plexus*.			
Chorda tympani	Facial	Parasympathetic Sensory		Sublingual and submaxillary glands Taste buds of anterior 2/3rds of tongue

Nerve	Origin	Branch	Type	Distribution
Ciliary, long (2 or 3)	Nasociliary		Sensory	Ciliary body; iris; cornea
Ciliary, short (2)	Ciliary ganglion		Motor	Sphincter pupillae; ciliaris; blood vessels of eyeball
			Sensory	Cornea; iris; choroid
Coccygeal	Coccygeal segment of cord	Anococcygeal	Sensory	Skin over coccyx
Cochlear	Spinal ganglion of cochlea		Sensory (hearing)	Organ of Corti
Cutaneous nerve of arm, lower lateral	Radial nerve		Sensory	Skin of lateral part of lower half of arm
Cutaneous nerve of arm, upper lateral	Axillary nerve		Sensory	Skin over lower part of deltoid and upper part of triceps
Cutaneous nerve of arm, medial	Brachial plexus		Sensory	Skin of medial side of arm
Cutaneous nerve of arm, posterior	Radial		Sensory	Skin of dorsal aspect of arm
Cutaneous nerve of calf, lateral	Common peroneal		Sensory	Skin of proximal part of leg
Cutaneous nerve, femoral, posterior	1st, 2nd, 3rd sacral nerves	Gluteal	Sensory	Skin over gluteus maximus
		Perineal		Skin of upper and medial side of thigh and scrotum (labium majus)
		Thigh and leg		Skin of back and medial side of thigh, popliteal fossa, and upper part of back of leg

Table of Nerves—*continued*

Name	Origin	Components	Branches	Distribution
Cutaneous nerve of forearm, lateral	Musculocutaneous	Sensory		Skin of lateral half of anterior surface of forearm
Cutaneous nerve of forearm, medial	Brachial plexus	Sensory		Skin covering biceps
			Anterior	Skin of front of medial side of forearm
			Posterior	Skin of back of medial side of forearm
Cutaneous nerve of forearm, posterior	Radial	Sensory		Skin of lateral side of arm and back of forearm
Cutaneous nerve, perforating	2nd, 3rd sacral nerves	Sensory		Skin covering gluteus maximus
Cutaneous nerve of thigh, intermediate	Femoral	Sensory Motor	Lateral	Skin of front of thigh; sartorius
Cutaneous nerve of thigh, lateral	2nd, 3rd lumbar nerves	Sensory		Parietal peritoneum of iliac fossa
			Anterior	Skin of anterior and lateral parts of thigh
			Posterior	Skin of lateral side of thigh
Cutaneous nerve of thigh, medial	Femoral	Sensory		Skin of medial side of thigh
			Anterior	Skin of medial side of thigh
			Posterior	Skin of medial side of leg

Nerve	Origin	Type	Branches	Distribution
Cutaneous nerve, transverse cutaneous, of neck	2nd, 3rd cervical nerves	Sensory	Ascending Descending	Skin of upper and front parts of neck Skin of side and front of neck
Digital nerves of fingers	Radial, ulnar, and median	Sensory		Skin of fingers
Digital nerves of toes	Medial and lateral plantar	Sensory		Skin of toes
Dorsal nerve of penis (clitoris)	Pudendal	Sensory		Skin of penis (clitoris)
Dorsal scapular	5th cervical	Motor		Rhomboids
Ethmoidal, anterior	Nasociliary	Sensory	Internal nasal External nasal	Nasal mucous membrane Skin of nose
Ethmoidal, posterior	Nasociliary	Sensory		Ethmoidal and sphenoidal sinuses
Facial (7th cranial)	Lower border of pons	Motor Sensory	Nerve to stapedius; chorda tympani; posterior auricular; stylohyoid; temporal; zygomatic; buccal; mandibular; cervical	*Motor* to muscles of face, scalp, and auricle; buccinator; platysma; stapedius; stylohyoid; posterior belly of digastric. *Sensory* (taste) to anterior 2/3rds of tongue; soft palate
Femoral	2nd 3rd, 4th lumbar	Motor Sensory	Muscular and articular; intermediate cutaneous of thigh; medial cutaneous of thigh; saphenous	*Motor* to iliacus; pectineus; sartorius; quadriceps femoris. *Sensory* to skin of anterior aspect of thigh, medial aspect of leg; hip and knee joints

Table of Nerves—*continued*

Name	Origin	Components	Branches	Distribution
Frontal	Ophthalmic	Sensory	Supratrochlear	Conjunctiva; skin of upper eyelid and lower forehead
			Supraorbital	Conjunctiva; skin of upper eyelid and scalp
Genitofemoral	1st, 2nd lumbar	Sensory	Genital	Cremaster; skin of scrotum (mons pubis and labium majus)
			Femoral	Skin over femoral triangle
Glossopharyngeal (9th cranial)	Medulla oblongata	Motor Sensory	Tympanic; carotid; pharyngeal; muscular; tonsillar; lingual	*Motor* to stylopharyngeus. *Secretomotor* to parotid gland. *Sensory* to pharynx, tonsils, posterior part of tongue
Gluteal, inferior	5th lumbar, 1st, 2nd sacral	Motor		Gluteus maximus
Gluteal, superior	4th, 5th lumbar, 1st sacral	Motor	Superior Inferior	Gluteus medius Gluteus medius and minimus; tensor fasciae latae
Hypogastric	Superior hypogastric plexus	Sympathetic	Inferior hypogastric plexus	Pelvic viscera
Hypoglossal (12th cranial)	Medulla oblongata	Motor		Intrinsic and extrinsic muscles of tongue

Iliohypogastric	1st lumbar	Anterior cutaneous	Skin of abdomen above the pubis
		Lateral cutaneous	Skin of side of buttock
Interosseous, anterior	Median	Motor	Flexor pollicis longus; flexor digitorum profundus; wrist joint: distal radio-ulnar joint
		Sensory	
Interosseous, posterior	Radial	Motor	Extensor carpi radialis brevis; supinator; extensor digitorum; extensor digiti minimi; extensor carpi ulnaris; extensor pollicis longus; extensor pollicis brevis; wrist joint
		Sensory	
Labial, superior	Maxillary	Sensory	Skin of cheek and upper lip; mucous membrane of mouth
Labial, posterior	Pudendal	Sensory	Labium majus
Lacrimal	Ophthalmic	Sensory	Lacrimal gland; conjunctiva; skin of upper eyelid
Laryngeal, recurrent	Vagus	Motor	Muscles of larynx except cricothyroid; laryngeal mucous membrane; trachea; oesophagus; cardiac plexus
		Parasympathetic	

Table of Nerves—*continued*

Name	Origin	Components	Branches	Distribution
Laryngeal, superior	Vagus	Motor Sensory	External laryngeal Internal laryngeal	Cricothyroid; inferior constrictor Laryngeal mucous membrane; pharyngeal mucous membrane; arytenoideus
Lingual	Mandibular	Sensory		Anterior 2/3rds of tongue; floor of mouth; mandibular gum
Lumbar	Five pairs of nerves that arise from the lumbar segments of the spinal cord. The dorsal rami are distributed to the muscles and skin of the lower back. The ventral rami form the lumbar plexus			
Mandibular	Trigeminal	Motor Sensory	Nervus spinosus; nerve to medial pterygoid; buccal; masseteric; deep temporal	Teeth and gums of mandible; skin of auricle, temporal region, lower lip, lower part of face; mucous membrane of anterior 2/3rds of tongue and floor of mouth; muscles of mastication
Masseteric	Mandibular	Motor Sensory		Masseter; temporomandibular joint
Maxillary	Trigeminal	Sensory	Meningeal; zygomatic; posterior superior alveolar; middle superior alveolar; ganglionic, superior	Dura mater; ala of nose; lower eyelid; skin and mucous membrane of cheek and upper lip; teeth of upper jaw;

Nerve	Origin	Type	Branches	Distribution
			alveolar, palpebral, nasal, and superior labial branches; anterior superior alveolar branch	maxillary sinus; nasal mucosa
Median	5th to 8th cervical nerves and 1st thoracic (brachial plexus)	Motor Sensory	Anterior interosseous; palmar cutaneous branch; muscular branch; palmar digital branches; articular and vascular branches	Pronator teres; superficial flexor forearm muscles (except flexor carpi ulnaris); flexor pollicis longus; flexor digitorum profundus; small muscles of thumb; 2 lateral lumbricals; skin of hand; elbow, wrist and hand joints
Mental	Inferior alveolar	Sensory		Skin of lower lip and chin
Musculocutaneous	5th, 6th, 7th, cervical nerves (brachial plexus)	Motor Sensory	Lateral cutaneous nerve of forearm	Coracobrachialis; triceps; brachialis; skin of radial side of forearm
Mylohyoid	Inferior alveolar	Motor		Mylohyoid; digastric
Nasal, lateral posterior superior (6)	Pterygopalatine ganglion	Sensory		Mucous membrane of posterior part of superior and middle nasal conchae, and posterior ethmoidal sinuses

Table of Nerves—continued

Name	Origin	Components	Branches	Distribution
Nasal, medial posterior superior (2 or 3)	Pterygopalatine ganglion	Sensory		Mucous membrane of posterior part of roof of nasal cavity, and of nasal septum
Nasociliary	Ophthalmic	Sensory	Anterior and posterior ethmoidal; long ciliary; infratrochlear; nasal branches	Eyeball; conjunctiva; lacrimal gland; nasal mucosa; mucosa of ethmoid and sphenoidal sinuses
Nasopalatine	Maxillary	Sensory		Mucosa of nasal septum and hard palate
Obturator	2nd, 3rd, 4th lumbar nerves (lumbar plexus)	Motor Sensory	Anterior branch	Skin on medial side of thigh; hip joint; adductor longus; gracilis; adductor brevis; pectineus
			Posterior branch	Obturator externus; adductor magnus; adductor brevis; knee joint
Occipital, greater	2nd cervical	Sensory Motor		Scalp of back of head Semispinalis capitis; splenius; longissimus capitis
Occipital, lesser	2nd cervical	Sensory		Scalp of side of back of head
Occipital, third	3rd cervical	Sensory		Skin of back of neck

Nerve	Origin	Type	Branches	Distribution
Oculomotor (3rd cranial)	Midbrain	Motor	Motor	All ocular muscles except superior oblique and lateral rectus; sphincter pupillae; ciliaris
Olfactory (1st cranial)	Olfactory bulb	Sensory (smell)		Nasal mucosa
Ophthalmic	Trigeminal	Sensory	Lacrimal; frontal; nasociliary	Eyeball; lacrimal gland; conjunctiva; nasal cavity; skin of nose, eyelids, scalp and forehead
Optic (2nd cranial)	Optic chiasma	Sensory (sight)		Retina
Palatine, anterior	Pterygopalatine ganglion	Sensory	Posterior inferior; nasal	Gums; mucous membrane and glands of hard palate; soft palate
Palatine, middle and posterior	Pterygopalatine ganglion	Sensory		Uvula; tonsil; soft palate
Palpebral	Maxillary	Sensory		Lower eyelid
Parotid	Auriculotemporal	Secretomotor		Parotid gland
Pectoral, lateral	5th, 6th, 7th cervical	Motor		Pectoralis major
Pectoral, medial	8th cervical, 1st thoracic	Motor		Pectoralis minor and major
Perforating cutaneous	2nd, 3rd sacral	Sensory		Skin over gluteus maximus

Table of Nerves—*continued*

Name	Origin	Components	Branches	Distribution
Peroneal, common	4th, 5th lumbar, 1st, 2nd sacral	Motor Sensory	Lateral cutaneous nerve of calf; deep and superficial peroneal	That of its branches
Peroneal, deep	Common peroneal	Motor Sensory		Tibialis anterior; extensor hallucis longus; extensor digitorum longus; peroneus tertius; ankle joint; extensor digitorum brevis; joints of feet
Peroneal, superficial	Common peroneal	Motor Sensory		Peroneus longus and brevis; skin of lower lateral aspect of leg and dorsum of foot
Petrosal, deep	Sympathetic plexus on internal carotid artery	Sympathetic		Lacrimal, nasal, and palatine glands
Petrosal, greater	Genicular ganglion	Sensory (taste) Parasympathetic	Mucous membrane of palate	Lacrimal, nasal and palatine glands
Petrosal, lesser	Tympanic	Parasympathetic		Secretomotor for parotid gland
Pharyngeal	Pterygopalatine ganglion	Sensory		Mucous membrane of nasal part of pharynx
Phrenic	4th cervical	Motor		Diaphragm

Plantar, lateral	Tibial	Motor	Flexor digitorum accessorius; abductor digiti minimi; flexor digiti minimi brevis; 2nd, 3rd and 4th lumbricals; abductor hallucis; interossei
		Sensory	Superficial; deep; skin of 5th toe, lateral side of 4th toe and lateral border of foot
Plantar, medial	Tibial	Motor	Abductor hallucis; flexor digitorum brevis; flexor hallicus brevis; 1st lumbrical; skin of sole of foot; tarsal and metatarsal joints
		Sensory	Cutaneous; muscular; articular; proper digital nerve of great toe; 3 common plantar digital nerves
Pudendal	2nd, 3rd, 4th sacral	Motor	Muscles and skin of perineal region
		Sensory	Inferior rectal; perineal; dorsal nerve of penis (clitoris)
Radial	5th–8th cervical 1st thoracic	Motor	Triceps; anconeus; extensor muscles of forearm; brachioradialis; skin of back of arm, forearm and hand; elbow, wrist, and hand joints
		Sensory	Muscular; cutaneous; articular; posterior interosseous
Rectal, inferior	Pudendal	Motor	Sphincter ani externus; skin around anus; lining and lower part of anal canal
		Sensory	
Sacral	Five pairs of nerves that arise from the sacral segments of the spinal cord		

Table of Nerves—continued

Name	Origin	Components	Branches	Distribution
Saphenous	Femoral	Sensory		Skin of medial side of leg and foot
Scapular, dorsal	5th cervical	Motor		Rhomboids
Sciatic	Sacral plexus	Motor Sensory	Tibial; common peroneal	Biceps femoris; semitendinosus; semimembranosus; adductor magnus; hip joint. See also its two branches
Spinal	The 31 pairs of nerves that arise from the spinal cord: 8 cervical, 12 thoracic, 5 lumbar, 5 sacral, 1 coccygeal			
Spinosus	Mandibular	Sensory		Dura mater; mastoid air cells
Splanchnic, greater	5th–10th thoracic	Sympathetic Sensory		Coeliac ganglion
Splanchnic, lesser	9th–10th thoracic	Sympathetic Sensory		Aorticorenal ganglion
Splanchnic, lowest	12th thoracic	Sympathetic Sensory		Renal plexus
Splanchnic, lumbar	Lumbar ganglia	Sympathetic Sensory		Coeliac, renal, intermesenteric, superior hypogastric plexuses
Splanchnic, pelvic	2nd–4th sacral	Sympathetic Sensory		Terminal ganglia in pelvic viscera

Name	Origin	Type	Division	Distribution
Subcostal	12th thoracic	Motor / Sensory		Abdominal muscles / Skin of lower abdomen
Subscapular (2)	5th–7th cervical	Motor		Subscapularis; teres major
Supraclavicular (3)	3rd–4th cervical	Sensory	Intermediate	Skin over deltoid and pectoralis major
			Lateral	Skin over upper and posterior parts of shoulder
			Medial	Skin over sternocleidomastoid
Supraorbital	Frontal	Sensory		Skin of upper eyelid and forehead; conjunctiva; mucosa of frontal sinus
Suprascapular	5th–6th cervical	Motor / Sensory		Supraspinatus; infraspinatus; shoulder and acromioclavicular joints
Supratrochlear	Frontal	Sensory		Conjunctiva; skin of upper eyelid and forehead
Sural	Tibial	Sensory		Skin of lateral side of leg and foot and back of leg
Temporal, deep (2)	Mandibular	Motor	Anterior; posterior	Temporal muscles

Table of Nerves—continued

Name	Origin	Components	Branches	Distribution
Temporal, superficial	Auriculotemporal	Sensory		Skin of temporal region
Thoracic	The 12 pairs of nerves that arise from the thoracic segments of the spinal cord			
Thoracodorsal	6th–8th cervical	Motor		Latissimus dorsi
Tibial	Sciatic	Motor Sensory	Articular; muscular; sural; medial calcanean; medial and lateral plantar	Muscles and skin of leg and foot; knee and ankle joints
Trigeminal (5th cranial)	Pons	Motor Sensory	Ophthalmic; maxillary; mandibular	See 3 branches for distribution
Trochlear (4th cranial)	Cerebral aqueduct	Motor		Superior oblique muscle
Tympanic	Glossopharyngeal	Sensory Parasympathetic	Tympanic plexus; lesser petrosal nerve	Mucosa of tympanic cavity and membrane; mastoid air cells; parotid gland
Ulnar	8th cervical, 1st thoracic	Motor Sensory	Articular; muscular; palmar cutaneous; dorsal; superficial terminal	Flexor carpi ulnaris; flexor digitorum profundus; adductor pollicis; muscles of hypothenar eminence; interossei; medial two lumbricals; skin of medial side of hand; elbow, wrist and hand joints

Vagus (10th cranial)	Medulla Oblongata	Motor Sensory Parasympathetic	Meningeal; auricular; pharyngeal; recurrent pharyngeal; cardiac; pulmonary; oesophageal; gastric, coeliac; hepatic	As shown by its branches
Vestibulocochlear (8th cranial)	Brain stem	Sensory (hearing and equilibration)	Vestibular; cochlear	
Vestibular	Brain stem	Sensory (equilibration)		Semicircular ducts, utricle and saccule
Zygomatic	Maxillary	Sensory	Zygomaticotemporal; zygomaticofacial	Skin over zygomatic bone and in temporal region

Table of Veins

Name	Tributaries	Area drained	Destination
Auricular, posterior	Stylomastoid vein	Posterior part of side of head	External jugular vein
Axillary	Basilic vein Brachial veins Cephalic vein		Subclavian vein
Azygos	Posterior intercostal veins of right side; hemiazygos and accessory azygos veins; oesophageal, mediastinal, and pericardial veins; right bronchial vein		Superior vena cava
Basal, of brain	Anterior cerebral, deep middle cerebral, and striate veins		Great cerebral vein
Basilic	Ulnar part of deep venous network of hand; median cubital vein		Axillary vein
Basivertebral veins		Vertebral bodies	Anterior internal vertebral plexuses
Brachial veins	Branches corresponding with branches of the brachial artery		Axillary vein. The right one may join the basilic vein
Brachiocephalic (innominate) veins	Internal jugular and subclavian veins		Superior vena cava
Brachiocephalic vein, left	Left vertebral, left internal thoracic, left inferior thyroid, left superior intercostal veins		

Brachiocephalic vein, right	Right vertebral, right internal thoracic, right inferior thyroid veins	
Bronchial veins		Larger bronchi and structures at roots of lungs	Azygos vein on right. Left superior intercostal or hemiazygos vein on left
Buccal			Pterygoid plexus
Cardiac, anterior		Front of right ventricle	Right atrium
Cardiac, great	Left marginal vein	Left atrium, both ventricles	Coronary sinus
Cardiac, middle		Diaphragmatic surface of the ventricles	Coronary sinus
Cardiac, small	Right marginal vein	Right atrium and ventricle	Coronary sinus
Cava, vena, inferior	Common iliac veins; lumbar, right testicular or ovarian, renal, right suprarenal, inferior phrenic, and hepatic veins	The body below the diaphragm	Right atruim
Cava, vena, superior	Brachiocephalic veins; azygos vein	Upper half of body	Right atrium
Central, of liver		Hepatic lobule	Hepatic veins
Central, of retina	Retinal veins		Cavernous sinus
Cephalic	Accessory cephalic vein	Radial part of dorsal venous network of head	Axillary vein
Cephalic, accessory		Back of forearm	Cephalic vein

Table of Veins—*continued*

Name	Tributaries	Area drained	Destination
Cerebellar veins, inferior		Inferior surface of cerebellum	Sigmoid, superior petrosal and occipital sinuses
Cerebellar veins, superior		Upper surface of cerebellum	Straight, transverse, and superior petrosal sinuses; internal cerebral veins
Cerebral, anterior		Area supplied by anterior cerebral artery	Basal vein of brain
Cerebral, great	Internal cerebral veins: left and right basal veins		Straight sinus
Cerebral veins, inferior		Undersurface of cerebral hemisphere	Superior sagittal, cavernous, superior petrosal and transverse sinuses
Cerebral veins, internal	Thalamostriate and choroid veins	Deep parts of the hemisphere	Great cerebral vein
Cerebral, middle, deep		Insula and neighbouring gyri	Basal vein of brain
Cerebral, middle, superficial		Lateral surface of hemisphere	Cavernous sinus
Cerebral, superior (8–12)		Superolateral and medial surfaces of hemisphere	Superior sagittal sinus
Cervical, deep	Occipital veins	Deep muscles at back of neck	Vertebral vein

Vein		Drains	Drains into
Choroid, of brain		Hippocampus, fornix, corpus callosum	Internal cerebral vein
Ciliary veins		Choroid	Ophthalmic veins
Colic, right and medial		Area served by corresponding arteries	Superior mesenteric vein
Cordis, venae, minimae		Myocardium	Atria and ventricles of heart
Cubital, median	Cephalic vein	Forearm	Basilic vein
Cystic		Gall-bladder	Hepatic veins
Digital, dorsal, of foot	Plantar digital veins	Dorsal aspects of toes	Dorsal metatarsal veins
Digital, dorsal, of hand		Dorsal aspects of fingers	Dorsal metacarpal veins
Digital, palmar		Palmar aspects of fingers	Palmar digital veins
Digital, plantar		Plantar surfaces of digits	Plantar metatarsal veins
Diploic (4)		Frontal, parietal and occipital bones	Supraorbital vein, sphenoparietal sinus, transverse sinus and occipital vein
Dorsal vein of clitoris		Clitoris	Vesical plexus
Dorsal vein, deep, of penis		Glans penis and corpora cavernosa	Prostatic plexus
Dorsal vein, superficial, of penis		Prepuce, and skin of penis	External pudendal vein
Emissary (10)		Establish communications between venous sinuses inside skull and veins external to it	
Epigastric, inferior		Venae comitantes of inferior epigastric artery	External iliac vein

Table of Veins—continued

Name	Tributaries	Area drained	Destination
Epigastric, superficial		Lower part of abdominal wall	Great saphenous vein
Facial	Supratrochlear and supraorbital veins		Internal jugular vein
Gastro-epiploic, left		Surface of stomach and greater omentum	Splenic vein
Gastro-epiploic, right		Greater omentum and lower part of stomach	Superior mesenteric vein
Femoral	Popliteal vein; vena profunda femoris; great saphenous, lateral and medial circumflex veins		External iliac vein
Gastric, left		Surface of stomach	Portal vein
Gastric, right	Prepyloric vein		Portal vein
Gastric, short (4)		Fundus and left part of greater curvature of stomach	Splenic vein
Gluteal, inferior		Venae comitantes of inferior gluteal artery	Internal iliac vein
Gluteal, superior		Venae comitantes of superior gluteal artery	Internal iliac vein
Hemiazygos		4th–8th left intercostal spaces	Azygos vein
Hemiazygos, accessory	Arises on left side in manner corresponding to origin of azygos vein on the right side		Azygos vein

Vein	Tributaries / Area drained	Drains into
Hepatic veins	Liver	Inferior vena cava
Ileocolic	Ileocolic	Superior mesenteric vein
Iliac, circumflex, deep	Venae comitantes of deep circumflex iliac artery	External iliac vein
Iliac, circumflex, superficial	Lower part of abdominal wall, and upper end of lateral parts of thigh	Great saphenous vein
Iliac, common (2)	External and internal iliac veins, iliolumbar and lateral sacral veins and median sacral vein	Inferior vena cava
Iliac, external	Femoral, inferior epigastric, deep circumflex iliac, and pubic veins	Common iliac vein
Iliac, internal	Gluteal, internal pudendal, obturator, lateral sacral, middle rectal, vesical, uterine, and vaginal veins	Common iliac vein
Intercapitular	Palmar digital veins	Dorsal digital veins
Intercostal, anterior (12 on each side)	Venae comitantes of anterior thoracic arteries	Internal thoracic and musculophrenic veins
Intercostal, posterior 11 on each side	Area served by posterior intercostal arteries, muscles and skin of back	Brachiocephalic, vertebral right superior intercostal, left superior intercostal, hemiazygos, accessory hemiazygos, and azygos veins

Table of Veins—*continued*

Name	Tributaries	Area drained	Destination
Intercostal, superior, left	2nd–4th left posterior intercostal veins, left bronchial veins		Left brachiocephalic vein
Intercostal, superior, right	2nd–4th right posterior intercostal veins		Azygos vein
Interlobar veins of kidney	Interlobular veins		Renal veins
Interlobular veins of kidneys		Intertubular capillaries	Interlobular veins
Intervertebral		Spinal cord, internal and external vertebral plexuses	Vertebral, posterior intercostal, lumbar and lateral sacral veins
Intralobular veins, of liver	Sinusoids of liver lobules		Sublobular veins
Jugular, anterior		Submandibular region	Jugular arch → external jugular vein
Jugular, external	Posterior division of retromandibular vein; posterior auricular, posterior external jugular, transverse cervical, suprascapular, and anterior jugular veins	Exterior of cranium and deep parts of face	Subclavian vein
Jugular, external, posterior		Skin and superficial muscles in upper and posterior neck	External jugular vein
Jugular, internal	Inferior petrosal sinus, facial, lingual, pharyngeal, and superior and middle thyroid veins	The brain, superficial parts of face, and neck	Brachiocephalic vein

Labial, inferior and superior		Facial vein
Labyrinthine	Internal ear	Inferior petrosal sinus
Laryngeal, inferior	Area served by inferior laryngeal artery	Inferior thyroid vein
Laryngeal, superior	Area served by superior laryngeal artery	Superior thyroid vein
Lingual	Tongue	Internal jugular vein
Lumbar (4 on each side)	Muscles and skin of loins, and walls of abdomen	Inferior vena cava
Lumbar, ascending		Connects common iliac, iliolumbar and lumbar veins
Marginal, lateral, of foot	Superficial part of sole of foot	Small saphenous vein
Marginal, medial, of foot	Superficial part of sole of foot	Great saphenous vein
Marginal, left, of heart	Myocardium	Great cardiac vein
Marginal, right, of heart	Myocardium	Small cardiac vein, or right atrium
Masseteric	Venae comitantes of masseteric arteries	Pterygoid plexus
Maxillary	Pterygoid plexus	Retromandibular vein
Meningeal, middle	Superior sagittal sinus, inferior cerebral veins	Pterygoid plexus and sphenoparital or cavernous sinuses

Table of Veins—*continued*

Name	Tributaries	Area drained	Destination
Mesenteric, inferior	Superior rectal, sigmoid, and left colic veins	Rectum, sigmoid and descending colon	Splenic vein
Mesenteric, superior	Jejunal, ileal, ileocolic, right colic and middle colic veins	Small intestine, caecum, ascending and transverse colon	Portal vein
Metacarpal, dorsal	Dorsal digital veins		Dorsal venous network
Metacarpal, palmar		Venae comitantes of palmar metacarpal arteries	Deep palmar venous arches
Metatarsal, dorsal	Dorsal digital veins		Dorsal venous arch
Metatarsal, plantar	Plantar digital veins		Deep plantar venous arch
Oblique, of left atrium		Myocardium of left atrium	Coronary sinus
Obturator		Adductor region of thigh	Internal iliac vein
Occipital	Venous network at back of skull		Variable: deep cervical and vertebral, internal or external jugular veins
Oesophageal		Oesophagus	Inferior thyroid, azygos, hemiazygos, accessory hemiazygos, and left gastric veins
Ophthalmic, inferior	Inferior palpebral, and lacrimal veins		Cavernous sinus or superior ophthalmic vein
Ophthalmic, superior	Nasofrontal vein		Cavernous sinus
Orbital	Lateral palpebral veins		Middle temporal vein
Ovarian		Ovary	Common iliac veins

Palatine, external	Tonsils and soft palate. The vein responsible for the severe haemorrhage that sometimes follows tonsillectomy	Facial vein
Pancreatic	Body and tail of pancreas	Splenic vein
Pancreaticoduodenal (4)	Head of pancreas and duodenum	Variable: superior mesenteric, mesenteric, gastroepiploic, or portal veins
Para-umbilical veins		Form anastomosis between veins of anterior abdominal wall and portal vein
Parotid	Parotid gland	Superficial temporal vein
Pericardiacophrenic veins	Pericardium and diaphragm	Internal thoracic veins
Pericardial veins	Pericardium	Left brachiocephalic and azygos veins
Peroneal veins	Venae comitantes of peroneal artery	Posterior tibial veins
Pharyngeal	Pharyngeal plexus	Internal jugular vein
Phrenic, inferior, left	Area served by the corresponding arteries in the diaphragm]	Left renal or suprarenal vein and inferior vena cava
Phrenic, inferior, right		Inferior vena cava
Plantar, lateral and medial	Deep plantar venous arch	Posterior tibial veins

Meningeal veins

Table of Veins—*continued*

Name	Tributaries	Area drained	Destination
Popliteal	Anterior and posterior tibial, small saphenous, and veins corresponding to the popliteal artery		Femoral vein
Portal	Superior mesenteric, splenic, left and right gastric, para-umbilical, and cystic veins	Abdominal part of digestive tube (except lower part of anal canal), spleen, pancreas and gall-bladder	Inferior vena cava
Prepyloric		Accompanies prepyloric artery	Right gastric vein
Profunda femoris	Medial and lateral circumflex femoral veins	Area served by muscular and perforating branches of profunda femoris artery	Femoral vein
Profunda linguae		Deep aspect of tongue	Sublingual vein
Profunda penis, deep		Glans penis and corpora cavernosa	Prostatic venous plexus
Profunda penis, superficial		Prepuce and skin of penis	External pudendal vein
Prostatic		Prostate	Prostatic venous plexus
Pubic		Connects the external iliac with the obturator vein	External iliac vein
Pudendal, external		The distribution of the external pudendal artery	Great saphenous vein

Vein	Tributaries	Region drained	Drains into
Pudendal, internal	Prostatic venous plexus and veins from bulb of penis, scrotal (or labial) and inferior rectal veins	Penis, scrotum (or labium), prostate, and lower part of anal canal	Internal iliac vein
Pulmonary (two from each lung)		Lungs	Left atrium
Radial	Deep veins of dorsum of hand	Venae comitantes of radial artery	Brachial vein
Rectal, inferior	External rectal venous plexus	Lower part of anal canal	Internal pudendal vein
Rectal, middle	External rectal venous plexus	Rectal ampulla	Internal iliac vein
Rectal, superior	Internal rectal venous plexus		Inferior messenteric vein
Renal, left	Left testicular (or ovarian), and left suprarenal veins		Inferior vena cava
Renal, right		Right kidney	Inferior vena cava
Retromandibular	Maxillary, and superficial temporal veins		Anterior branch unites with facial vein; posterior branch joins with posterior auricular vein to form external jugular
Sacral, lateral		Area served by lateral sacral arteries	Internal iliac vein
Sacral, median		Area served by median sacral artery	Left common iliac vein
Saphenous, accessory		Medial and posterior parts of thigh	Great saphenous vein

Table of Veins—*continued*

Name	Tributaries	Area drained	Destination
Saphenous, great	Medial marginal vein of foot, accessory saphenous, superficial epigastric, superficial circumflex iliac, and external pudendal veins	The longest vein in the body	Femoral vein
Saphenous, small	Lateral marginal vein of foot		Popliteal vein
Splenic	Short gastric, left gastroepiploic, pancreatic, and inferior mesenteric veins		Portal vein
Stellate, of kidney		Superficial renal cortex	Interlobular vein of kidney
Striate		Anterior perforated substance of brain	Bassal cerebral veins
Stylomastoid		The tympanum	Posterior auricular vein
Subclavian	Axillary and external jugular veins; thoracic duct joins left, and right lymphatic duct joins right subclavian vein		Brachiocephalic vein
Subcostal veins		Vena comitans of subcostal artery	Left vein ends in hemiazygos vein; right vein ends in aygos, vein
Sublingual		Sublingual gland	Vena comitans of hypoglossal nerve
Sublobular veins of liver	Intralobular veins		Hepatic veins
Submental		Distribution of submental artery	Facial vein
Supraorbital		Front of scalp	Facial vein

Vein	Drains	Tributaries	Ends in
Suprarenal, left	Left suprarenal gland		Left renal vein
Suprarenal, right	Right suprarenal gland		Inferior vena cava
Supratrochlear		Nasal arch	Anterior facial vein
Temporal deep	Deep portions of temporal muscle		Pterygoid plexus
Temporal, middle	Temporal muscle		Superficial temporal vein
Temporal, superficial	Lateral part of scalp	Middle temporal vein	Retromandibular vein
Testicular	Testis and epididymis		Left vein ends in left renal vein; right vein ends in inferior vena cava
Thalamostriate	Caudate nucleus and thalamus		Internal cerebral vein
Thoracic, internal	Venae comitantes to lower half of internal thoracic artery	Pericardiacophrenic	Brachiocephalic vein
Thoracoepigastric			Connects superficial epigastric vein, or femoral vein, with lateral thoracic veins
Thymic	Thymus		Left brachiocephalic, internal thoracic, and inferior thyroid veins
Thyroid, inferior (2)	Isthmus and lateral lobe of thyroid	Oesophageal, tracheal, and inferior laryngeal veins	Brachiocephalic veins
Thyroid, middle	Lower part of thyroid, larynx and trachea		Internal jugular vein

Table of Veins—*continued*

Name	Tributaries	Area drained	Destination
Thyroid, superior	Superior laryngeal, and cricothyroid veins	Upper part of thyroid, and larynx.	Internal jugular or facial vein
Tibial, anterior (2)		Accompany anterior tibial artery	Popliteal vein
Tibial, posterior (2)	Peroneal veins	Accompany posterior tibial artery	Popliteal vein
Tonsillar		Tonsils	Paratonsillar vein
Tracheal		Trachea	Inferior thyroid vein
Ulnar	Deep palmar venous arch	Venae comitantes of ulnar artery	Brachial vein
Uterine	Uterine plexuses		Internal iliac vein
Vaginal	Vaginal plexuses		Internal iliac vein
Ventricle, left, posterior vein of		Posterior surface of left ventricle	Coronary sinus, or great cardiac vein
Vertebral	Internal vertebral plexuses; anterior vertebral and deep cervical veins	Plexus around vertebral artery	Brachiocephalic vein
Vertebral, accessory			Brachiocephalic vein
Vertebral, anterior	Plexus around transverse processes of upper cervical vertebrae		Vertebral vein
Vesical	Vesical plexus		Internal iliac vein

APPENDIX II—WEIGHTS AND MEASURES

Metric System
Mass (weights)

1 kilogram (kg.)	=	1000 grammes
1 gramme (g.)	=	1 gramme
1 milligram (mg.)	=	0·001 gramme
1 microgram (µg.)	=	0·000001 gramme

The *British Pharmacopoeia* recommends that, for the purpose of writing prescriptions, the symbol 'G' should be used as the contraction for gramme. This divergence from international practice is recommended to avoid the possibility of confusion between 'g' and 'gr' (the abbreviation for grain). It is also recommended for prescribing purposes that the word 'microgram' should be written in full; if not, 'mcg' should be used as the contraction. This divergence from international practice is recommended to avoid the possibility of confusion between 'µg' and 'mg'.

Capacity (volume)

1 litre (l.)	=	1000 millilitres
1 millilitre (ml.)	=	0·0001 litre

Length

1 metre (m.)	=	1000 millimetres
1 decimetre (dm.)	=	100 millimetres
1 centimetre (cm.)	=	10 millimetres
1 millimetre (mm.)	=	0·001 metre
1 micron (µ)	=	0·001 millimetre
1 nanometre (nm.)	=	0·00001 millimetre

Imperial System

Mass (weights)

1 pound (avoirdupois)	=	7000 grains	=	453·6 grammes
1 ounce (avoirdupois)	=	437·5 grains	=	28·35 grammes
1 ounce (apothecaries)	=	480 grains	=	31·10 grammes
1 grain			=	64·8 milligrams

Capacity (volume)

1 gallon	=	8 pints	=	4·55 litres
1 pint	=	20 fluid ounces	=	568 millilitres
1 fluid ounce	=	8 fluid drachms	=	28·5 millilitres
1 fluid drachm	=	60 minims	=	3·5 millilitres
1 minim			=	0·59 millilitre

Length

1 mile	=	1760 yards	=	1·61 kilometres
1 yard	=	3 feet	=	0·914 metre
1 foot	=	12 inches	=	30·479 centimetres
1 inch			=	25·4 millimetres

Equivalents of Imperial and Metric Weights and Measures

Imperial to Metric (*Length*)

Imperial	Metric
1 inch	25·399 millimetres
1 foot	30·479 centimetres
1 yard	0·914 metre
1 chain (22 yards)	20·116 metres
1 furlong (10 chains)	201·164 metres
1 mile	1·609 kilometre

Metric to Imperial (*Length*)

Metric	Imperial
1 millimetre	0·0394 inch
1 centimetre	0·3937 inch
1 decimetre	3·937 inches
1 metre	39·3708 inches
1 hectometre	0·0621 mile
1 kilometre	0·6214 mile

Imperial to Metric (*Mass*)

Imperial	Metric
1 grain	0·0648 gramme
1 ounce	28·349 grammes
1 pound (avoirdupois)	454 grammes
1 pound (troy)	373 grammes
1 cwt.	50·8 kilograms
1 ton	1016 kilograms

Metric to Imperial (*Mass*)

Metric	Imperial
1 decigram	1·543 grains
1 gramme	15·432 grains
1 decagram	0·353 ounce
1 hectogram	3·527 ounces
1 kilogram	2·2046 pounds
1 tonne	2204·6 pounds

Imperial to Metric (*Capacity*)

Imperial	Metric
1 pint	0·568 litre
1 quart	1·136 litres
1 gallon	4·545 litres
1 peck	9·092 litres
1 bushel	3·637 decalitres
1 quarter	2·909 hectolitres

Metric to Imperial (*Capacity*)

Metric	Imperial
1 centilitre	0·070 gill
1 decilitre	0·176 pint
1 litre	1·7598 pints
1 decalitre	2·2 gallons
1 hectolitre	2·75 bushels

Apothecaries to Metric (*Capacity*)

Apothecaries	Metric
1 minim	0·059 millilitre
1 fluid scruple	1·184 millilitres
1 fluid drachm	3·552 millilitres
1 fluid ounce	2·842 centimetres
1 pint	0·568 litre
1 gallon	4·545 litres

Metric to Apothecaries (*Capacity*)

Apothecaries	Metric
1 grain	0·0648 gramme
1 scruple	1·296 gramme
1 drachm	3·888 gramme
1 ounce	31·1035 gramme

Thermometric Equivalents

Centigrade to Fahrenheit:
$(\frac{9}{5} \times {}^\circ C) + 32$

Fahrenheit to Centigrade:
$\frac{5}{9}({}^\circ F - 32)$

Prefixes for SI* Units

Prefix	Symbol	Multiple or fraction	
Mega	M	10^6	$= 1,000,000$
Kilo	k	10^3	$= 1,000$
Hecto	h	10^2	$= 100$
Deca	da	10^1	$= 10$
Deci	d	10^{-1}	$= 0{\cdot}1$
Centi	c	10^{-2}	$= 0{\cdot}01$
Milli	m	10^{-3}	$= 0{\cdot}001$
Micro	μ	10^{-6}	$= 0{\cdot}000001$
Nano	n	10^{-9}	$= 0{\cdot}000000001$
Pico	p	10^{-12}	$= 0{\cdot}000000000001$

* Système International d'Unités.